To Prof. Bor

with
admiration for his
strength

Giuseppe Zerbotti

Advanced Materials for Joint Implants

Giuseppe Pezzotti

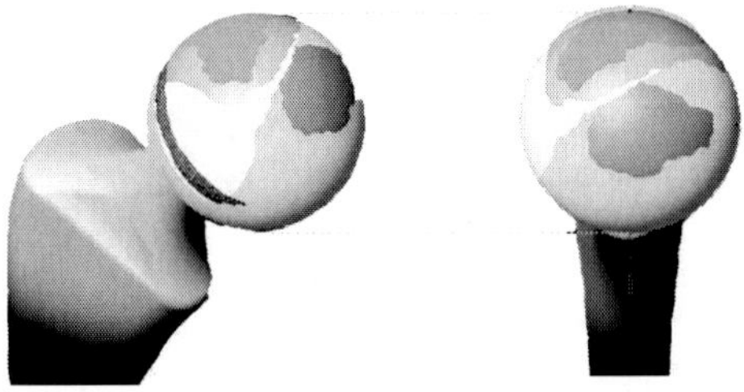

Advanced Materials for Joint Implants

Pan Stanford Publishing

Published by

Pan Stanford Publishing Pte. Ltd.
Penthouse Level, Suntec Tower 3
8 Temasek Boulevard
Singapore 038988

Email: editorial@panstanford.com
Web: www.panstanford.com

British Library Cataloguing-in-Publication Data
A catalogue record for this book is available from the British Library.

Advanced Materials for Joint Implants

ISBN 978-981-4316-88-0 (Hardcover)
ISBN 978-981-4364-39-3 (eBook)

Printed in the USA

To the young samurai, Iori

Reviews

"This book presents the most updated and basic knowledge about the biomechanics of artificial hip and knee joints from the macroscopic to the molecular scale. It covers advanced biomaterials, including alumina and zirconia ceramics and their composites and ultra-high-molecular-weight polyethylene. The latest developments in methods of characterizing these biomaterials are also explained at the outset so that readers get updated with new analytical techniques. The book will help young doctors and researchers to better understand the past failure patterns, and it proposes innovative ideas in the field of joint arthroplasty, thus giving fundamental hints for realistic breakthroughs in the time to come."

Prof. Nobuhiko Sugano, MD, PhD
Osaka University Graduate School of Medicine, Japan

"This book is an excellent review of the ceramic and polymeric materials that constitute advanced orthopaedic prosthetic materials. After an introduction, a chapter is devoted to characterisation techniques, which is exceptionally well written and, like all the chapters, is very well referenced with sufficient illustrations to highlight the basis of the technique. The following chapters deal with alumina, zirconia, alumina–zirconia composites and, most important, ultra-high-molecular-weight polyethelene (UHMWPE). The detail the author devotes to these different systems considering their intrinsic properties, factors that determine the strength, toughness and wear behaviour and, in the case of zirconia, the polymorphic transformations is impressive. The author highlights the critical need for more research on the properties of and means for reliably improving UHMWPE. This is a substantial and excellent text and should be on the bookshelf of every orthopaedic surgeon and medical library. I am unaware of any other text that matches the thoroughness of this contribution."

Prof. Michael Swain, PhD
University of Otago, New Zealand

"This book is the most comprehensive and informative source of information on implants for orthopaedic prostheses yet available. It draws on Prof. Pezzotti's extensive knowledge covering fracture mechanics of ceramics and environmentally induced chemical changes of ceramics and their subsequent interactions. It also includes Prof. Pezzotti's excellent insights into the chemical and structural characterisation of materials. The importance of bringing these factors together to understand the issues associated with biomedical implants is key and has never been properly addressed to date. I am sure this publication would be of great interest to surgeons, students, prostheses designers and scientists."

Prof. Mark Hoffman, PhD
The University of New South Wales, Australia

"This book, written by one of the most recognized authors in the field, represents an outstanding review of state-of-the-art and future trends concerning materials for joint prosthesis applications. With more than one thousand references, the book covers the fields of ceramic and polymer materials, with emphasis on their characterization from the nano- to the macro-scale, microstructure-properties relations and lifetime. It gives clear features of what the future could be in this important societal area. This is an excellent reference for university teachers and a source of inspiration for students and engineers."

Prof. Jérôme Chevalier, PhD
University of Lyon—INSA Lyon, France

"This book is an invaluable guide to the physical and chemical features of bioceramics as applied to implants for joint replacement. Improving the longevity of implants on active, aging population is a priority, and the beneficial cross-talk between material scientists, biologists and clinicians should reflect a thorough knowledge of novel materials. The advanced analytical methods described here unveil significant insights into the intimate structure and properties of bioceramics and offer a powerful tool to all scientists and clinicians who are involved in this promising field of translational research."

Prof. Nicola Baldini, MD, PhD
University of Bologna, Italy

"Readers will definitely enjoy the fruits of dazzling progress in biomaterials science and spectroscopic technology vividly described in this book by Prof. Giuseppe Pezzotti. The deep scientific knowledge reported in it will further promote new studies for scientists as well as for clinicians working in the field of joint arthroplasty. This book could effectively contribute to the future developments of next-generation products responding to the increasing expectations of patients and orthopaedic surgeons. In addition, I have great expectations that the introduced novel spectroscopic approaches could provide the final deterministic evaluation tool needed for screening individual joint implants before being delivered to the surgery room, a process which is definitely needed for strengthening and completing the regulatory procedures of new products made by the PMDA in Japan and the FDA in the United States."

Prof. Kengo Yamamoto, MD, PhD
Tokyo Medical University, Japan

About the Author

Giuseppe Pezzotti is a full professor (tenure) at the Ceramic Physics Laboratory of the Kyoto Institute of Technology, Japan, since 2000. He graduated *summa cum laude* in mechanical engineering from Rome University "La Sapienza", Italy, in 1984 and holds two doctoral degrees in engineering and in medical sciences, both obtained in Japan, the country where he has steadily lived for 25 years. From 2002 to 2012, Prof. Pezzotti served as the director of the Research Institute for Nanoscience at Kyoto Institute of Technology. Since 2005, he is an adjunct professor at the Department of Orthopaedic Research of Loma Linda University, Loma Linda, CA. Since 2009, he has held an invited professorship at the Department of Medical Engineering of Osaka University and since 2010 has been visiting professor at the Department of Molecular Cell Physiology of Kyoto Prefectural University of Medicine. Prof. Pezzotti has published around 550 scientific papers and 10 book chapters and holds 8 patents, including a world patent regarding nanoscale stress microscopy in the scanning electron microscope. The spectroscopic methods and algorithms developed by Prof. Pezzotti have been so far transferred to more than 20 major industries around the world. Among other numerous awards and prizes, he was twice recipient of Official Gratitude Awards from the Chinese Embassy in Tokyo. In 2010, he was chosen as one of the 80 most successful Expatriate Italians in the World by the Ministry of Foreign Affairs of Italy. He received the 2011 "150 Years of Italian Science in the World" award on occasion of the 150th anniversary of the Italian Republic. In 2013, he became a member of the Academy of Science of Bologna Institute in appreciation of his advanced studies linking quantum mechanics to medical sciences.

Contents

Preface

Just around ten years ago, when I occasionally met Prof. Ian C. Clarke at a meeting of the American Ceramic Society, I had not even imagined that I would author a book on biomaterials ten years later. At that time, I was deeply involved with some basic issues related to the grain boundary structure and the viscosity of polycrystalline ceramics and was definitely more concerned with the effect of temperature rather than the biological environment. Besides the charismatic leadership of Prof. Clarke, who guided me through the new scientific path, I could obtain fundamental strength from what initially seemed like the clarification of a scientific curiosity rather than a useful discovery: the stress dependence of the cathodoluminescence emission from oxygen vacancy sites in ceramic oxides. The more I investigated this effect, the more I wondered about the bold and intrinsic non-stoichiometric nature of ceramic surfaces, as well as the related vacancy site multiplication or annihilation in the biological environment. I also realized that this somewhat obvious piezospectroscopic effect could have a profound impact on the existing biomaterials science and represent a first clue toward a quantitative molecular-scale approach to the tribological evaluation of modern artificial joints.

This book is the culmination of ten years of research that I have mainly undertaken to develop a consistent and feasible procedure for the quantitative assessment of ceramic surfaces in joint implants on the molecular scale. Many experiments, including Raman assessments not only of ceramic but also of polyethylene bearings, were originally carried out to support and complement the cathodoluminescence approach, although they now represent a substantial part of this book. Honestly, I had never expected it would take so long to actually finish this book, but investing such a large amount of time on this topic was the fruit of a necessary decision, since I gradually came to realize that technical papers scattered across journals, no matter how many they be, could never successfully communicate the entireness of my findings. Yet, I hope that the ideas presented in this book will sometimes come to permeate biomaterials science, with the newly shown spectroscopic methodologies eventually becoming a standard. I feel happy about the idea that through the logical structure built in this book, the joy and the excitement I obtained from my little discoveries could be shared with those courageous readers who had the patience to go through it.

Giuseppe Pezzotti

Kyoto, July 2013

Acknowledgments

The author offers his most grateful thanks to Prof. Ian C. Clarke, PhD, at Loma Linda University, CA, for picking him out of a crowd of physicists and engineers, introducing him to the field of joint arthroplasty, and teaching him how to concurrently manage basic research and industrial outcomes. Partnerships with Prof. Nobuhiko Sugano, MD, PhD, at Osaka University Medical School, and Prof. Kengo Yamamoto, MD, PhD, at Tokyo Medical University, greatly accelerated research on biomedical implants and linked it to actual medical needs; for all this, the author conveys them his deep gratefulness. Professor Masahiro Hasegawa, MD, PhD, at the Graduate School of Medicine of Mie University, and Dr. Masaaki Matsubara, MD, PhD, at Nissan Tamagawa Hospital, Tokyo, are acknowledged for sharing their precious retrievals and new samples and for constructively discussing the related research outcomes. Many valuable contributions and constructive criticisms were received from Prof. Jérôme Chevalier, PhD, at INSA-Lyon MATEIS, CNRS, Prof. Mike Swain, PhD, at Otago University, and Prof. Mark Hoffman, PhD, at the University of New South Wales. Their favorable opinions on this research were vital to getting this book published. Special appreciations are due to Prof. Mark Rainforth, PhD, at the University of Sheffield, for his inspiring high-resolution microscopy work on worn ceramic surfaces. The author is deeply indebted to his former students and present co-workers, Wenliang Zhu, Dr. Eng.; Andrea Leto, Dr. Eng.; Yasuhito Takahashi, Dr. Eng.; Leonardo Puppulin, Dr. Eng., and Kyoju Fukatsu, Dr. Eng., for their fundamental contributions during the development of the Raman and cathodoluminescence algorithms for stress, molecular orientation, and oxygen off-stoichiometry analyses, for their patient proofreading of several chapters of this book, and for their kind help in the preparation of its figures. This book would not have been possible without the research contributions of all the Japanese and foreign students and researchers who have belonged in the past and those who presently work at the Ceramic Physics Laboratory of Kyoto Institute of Technology in Japan. Sincere gratitude is finally given to Ms. Manami Tanaka for her stoic help with nasty administration issues at Kyoto Institute of Technology, thus pledging me with the freedom and the concentration to write this book.

Chapter 1

General Introduction

1.1 Recent Trends in Joint Arthroplasty and the Scope of This Book

The continuously increasing demand for artificial joint prostheses (Fig. 1.1) [1] represents the composite result of an increasing world population and increasing human average lifetime, as well as a consequence of the changes in our habits and lifestyle. Since people nowadays live longer and get increasingly overweight due to overeating and lack of exercise, eventually the protective tissue lining on the acetabular cup wears away, friction increases, and inflammation, pain, and finally immobilization will result. It should be considered that a healthy average person walks about one million steps per year (with a frequency of about 1 Hz), which results in a walking distance of approximately twice the circumference of the Earth if an average lifetime of 75 years is assumed. During walking, the load on the joints can rise up to two or three times the body weight. This certainly represents an extremely severe engineering performance for any structural material. Total joint replacement might be the only reasonable option to maintain mobility, freedom from pain and hence a rewarding life in old age for those who suffer from joint problems. Furthermore, unfortunately with increasing frequency, younger people require such a surgery because their lifestyle, including aggressive (and

Advanced Materials for Joint Implants
Giuseppe Pezzotti

ISBN 978-981-4316-88-0 (Hardcover), 978-981-4364-39-3 (eBook)
www.panstanford.com

damaging) sports activities, might promote premature wear on their joints. In such cases, a problem arises since younger patients might outlive the average lifetime of the available artificial implants so that a revision surgery might be required, with substantial additional costs, pain, and associated mental stress. However, as mentioned above, nowadays it is an undeniable fact that an increasing fraction of patients will outlive the expected lifetime of artificial joints, which presently can be set to 15~20 years in case of a successful surgery. Consequently, research is continuously ongoing worldwide to provide improved biomaterials with increased mechanical, chemical, biological, and frictional properties, which will result in a longer lifetime in the body environment.

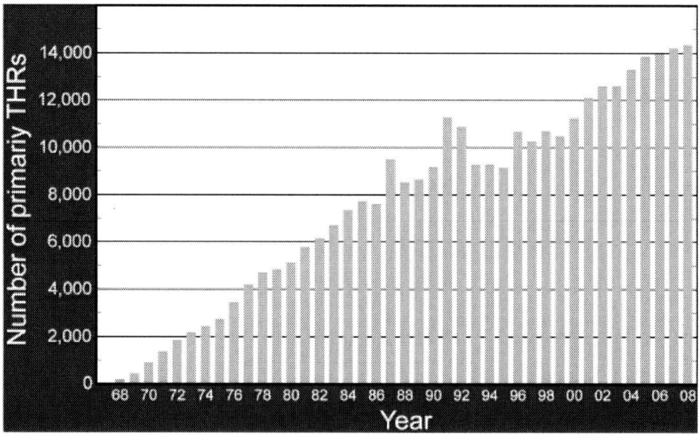

Figure 1.1 Numbers of primary total hip arthroplasties (THA) performed in Sweden during the last four decades [1]. Note the tremendous increase between 1967 (6 surgeries) and 2008 (14,105 surgeries).

For these reasons, decisional and research directives in the field of joint arthroplasty reveal a quite peculiar trend as compared to other fields in modern emerging technologies. While the technology of total joint replacement has been clinically solidly established and surgical procedures have already reached quite successful statistics, unique effectiveness, and high marketing efficiency, biomedical companies continue to invest a large capital in research and innovation following an unceasing pattern of materials innovation [2]. Undoubtedly, the replacement of diseased joints (especially hips and knees) definitely marks one of the most successful surgical inventions of this century; however, efforts are continuously made in developing new materials and in refining the design of joint implants already existing in the market. Excellent performances, systematically reported for implant systems [3, 4], seem to be paired with a relentless call for new goals of improved functionality and lifetime elongation. The reason for such a peculiar situation is twofold: on the one hand, there are both need and belief that human welfare should always progress, which will unavoidably push human beings to develop improved implants (and to search for the inherently high profits involved); on the other hand, there is always the risk of a dramatic drop in the market share when companies do not timely accomplish their market strategy with incorporating in their production the latest cutting edge technologies. These peculiar circumstances make the field of biomaterials for orthopedic applications extremely active and innovative. Nevertheless, the historical evolution toward the perfect joint implants has traditionally been slow and is idiosyncratically lagging behind innovative findings. This is mainly due to the fact that only a quite limited number of patients, voluntary participants in controlled trials, can be subjected to novel, yet unproven surgical principles. Except for those patients, joint surgeries should be made according to the "standard" existing knowledge, with selecting prostheses that have been known for their good long-term results.

It should be noted at the outset that the ideal social scheme based on voluntary clinical trials for new materials and joint designs, lying behind the introduction in the market of innovative solutions, has not always been successful. Even after successful clinical trials, disputations have often occurred all across the world. Systematic statistics teach us that joint loosening and osteolysis have been over the past years the most detrimental issues in joint arthroplasty (see, for example, Ref. [5]), which thus require prompt actions to be counteracted and to further improve the overall clinical outcomes. However, historical disputations have been dealing with a significantly wider spectrum of reasons as, for example, the premature wear failure of polyethylene liners, the catastrophic fracture of defective ceramic zirconia femoral heads, and the *in vivo* fracture and/or rim chipping of alumina acetabular cups These are the cases of defective implant components, which have circulated the market in the past and, unfortunately, will most probably also be sold in the future; but the way to counteract those failures resides in a better way to manage quality control, which should be concurrently challenged by both manufacturers and hospitals.

Looking at the main path of development of load-bearing components in artificial joints, one can recognize the great efforts made towards the reduction of the number of cases of polyethylene wear failure, which in turn have triggered the development of advanced acetabular cups and femoral inserts made of ultra-high molecular weight polyethylene materials with a highly cross-linked molecular structure. These latter materials represent a new family of polymeric materials engineered down to their molecular scale. On the other hand, ceramics have been the object of deep consideration as ideal candidates for realizing ultra-low-wear components, given their superior sliding behavior and the high inertness of their wear debris. With their high bioinertness, ceramic materials also allow eliminating blood contamination by release of metal ions and fully counteracting hypersensitivity and allergy. It should be also noted that as wear rates in ceramic components result significantly reduced in comparison to metallic components, larger femoral heads could be used with a higher safety margin. In hip joints, for example, such circumstance involves additional advantages, such as allowing the patient a greater range of motion, minimizing impingement of the femoral neck on the liner, thus greatly reducing incidence of dislocation and increasing safety margin during surgery in correctly positioning the acetabular component. According to these arguments, future trends in joint arthroplasty can be foreseen that lead to a statistical increase in the use of ceramic materials (to replace metals), despite their inherent brittleness. A concurrent tendency will most likely develop in manufacturing ceramic components of larger sizes for both better functionality and safety reasons.

Nowadays, surgeons and technologists make daily efforts in improving the outcomes of joint surgeries, with the ultimate goal of creating prostheses that reliably last longer than a human lifetime. While the results of primary joint arthroplasty (i.e., the surgery in which a joint is replaced for the first time) are generally very good, revision surgeries (i.e., the surgery in which part of or the entire prosthesis is exchanged or removed from the patient) might score variable success with regard to their clinical outcomes [6]. In addition, they invariably represent an expensive procedure and a severe burden to the patients. Thus, even a reduction of the failure rates of only a single unit percent can, due to the large number of patients yearly involved with surgical procedures, have a vast influence on the accumulated costs and the patient suffering. The key issue in arthroplasty resides in improving the prosthesis performance with regard to its long-term *in vivo* reliability. In this context, the most innovative trends in joint arthroplasty nowadays focus on the improvement of the tribological performance and naturally challenge the achievement of a longer joint durability with the potential for a service-life spanning several decades. While, as already mentioned, such trends have naturally led to an increase in the use of ceramic materials, we are all aware that ceramics are not "user friendly" materials for joint surgeons. For example, ceramic-on-ceramic articulations strongly require high precision in setting the orientation of the components during surgery, in order to avoid excessive loading on the bearing surface. Clearly, ceramic components offer a very high potential for further improving both structural performance and lifetime of hip joints but, being made of fragile materials, they also require the achievement of significant progress in surgery technique, advancements in joint design and materials manufacturing processes, as well as a peer preventive and non-destructive control of their structural reliability. The inherently high fracture strength of the most recently manufactured ceramic biomaterials and the consequent low percentage of fracture incidence of the ceramic components are encouraging; however, the achievement of such a high strength necessarily involves a ceramic component being conspicuously flawless after manufacturing, properly installed and precisely placed with the proper geometrical orientation. Therefore, the inherently brittle behavior of ceramics may involve additional guidelines during surgery in order to reduce the risk of post-operative complications and revision. Several intraoperative factors may also have an impact on the clinical outcome and play a crucial role on the survival time of a ceramic artificial implant. Advanced alumina, zirconia, and their optimized composite materials are nowadays of remarkably higher quality as compared to the corresponding materials manufactured in the past. Such improvement is due to concurrent progresses in microstructural material design, manufacturing, and non-destructive proof testing [7, 8]. Undoubtedly, the wear characteristics of ceramic-on-ceramic articulations are extremely favorable and, in most of the published reports, mechanical failures of modern ceramic bearings have been found to be exceedingly rare. However, shortcomings related to their inherent brittleness as, for example, chipping of acetabular liners due to *in vivo* edge loading and/or to impingement, as well as damage due to manipulation during surgery will always remain standing issues.

In discussing the most recent technological trends in biomaterials for arthroplastic applications, special attention should be paid to polyethylene, the biomaterial with structure and mechanical properties most similar to the human cartilage. It is quite intuitive that the presence of a "soft" component in the joint makes immensely less severe the positioning of the joint components during surgery as compared with all-rigid systems. While polyethylene is (and will probably continue to be) the most used biomaterial in joint arthroplasty, its history is spangled with dramatic and often large-scale failures [9, 10]. Comprehensive reports on the long-term clinical performance of advanced polyethylene materials with improved molecular structures are available in the recent medical literature [11–14]. However, viewed on a deterministic base, biomedical polyethylene components may intrinsically differ from each other and, more remarkably, even from piece to piece in the same production batch. This is due both to polyethylene being prone to quick oxidation and relatively easy deformation, and to a somewhat stagnant technological development of quantitative methods of non-destructive quality control for polyethylene bearings after irradiation by γ-rays or after being subjected to other types of sterilization process. Recent concerns arose from the finding that even in presence of a clear reduction in the amount of worn volume upon irradiation/cross-linking, the amount of polyethylene debris particles with finer size (i.e., comprised in the osteolytic potential range) might remain high [15]. Thus, the potential for a reduction in clinical cases of osteolysis could be possibly lower than theoretically expected from the lowered volumetric wear rate. Furthermore, poor control of the sterilization process may also trigger the presence of free residual radicals on the irradiated surface of the polyethylene structure after cross-linking, thus causing local oxidation gradients with subsequent material embrittlement [16]. In this latter context, retrieval studies of explanted highly cross-linked acetabular cups after short-term *in vivo* service have eventually shown wear trends that could be not predicted by exposing the components to several million cycles in joint simulators [14, 17–19]. Besides, reports on explanted polyethylene components clearly show that testing in joint simulators cannot be seen as a means for a fully predictive lifetime performance of the artificial joint. Technological improvements are needed for screening in real time the oxidation state of polyethylene components on a deterministic base (i.e., piece by piece) before implantation in order to remove the fraction of surgery failures related to poor manufacturing or oxidation during storage on shelve.

Looking back to statistics over the all span of history in joint arthroplasty, one might realize that the main problems encountered by patients are almost systematically related to the performance of the employed biomaterials [20, 21]. Therefore, any discussion about newly emerging technologies in joint arthroplasty can neither rescind deep investigations down to the molecular scale nor neglect focusing on the improvement of both structural and environmental reliability of advanced biomaterials. New perspectives should be, accordingly, given in terms of both microstructural material design and characterization techniques spanning several orders of magnitude, from the molecular to the macroscopic size. Furthermore, the attention of patients, surgeons, and technologists should be brought to deeper contents and the public opinion should be educated and oriented toward more meaningful biomaterial parameters. This book, written from a materials science perspective, is indeed dedicated to refresh and update those aspects of biomaterials science that are too easily stereotyped in the current scientific literature. It is believed that misleading assertions are spread throughout information networks that might induce even an expert audience to retain inexact understanding. For example, all of us had the chance to read in scientific papers or to hear in podium presentations standard phrases such as "alumina is a fully bioinert material" or "a femoral head containing monoclinic zirconia polymorph will fracture" or "one *in vitro* cycle in a joint simulator corresponds to a patient's step *in vivo*". Expert physicists, chemists, or tribologists could reply that all such "axioms" are untrue and rely on a poor understanding of material stoichiometry, micromechanics, and molecular physics. In other words, there is a tendency to oversimplify the real situation in search for a wider consensus from the less specialized audience. The most detrimental outcome of this "conventionalization" process of the notions related to biomaterials is that biased concepts become vehicles for marketing strategies and important hints are lost for future scientific and technological improvements.

In this book, a detailed description is attempted of the most recent technological approaches to tailor biomaterial micro-structures, to understand their behavior *in vitro* and *in vivo*, and to control their reliability through non-destructive analyses before and after their exposure to human body environment. The main aim here will be to drive the attention of the international orthopedic community on the need for a highly interdisciplinary approach to joint arthroplasty, which will hopefully contribute to minimize inexactness of the given information and trigger a faster development of new biomaterials with better performances, according to innovative approaches. Experimental evidence will be shown that directly hint at how newly developed technologies may provide final solutions to historical problems related to both chemical stability and structural reliability of biomaterials employed in joint arthroplasty.

1.2 Basic Background on the Biomechanics of Artificial Joints

Advanced studies on the mechanics of the human hip joint (schematically represented in its artificial configuration in Fig. 1.2) have revealed the complexity of the load-distribution mechanisms on the femoral head [22–25]. The hip joint consists of concave (acetabulum) and convex (femoral head) parts that are symmetrical, the joint space being equal at all points with slight deviation to permit adequate lubrication. This symmetry allows for rotation about a fixed axis and simplifies the muscle action on

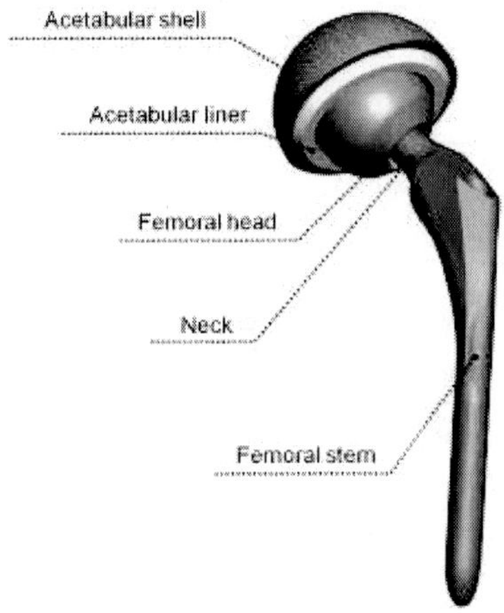

Figure 1.2 Schematic draft of an artificial hip joint with its composite structure and the definition of its components.

the joint. The femoral head articulates within the acetabulum, which is horseshoe-shaped and coated with cartilage around most of its periphery. The center is free of cartilage. The head of the femur fits into the acetabulum, where it is held firmly by a thick capsule, which is divided into thickened layers forming the hip ligaments. The head of the femur is coated by cartilage that acts to cushion compressive forces, lubricates the joint during compression, and, when not bearing weight, imbibes nutritional fluid. It has also been shown that the inter-cartilaginous space is variable in size and location [26, 27], and that it changes in shape with different positions of the joint [28]. In addition, the pressure distribution in the hip at the cartilage interface has been measured during load bearing, according to either direct or indirect methods. Measurements have mostly involved the insertion of piezo-electric transducers in the acetabulum [29, 30], as well as the use of pressure-sensitive films [23, 24, 31, 32] or instrumented endoprostheses [22, 25, 33, 34], in order to obtain the pressure contours developed on the cartilage when the hip was loaded. An area of high pressure could be identified in the anterosuperior segment of the joint, a site that coincides with the most usual location of the progressive cartilage loss seen in osteoarthritis. Most joints of the older population show this pattern, with a 3% prevalence of osteoarthritis of the hip, with a detrimental factor being the pressure gradient around the high-pressure sites. Experimental contour maps usually show tortuous shapes, which may be influenced by surface irregularities; an alternative explanation has been given that when a spherical head mates with a spherical acetabulum, unusual contour patterns arise through local differences in stiffness of the cartilage or underlying cortical bone. It is presently believed that a combination of both phenomena should be responsible for the observed patterns. The contact pressures experimentally measured are steeply graded and represent the radial stresses developed perpendicular to the contact surface between femoral head and acetabular cup. The application of external load also generates secondary stresses acting parallel to the joint surface, which are difficult to measure. Such secondary stresses can be of greater or smaller magnitude than the radial ones, depending on local geometry and stiffness of the cartilage. The most relevant issue here is that pressure differences within the area of steep pressure gradients would set up forces within the cartilage, thus producing tensile stresses in the collagen fibers running in the direction of the pressure gradient (i.e., lateromedial in the case of the hip joint). Afoke *et al.* [31] have estimated that the tensile stress induced in the collagen fibers experiences a magnitude of about 12 times the applied pressure (peak value of about 10 MPa); thus, the maximum tensile stress that the collagen fibers should sustain is about 120 MPa. Although at present it is not possible to relate this stress to the ultimate tensile strength of collagen fibers, it would seem natural that the structure of cartilage can cope with pressure gradients in the lateromedial direction since the collagen fibers in its superficial layer are observed to predominantly align along the lateromedial direction.

The biomechanical characteristics of the knee joint (schematically represented in its artificial configuration in Fig. 1.3) are perhaps even more complex than those of the hip joint. The knee joint is a site for the femur and tibia meeting together and it is composed of two main parts: the tibiofemoral and the patellofemoral part. Being a synovial joint, the knee joint is surrounded by a ligament capsule filled with synovial fluid as a lubricant. A patella, or kneecap, sits in the anterior side of the knee. The knee joint is stabilized by a complex arrangement of ligaments, tendons, and muscles, which provide anterolateral and posterolateral stabilization.

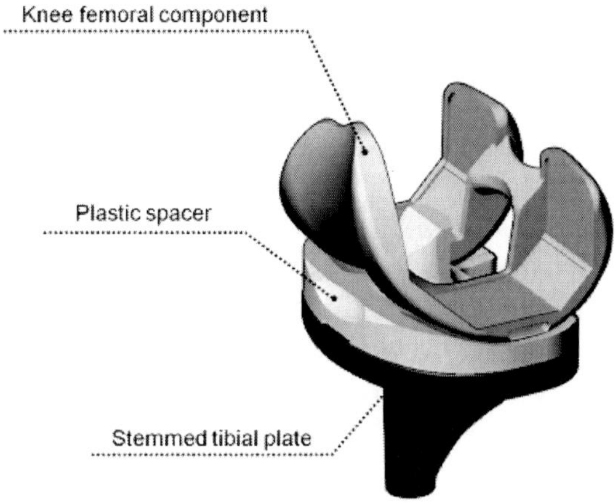

Figure 1.3 Schematic draft of an artificial knee joint with its composite structure and the definition of its components.

The underside of patella is covered by articular cartilage, which is made of hyaline cartilage to provide a smooth surface and absorb shock. This smooth surface at the back of the patella allows the patella to glide smoothly within the groove on the anterior portion of the femur during flexion and extension of the leg. Two femoral condyles are found on the rounded end of distal portion of the femur, which are covered by articular cartilage. The smooth cartilage surface allows the femur to move with minimum friction over the tibia's meniscus. The medial and lateral menisci cover the surface of the tibia acting as a cushioning system to distribute the load or stress of the femur over a wider area of the tibial plateau. Being the menisci thicker at the outside, they can help the rounded condyles from rolling smoothly on the flat tibial plateau and to distribute the load or weight from the femur on a larger contact surface, thus reducing the compressive stress and the damage and degeneration of articular cartilage over time. It is also known [35] that collagen fibrils networks in knee cartilage change in content and structure from a region to another. While resisting tension, they influence global joint response as well as local strains particularly at short-term periods. Deep vertical fibrils network in cartilage play a crucial role in stiffening the global response of the knee and protecting cartilage by reducing large strains, in particular at subchondral junction. Superficial horizontal fibrils protect the tissue mainly from excessive strains at superficial layers. Local cartilage splitting disrupts the normal function of vertical fibrils at the affected areas resulting in higher strains, the collagen fibril networks thus playing a fundamental role in the demanding mechanical environment of the tissue. The organization of the collagen network is different in healthy and in osteoarthritic cartilage, the structure and properties of collagen network of cartilage modulating stresses in an altered and less functional way in a knee joint with osteoarthritis. Based on magnetic resonance imaging, Mononen *et al.* [36] recently conducted a study on male knee joints in which the knee joint stresses were simulated under impact loads by implementing the structure and properties of healthy and osteoarthritic cartilage in the models. During the progression of osteoarthritis, characterized especially by the progressive increase in the collagen fibrillation from the superficial to the deeper layers, the stresses were found to reduce in the superficial zone of cartilage, while increasing in and under menisci. High collagen fibril strains were indicative of stress concentration areas in osteoarthritic cartilage, thus providing the rationale according to which collagen network orientation and stiffness control stress distributions in healthy and osteoarthritic knee joints. Again, the intrinsic properties of the natural biomaterials (e.g., collagen) appear to play a fundamental role on the functionality of the joint, which clearly evidences how deep and delicate are the factors contributing to a correct functionality of the human joints.

While advanced biomechanics studies seem to unequivocally remind us how even the most advanced designs of hip and knee joints are yet far behind in thoroughly reproducing the natural working conditions of hip bearing surfaces, they also provide us with basic observations and quantitative parameters for evaluating new synthetic materials. Concerning the intrinsic strength of a synthetic ceramic crystal, it can be estimated as more than one order of magnitude larger than the maximum tensile stress piled up that can be supported by collagen fibers in a femoral head [37, 38]. However, in contrast to the high intrinsic strength of a synthetic ceramic crystal, the actual strength of a ceramic polycrystalline body typically experiences significantly lower values and also fluctuates with a relatively high statistical scatter from piece to piece of the same material [37]. It is important in this context to understand that failure in a polycrystalline ceramic is always triggered by imperfections in its microstructure arrangement [39, 40], as we shall discuss more in details in a forthcoming section. Owing to their intrinsic brittleness, ceramics with high structural performance can only be achieved when the size of inherent defects in the material microstructure is very small. Typical relevant imperfections in advanced ceramics are comprised within a range of 5~50 μm in size. Accordingly, the available strength might be lowered by at least one order of magnitude with respect to the inherent strength of the corresponding (unflawed) ceramic crystal. The scatter in size of inherent defects directly matches the scatter in strength, which should be in turn inferred through statistical parameters. Thus, a low scatter in strength data collected on a series of samples obtained from the same ceramic material directly represents a high degree of structural reliability, also implying that the knowledge of statistical strength scatter for a given ceramic component is an experimental datum as important as the average strength value in designing a load-bearing ceramic component.

We have mentioned how the ability of the joint collagen structure of internally re-distribute and thus relieve high stresses plays a fundamental role in the mechanics of healthy joints. Interestingly, the orientation of crystalline lamellae in advanced polyethylene for biomedical joint applications after tribological loading resembles very much the orientation of collagen fibrils in human articular cartilage. This phenomenon was first observed by Benninghoff [41] and, later on, approved by a wide community of researchers [42–45]. Benninghoff introduced the partition of articular cartilage into different layers or zones and used polarized light microscopy to examine the orientation of collagen fibers in human articular cartilage. The most external zone, which represents up to 10~20% of the full thickness of articular cartilage, also experiences a strong degree of orientation in the plane of articulation sliding and a highly interconnected (cross-linked) structure. The middle zone contains collagen fibers that are randomly oriented, although this randomness can also be regarded as a transition state from a fully tangential orientation in the most external layer to a radial (i.e., fully vertical to the plane of sliding) orientation in the bulk zone. In this deep zone, collagen fibers extend radially down into a calcified zone, which is classified as the final zone of the graded structure including processes of mineralization. Amazingly, in the in-plane-oriented layer at the very top, as well as in the intermediate layer and in the radial layer in the bulk, polyethylene lamellae of artificially made acetabular cups can be shown to experience the same zonal arrangement and orientation as those observed in joint collagen. Although such important structural features have not been intentionally achieved by a systematic molecular design of the synthetic polyethylene structure (but rather serendipitously found out by *a posteriori* observation), it might serve to inspire in the near future advanced designs of polyethylene components for hip and knee joints. One could foresee, for example, surface treatments of the polyethylene structure (e.g., γ-ray irradiation) for tailoring the initial structural gradient in newly implanted components, in order to minimize degradation and, thus, to maximize *in vivo* lifetime.

1.3 Statistics, Past Failures, and the Need for Basic Scientific Understanding

Statistics became recently available that can be used to clarify the reasons for revision in total hip arthroplasty (Figs. 1.4 (a) and (b)). Such reasons are various and differentiated [5], and they mainly include aseptic implant loosening, osteolysis, pain, deep infection, instability, and wear damage. Noticeably, fracture of the prosthesis components or of the periprosthetic bone cover a quite low fraction of cases. Uncemented acetabular cups have been most commonly revised due to substantial wear of the liner, or owing to other (polyethylene) debris-related problems such as osteolysis, or aseptic loosening. However, due to the considerable heterogeneity of patients and operative procedures, as well as to a substantial lack of massive comparative trials, proofs to support a specific procedure above another in any specific trend of patient may be hardly found in the available literature. From a general perspective, the statistical plot in Fig. 1.5 [5] shows the number of hip operations by type as categorized into primary and revision in the period of time 2003~2008. Two main features can be envisaged in the plot, (a) the number of hip surgeries follows an increasing trend year after year; and, (b) the ratio of revisions to the total number of primary surgeries appears to be approximately constant. Nevertheless, it follows from (a) and (b) that the absolute number of patients undergoing revision surgery is increasing year after year. Besides this statistical panorama, which can be considered to be a standard state of art in modern hip arthroplasty, in recent history, there have been dramatic patterns of failure either related to material or to design mismanagements, but nonetheless related to technological rather than surgical reasons. We shall briefly review here such failures, because they represent a unique source of technological information and should serve as "experimental" data to guide surgeons in the choice, and scientists and technologists in the development of better prostheses designs and new materials.

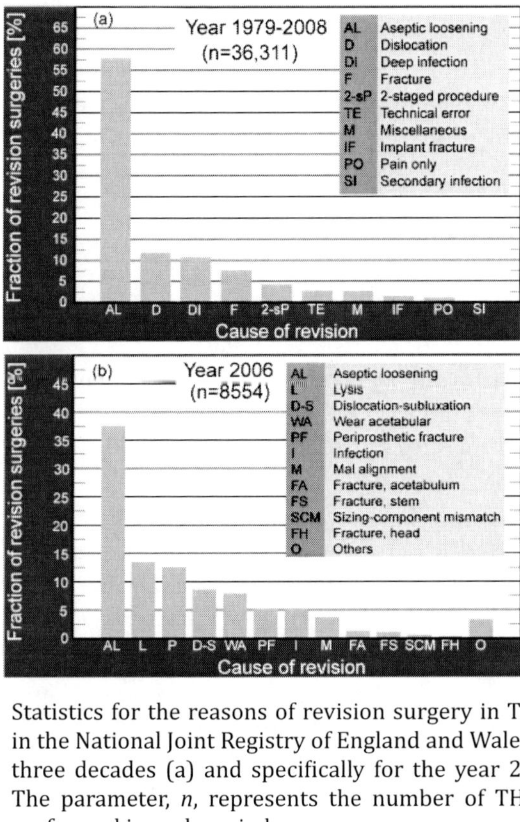

Figure 1.4 Statistics for the reasons of revision surgery in THA as listed in the National Joint Registry of England and Wales for the last three decades (a) and specifically for the year 2006 (b) [5]. The parameter, *n*, represents the number of THA surgeries performed in each period.

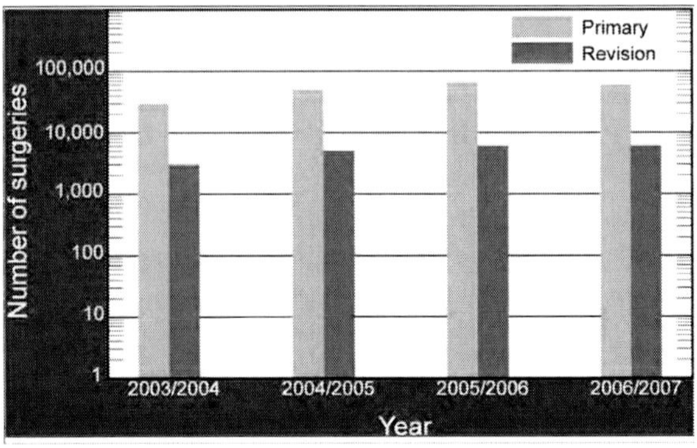

Figure 1.5 Number of hip surgeries by type as categorized into primary and revision in the period of time 2003~2008, according to the National Joint Registry of England and Wales [5].

The polyethylene part of hip prostheses, referred to as a liner, is responsible for absorbing the impacts experienced by the implant during its lifetime and may become subjected to extensive wear (i.e., resulting in the release of foreign debris into the patient). One can obviously expect that sooner or later oxidation of a polyethylene liner will unavoidably take place *in vivo*, but the ultimate goal should be that such a process does not affect the structural integrity of the liner over a reasonable lifetime, because extensive wear of the liner will result in the need for a revision surgery. Modern liners are manufactured from ultra-high molecular weight polyethylene, a material with extreme durability in its non-oxidized state [46, 47]. Orthopedic companies often employ a sterilization method involving the exposure of the liner to γ-radiation. However, when this method has been applied in air or in a non-completely controlled inert atmosphere, it has been found to cause severe oxidation of the polyethylene surface, with the liner becoming highly brittle, defective, and with a surface highly prone to wear [48]. One also expects that these negative effects be strongly amplified when irradiation in presence of air is coupled with an extended shelf life [49]. In 1987, a modified polyethylene developed to reduce wear in total joint replacement components, including hip, knee, shoulder, and elbow joint replacements, was introduced in the market. Initially, a γ-ray process in air was used to sterilize all components, while subsequently the components were sterilized by different processing methods, including γ-sterilization in nitrogen environment and gas plasma. In the late 1990s, a large number of defective products were with drawn from the market. In 2001, the British Government's Medical Devices Agency issued a voluntary recall of liners sterilized by γ-irradiation in air. Following a review of hip patients at sites with exceptionally high failure rate (up to more than 13 times higher than the expected rate), a warning was also issued and patients instructed to proceed to a peer check of their implanted liners. It is now generally known that γ-ray sterilization of ultra-high molecular weight polyethylene can induce oxidative degradation and that this effect increases during both shelf storage and implantation, significantly shortening the clinical life span of the prosthesis [50, 51]. Analytical studies of polyethylene wear debris, recently published for a statistically meaningful number of patients who received defective polyethylene implants sterilized by γ-rays in air and had successively suffered prosthetic loosening [52], showed a comparison between those implants and implants made of traditional polyethylene and sterilized by the same method. Interestingly, the frequency distribution of globular and fibrillar particles was similar in both groups, but the globular particles of the defective samples had a mean surface area significantly lesser than that of the implants used for comparison. In other words, the two materials, despite undergoing the same type of sterilization, produced wear debris with significantly different morphologies. Such a difference triggers a more intensive biological response and thus an earlier and more massive osteolysis. In other words, we have learnt that the oxidative degradation of polyethylene joint components is a very complex phenomenon, strongly affected by the intrinsic molecular structure of the material. While some manufacturers prefer to sterilize their implants using ethylene oxide, gas plasma, or electron beam irradiation, others continue to use γ-irradiation, but with the implant sealed in a low-oxygen package [53]. Enormous progress has been made in material processing since the disclosure of the failures of liners sterilized by γ-irradiation in air. However, clinical reports continue to show that the problem of oxidation in polyethylene liners still matters, depending on type of resin, atmosphere in which the component was irradiated and subsequently stored, duration of shelf storage, and duration of use *in vivo* [54]. In other words, an open issue yet remains on how can we be assured on a deterministic basis, namely with respect to each very piece of polyethylene implanted in the human body, about safety and lifetime concerns. A comparison between Figs. 1.1 and 1.5 shows that these concerns are particularly true because, even assuming that the revision rate will not significantly increase during the next decade, an overall increase in the total number of revisions can be promptly foreseen. In this perspective, an even minimum reduction of failure rates can have a vast influence on the reduction of the number of patient suffering. This observation should represent the main driving force for deepening our knowledge of polyethylene structures and for pursuing further improvements in manufacturing processes.

The most dramatic and massive failure of zirconia ceramic femoral heads happened in 2001 with a French manufacturer recalling batches of femoral heads fracturing at a higher rate than expected. This manufacturer recall applied to nine batches of zirconia heads produced since early 1998 after the company changed part of its manufacturing process. The US Food and Drug Administration subsequently issued a voluntary recall for these zirconia components, advising surgeons not to continue the implantation of artificial hips with zirconia femoral heads manufactured by this French maker between early 1998 and 2001. Patients who already had these hip implants were also recommended to contact their surgeons for any question or concern, although no surgery was recommended to replace hip implants that have not fractured. An external panel of zirconia experts was then formed to study femoral head fractures in the United States. According to those experts, a conclusion was reached that the majority of the fractures were from two lots produced early in 1988 and that fractures generally originated near the upper taper-crown regions of the machined area. The femoral heads fractured into many small fragments and their fracture surfaces showed numerous large flaking structures and multiple cracks through poorly consolidated areas. Significant phase instability, namely phase transformation from the tetragonal to the monoclinic polymorph, was found nearby the fracture origin and on the ball surface. Post-mortem analyses showed numerous potential fracture origins, which were also observed on the ground taper surface. Autoclaving unused femoral heads of the same type resulted in a very high degree of monoclinic phase transformation, with monoclinic volume fractions up to 70%. In other words, the femoral heads were found to be in a highly "metastable" state. It should be noted that the first 12 years of clinical experience with zirconia femoral heads provided an excellent safety record, with very small incidence of fracture. This result could be achieved when a batch furnace was used for production, in which an oven was set through one complete heating and cooling cycle to sinter the ceramic femoral heads. Only 28 fracture cases were reported for this sintering process over that time and represented a fracture rate as low as 0.0085% (i.e., 1 per 11,000 units). With the use of the proof test on every head produced, the fracture rate fell down further to 0.002%. In January 1998, a crucial change was made to the manufacturing process with the introduction of a "tunnel" furnace in order "to optimize" the production process. After thorough consultations, the expert study group concluded that the combination of the tunnel-sintering and subsequent machining operations had probably negatively interacted to make the femoral heads extremely vulnerable to transformation into monoclinic phase in patients. Clarke *et al.* [55] noticed that since their inception 18 years ago, the performance of zirconia ceramic balls has been both confusing and controversial. Grouping all zirconia materials as the same product, in the absence of a rigorous scientific clarification of individual chemical and physical properties, has led to confusion and to misleading generalizations. As in the case of oxidized polyethylene, the degree of metastability of zirconia materials *in vivo* as well as the increased probability of fracture strongly depends on the microstructural characteristics of the very individual material, and thus strongly on the manufacturing process. In this context, for example, it can be interesting to follow the clinical history of partially stabilized zirconia ceramics, which has been quite controversial. *In vivo*, a combination of hydrothermal and mechanical exposure may selectively trigger detrimental changes on the surface of femoral heads that have inferior phase stability [56, 57]. Transformation from the tetragonal to the monoclinic phase may be influenced by the effect of body fluid and impingement conditions. Since hydrothermal processes are the most salient to material stability, the implant can be very sensitive to the adopted lubrication mode;

for example, for zirconia ceramic-on-ceramic bearing systems tested in a hip simulator, early catastrophic failure was found when run in water but implants survived as long as 20 million cycles when run with calf serum lubrication [58]. This observation suggests that tribological conditions under the cup are the trigger for a metastable behavior. Most of the early implanted zirconia femoral heads, independent of bearing counterparts, showed transformation areas after *in vivo* exposure, especially in areas of contact. However, some femoral heads were found to be completely stable and untransformed, showing that yet little is understood of the actual hydrothermal conditions operating in the hip joints *in vivo*. Despite the numerous queries and worries on zirconia implants, it should be noted that all cases of fracture and premature retrievals in such implants refer to early generations of this material. In particular, the above-mentioned fracture recall, although representing a catastrophic experience, was contained and unique to the defective manufacturing process. But, again, what is of considerable importance here is that there is little (or nothing) of predictive in the present approach to the analysis of hip failures; quality control in this field, however accurate, is yet of a statistical and not of a deterministic type in its ultimate nature. This circumstance calls for a better understanding of critical material parameters and of their actual role in the lifetime elongation of prosthetic implants. Concurrently, we also need to emphasize the urgency in the development of improved analytical methods, which can clarify and help makers to predict with high exactness and in a non-destructive manner the expected lifetime of individual hip components to be implanted in the human body, *before* they actually fail.

The incidence of fracture among the causes for revision of alumina ceramic hip joints has been historically low. Heros and Willmann [59] published a milestone report on alumina fracture incidence in 1998. According to their publication, clinical data published in the early 1990s (representing the 1980s) gave a fracture incidence ranging from 0 to 0.8%, namely a maximum of 8 fractured femoral head per 1000 cases. Statistical data for the early 1990s showed already a fracture incidence reduced to 2 balls per 10000 cases. Most recent clinical statistics, according for example to the National Joint Registry for England and Wales and pertaining to the cause of hip revision in 2006, report a percent of head and acetabulum fractures of 0.27% and 1.14%, respectively (on a number of revision surgeries n = 8554) (cf. Fig. 1.4 [5]). Among the cases of acetabular fracture, surgeons in Europe, Asia, and the United States, have concurrently reported rim chipping and fracture of ceramic inserts [7, 8, 60–62]. However, it should be noted that the polycrystalline materials, of which modern alumina implants are made, are strongly improved over the previous generations, being treated by hot isostatic pressing, laser engraved, having a smaller grain size, fewer impurities, and being subjected as individual components to proof-testing after manufacturing. One of the early reported issues, dealing with ceramic acetabular inserts, involved the intraoperative chipping of ceramic inserts as the surgeon seats into a metal shell the alumina acetabular insert during total hip arthroplasty. These kinds of problem can be analyzed in a quite straightforward manner from a biomechanical viewpoint: if not properly handled or aligned with the metal shell, a piece of ceramic can chip off in correspondence of the insert edge. However, the problem is clearly technique-related since it mainly occurs if the surgeon, unaware of the brittleness of ceramics, impacts an eccentrically placed insert into a metal shell. While chipping likely damages only a small part of the edge, significant stress intensification can be created in the material, and the chipped insert must be mandatorily replaced with a new one [20, 21, 63]. With special emphasis placed on Asian patients, design concerns have recently arisen about ceramic-on-ceramic bearings including a sandwich-type ceramic liner, given the pronounced attitude to squatting, which in turn results in hyperflexion and wide hip abduction. Early fracture of ceramic liners has been thus associated with impingement from excessive anteversion of the acetabular cup. However, unlike the cases of polyethylene and zirconia materials described above, the origin of these failures should be mainly identified with the choice of a defective design rather than dealing with the poor structural quality of the selected material. Unlike material defective cases, solutions for design-related surgical failures should become promptly available upon shifting the hip design concept toward more advanced perspectives and/or appropriately selecting design parameters, as for example allowing larger head diameters [64–69]. As far as future developments of alumina joint components are concerned, their brittleness and tribological performance become thus the main issues. Tailoring new material microstructures with considering both the addition of secondary phases and of alloying elements seems to be the key for future improvements. While the former (e.g., zirconia dispersoids [70]) might produce crack-tip toughening mechanisms that increase the reliability of the joint components, selected dopant elements might alter the mechanochemical performance of the bearing surface by affecting the stoichiometry of the material at its sliding surface [71], as we shall explicitly show in a forthcoming chapter.

1.4 Linking Molecular Scale Phenomena to Macroscopic Performance

Unlike natural bone, which can remodel and adapt itself to the externally applied mechanical environment (so that, for example, the application of higher stress naturally results in a more dense bone [72–76]), artificially made biomaterials lack of such inherent "smartness"; accordingly, biomaterial microstructures should be designed with taking into account their evolution during service and to match the desired performance over the entire *in vivo* lifetime. Additionally, the axiom "a chain is as strong as its weakest link" may explain in what it might consist the striking vulnerability of the overall artificial joint implant to the brittleness of its ceramic parts or to the proneness to oxidation (and subsequent wear) of internal polyethylene surfaces. In other words, the macroscopic performance (and lifetime) of the overall artificial joint ultimately depends on phenomena occurring on the molecular scale and no substantial improvement is possible without understanding the microscopic mechanisms governing the physical, mechanical, and chemical interactions between the biomaterial and the human body environment. However, the functionality of an artificial joint composed of various parts of complex shape and made of different materials, is a formidable challenge and the intricacies of the coupled motions of the joint components have made development of new materials and joint designs becoming a field in continuous evolution. For example, there have been many design attempts to create hip and knee joints that recapitulate normal motion while providing significant longevity, a low incidence of complications and no possibility of catastrophic failure. On the other hand, better basic understanding of the biomechanics of hip and knee joints, and improvements in implant materials have made successful joint replacements a likely reality, and now several new materials and designs are ready for clinical trials. But, again, looking at the overall problem on the microstructural scale, how much of empiricism has been lain (and yet lies) behind those improvements? To which extent can we yet control what is going on in the tiny nanometer scale where molecules are stretched and torn at load-bearing surfaces to their ultimate strength under such an aggressive environment as the human body? Regrettably, the answer to those questions is that when things are seen on the scale of single molecules, our knowledge is yet too poor to fully understand the complex cascade of interactions between biomaterials and the human body. In other words, it is likely that at the present stage only a fortunate empiricism (mainly based on macroscopic analyses) might enable successful surgeries and that, consequently, there is room for further substantial improvements.

The focus now shifts on how we can improve our understanding of local phenomena taking place in artificial joints, especially at their highly stressed and environmentally loaded interfaces. The answer to this challenge resides in the development of new characterization tools that involve multiple complementary metrology approaches. While correlating results obtained from newly developed analytical tools has traditionally been very time consuming and has led in the past to ambiguous conclusions, the challenge must be taken. The use of new advanced analytical equipments becomes a serious need. Confocal/polarized Raman spectroscopes with their potential to rapidly screen and evaluate in three dimensions chemical, crystallographic and mechanical properties of environmentally exposed biomaterials can partly provide new answers. Polarized Raman microspectroscopy has already been widely employed to gain knowledge of bone chemistry [77], of the organization of the components of bone [78–84], of bone fracture mechanisms [84, 85], which in turn is of primary importance in understanding how the bone tissue responds to external stresses, and provides a starting point for the design and development of artificial biomaterials. Raman spectroscopy has greatly contributed, for example, to clarify that the mineralized fiber arrangement in cortical bone is either a twisted or an orthogonal plywood structure, both mineral models coexisting in compact bone. Polarized Raman spectroscopy offers definite advantages in the study of biological samples, enabling the simultaneous analysis of mineral and organic components, and the determination of molecular orientation through the polarization properties of the Raman scattering. The Raman polarization approach has been used to simultaneously investigate the orientation of collagen fibrils and apatite crystals in human cortical bone [86]. The measurement principle is based on the fact that Raman band ratios can be monitored as a function of sample orientation, which show quite high sensitivity to apatite crystal and collagen fibril orientation. Based on this research approach, spatial changes can be locally monitored as a function of in-plane distance and depth, which reveal simultaneous tilting in intra-lamellar collagen-fibril and mineral crystal orientations, consistent with a twisted plywood organization. At the molecular level, more or less degree of co-alignment of collagen fibrils and apatite crystals has also been observed depending on the investigated bone region, thus highlighting the interest in Raman microprobe spectroscopy for multiscale investigations of bone structure. Now, the challenge is shifted to understand how such a precious body of information can be translated to the micro-structural design of new and improved artificial biomaterials.

Beyond mere topological visualizations of biomaterials surfaces, the electron beam is becoming a precious tool in spectroscopic assessments of biomaterials. Auger electron spectroscopy together with scanning electron microscopy has long been used, for example, to study the interface between stainless steel implants and human tissue [87, 88]. Through such spectroscopic studies, it has been clarified that the thickness and the nature of the oxide layer on the implants greatly depend on the location of the implants in the body. In the case of implants located in cortical bone the thickness of the interfacial chromium oxide layer remains unaffected, while it increases in three to fourfold fashion in samples located in bone marrow. Furthermore, implants located in soft tissue eventually incorporated sulfur in the oxide layer. Understanding the interactions between biomedical implants and human tissues by observing spectroscopic changes of the implant surfaces thus revealed the important role of oxygen pressures and metabolic activity in the chemical behavior *in vivo* of metallic materials. Efforts in expanding the analytical outputs obtainable from using an electron probe as, for example, the collection of cathodoluminescence spectra [71] or of backscattered diffraction patterns [89] on biomaterials should soon lead to a new vision of lattice strain and stoichiometry gradients developed at the articulating joint surfaces. An expanded spectroscopic approach could greatly help to spread new trust in advanced materials, through the process of their integration in the market. The end results could eventually lead to the obtainment of safer products while shortening both material development efforts and time lag to marketing (i.e., due to unclear filing of marketing applications and consequently lengthy approval procedures).

It is beyond the scope of this book to provide conclusive statements on how and how long the lifetime of the bearing components of artificial joints can be ultimately elongated. However, one main attempt here will be to inform the readers of the new possibilities that non-destructive analyses, such as confocal vibrational spectroscopy, atomic force microscopy, and scanning electron microscopy (and related analytical attachments) can offer in terms of understanding biomaterials on the molecular scale. Newly developed algorithms for microscopy and spectroscopic techniques, which allow visualizing with a spatial resolution down to the nanometer scale the salient characteristics of biomedical materials, make it easier visualizing and, thus, understanding the complex phenomena occurring on the molecular scale. In past years, for example, Fourier-transform infrared spectroscopy, a technique mainly operating in transmission mode and thus requiring thin slicing of the sample, has been extensively used to characterize the hydroperoxide concentration and distribution in polyethylene biomedical samples [90–97]. According to such a spectroscopic method, different oxidation behaviors and mechanisms have been identified and discussed in correlation with processing, sterilization, and packaging conditions. Nowadays, Raman spectroscopy enables one to make the same quantitative assessments of ultra-high molecular weight polyethylene (UHMWPE) but in a non-destructive manner [98–100]. Raman spectra can also identify crystalline and amorphous phase fractions, oxidation state and residual strain in polyethylene materials. In other words, through Raman spectroscopic experiments, it is possible to verify the actual structural changes that occur during sterilization by γ-radiation in UHMWPE; but, more important, by taking advantage of its fully contactless character, its high scanning flexibility, and non-destructiveness, it becomes possible to deterministically scrutinize each single polyethylene component according to a fast procedure before implantation. According to this practice, a new possibility might be opened to introduce an advanced quality control procedure for biomedical implants on their molecular scale. Such a monitoring of deterministic nature should fully eliminate the inability of randomized (i.e., statistically) controlled trials to detect infrequent events and unexpected side effects.

Nowadays, national registers have developed in many countries for follow-up and surveillance of joint replacement surgery. Registers are primarily intended to function as quality control systems, their main objective being that of detecting inferior prosthetic implants, bone cements, routines, and procedures as early as possible after their introduction to the market. The intrinsic quality of joint devices and replacement surgeries can be promptly assessed owing to hospital-specific results that are in turn reported yearly to all hospitals involved with joint replacement surgery. Statistical methods are commonly used in the evaluation of the data, which typically include survival analyses and sample regression. The end-point in these analyses usually is the revision of prosthetic components. However, it should be noted that all those kinds of macroscopic "quality control" methods only work *a posteriori* and strongly rely on a statistical sampling rather than on a control of deterministic nature. It is evident that inferior quality as well as defected implants have been used, still are used, and will continue to be used in the lack of an obligatory system not only for the introduction but also for the *a priori* quality control of each individual prostheses implanted in the clinical practice. Severe lessons from the past teach us that regulations should allow not only future revisions in the same hip of the same patient to be linked to the corresponding primary procedure, but also the initial quality of the implanted components to be systematically measured, followed up and evaluated in terms of reliability parameters and residual durability. Therefore, there is a clear hint for the health authorities to start engaging in the development of fully deterministic quality control procedures, including advanced spectroscopic screening especially for those components subjected to high risk of degradation (e.g., polyethylene). Concurrently, the research community together with orthopedic associations should strive to widely spread deeper understanding of biomaterials on the molecular scale and to influence this process with clear research outputs and outline suggestions for the selection of more advanced evaluation methods. With the aid of modern technologies, non-destructive evaluations, deterministic proof testing and meticulous intraoperative techniques, artificially made joint components should become available and be used with a significantly improved degree of reliability. With a substantial control of the behavior of bearing surfaces (i.e., "the weakest link in the chain") *in vivo*, reduction in wear rates and fracture events will likely lead to significantly durable joint replacement with the potential for a service life spanning several human lifetimes. It is hoped that the contents of this book contribute to this cultural and technological evolution with shifting the paradigm of research in the biomaterials field toward deeper studies of their complex but intriguing behavior on the molecular scale.

Chapter 2

Characterization Methods

2.1 Characterization Techniques in Biomaterials for Artificial Joints

In the past decade, substantial advances in biochemistry and materials science, including surface science, have occurred, allowing a comprehensive description of processes and mechanisms on the molecular scale and, thus, a deeper understanding of the interactions between artificial implants and the host human body. From the manufacturing viewpoint, an integrated approach by physicists, chemists, materials scientists, biologists, and physicians has successfully led to the development of a large variety of devices implantable in the human body that use many different materials, including metals, polymers, and ceramics. An entirely new generation of biomaterials has thus been developed, which shows suitable physical properties, including acceptably high responses in terms of biocompatibility and overall structural reliability. However, while extensive research has so far detailed substantial improvements in biocompatibility, this enhanced property has been strongly correlated with surface topography and yet less with surface chemistry and mechanics. An increased capability to measure surface roughness down to the nanometer scale, as produced by tribomechanical processes occurring during

Advanced Materials for Joint Implants
Giuseppe Pezzotti

ISBN 978-981-4316-88-0 (Hardcover), 978-981-4364-39-3 (eBook)
www.panstanford.com

frictional exposure of artificial joints *in vivo*, has not yet been sufficiently matched with the necessary links to a full clarification of the elementary chemical and physical processes behind its occurrence. Therefore, it is now expected that the major emphasis on wear-resistance issues given so far in the field of load-bearing biomaterials should naturally result in a shift toward further understanding of the complex boundary conditions imposed by the living environment. When reviewing, for example, the development of ceramic biomaterials, the most commonly employed one is found to be alumina, which can certainly be regarded as a highly bioinert material. However, the alumina microstructure is highly dependent on the applied manufacturing process (e.g., maximum temperature during sintering, duration of the thermal steps, purity of the raw powder, size, and distribution of the grains, and porosity) and this might have a clear and direct impact on both mechanical and biological properties. It is also well known that both wear and friction behaviors of alumina ceramics are significantly better in water than in a dry atmosphere. However, the effect of the pH of the aqueous media on wear and friction behavior is also known to play a key role in reciprocating sliding tests. It has been found that the wear resistance can vary up to one order of magnitude and that the coefficient of friction increases by a threefold factor, depending on the pH environmental conditions [101]. Furthermore, significantly different wear surfaces can be generated for different pH values, and the cumulative development of these surfaces in turn exerts a diverse effect on long-term wear and friction behavior. Clearly, chemical and electrochemical effects associated with the selected tribological conditions should be invoked in order to explain the observed behavior since, by varying the pH of the sliding environment, one might obtain low-wear or high-wear counterparts with exactly the same alumina ceramics. Despite such evidence, there have been so far no attempts to classify the pH environment naturally existing in human joints, nor has been the pH chemical effect introduced among the variables of *in vitro* wear simulation in artificial joints.

Since all the human-made biomaterials are unequivocally employed at the interface between organic and inorganic functions, it is quite intuitive that surface properties impact enormously on the success or failure of a selected biomaterial. Accordingly, the search for new instrumental approaches is quite demanding and advanced analytical techniques of surface analysis are continuously updated in the field of biomaterials [102]. There is also a great need to provide quick and non-destructive detection of biomaterial damage at their early stage and to quantify degradation at the micro-structural level in order to both assess residual life *in vivo* and as an aid to material development. In this latter context, analytical techniques have been developed and employed for measuring surface properties, including chemical and phase structures, bioinertness, morphology, and topography, and for correlating those properties to the macroscopic joint performance. Methods of surface analysis can be also systematically used for the verification of intentionally produced surface modifications *in vitro*, as well as for differentiating sliding responses of different bearing couples upon exposure in body environment. Surface analyses also play key roles in understanding the effects of different lubricants, especially useful in characterizing the intrinsic differences between *in vivo* and *in vitro* exposure. Since even slight stoichiometric changes and/or topological modifications can greatly alter the performance of a joint bearing surface, the characterization tools should be highly sensitive and effective in correlating any of such modifications with changes in biological and frictional performance. Accordingly, the detailed information gained may allow one tailoring biomaterial microstructures that can significantly elongate the joint lifetime or even favor specific biological responses [103–106].

A combination of several surface characterization methods is usually necessary to provide the comprehensive information necessary for judging about the performance of a biomaterial to be used in artificial joints. The most basic assessment is that of the morphology and of the topography of the load-bearing surface (i.e., surface roughness, planarity, etc.), which can be measured with different resolution and degrees of precision by optical (or stylus) profilometry [107–109] or by atomic force microscopy (AFM) [110, 111]. The choice of the analytical instrument should be made depending on the scale on which surface roughness has to be measured (i.e., on the micrometer and on the nanometer scale for optical profilometry and AFM, respectively). Spectroscopic techniques such as Raman, infrared (IR), and luminescence spectroscopy are often used to broaden knowledge about oxidation [91, 112–116], phase composition [117–119], elastic or plastic state of strain [92, 116, 120–123], and texture on the molecular scale [123, 124]. Nowadays, the ease, rapidity and non-destructiveness with which spectroscopic techniques can be applied make them more and more frequently used in combination with optical microscopy methods. Nevertheless, care should be taken in interpreting spectroscopic data when steep gradients are present along the immediate subsurface of the biomaterial. As a matter of fact, many biomaterials are quite transparent to visible light and a laser beam focused on the biomaterial surface might probe significantly deep portions of materials. Under such circumstances, the spectroscopic output becomes an average between the surface and the bulk state of the biomaterial, thus making it difficult understanding the actual state of the biomaterial surface. Substantial improvements of in-depth resolution can be obtained by means of confocal pinholes placed in the optical circuit of the measurement device [92, 125–127]. The pinhole aperture can be modulated to allow a controlled depth, in the scale of the single micron, to be monitored. However, when nanometer-scale shallowness is required for the measurement the choice of the probe unavoidably shifts to electrons. The success of using electron microscopy methods (especially in terms of spatial resolution) to characterize biomaterial surfaces is well established [122]. A microscopy technique historically well established and most frequently found in the biomaterials literature is scanning electron microscopy (SEM) [128–136]. This technique makes use of a primary beam of electrons that interact with the specimen of interest, in a vacuum environment, resulting in different types of electrons and electromagnetic waves being emitted. The secondary electrons discharged from the specimen surface are collected and displayed to provide a high-resolution micrograph. Unlike optical microscopy methods, SEM involves a sample preparation procedure for coating the (usually) electrically non-conductive biomaterial with a metal prior to data collection. The thin metallic coating, which can be applied by sputter coating, is typically kept to an extent of few nanometers in thickness. Common conductive metals used for coating include gold, platinum, or gold/palladium alloys. Upon insertion of the sample into the SEM, acquisition of the micrographs can be quickly done allowing for a series of images to be obtained with increasing resolution. Modern SEM devices can easily resolve features in the nanometer range, while computerized image acquisition provides a permanent record of them. In addition to imaging the surface morphology of biomaterials, the SEM can be combined with other analytical methods such as energy dispersive X-ray analysis (EDX) to determine the elemental distribution on the biomaterial surface [137, 138], electron backscattering diffraction (EBSD) for highly localized crystallographic assessments [139–141], and cathodoluminescence (CL) spectroscopy for monitoring surface modifications in terms of stoichiometry, lattice defects and elastic strain [71, 121, 142–144]. EDX, EBSD, and CL thus provide a set of complementary data of various nature that are typically obtained from sampling depths ranging from few nanometers to few micrometers, depending on the acceleration voltage used for generating the primary electrons. In other words, an increase in acceleration voltage can be seen as a means for collecting data that are more representative of the bulk material rather than the surface and vice versa [145, 146]. Obviously, the choice of surface characterization methods can be influenced by numerous factors, including not only the type of measurement required but also the extent of the analyzed surface region, the required spatial resolution, precision and accuracy, the influence, and the eventual damage induced by the selected probe on the biomaterial surface, namely, the bias that such probe can introduce in the output of the measurement itself. Further criteria for the choice can be the degree of manipulation to which the sample must be subjected before being analyzed and the ease of use of the analytical instrument.

The remainder of this chapter is conceived to provide a succinct yet comprehensive overview of emerging characterization techniques in the field of biomaterials for artificial joints. For reasons of available space, only a limited selection of information can be given here, but emphasis is placed on those new aspects that have recently come to the forefront of biomaterials research, including the applications and limitations of each technique. While the main aim of this chapter is to provide a brief synopsis of some of those less known (but newly developed or newly extended) analytical techniques, a number of references are also listed that detail how those technique are specifically applied to the characterization of biomaterials. In addition, some discussion is also included to more common characterization methods such as fracture mechanics [147–149] that have been long performed in biomaterials research but require updating. A subchapter is also dedicated to methods of surface tribology characterization [150, 151] updated with the use of *in situ* laser spectroscopy in a specially designed tribometer. These latter two characterization methods are important because they provide direct outputs about the intrinsic structural resistance of joint biomaterials when loaded under extreme environmental conditions.

2.2 Atomic Force Microscopy

The AFM device can be considered a modern and highly technological update of the more traditional stylus profilometer. In its original version, the stylus profilometer employs a sharp cantilever-mounted probe affixed with a mirror to magnify surface profile features onto photographic paper. A light source is shined into the mirror, which reflects onto the paper. As the cantilever scans across the surface, it deflects upon interacting with various surface features. Deflections are then translated into the photographic paper by changes in the intensity of the light from the mirror. Under optimized conditions, the stylus profilometer is capable of resolutions in the single micrometer scale [152, 153]. This is the case of a profilometer using electronic amplifications or non-contact optical profilometers based on the principle of two-beam optical interferometry, for some of which an in-depth spatial resolution in the sub-micrometer range has also been reported [154–158]. Although using the same measurement principle, the AFM allows for further enhancing spatial resolution down to the atomic scale [159–161]. The AFM relies upon a very sharp tip held by a cantilever and brought in contact with the sample surface. As the tip is scanned across the sample, variations in the deflection of the cantilever appear as the sample profile changes. These variations are used as the error signal arises from the deflection of the probe assembly as it moves in response to features on the sample surface. This deflection is captured by reflecting a laser beam from the back of the probe into a detector, which in turn measures the voltage change as the laser moves across its surface.

If the horizontal raster motion is stopped, then the error signal arising from cantilever deflection represents motion in the vertical direction only. Applying a voltage ramp to a piezo-actuator (controlled by the error signal in a feedback loop) then displaces the probe downward, into contact with the sample, and eventually pulls the probe back to its initial position. By recording the deflection of the cantilever across this ramp, a one-dimensional profile of the tip interaction is generated as the tip approaches to, contacts with, and retracts from the sample surface. A schematic of the AFM device is shown in Fig. 2.1(a). A solid-state laser diode is used to impinge a beam on the scanner head to be then reflected from the back of the cantilever onto a split photodiode sensor Fig. 2.1(b). Then, as already mentioned, data recorded by the photodiode are translated into deflection voltages and piezo-actuator displacements that describe the statistical texture of the sample surface (Fig. 2.1(c)). Computer software allows maintaining a feedback loop based on constant cantilever deflection/interaction

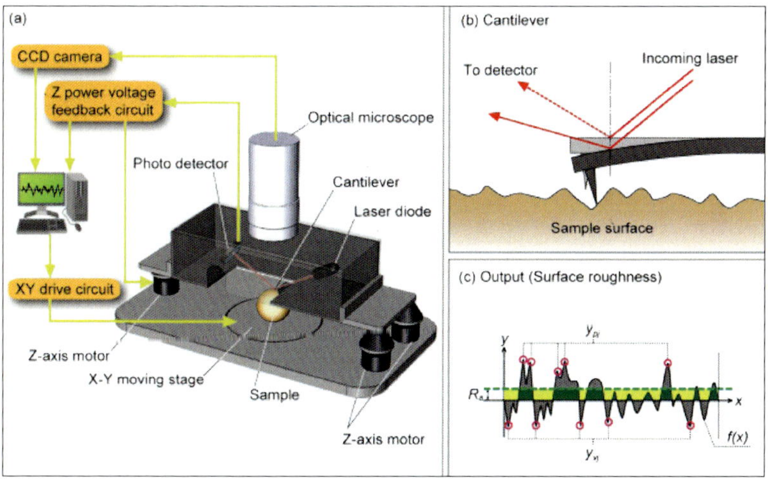

Figure 2.1 Schematic drafts of: (a) the AFM device; (b) a laser beam impinging on the scanner head and to be reflected onto a detector; and, (c) output data recorded by the laser that are successively translated into deflection voltages and piezo-actuator displacements to describe the statistical texture of the sample surface. The vertical displacements y_{pj} are heights detected from the peaks, while y_{vj} are depths detected from the valleys encountered along the scanning profile.

force (for contact mode) or on constant cantilever oscillation amplitude (for intermittent contact mode). The latter measurement mode is also referred to as the "tapping" mode, its main characteristic being that the cantilever is displaced laterally at the peak of the oscillation. The tapping mode might involve several benefits when applied to biomaterials; for example, it allows for increased lateral resolution of soft and/or hydrated samples, and decreased damage to the sample surface. However, the use of tapping mode with compliant samples might also introduce artifacts into the collected data [162, 163], for the amplitude signal could be damped as it rapidly indents into the sample.

By AFM method, topographical images of the sample can be created at extremely small lateral resolutions, in the order of the single angstrom [159–161]. Applying equilibrium relationships, according for example to Hooke's law, between cantilever deflection and force, the deflection profile can eventually be translated into a map of the force of an interaction across some distance associated with the voltage ramp. These data may be used to determine physicochemical and physicomechanical properties of the samples [164–170], including hardness, stiffness, and adhesive/tensile strength. In conjunction with appropriate mathematical models, so-called force cycles may be used for assessing the relative importance of electrostatic, dispersion, London–van der Waals and electromagnetic forces in producing the interaction profile [171, 172]. While specifically designed for applications to the semiconductor and electronic materials, the AFM has been applied to a variety of fields, including microbiology and biomedicine. Examples of these applications include, for example, the measurement of atomic bond rupture-forces between organosilane monolayers [164], the study of the molecular interactions and mechanical properties of microbial cell surfaces [173], the characterization of lectin-carbohydrate interactions at the nanometer scale [174], measurement of interaction forces between complementary DNA strands [175], biomedical characterizations through mechanically or chemically modified probes [176–178], just to cite a few of those applications. Being the AFM a highly sensitive tool, it must be operated with a degree of expertise to produce reproducible results. Of primary importance to reproducibility is knowledge of the state of the machine as it operates, which is obtained through careful calibration of the instrument. Specifically, three quantities are concurrently measured: the AFM laser wavelength, the ratio between actual and software-reported piezo-actuator displacement, and the spring constant of the cantilevered probe. The precision of such measurements determines the reliability of height, force, and separation data. Additionally, the radius of curvature of the tip probe has a profound effect on the interpretation of AFM data [161, 163, 179], in terms of the degree of dilation present in topographical images, the available contact area in a force-separation interaction, and the error propagated when using the radius as a parameter in mathematical models. A more precise description of each parameter to be measured during instrument calibration is beyond the scope of this book and a broader description of the technique, including the calibration involved with the use of the AFM, is left to more specific publications [166, 180–183].

In artificial joint applications, topography represents the main external features of bearing surfaces, for which the surface smoothness and texture can be very important. Besides the clear influence of these parameters on the mechanical stress distribution on the bearing surface, the smoothness/texture are expected to affect protein adhesion, friction and, ultimately, wear and thus the clinical performance of the joint. Roughness is represented by the finer irregularities of the surface that originally result from the inherent action of the production process or material condition and overlapped by the effect of wear between the sliding surfaces during service in the human body. In biomaterials for artificial joints, roughness gains great attention as its spatial scales are close to the scales of chemical, biological, and mechanical processes that take place on the load-bearing surfaces. However, although surface roughness (i.e., the arithmetic average of the absolute values of the profile height deviation recorded within the evaluation length and measured from the mean line (cf. Fig. 2.1(c))) is the traditional parameter that has been used to evaluate joint bearing surfaces before and after implantation, it might not represent a parameter of merit, and frequently its value does not produce good correlation with the expected wear behavior. In this sense, hip joint surfaces with similar roughness values may have different behavior in surgical success [184–186]. This situation points out the necessity of other statistical parameters to express correctly the surface nature [187–189]. For example, the effects of kurtosis and skewness of the surface roughness distribution have been investigated and modeled to calculate frictional forces and friction coefficients [187]. It has been predicted that surfaces with high kurtosis and positive skewness exhibit lower static friction coefficient compared to the Gaussian case. More important, for high kurtosis values, the static friction coefficient decreases with decreasing external force rather than increasing as seen with increasing skewness. Predictions can be used to determine the optimal characteristics of joint devices in order to achieve lower friction in terms of surface roughness, apparent contact area, and operational environment. It should be also noted that the evaluation of smoothness in a joint prosthesis surface (i.e., especially in prostheses made of ceramics) requires to be measured down to the nanometer level in order to monitor wear and pit distribution, for which the spatial resolution of a stylus profilometer (about 1 μm) is insufficient. In such cases, an AFM has to be mandatorily employed. These characteristics naturally select the AFM as the most suitable technique to quantify topography in highly wear resistant materials like as ceramics and advanced polyethylene grades, for which surface damage lies on the sub-micrometer scale. Unfortunately, neither stylus profilometry nor AFM gives additional information on the chemical and stress states of the surface, so these techniques must be coupled with chemical and mechanical investigations on the nanoscale, with the use of different spectroscopic methods.

2.3 Raman and Infrared Spectroscopy

Raman spectroscopy is a technique nowadays widely used in condensed matter physics and chemistry to study vibrational, rotational, and other low-frequency modes in a material system [190]. The Raman effect (first predicted by Smekal in 1923 and then observed by Raman in the 1928) relies on inelastic scattering (or Raman scattering) of monochromatic light, usually from a laser in the visible, near infrared, or near ultraviolet range. The laser light interacts with phonons or other excitations in the system, resulting in the energy of the laser photons being shifted up or down, according to the phonon modes present in the system. Infrared spectroscopy yields similar but complementary information. Both Raman and IR can be used in backscattered and transmission collection modes. However, due to a possibly lower efficiency in signal detection as compared with visible light, IR signals might need to be collected in transmission mode. In case of joint biomaterials, this might represent a serious disadvantage as compared to Raman spectroscopy, especially because sample manipulation during cutting the sample in thin slices might alter the original structure of the biomaterial or because the sample, for reasons extraneous to the spectroscopic experiment, can only be treated in a non-destructive way (e.g., joint retrievals obtained from hospitals). In order to confine the collection of the Raman emission to a micrometer scale, an optical microprobe can be used. After illuminating the sample with focusing the laser through an optical lens, the light scattered from the illuminated spot is collected back through the same lens and sent to a monochromator (Fig. 2.2(a)). Wavelengths close

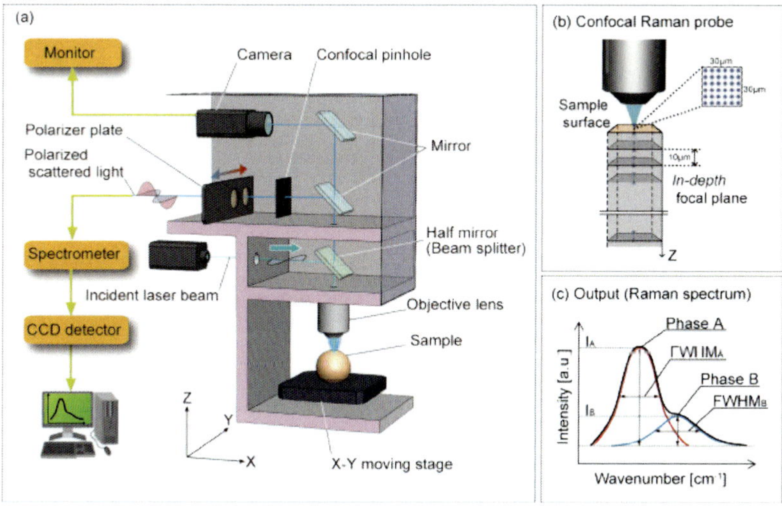

Figure 2.2 Schematic drafts of: (a) the Raman microprobe device; (b) a laser beam impinging on the sample and mapping it in plane and in depth using a confocal probe configuration; and, (c) example of an output spectrum recorded by the Raman device that is successively deconvoluted into different sub-band components. Note that polarization filters might allow crystallographic analysis. The draft in (b) refers to a typical Raman characterization of biomedical UHMWPE, as described in a forthcoming chapter.

to the laser line (due to elastic Rayleigh scattering) are filtered out and those in a selected spectral window, away from the laser line, are dispersed onto a CCD camera and displayed as a spectrum. In the past, pioneering Raman experiments were carried out using focused sunlight and filters, while the output of such experiments relied on visual observation of color changes in the scattered light. Raman spectra of several liquids were successively recorded using a mercury lamp and a spectrograph until, in the 1960s, a major improvement occurred with the development of visible lasers. Suddenly after the introduction of such monochromatic, coherent, narrow-beam, and high-intensity light sources, Raman spectra could easily and precisely be recorded from very small sample volumes, including solids, liquids, and gases in a variety of nonstandard conditions. In recent years, microelectronics has further improved the technique such that stepper motor drives, photon counting, digital data acquisition and computer processing have provided chemists, physicists, and analysts with a technique, which many claim being more useful and versatile than IR. Upon coupling the Raman device with an optical microscope, thus obtaining a Raman microprobe, the study of chromophoric species at very low concentrations has become possible and now plays an important role in the study of biologically significant molecules. Nowadays, Raman spectroscopy and its related techniques are finding a large number of applications across a wide range of research activities in the biomedical field [86, 98, 191–196]. Concurrently, there concurrently exists extensive effort in describing new developments of the Raman theory [197–201].

The Raman effect can be generally described as the inelastic scattering of light by matter. When a photon, too low in energy to excite an electronic transition, interacts with a molecule it can be scattered in one of the two following ways: elastically, thus retaining its incident energy; or, inelastically, by either giving energy up to or by removing energy from the molecule. Photons undergoing inelastic loss of energy give rise to Stokes scattering whilst photons undergoing inelastic gain of energy give rise to anti-Stokes scattering. The energy gained by the molecule in Stokes scattering appears as vibrational energy; then, such same excess in vibrational energy above the ground state is lost to the anti-Stokes scattered photons. Note, however, that only a very small percentage of the excited molecules relax back to a vibrationally excited state, hence the emitted photons are smaller than the exciting photons. Since only a very small fraction of molecules use this relaxation pathway, Raman scattering is generally of a quite low intensity. Therefore, its investigation requires high-quality instrumentation, with the main difficulty in Raman spectroscopy consisting in separating the weak inelastically scattered light from the intense Rayleigh scattered laser light. Modern Raman spectrometers typically use holographic diffraction gratings and multiple dispersion stages to achieve a high degree of laser rejection. The recent use of CCD detectors has made dispersive Raman spectral acquisition much more rapid and efficient.

In Raman microscopy, a research grade optical microscope is coupled to the excitation laser and the spectrometer thus producing a platform capable of obtaining conventional visible images and, in addition, generating Raman spectra from sample areas approaching the diffraction limit (i.e., lateral resolutions of ≈1 μm). The combination of a Raman microscope and a motorized *x*, *y*, and *z* stage allows for the generation of 2-D or even 3-D maps that can yield information on the distribution of materials in a heterogeneous sample over a defined area. When a laser is focused in air, a beam waist and beam length, related to the numerical aperture of the lens and wavelength of radiation, is produced. If a laser is instead focused onto surface of a condensed phase material, then the beam length below the surface will be strongly affected by the refractive index of the material and by the material absorption characteristics. Raman scattering will thus occur along the axis of the beam length and the collection lens will collect the entire radiation. Therefore, the spectrum measured from a single (*x*, *y*) point on a surface will be the result of a convolution of information from several *z* planes (below the "surface") [126, 202–204]. By employing a technique known as "confocal spectroscopy", it is possible to probe discrete *z* planes (Fig. 2.2(b)). In this technique, a conjugate aperture (i.e., a pinhole) is used to reject out of focus radiation originating from different *z*-planes from reaching the detector [205, 206]. The radiation originating from above the sample surface is not brought to a focus before the pinhole and, thus, the measured signal from this layer might result significantly attenuated by the aperture. The principal advantage in using a confocal aperture is the possibility of spatial discrimination to a well-defined area of a heterogeneous sample and, thus, the possibility of screening the sample non-destructively in its bulk volume. However, even in confocal configurations, the study of highly graded sample features might requires deconvolution of Raman maps over individual z planes inside the sample, which in turn require the precise knowledge of the response function of the microprobe (i.e., the morphological function characterizing the laser probe geometry when the probe interacts with the sample) [125, 207, 208]. The probe function should be experimentally determined case by case for each individual material, as shown in the forthcoming chapters. The knowledge of the probe response function enables one to characterize the amount of signal contributed by each portion of volume within the overall irradiated volume. Experimental practice teaches that probe calibrations should be performed not only on each investigated material but also on each individual Raman band of the investigated material, and on individual materials with the same chemical composition but different microstructures [208].

In principle, it is possible to separate the energy of an atom (or a group of atoms) embedded in a crystal into three additive components: (i) rotational (for molecules), (ii) vibrational (referred to vibrations between the constituent atoms), (iii) electronic (due to the electronic motion inside atoms). The basis for this separation lies in the fact that the velocity of electrons is much greater than the vibrational velocity of nuclei, which is in turn much greater than the velocity of molecular rotation. If a crystal is analyzed under incident light, a transfer of energy from the electromagnetic field of light to the atom will occur, which equals the energy gap between two quantized states. Furthermore, using polarized light, it is possible to inquire about the structure of individual vibrational modes [209]. Polarization analysis in Raman spectroscopy provides a powerful tool in chemical physics to identify the symmetry of the vibration modes of molecules, macromolecules, and crystals, according to their crystallographic structure, texture, and local spatial orientation. The joint use of parallel and crossed polarization data yields accurate source separation results and improves the uniqueness properties of the solution in blind non-negative source separation algorithms.

Polarized Raman approaches have been validated for a large number of crystals [210–212] and, according to such approaches, information about the local orientation of the sample under the microscope objective has been obtained through systematic sample rotation and the retrieval of the local components of the Raman polarizability tensor. A schematic of the spectral output of a Raman experiment and related spectral deconvolution is given in Fig. 2.2(c). As shown, typical parameters used in Raman spectroscopic analyses are band intensity, *I*, and band full width at half maximum, FWHM.

A main contribution of Raman spectroscopy to the analytical biomedical issues has been made in the area of biomaterials, especially in the identification of biodegradation and deterioration [213, 214]. The impact of Raman spectroscopy on the study of biomaterials has been extensive, in particular for those biomaterials widely employed as load-bearing components in artificial joints [215–217]. Important case studies have also been presented in the literature [218–221] that illustrate the power of the Raman technique to answer key questions of broad medical, scientific, and technological interest. The analytical and physical science lying behind the Raman effect can be thus shown to contribute to the accumulation of a wealth of fundamental information about the medical and technical achievements of biomaterials makers. It should be also emphasized that Raman microprobe spectroscopy offers, via the double approach of spectral and spatial deconvolution, the possibility of non-destructively testing the reliability of biomaterials, a matter of great concern to patients, surgeons, implant makers, and technologists.

Raman spectroscopy also offers the possibility of performing highly localized assessments of mechanical stress. This can be made by exploiting the so-called piezo-spectroscopic (PS) effect, simply defined as the shift in frequency of a spectroscopic transition in response to an applied strain or stress. The definition of the PS effect can be stated independent of spectrum arising from luminescence [222], or from Raman scattering [223]. The PS effect usually obeys a linear relationship between the second-rank stress tensor and the observed Raman shift [224–226], and in the experimental practice, all the components of the PS tensor need to be directly measured. In addition, various kinds of quantitative information can be achieved by Raman inspection of biomaterials as, for example, surface modifications in terms of phase transformation upon exposure to biological environment, the associated residual stress state stored within different phases, and the amount of oxidation and other chemistry-related alterations of the bearing surfaces. Clear correlations can be found between the degree of phase transformation, the residual strain magnitude, and the oxidative phenomena, which are in turn related to the complex, environmentally assisted wear interactions occurring in artificial joints, (e.g., between the femoral head and its bearing counterpart acetabular cup). It should be noted that the interpretation of Raman spectra in the presence of overlapping phases might be not straightforward; however, it has been shown [117] that an assessment of the surface Raman response of relevant zirconia bands is possible with the aid of confocal spectroscopy. Phase transformation fractions in the early nucleation stage of the monoclinic phase (and related residual stress fields stored within both tetragonal and monoclinic phases) on the surface of ZrO_2 femoral heads can be, for example, characterized by Raman spectroscopy. The monoclinic phase content can be quantitatively evaluated from the relative intensities of Raman bands arising from different polymorphs, namely the tetragonal phase and the monoclinic phase [227]. Evaluations of phase fractions are accurate to about ±0.1 vol.%. Intensification of elastic stress fields are expected on the surface of ceramic hip joints and they may be rather severe owing to the overlapping of several factors, including pre-existing defects, wear, and machining effects. Elastic residual stress components arising from phase transformation are also expected in metastable materials, with the formation of severe, highly localized stress gradients on the biomaterial surface.

Raman spectroscopy characterizations are also very important for biomedical polyethylene and ultra-high molecular weight (UHMWPE), which are materials of wide use in joint arthroplasty. γ-Ray irradiation is commonly used for the sterilization of medical devices. Cobalt 60 γ-sterilization has become the industry's method of choice because of its reliability in sterilizing thoroughly throughout the entire sample, the absence of chemical residues after sterilization, its flexibility, and its cost effectiveness. However, no fully conclusive verdict has been reached about the optimum radiation dose and the method of sterilization, yet represents a primary concern in total joint replacements. In this context, the goal of Raman spectroscopic experiments can be pivotal in verifying the actual structural changes that occur during irradiation of UHMWPE, specifically with regard to their impact on wear properties [228–231]. Evaluations of the extent to which structural changes influence the lifetime of the joint with respect to creep deformation and oxidation can be made by Raman spectroscopy by means of quantitative assessments of molecular structures, orientation patterns and residual plastic strain.

2.4 Cathodoluminescence Spectroscopy

The interaction of the electron beam with the sample gives rise to a number of concurrent effects, including the emission of secondary electrons, backscattering of electrons, electron absorption, and emission of light and characteristic X-rays. The term CL designates the luminescence induced by electron irradiation, which can be measured by means of additional equipment attached to the SEM as shown in Fig. 2.3(a). The penetration depth of electrons, and accordingly the excitation depth, depends on the energy of the impinging electron beam; therefore, using low acceleration voltages, the probing depth can be confined to the nanometer range, thus obtaining a spatial resolution several orders of magnitude higher as compared to laser probes [145, 232–234]. From the point of view of spatial resolution, CL is thus the most appropriate analytical method for screening the very surface of the inorganic materials employed in joint arthroplasty. The electron-stimulated luminescence can be divided into two types, the intrinsic CL, which is characteristic of the host lattice, and the extrinsic CL, which results from impurities or dopants intentionally introduced in the host lattice. The former type of CL is enhanced by non-stoichiometry (e.g., vacancies) and other structural imperfections that distort the crystal lattice. Impurities or dopants, responsible for the extrinsic luminescence, are called activators. Elements are also referred to as sensitizers when their presence is necessary to create a luminescence center with an activator. Impurities and dopant elements can either be super-, sub- or isovalent with their host lattice. Super-valent impurities are called donors as they contribute electrons to the conduction band, while sub-valent impurities, which supply

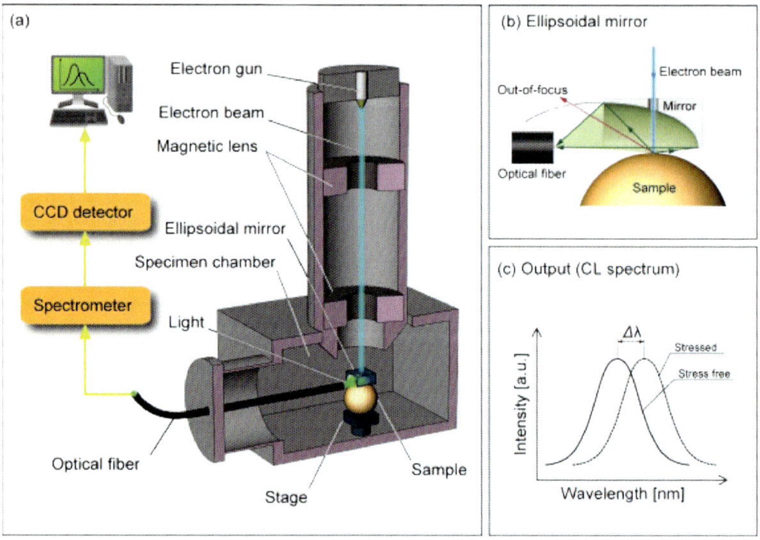

Figure 2.3 Schematic drafts of: (a) the cathodoluminescence device attached to an SEM; (b) an electron beam impinging on the sample that in turn emits a characteristic light collected by an ellipsoidal mirror and sent to the spectrometer; and, (c) example of an output spectrum recorded by the cathodoluminescence device that shows the effect of stress on the spectrum.

holes to the valence band, are known as acceptors. The luminescence center is eventually transferred into an excited state, which results in a sensitized luminescence [235, 236]. In this latter case, the CL properties are mostly the result of luminescence-activating ions such as transition metals, rare-earth elements or actinides. Changes of the crystal field properties, i.e., field strength, site symmetry, and coordination number, cause differences in the magnitude of the energy levels of the activator elements and also the splitting of closely spaced levels. Therefore, the CL spectrum is not a characteristic property of the activator but it should be regarded as a material property. Furthermore, some trace elements in the host lattice may induce (or quench) both intrinsic and extrinsic CL. CL emission can be considered to form in three successive steps: the absorption of excitation energy and consequent stimulation of the atoms into an excited state, the transformation and transfer of the excitation energy, and the emission of light and relaxation to a non-excited state [237]. Note that the majority of bioceramics, such as alumina (Al_2O_3), are insulators, thus possessing a broad gap (i.e., also referred to as the "forbidden" gap) between the valence band and the conduction band. In those materials, a precondition for CL is the existence of activators (impurity ions, lattice defects), which cause and occupy discrete energy levels in this forbidden zone. Luminescence centers can then be differentiated by their energy position within the forbidden gap and be divided into electron traps near the conduction band (donor level) and recombination sites in the vicinity of the valence band (acceptor level) [238].

The SEM is nowadays, along with optical and laser microscopes, the most widely employed imaging instrument. The scanning electron microprobe utilizes a scanned electron beam with a small spot size normally in the order of the single nanometer in diameter. By scanning with an electron beam, synchronized with the in-plane deflection of a display oscilloscope, and by modulating the display oscilloscope intensity with the photomultiplier output, localized CL spectra and a magnified map of the CL emitted from the specimen can be obtained. CL equipment attached to an SEM offers advantages over conventional laser spectroscopy, the main advantage being the larger spatial resolution in the nanometer range. Another advantage is the possibility of combining CL/SEM investigations with electron backscattering spectroscopy and imaging (as described in the next section) for local crystallographic analyses and elemental analyses from the very same area. In the CL equipment, an aluminum parabolic mirror is placed between the sample stage and the electron source (Fig. 2.3(b)). Through a hole in the mirror, the sample is irradiated with electrons and the luminescence is collected. For the most efficient collection, the sample must be in the focal point of the mirror, which is typically 1 mm or less below the mirror itself. Owing to of its parabolic shape, the mirror reflects the light as a parallel beam into a waveguide. The detection of the emitted light can occur in two modes: either the light is led through a monochromator and a CCD camera, which allows one to collect a CL spectrum, or a CL image is built up by photon counting at a given particular wavelength. While the collection of the full CL spectrum is a fundamental prerequisite for detailed analyses of band shift and width, photomultiplier maps of CL intensity provide a fast screening and a quickly collected visual output that can be thus promptly applied to relatively large areas of the sample.

As mentioned above, CL arises from and, thus, can be used for visualizing a wide variety of lattice defects. These defects can be vacancies, interstitials, anti-site defects, and their complexes, dislocations, stacking faults, grain boundaries, or precipitates. Unfortunately, no universal theory is available to take into account and predict CL emission for all these cases. Nevertheless, the optical activity of lattice defects, especially that of vacancies, can be shown to cover a fundamental importance in unfolding tribological effects occurring both *in vitro* and *in vivo* on the load-bearing surfaces of oxide ceramics used in joint arthroplasty. The CL spectrum of oxide bioceramics indeed contains plenty of invaluable information. A number of parameters determine the morphology of individual bands in the CL spectrum: the nature of the CL emission, the degree of electron-phonon coupling with the lattice (a measure of the number of phonons emitted during the electronic transition), the specimen temperature and electron beam excitation conditions, the strain magnitude and gradients in the probed volume. A schematic of the spectral output of a CL experiment and the effect of stress on the spectrum are shown in Fig. 2.3(c).

Not only the knowledge of the influence of each of these parameters on the peak shape greatly assists us in the assignment of the CL emission peaks to particular lattice features, but also experiments can be undertaken to identify local temperature and strain fields. In practice, CL identification requires precise preliminary calibrations to be performed over a selected range of known parameters and with fixed electron probe excitation conditions [211, 239–241].

As far as load-bearing biomaterials are concerned, CL becomes a fundamental tool for unveiling the role of surface stoichiometry on wear behavior, for quantifying the tribochemical differences between *in vitro* and *in vivo* environments and, more generally, for assessing the environmental resistance of ceramic oxides. While the majority of ceramic oxides have long been considered to be completely bioinert in the human body [242], observation on the molecular scale might reveal significant stoichiometric differences for environmentally exposed surfaces as compared to the respective as-manufactured ones. For example, the oxygen vacancy levels in Al_2O_3 have been recently calculated using first-principle methods [243]. They have been found to lie just below midgap in the oxide, such low energy conceivably accounting for the highly inert behavior of Al_2O_3 in aggressive biological environment. However, the destabilizing effect of body environment, especially of divalent cations contained in the body fluid, cannot be neglected under the extreme mechanochemical conditions of frictional contact between joint surfaces. The combined action of highly localized surface strain and the aggressive chemical activity of the tribolayer might lead to marked off-stoichiometry on the Al_2O_3 bearings, with severe consequences on its wear behavior. Vacancies in the oxygen sub-lattice also greatly facilitate ionic conductivity toward the in-depth direction, thus establishing a detrimental cycle that accelerates wear rate.

The effect of lattice defects is even more striking in zirconia (ZrO_2) bioceramics. The addition of trivalent dopants and oversized/undersized tetravalent dopants into ZrO_2 is known to stabilize the tetragonal metastable phase of this oxide bioceramic by creating oxygen vacancies to energetically favor such structures. The cubic phase of ZrO_2 can be also produced by the addition of up to 20% trivalent stabilizer oxides such as yttria or ceria [244]. However, the mechanical properties of such ZrO_2 material deteriorate with large concentrations of stabilizing oxides [245]. In addition, the possibility of stabilizing metastable phases of zirconia materials through the direct formation of oxygen vacancies in its nanostructures has been theoretically predicted [246] and experimentally verified [247]. Vacancies in ZrO_2 crystallites can be induced by a thorough control of the sintering atmosphere [248]. Furthermore, nanocrystalline zirconia with grain sizes in the order of the tens of nanometer and, thus, with large surface area and surface to volume ratio can stabilize the cubic phase through formation of oxygen vacancies [249]. This effect is equivalent to the effects of chemical trivalent stabilizers such as yttria and ceria and has been adopted to produce zirconia femoral heads with improved stability in body environment [250, 251]. However, despite some clear experimental evidence on the role of processing parameters in oxide ceramics, a full understanding of the origin of zirconia metastability induced by exposure in the human body appears to necessarily require further investigations.

In this context, CL spectroscopy, being capable of visualizing surface vacancies through their optical activity, plays a pivotal role in such a process of scientific and technological understanding.

2.5 Electron Backscattering Diffraction

EBSD, also known as backscattered Kikuchi diffraction, is a microstructural-crystallographic technique enabling the quantitative assessment of crystallographic textures or preferred orientations of crystalline materials [252]. This technique can be used to index and identify crystal systems and can be applied to crystal orientation mapping, phase identification, domain-like heterogeneity investigations, and phase patterning. EBSD is conducted using a SEM equipped with a backscatter diffraction camera (Fig. 2.4(a)), which is essentially a focal plane CCD coupled with a phosphor screen (inserted into the specimen chamber of the SEM at an angle greater than or equal to 90° to the pole piece). A flat/polished crystalline specimen is placed into the normal position in the specimen chamber, but is highly tilted (~60° from horizontal) toward the diffraction camera. When the electrons impinge on the specimen they interact with the atomic lattice planes of the crystalline structures, many of these interactions satisfy Bragg conditions and undergo backscatter diffraction. Due to the angle of the specimen these diffracted electrons are directed toward and impinge upon the phosphor screen of the diffraction camera causing it to fluoresce, the fluorescent light being then detected by the CCD. According to this mechanism, the diffracted electrons form an image termed a diffraction pattern that is unique to the microstructural-crystallographic properties of the material. Using a computer-aided procedure, one can obtain precise indexing of the investigated surface in terms of diffraction patterns consisting of several intersecting lines termed Kikuchi bands. Since the Kikuchi bands correspond to the lattice diffracting planes, they can be individually indexed by the Miller indices of the diffracting plane from which they originate. Indexing allows for identification of the microstructure or orientation at a given point on the sample from which the pattern is collected. Pattern bands are usually detected via a mathematical routine in which every pixel denotes a unique line in the EBSD pattern. The detection principle is based on the fact that angles between bands correspond to angles between lattice planes, when the position/angles between three bands are known an orientation solution can be determined [253].

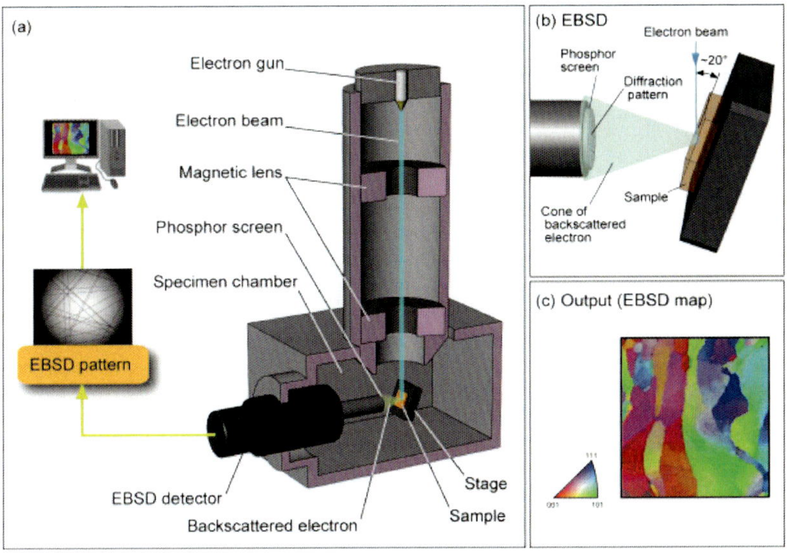

Figure 2.4 Schematic drafts of: (a) the EBSD device attached to an SEM; (b) diffraction pattern collected by the phosphor screen; and (c) example of an output crystallographic map recorded by the EBSD device.

EBSD patterns are generated in a two-step process: in the first step the electrons enter into the crystal and are quasi-elastically but incoherently scattered. This process can be regarded as the formation of an electron source inside of the crystal, namely as emerging from a small area in the crystal and consequently diffracted at the crystal lattice according to the Bragg equation. In order to clearly observe the diffraction pattern, it is necessary to tilt the sample by about 60° or 70°, which will increase the amount of electrons which can reach the detector (Fig. 2.4(b)). The quality of an EBSD measurement depends on the signal-to-noise ratio observed in the pattern and on the spatial resolution of the electron probe, which in turn depend on the investigated sample. As far as the equipment is concerned, the quality of the pattern is controlled by a number of factors, including beam size and current (and its mechanical and electronic stability), the EBSD camera (light sensitivity, pixel resolution, read-out time), and the software. A detailed treatment about the incidence of such factors on the EBSD measurement can be found in the work published by Humphreys [254, 255]. As far as the sample is concerned, the image quality of the EBSD patterns, i.e., the sharpness of the Kikuchi lines, mainly depends on the distortion of the lattice (i.e., due to dislocations or lattice deformation) and on surface artifacts. In the latter case, the effect can be very critical because electron backscatter diffraction only occurs in a region very close to the surface (10~50 nm in depth). For example, a diffuse (noise) pattern might result from a foreign surface layer such as carbon of excessive thickness (which may have been deposited by intention to avoid specimen charging), a contamination layer due to poor vacuum conditions, or an insufficiently focused beam spot. In other words, since EBSD is a surface-sensitive technique, it does not give volume information. EBSD is now widely accepted since it enables crystallography of small grains in the surface of bulk specimens to be studied in the SEM in a much easier and efficient way than was previously possible by the acquisition of electron spots and by channeling patterns in (transmission or reflection) electron diffraction.

Crystal lattice orientation measurement grain-by-grain might yield information on the biomaterial microstructure that is not easily obtainable by any other technique. It should be considered that load-bearing medical implants such as the hip and knee joints undergo highly variable loading in aggressive physiological environment. The implant materials are thus required to have appropriate mechanical, physical, chemical and biological properties. Corrosion issues are particularly relevant to metallic materials, among which Co–Cr alloys are amongst the few materials that can fulfill suitable requirements [256, 257]. The quality of Co–Cr castings has been improved through substantial advances in manufacturing techniques over the years. However, wear rate are yet a concern in metal-on-metal-type implants as well as rare incidences of fracture still occur in service. SEM can reveal facets on the fatigue fracture surface and zigzag shaped secondary (grain-boundary) cracking on the adjacent fracture surface but lacks in the quantitative analysis of crystallographic slip and primary deformation planes. Convergent beam electron diffraction in a transmission electron microscope can be used for conducting quantitative crystallographic analyses [258–260] by tilting the grain-boundary plane to the edge-on condition and determining the diffraction vector perpendicular to the grain-boundary trace line but in such assessments it is difficult to keep the cracks intact during electro-polishing. On the other hand, quantitative crystallographic information on the very surface of the load-bearing joint surface can be achieved in a fully non-destructive manner by EBSD analyses conducted in the SEM [261]. In a recent paper [261], Sun *et al.* have applied EBSD to the study of micro-abrasion mechanisms in cast CoCrMo alloys (i.e., commonly used for metal-on-metal hip replacement due to their superior wear and corrosion resistance) when lubricated with simulated body fluid. EBSD analysis clarified that the face-centered cubic phase of the cast alloys partially transforms into a stable (and harder) hexagonal close-packed phase (ε-martensite) during abrasive contact. This suggests that this newly formed phase undergoes coarse slip bands, which may in turn contribute to fracture line formation. The initiated cracks may subsequently lead to detachment of material upon multiple abrasive cycles.

Apart from the above study, EBSD studies of ceramic biomaterials are yet conspicuously lacking in the available literature. Some of the problems associated with characterizing ceramics by EBSD include charging due to the low electrical conductivity of many ceramics, polishing-induced surface damage that degrades EBSD image quality, and the low backscatter yield of some ceramics that have low average atomic weights (due to the large amounts of oxygen, nitrogen, carbon, etc., present). The most critical issue is perhaps charging, because distortion in the EBSD data due to charging will make it impossible to align and register adjacent slices in the serial section, and may make the data unusable. Fine surface preparation of materials with high bond strength, like ceramics, can take considerably longer time than materials with much lower bond strengths (e.g., metals). While many ceramics may be non-ideal candidates for EBSD, the interest in characterizing them is considerable. Despite the experimental difficulties, EBSD studies of ceramic biomaterials used in artificial joints are indeed very promising. In particular, it will be shown in this book how the study of correlations between EBSD orientation parameters enables a precise determination of the lattice strain developed in alumina-based bioceramics after exposure in water-vapor environment. Such a determination is possible with high spatial resolution in the SEM in combination with CL spectroscopy [71, 122].

2.6 Fracture Mechanics and Toughening Mechanisms

The structural characterization of joint biomaterials is mainly based on fracture mechanics investigations. Brittle materials (e.g., ceramics), unlike metals, do not allow for blunting of a propagating crack and, thus, for the consequent relaxation of concentrated stresses. Consequently, a fracture path, initiated under a threshold load at the most critical flaw, is expected to propagate almost instantaneously and, thus, catastrophically through the component. Note that the assumption that failure is catastrophic above a given threshold load is, in principle, always acceptable for brittle materials because it leads to the estimate of a "minimum" value for the structural resistance of the component. However, the problem resides in the fact that the critical load for fracture will depend not only on the intrinsic properties of the material (measurable) and on the size and shape of the component (changeable by design) but also on the size (and the morphology) of the critical defect, which is unknown. One can see the problem from an inverse viewpoint and state that the component will stand unbroken under a given load only if its internal flaw population does not include any flaw above a certain "critical" size. In other words, the strength of a component made of a brittle material is mainly governed by the probability that a defect of size larger than a threshold value be encountered. The close link between the presence of defects in brittle materials and their unpredictable catastrophic fracture makes the structural performance quite unpredictable and sensitive to processing conditions. Note that besides the importance of a statistical approach to component reliability [262], this circumstance leads to a lack of correlations even among materials obeying the same chemical formula. Predictability of the structural properties is thus irremediably compromised, the strength of a ceramic joint component being a parameter greatly dependent on the manufacturers' ability to minimize the inherent flaw size. A reaction to such an unacceptable situation of "maker dependency" of the selected ceramic component may well explain the shift in focus of the biomaterials research community over the past 10~15 years toward the improvement of flaw-tolerance ability (i.e., the fracture toughness) in structural bioceramics, as well as the efforts toward the application of fracture mechanics methodologies for its reliable characterizations [263–265]. Starting from theoretical considerations that comply with assumptions of the theory of elasticity and with conditions of plane strain that minimize the effects of departure from elasticity [266], studies of the intrinsic fracture toughness of ceramic biomaterials have flourished and gradually expanded in search for deeper understanding of toughening mechanisms activated during crack initiation and successive propagation [267–272]. Accordingly, the interest in fracture mechanics characterizations of bearing biomaterials has also shifted toward advanced methodologies to characterize crack propagation in semi-brittle biomaterials. Under these circumstances, it has been possible through many years of research clarifying important phenomena, like as crack shielding by the occurrence of local phase transformation [273–275] and the enhanced resistance to crack propagation with increasing crack length associated with crack-face bridging by unbroken ligaments or elongated grains [276–278]. Note that both mechanisms result in a tougher response of the biomaterial to *in vivo* crack initiation and, especially, propagation of fatigue cracks. Nowadays, the newest microstructural design concepts and the predictions of structural performance of modern ceramic joint components are based on these innovative (microscopic) aspects of fracture physics.

In the following description, we shall leave aside the positive effect on fracture toughness of a fractional addition of a metallic phase to the ceramic matrix that, although obviously effective, could, however, introduce problems in hip surgery similar to those reported for metallic implants [279–281]. As mentioned above, two major mechanisms have been discovered that can lead to significant toughening in sintered bioceramic components: (i) crack-face bridging [276–278] and, (ii) transformation toughening [273–275]. These two mechanisms are schematically drawn in Figs. 2.5(a) and (b), respectively. The former mechanism arises from the presence of elongated microstructural features

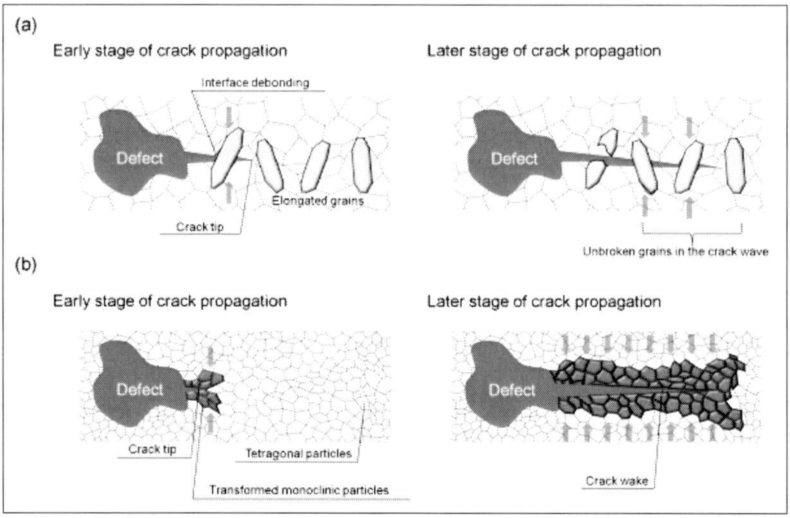

Figure 2.5 The most effective toughening mechanisms so far discovered in artificially made ceramic materials: (a) crack-face bridging; and, (b) transformation toughening. Mechanistically speaking, both toughening effects exploit crack-wake shielding behind the crack tip; however, in transformation toughening some positive effect is also foreseen ahead of the crack tip, which is not possible by crack-face bridging.

(i.e., grains or secondary-phase dispersoids) that are left unbroken behind the advancing crack front. Precursor to crack bridging is interface debonding in front of the crack tip, which actually impedes cleavage fracture of the bridge. Unbroken sites can act (up to their ultimate strength) as "bridges" against further opening of the crack faces, thus exerting a shielding effect on the advancing crack through the action of localized closure forces on the crack faces. The distribution of such forces along the crack path is of a discrete nature and depends on the volume fraction of the bridging sites. The latter mechanism instead is a consequence of the peculiar capacity of some ceramic phase (e.g., zirconium oxide, ZrO_2) to undergo a polymorphic transformation with a volume expansion (i.e., density reduction) in the order of ≈3%, under the high tensile stress field developed at the tip of the advancing crack. Volume expansion is, however, locally impeded by the constraint of the surrounding (untransformed) material and, thus, it causes a shielding effect on the advancing crack. Unlike crack bridging, the closure stress distribution operated by a transformed zone surrounding the crack path is of a continuous nature and depends on the size of such zone: the larger the size the stronger its shielding action. Note that from a mechanistic viewpoint, the two above toughening mechanisms are similar in the fact that they both result in closure forces on the faces of the propagating crack, such forces being additive and cumulatively effective with increasing crack length. This is in fact the physical origin of the observed increase of fracture resistance with increasing crack length, often referred to as "rising *R*-curve behavior". Note, however, that effective crack-face bridging contributions have so far been found only in non-oxide ceramics such as silicon nitride [282, 283] and silicon carbide [284], which are yet almost unexplored as biomaterials. Thus, the main toughening mechanism so far exploited in load-bearing biomedical components is the transformation toughening effect occurring in partially stabilized (monolithic) zirconia ceramics as well as in composite ceramic oxides containing metastable zirconia dispersoids.

Since fracture toughness, unlike fracture strength, is an intrinsic material property that describes the ability of a material to withstand unstable crack propagation, its determination represents an important aspect in the characterization of load-bearing biomaterials. The determination of fracture toughness constitutes the focus of several international standards, which have been recently updated and specialized to materials for artificial joints [285–287]. The main scope of standardization is to ensure that the results obtained represent true, reproducible, and comparable fracture resistance values. The standards provide detailed descriptions of specimen configuration and rigorous requirements as to the specimen size necessary to ensure stress conditions at the crack tip, along with details regarding testing parameters and data interpretation. Several specimen configurations have been commonly used for the characterization of joint biomaterials. The two most popular configurations are the single-edge-notched beam (SENB) test in three- or four-point bend specimen configuration (Fig. 2.6(a)), and the micro-indentation test (Fig. 2.6(b)) [288]. One of the main difficulties in determining the fracture toughness of ceramics is the introduction of a stress-free pre-crack that assures a square root singularity at the crack tip, namely the most severe testing configuration to ensure measuring the "worst" material

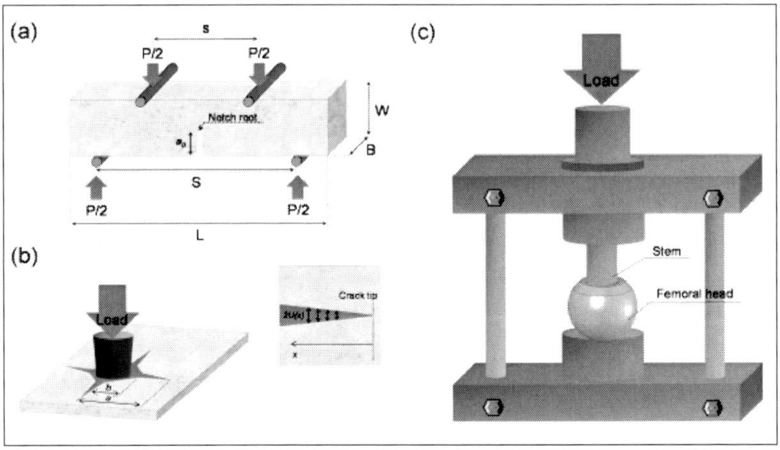

Figure 2.6 (a) Single-edge-notched beam test in four-point bend specimen configuration: a parallelepiped sample ($B \times W \times L$, in dimension) is placed under a load P; a_0 is the notch length, while S and s are the lower and the upper spans, respectively; (b) micro-indentation test: $2U(x)$ represents the crack COD profile, and a and b are the crack length and the print diagonal, respectively; (c) schematic of the burst strength test on hip implants as regulated by ISO 7206-10 [286].

performance. The difficulties are a consequence of the lack of crack arrest mechanisms; hence catastrophic crack propagation follows crack initiation. As a usual procedure, a thin notch is introduced by means of a diamond-cutting saw, as thin as 3 μm, which is used as a starter notch (i.e., in the SENB test). The stress singularity in this case is not certain, although it has been suggested that notch-tip flaws generated during cutting may eventually result in a stress singularity at the root of the starter notch [289]. Nevertheless, notch root radii larger than the single micron might lead to overestimate the fracture toughness of the material [290]. Because of its relative simplicity, the Vickers indentation method is widely used to evaluate the toughness properties of brittle materials [291–293]. Toughness is most easily estimated from the length of surface radial cracks around indents as a function of indentation load according to semi-empirical equations [294–296]. The indentation method is widely used for small specimens or in those cases, as in environmentally exposed artificial joints, for which the local toughness value at the material surface is a main object of investigation, since it might impact on the wear resistance of the biomaterial and be lower than the bulk toughness of the material [70]. Another, similar but somewhat more laborious way of evaluating toughness from indentations is to measure crack-opening displacements close to the crack tips in high magnification, e.g., by SEM [296–298] or AFM [299] observation. In this latter case, toughness is determined from the crack profile and the method only requires that the crack remain in quasi-equilibrium, i.e., on the verge of extension, which is the case immediately after indentation with sharp indenters [300]. Such a modified indentation method provides a means for examining intrinsic toughness properties in a direct manner. Recent work by Burghard *et al.* [301] has demonstrated that the crack opening displacement method provides more reliable estimates of the intrinsic material toughness as compared to the crack-length indentation method.

Nowadays, besides extensive research being performed on toughening of bioceramics, quite systematic efforts are also made to statistically analyze the strength properties of advanced biomaterials, especially in the field of artificial joints. Statistical analyses are routinely performed not only on different types of material but also by screening individual batches of joint components (or raw ceramic powders), directly taken from the production line. It is nowadays established that the strength properties of load-bearing components in artificial hip joints should be determined according to the standard ISO 6474-1 [302], which specifies the characteristics of and the corresponding test methods for high-purity alumina for use as components of orthopedic joint prostheses. This standard is currently being extended to composite materials (ISO 6474-2 [303]). Among other aspects, the standards take into account that the strength of a joint component depends not only on the intrinsic material properties but also on the design and manufacturing quality of its components, on external load, and on environmental conditions (i.e., leaving aside the quality of surgical operations, such as joint mounting and installation). Obviously, the adoption of high-strength materials can greatly ameliorate the performance of an artificial joint system; however, other factors may be even more decisive for its success. Therefore, design analyses, modeling, simulations, non-destructive evaluations, and risk analyses must be concurrently used to evaluate all those complex factors that determine the structural performance of a joint component and its reliability under service conditions. The most basic assessments of materials and systems for hip joints rely on the setup of a 4-point bending test (Fig. 2.6(a)) (i.e., also recommended in the ISO 6474-2 [303]). Following the early publication in 1995 by the FDA of a guidance document for "Ceramic ball hip systems," which adds the further requirements of ball head burst strength and ball head fatigue strength tests (cited in [304]), burst strength is now also tested according to ISO 7206-10 [286]) (Fig. 2.6(c)). The bending test reveals the intrinsic (statistical) strength of the material whereas the burst test is designed in order to simulate the *in vivo* loading conditions of a ceramic ball head. Unlike early ceramic acetabular components, which were not the subject of widespread use due to their poor structural reliability and fixation problems [305], the newest generation of ceramic materials guarantees an improved quality due to progress in material and system design, manufacturing, and proof testing [306, 307]. All those aspects are being continuously updated in the field of ceramic joint components. Accordingly, ceramics for both acetabular and femoral bearing parts are becoming increasingly popular. In most statistical reports, mechanical failure of the ceramics is exceedingly rare when modern ceramic microstructures are employed (cf. also recent statistics, as shown in Figs. 1.4(a) and (b)).

The remarkable statistical reduction in the number of fracture events in ceramic hip joints obtained in the last decade has been possible mainly due to two key factors: (i) the significant improvement achieved in ceramic manufacturing processes, including sintering, machining techniques, and microstructural optimization in achieving toughened microstructures [308, 309], and (ii) the widened understanding of joint mechanics in presence of ceramic components and the introduction of a deterministic proof-testing procedure, according to which each individual component is tested with respect to its structural reliability before being released to the market [306, 307, 310–312]. In order to ensure on a fully deterministic scale the structural reliability of the femoral heads made of ceramics, proof tests in burst loading geometry are nowadays systematically performed on any individual femoral head produced, before it being released to the market. In proof testing, a static load of a sub-critical level is applied to the femoral head, which is comparable in magnitude but higher than the expected maximum load under physiological conditions. Femoral heads with internal flaws, and thus with low strength, fracture and can be thus systematically eliminated. Such a test represents a quite severe structural check. In particular, it allows eliminating from the production batches the minimal fraction of pieces that were already flawed since the manufacturing procedure. At the present stage of development in manufacturing and in non-destructive evaluation, new ceramic materials appear to have achieved their maturity as structural components to be fully and safely employed in hip arthroplasty. From a statistical point of view, it is thus possible to conclude that the reliability of advanced load-bearing ceramics for arthroplastic use has been pushed toward values that exceed by far the standard requirements needed by reliable surgical components for artificial joints, although further material development in quest of tougher bioceramics will continue to be an hot topic in the arthroplastic field. Concerning this latter aspect, it is believed that there is yet quite a large margin for future improvements. The next step should rely on the development of a fully deterministic assessment.

2.7 Tribology Assessments and Their Recent *in situ* Developments

Tribological analyses are usually carried out by means of tribometers, devices used to simulate wear and friction that occur when two surfaces in contact slide over each other under an applied normal load. Such devices are continuously advanced to achieve higher precision and ameliorated with introducing in them additional functions [313–316]. On the other hand, mechanical hip and knee simulators are designed to conduct wear tests on femoral heads and acetabular liners used in total hip and knee replacements [317–320]. Hip joint simulators have been widely used for modeling wear and for providing accurate predictions of *in vivo* wear in a broad spectrum of bearing materials, including cross-linked polyethylene, metal-on-metal, and ceramic-on-ceramic couples. Owing to the most recent technical developments, more complex and severe wear conditions have been successfully modeled, including jogging, stair climbing, ball–cup micro-separation, third-body abrasion, and neck-socket impingement (for a review, see Ref. [320]). Such improved tests have contributed to establish a comparative scale of performance among different materials, thus helping eliminate those with inadequate wear resistance prior to their clinical use. On the other hand, simulation of the knee joint, which is inherently more complex than that for the hip, has certainly encountered more difficulties when researchers have attempted to compare the results of laboratory tests with actual clinical performance. Nevertheless, some types of surface damage occurring *in vivo* (e.g., scratching and pitting) have been successfully reproduced also in knee simulators. Besides optimal sliding condition, also more severe wear modes in the knee joint have been successfully reproduced *in vitro*, such as misalignment, higher loading, higher activity levels, and third-body roughening. Hip and knee joint simulators differ from one another in the type of motion produced, apart from other variables such as type of lubricant and positioning of the sliding components. Due to the variation in kinematics between the machines, the paths traced by the contact points on the femoral head against the acetabular liner or by the femoral condyle on the tibial plate might range from simple linear traces to elliptical paths during a single simulator cycle [321]. In addition, also the distances traveled by the contact points might vary appreciably among different simulator designs. While these results are important in showing how kinematics can play an important role in the outcome of *in vitro* wear experiments, they also prove that kinematic differences might originate substantial differences in wear data reported from different simulator designs, which in turn underscore the usefulness of the technique in judging the results from different simulator experiments. In other words, hip and knee simulators provide the closest testing procedures to real joints but they might provide insufficient information on the intrinsic wear properties of the sliding biomaterials. This latter information, more related to the intrinsic properties of the reciprocating surfaces, should be made available by testing individual sliding couples in a suitable tribometer under standardized wear conditions (also described in the standard ISO 6474-1 [302]).

According to the geometry of the two materials in contact, there are many standard configurations for tribometers: ball-on-disk [322], pin-on-disk [323], ring-on-disk [324], etc. For example, in the ball-on-disk the sliding contact is obtained by pushing a ball specimen on to a rotating disc under a constant load. Tribological studies of *in vivo* exposed joint load-bearing surfaces usually rely on *post mortem* phenomenological parameters for describing the essence of wear effects, such as surface roughness and material loss rates [325–331]. However, more accurate characterizations of tribological parameters, as frictional forces and wear rate, can only be characterized by *in vitro* testing. Kerkwijk *et al.* [332, 333], as well as other authors [334–336], investigated the friction and wear characteristics of alumina, zirconia, and their composites by using classic frictional testers. Conoci *et al.* [337] published an interesting wear study of tetragonal zirconia polycrystals, in which the effects of residual stresses and phase transformation on wear resistance were particularly emphasized. In the most recent developments, the interest of researchers has gradually shifted toward the nanometer scale and, in particular, on understanding plastic phenomena occurring in their basics at the molecular scale. Agraït *et al.* [338] used a combination of scanning force and tunneling microscopy techniques to study of plastic deformation in the nanometer scale with unprecedented spatial resolution. In their experiments, retraction of the tip after indentation produced a connective neck, which deformed in alternating elastic and yielding stages in agreement with theoretical predictions using molecular dynamics simulations. Although this process is not directly related to sliding wear conditions, the outcomes of this novel approach prove that a description can be given of the plastic deformation process in terms of a simple model based on continuum contact mechanics, which in turn makes it possible a quantitative analysis in connection with the bulk properties of the material. In a way more directly related to sliding wear, Guicciardi *et al.* [339] studied the extent to which the mean grain size of polycrystalline ceramics influenced the steady state friction coefficient. The mean grain size was found to clearly affect the wear rate, the finer the grain size the lower the wear rate, the basic wear mechanisms being grain fracture and fine abrasion. By means of depth-sensing indentation, a possible explanation could be given that the observed differences in wear behavior between micro- and nano-sized ceramics arose from their different values of mechanical properties, especially hardness, when measured on volumes scaling with the material microstructure.

Nakayama and Martin [340] have recently presented an interesting overview concerning the various possible chemical reactions taking place in the vicinity of the sliding contact point. It should be noted that tribological assessments enable to scrutinize different couples of materials and provide one with a means to compare their contact damage resistance, but the physical, chemical and mechanical state of the biomaterial at the contact point is very difficult to monitor. As discussed in Section 2.2, Raman and other spectroscopic analyses can be useful to obtain a deeper understanding of the mechanisms and kinetics behind the wear behavior of ceramics, which typically occurs on the micrometer range. This additional knowledge is particularly relevant to ceramic-on-ceramic bearings, the most recent protagonists in the new generation of low-friction materials for arthroplastic applications. Optical microspectroscopy, due to its high spatial resolution, might be thus considered a suitable technique to evaluate the temperature gradient rising in the vicinity of the contact spot. *In situ* surface characterization combined with Raman spectroscopy during tribological tests has also been reported, although less extensively. This composite spectroscopic method is an effective non-destructive tool to assess temperature, stress, and microstructural features in ceramic materials such as alumina and zirconia. Singer [341] first drew attention to surface modifications during wear, which successively led to an *in situ* Raman spectroscopy approach of third body processes and friction during sliding of different counterparts [342]. This author and co-workers placed the accent on the fact that friction should not be merely treated as a two-body problem but emphasized that at some scale "third bodies" play an important role in friction. Third bodies are often born in the sliding contact, detach from one surface, transfer to the counterface, and eventually agglomerate as macroscopically visible debris particles. When ejected from the contact, they are recognized as wear particles as extensively described in friction and wear literature. However, entrapped in the contact, third bodies strongly influence sliding motion. The main reasons for which frictional processes are difficult to be understood is that the buried sliding interface is not easily accessible *in situ*. To study such interface, tribologists used to separate the contacts before analyzing them, such *ex situ* approach providing useful clues about the chemistry and the structure of third-body particles, and how they participate in the sliding process. However, an *in situ* approach is necessary when the chemistry of surface films occurs to play an important role, as it is the case of artificial hip joints. The buried interface can be accessed in real time by probing the location of sliding contact directly, via electrical [343], thermal [344], spectroscopic [345, 346] or optical techniques [347–350]. When optical spectroscopy is combined with optical microscopy, this *in situ* approach allows one to identify the composition of the sliding interface while locating the formation of third bodies at the contact point. Donnet has given a comprehensive paper that reports about *in situ* approaches to tribological assessment [351]. Joly-Pottuz *et al.* [352] also performed *in situ* experiments to study modifications of nanoparticles used as lubricant additives such as inorganic fullerenes and carbon nanotubes. *In situ* analyses require a configuration that allows the tribometer be placed under the microscope of the spectrophotometer has usually been that of a pin-on-disk, with the pin (or the disk) made of a transparent material (e.g., glass or sapphire) and, thus, allowing one to focus the laser at the contact point with the counter-surface. It appears immediately clear that for such configuration of the tribometer, sapphire with its high transparency is one of the very few crystalline material choices for the pin (or for the disk), which represents a clear limitation in setting a comprehensive study on advanced devices. Note that the absence of grain boundaries in a single-crystalline sapphire material does not allow one to obviously extend the obtained tribological results even to polycrystalline alumina biomaterials, which have the same chemical composition. Cherif *et al.* [353] investigated the wear of alumina–zirconia composite and measured the temperature in the mid-thickness of the disk during the tribological test using a *K*-type thermocouple fixed by alumina cement in a hole drilled in the disk. Nevertheless, it should be noted that temperature gradients at the sliding contact point decade very sharply in space. Therefore, even this latter result is far from being considered accurate in reporting the real temperature at the contact point between the two sliding surfaces. In other words, despite the large number of available investigations regarding wear and friction of biomaterials, no successful attempts could be so far made to directly investigate the behavior of materials used in biomedical implants *in situ* during frictional sliding tests. As a result, the actual physical and chemical state of the bearing surfaces at the contact point yet remains conspicuously unknown. In order to improve this unsatisfactory situation, in this book we propose the use of optical microspectrometry *in situ* through a specially designed configuration for the tribometer device, which gives no limitation on the type of material investigated (Figs. 2.7(a)). This novel instrument can be used to perform wear tests and to concurrently collect Raman and fluorescence spectra at the contact point on a femoral head. The peculiar design of this *in situ* tribometer was specifically conceived to place the device under an optical microscope attached to a spectrophotometer, and to enable one to focus the laser at the contact point between a pin and the femoral head and collecting the backscattered signal during the tribological test. The used configuration corresponds to that of a pin-on-ball geometry (Figs. 2.7(b)), but the diameter of the pin can be eventually increased so that a femoral head can be used as pin, with the configuration thus becoming that of a ball-on-ball tribometer device. Forces can be then calibrated to reproduce standard parameters for tribological tests [354–356]. The concurrent collection of Raman or photoluminescence spectra from the contact point requires a precise knowledge of the geometrical configuration of the focused laser probe, which represents the most challenging among the innovative features characterizing this new instrument. Nevertheless, despite such computational difficulties, clear advantages arise from the possibility of testing the actual joint materials while preserving standard test conditions. In this specially designed tribometer, pin and femoral head are mounted into their respective holders, while the eccentricity of the rotating ball is checked using profilometry. Pin and ball are then brought into contact with the desired contact angle (e.g., 45°). The entire tribometer device is set into the Raman equipment and the laser beam focused through the objective lens at the contact point between pin and ball. A selected load (up to several tens of N) is applied to the lever-arm device and the sliding velocity set on the tribometer controller. The tribological test starts when the drive engine is started and, during sliding, the magnitude of lateral and vertical forces on the sample can be recorded while Raman or luminescence spectra are collected *in situ* as a function of sliding distance. The tribological test usually experiences an initial transient period of time, in which the wear parameters monotonically vary to reach stable values, namely a regime state that ends when a predetermined sliding distance is reached (Fig. 2.7(c)).

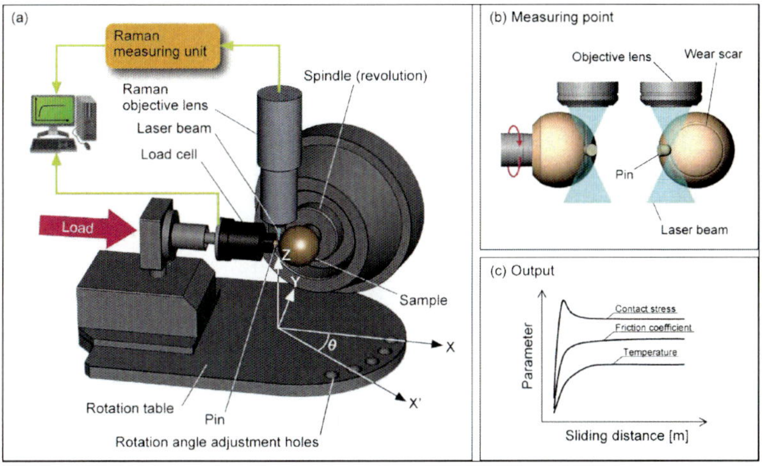

Figure 2.7 Schematic drafts of: (a) tribometer device that can be used to perform wear tests and concurrently collect *in situ* Raman or fluorescence spectra at the contact point on a femoral head; (b) sliding configuration corresponding to that of a pin-on-ball geometry; and, (c) typical outputs of the tribometer device, including contact stress, friction coefficient, and contact temperature.

In situ spectroscopic experiments are conducted with focusing the waist of the laser beam on the material through a 50 × optical lens (i.e., with a lateral resolution of about 2 μm). The backscattered light is then re-focused onto a confocal pinhole, transmitted into the spectrometer through the same optical lens used to focus the incoming laser, and dispersed onto a CCD camera to produce Raman or luminescence spectra. The pinhole aperture affects the spatial resolution of the measurements. While reducing the pinhole diameter enables to improve spatial resolution by cutting out the light scattered from portions of the probed volume above and below the focal plane, the use of a small pinhole can severely reduce the signal intensity. Therefore, a compromise should be found between spatial resolution and efficiency in the collection of the scattered light. A lower limit for confocal pinhole aperture (i.e., an upper limit for spatial resolution) can be obtained by setting the pinhole diameter at 100 μm. The additional information obtainable from the *in situ* spectroscopic characterizations can be summarized in: (i) possible changes in phase composition of the biomaterials due to the concurrent effect of highly localized stresses and chemical triggers from the environment, and its evolution with sliding distance; (ii) assessment of local temperature at the contact point; and, (iii) determination of the elastic stress field at the contact point. After wear testing being completed and the worn femoral head and pin ultrasonically cleaned to remove debris, the respective masses can be measured and compared with those measured before the wear treatment to obtain the worn volumes. The characteristic dimensions of the longitudinal scar on the femoral head and of the elliptical scar on the pin (Fig. 2.7(b)) can also be measured using conventional SEM observation and the topological characteristics of the worn surfaces characterized by AFM.

Nowadays, conventional wear analyses in standard hip and knee joint simulators unfortunately yet conspicuously lack of final statements on chemical and other kinds of local phenomena occurring at the very surface of the sliding components. While deep analyses of the chemical reactions that can occur *in vivo* between the sliding joint counterparts are yet missing in the available literature, important improvements have been achieved in understanding plasticity effects that occur in metallic materials and, to some extent surprisingly, even in the immediate neighborhood of ceramic bearing surfaces. The main driving force in the field of metal-on-metal joints has been that of controlling and of minimizing wear through a deep understanding of the mechanisms of debris generation. *In vivo*, mainly nanometer-sized globular and needle-shaped debris particles are found, for example, in CoCrMo alloys [357–363], taken as paradigm metallic joint biomaterials. Such debris could neither stem from the action of abrasion nor from tribochemical reactions. Through observing the subsurface regions of explanted joints using a transmission electron microscope [357], it is revealed that at some distance from the surface, a network of stacking faults and hexagonal ε-martensite phase is formed, which strengthen the bulk material. However, this microstructure changes into a nanocrystalline type moving closer toward the surface. Upon comparing *in vivo* debris size and grain size of the explanted joint surface, it can be revealed that globular wear particles result from torn off nanocrystals, while the needle shaped particles are generated by fractured crystallites of the ε-martensite phase. The process of debris formation is obviously assisted by microcracks that propagate through the brittle nanocrystalline layer and the dominating mechanism of particle generation for metal-on-metal joints is surface fatigue within the nanocrystalline surface layer. The high defect density within dislocation cells can indeed initiate fatigue microcracks, which successively propagate parallel to the contact surface through the bulk. When these microcracks attain a critical length, they might finally break to the surface and form large, flake-like particles [364]. Transmission electron microscopy studies of surface damage accumulation mechanisms that follow *in vitro* tested worn alumina-on-alumina hip replacement prostheses also indicate extensive surface dislocation activity [365–367], which is, however, restricted to a rather thin outer surface layer. Quite interestingly, dislocation slips are found to develop on pyramidal planes, while both inter- and transgranular cracks are observed in regions of high wear. The most extensive dislocation activity is found in correspondence of grooves, largely associated with third-body abrasion. Wear debris also form from the worn surface as granular, nanocrystalline, and needle-shaped particles. The process of debris formation in alumina ceramics mainly arises from the concurrent effects of grain pulling-out and severe plastic deformation at the surface. Given the quite anomalous dislocation slip behavior (i.e., as compared to high-temperature creep [368–370]), it is likely that plastic deformation during wear might be assisted by a sequence of tribochemical reactions occurring between alumina and lubricant. Such reactions might significantly weaken the alumina lattice through a conspicuous formation of oxygen vacancies, and even alter locally its phase composition. It is indeed toward this research direction that we shall orient our novel studies on the wear behavior of retrieved alumina femoral heads, which will be described in a forthcoming chapter of this book.

Chapter 3

Polycrystalline Alumina for Joint Replacement

3.1 Alumina as a Load-Bearing Biomaterial

In artificial joints, biomechanical loading and load transfer over time are strongly affected by the choice of the bearing materials. Regarding such issues, the orthopedic literature contains a myriad of studies that consider material-related effects on joint performance and lifetime, such as surface chemistry and roughness, fretting, brittle or fatigue fracture, and so on. Particularly concerning ceramic biomaterials, it is well established that wear properties and structural reliability of these materials are drastically influenced by both material properties and manufacturing processes. However, multiple confounding conditions (e.g., patient-related factors, surgical techniques, differences in raw materials and processing) greatly limit the identification of simple cause–effect relationships [371–373]. Such a plethora of conditions necessarily makes the incorporation of any new material in the joint design a cumbersome and difficult issue. The most striking consequence of the above situation is that the design choices among available biomaterials are quite limited. Among commonly accepted biomaterials, alumina is by far the most popular ceramic employed in joint arthroplasty [374]. The use of alumina in ceramic-on-ceramic bearings is logical and appropriate if one just think that wear debris and debris-associated osteolysis are the most common (and severe) problems affecting

Advanced Materials for Joint Implants
Giuseppe Pezzotti

ISBN 978-981-4316-88-0 (Hardcover), 978-981-4364-39-3 (eBook)
www.panstanford.com

total hip arthroplastic surgery in the presence of polyethylene. Among various types of bearing material developed to reduce wear rate, alumina ceramic-on-ceramic bearing couples definitely have the greatest scientific and clinical support. In this context, it is interesting to note that, ironically, cross-linked polyethylene overcomes alumina in popularity, stemming as the most used material in hip arthroplasty. However, polyethylene possesses the shortest clinical experience (only since 1998) and the highest wear rate among biomaterials used in hip implants. So, why does such a mismatch between performance and popularity arise for alumina ceramics? This is the main question that we will try to answer in this chapter.

The first use of alumina as a biomaterial can be traced back (from German patent activity) to 1930 [311]; however, Boutin was unequivocally the first to use alumina in orthopedic surgery, with successfully implanting alumina joints since 1970 [375]. During the following 40 years of clinical use, millions of alumina femoral heads have been implanted in patients worldwide and, nowadays, a very large family of orthopedic surgeons considers alumina femoral heads the best choice in hip arthroplasty [376–378]. The alumina ceramic used in biomedical applications is the so-called α-phase Al_2O_3, which possesses a hexagonal (corundum-type) crystallographic structure. Its strong ionic bond and oxygen-rich stoichiometry make alumina exceptionally stable in the human body, leaving its structure conspicuously unaffected by corrosive processes. Such stability is a key property in impeding Al-ion release from the bulk material and from wear debris. Alumina is quite strong under compressive load, but possesses limited tensile strength and is quite brittle under tension, showing no trace of plastic deformation at the onset for fracture at room temperature.

Prosthesis components are made of polycrystalline alumina and, according to a general trend observed in ceramic polycrystals, also in alumina the tensile strength increases when fully dense microstructures are produced with an increasingly smaller grain size. Therefore, alumina manufacturers carefully select raw materials and strictly design the production process in order to minimize grain size, thus maximizing strength. However, the obtainment of dense alumina components with sub-micrometer grain size definitely does not represent an easy task and minimizing grain size in alumina has long been a main target for material technologists. The fabrication of dense alumina bodies with a grain size in the order of the single micrometer has indeed become possible through years of technological improvements owing to two important findings:

(i) The addition of a small fraction of magnesia (MgO) to the raw alumina powder: Such addition enhances mass transport during solid-state sintering, thus allowing the ceramic body to reach full density at relatively low sintering temperatures, which in turn enables to control grain growth during sintering (i.e., with a beneficial effect on strength).

(ii) The use of hot isostatic pressing (HIPing) at some step of the production process. Such improved processing procedure provides the essential driving force for closing internal pores and pushes the density of the polycrystal close to its theoretical value at relatively low sintering temperatures (i.e., in turn improving both the strength and the reliability of the material).

It should be noted that as a consequence of the high asymmetry (and anisotropy) of its crystalline corundum structure, alumina grains possess a pronounced thermal expansion mismatch between the *c*-axis and the *a*- (or *m*-) axis lying on its basal plane. The linear thermal expansion coefficients at room temperature are 5.3×10^{-6}/K and 4.5×10^{-6}/K for directions parallel and perpendicular to the *c*-axis of the crystal, respectively [379]. The main consequence of such anisotropy is that upon cooling from sintering temperature, a higher thermal expansion coefficient along the *c*-axis involves larger (and faster) shrinkage as compared to axes in the basal plane [380–383]. Therefore, even in a random distribution of grain orientation, there will always be a finite fraction of particularly weak grain boundaries (e.g., those comprised between grains sharing a common *c*-axis orientation) affected by high residual stresses of tensile nature. In this context, it has been demonstrated that the residual stress magnitude increases with increasing grain size [382]. Grain boundaries thus become the "weak points" in the polycrystalline array and they might eventually crack upon cooling from sintering temperature [384] or act as preferential sites for the fracture origin when an external stress is applied. Note also that grain growth during sintering involves not only a statistically larger length of (weak) grain boundaries but also a statistically larger probability of finding them in the polycrystalline array, since boundaries comprised between grains with similar orientation are the most stable and, thus, also the last to disappear upon grain growth [385]. In alumina, anisotropic (i.e., also referred to as abnormal) grain growth can be observed, which refers to the sporadic growth of grains with a large aspect ratio as opposed to equiaxed grains. This occurs because certain crystallographic planes grow faster than others, with the higher growth rate being due to a relatively low interfacial energy (i.e., providing them with a higher driving force for growth). Therefore, abnormal grain growth refers to the presence of very large grains growing in a matrix of grains that are finer by at least one order of magnitude. Under these conditions, grain boundary mobility might exceed pore mobility; also resulting in trapped pores in the final product (i.e., an additional source of defective locations). Abnormal grain growth (and, in general, grain growth) has proved quite detrimental to the mechanical properties of sintered materials. If one looks at the histogram of internal residual stresses piled up in alumina polycrystals, significant broadening can be found for materials with larger grain sizes (as we will explicitly show in a later section of this chapter), which possess grain boundaries stressed to higher magnitudes. The extreme tensile "wing" of the residual stress histogram refers to a population of microscopic locations highly stressed after manufacturing and, thus, intrinsically weak (i.e., much weaker than the alumina lattice structure). Any of those locations can easily originate a catastrophic fracture path under relatively low external stresses. It is exactly from the aforementioned physical circumstances that a consistent drop down in strength unavoidably strings along with a poor microstructural control during sintering. It should be noted that, also from the point of view of wear resistance, the extreme compressive and tensile "wings" of the residual stress histogram, represent preferential sites prone to wear damage on the surface of the polycrystal. Surface locations subjected to highly compressive residual stresses easily undergo grain spalling and are thus subjected to subsequent grain detachment under localized frictional loading [386].

Figure 3.1 (a) shows a schematic draft that illustrates the formation of grain-boundary residual stresses in alumina polycrystals during cooling down from sintering temperature. Helpful in understanding the phenomenon in mechanistic terms is a graphic

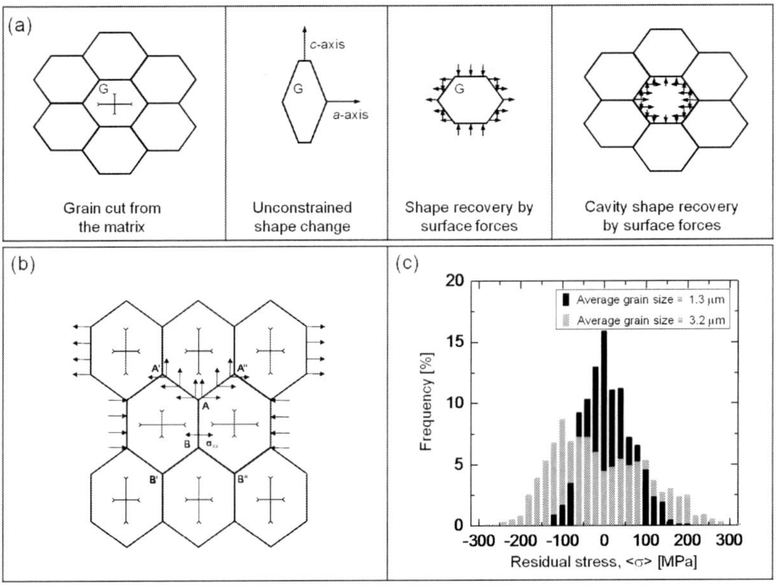

Figure 3.1 (a) Eshelby procedure for visualizing grain-boundary residual stresses due to thermal expansion anisotropy in polycrystalline alumina; (b) schematic of one of the "worst" configurations of alumina grain array for the development of grain-boundary residual stresses; and, (c) residual stress histograms collected by CL piezo-spectroscopy on the surface of biomedical alumina materials with different grain sizes.

procedure, which was first proposed by Eshelby [387–390]. A grain element, G, is first extracted from the surrounding polycrystalline matrix array and allowed undergoing an unconstrained shape change during cooling. Then, surface forces should be applied to the unconstrained grain in order to achieve shape compatibility and for being reinserted into the original matrix cavity. Finally, interface forces should also be applied to the cavity, which provide continuity of stress across the interface. As already mentioned, the highest tensile stress that can develop in a polycrystalline array with thermal expansion anisotropy occurs for neighboring grains with a close crystallographic orientation. Such "worst" local array configuration is considered to trigger catastrophic fracture in the polycrystal, which in turn originates from the "weakest" grain boundary as the fracture origin. Theoretical studies [382, 389] indicated that a hexagonal grain array is liable to maximum stress intensification at grain boundaries because its characteristic geometrical angle (i.e., 30°) maximizes the magnitude of an externally applied (tensile) stress field. A grain array is schematically represented in Fig. 3.1(b) that can be considered as one of the "worst" multigrain configurations leading to grain-boundary weakening in polycrystalline alumina. This array configuration is the one experiencing the maximum tensile and the maximum compressive residual stresses on the grain boundaries labeled as segment "AB" and the oblique grain boundaries (i.e., "BB′" and "BB″") in Fig. 3.1(b), respectively. In Fig. 3.1(c), residual stress histograms are compared, which were collected by a nanometer-sized CL probe on the surface of unused ceramic femoral heads. The two histograms shown in this latter figure correspond to alumina materials with different grain sizes (i.e., alumina microstructures manufactured before and after 1995, respectively [391]). As can be seen, both "wings" of the stress histograms reach relatively high magnitudes, which consistently increase with increasing grain size. At this stage of our description, we only want to qualitatively emphasize the conceptual meaning expressed by the above Fig. 3.1, from which one can easily understand why modern alumina materials, with finer microstructures, perform better in hip joints from the viewpoint of both structural and wear resistance.

Unlike MgO, which, as mentioned, has a quite beneficial effect on the mechanical behavior of alumina [392, 393], there are other oxides that need to be accurately eliminated from medical-grade alumina materials. Special care should be paid in eliminating any calcia (CaO) impurity from the alumina microstructure since this oxide can severely compromise the mechanical properties of alumina in wet environment, with significantly weakening its grain boundaries [394]. Also the presence of traces of Na and other subvalent (i.e., with valence <3) impurities, eventually stemming from the raw powder, make the dense alumina body unsuitable for structural biomedical applications. For these reasons, continuous efforts are made by manufacturers to improve the purity of the alumina raw material and to avoid contaminations during processing. On the other hand, there have also been discovered some elements, especially rare earths (e.g., lutetium [395]) or nanometer-sized dispersoids (e.g., SiC particles [396, 397]), which added in low fractions to the raw alumina powder contribute to refine its grain size and to strengthen its grain boundaries by conspicuously suppressing the weakest locations [398, 399].

Strengthening mechanisms, based on the engineering of residual stress fields at the sub-micrometer scale by means of adding a secondary phase to the Al_2O_3 matrix, have been widely reported in the literature [400–403]. These studies show the importance of controlling thermal expansion mismatches in the obtainment of a strengthening effect. Based on the Eshelby procedure, we can repeat the same exercise made for monolithic alumina in Fig. 3.1(a) for an array of alumina grains containing intragranularly located (nano-sized) particles whose linear coefficient of thermal expansion is lower than that of the alumina matrix (e.g., β-SiC particles). Note that the thermal expansion mismatch between the β-SiC particles (linear thermal expansion coefficients at room temperature equal to 2.8×10^{-6}/K) and the Al_2O_3 matrix is much larger than that arising from the internal anisotropy of the corundum structure, so that the effect of this latter mismatch can be neglected in first approximation. In addition, being β-SiC a cubic structure, no anisotropy is expected during its shrinkage to room temperature. Figure 3.2(a) shows an ideal array of Al_2O_3 matrix grains all containing a β-SiC particle with lower thermal expansion. We can then extract the Al_2O_3 grain, G, from the array and separate it from its internal particle, P, letting both the grain (with a holed core) and the particle free to undergo unconstrained shape change during cooling. According to a shape-recovery process on grain, particle and related cavities, a grain-boundary "tightening" effect can be envisaged. Note that this positive effect only occurs when particles are intragranularly located and possess a linear coefficient of thermal expansion lower than that of the matrix. On the other hand, the location of nanometer-sized particles with a lower thermal expansion coefficient at grain boundaries of the alumina matrix grains might be detrimental to the strength of the material, since such particles might operate a wedge-like opening effect on the boundary itself. Figures 3.2(b) and (c) represent drafts of alumina microstructures with intra- and intergranularly located SiC particles, respectively. From force balance, as shown in the two latter figures, one can easily recognize a tightening effect in the former case versus a wedge-opening effect in the latter one. One can immediately foresee a problem in the strengthening approach by mismatched particles: how can the material manufacturer be sure that *all* the nano-sized added particles are located inside the matrix grains? Is the probability of finding a mismatched particle at the grain boundary of the composite material lower than that of finding a grain boundary "weakened" by thermal expansion in the monolithic array of grains? The actual impossibility of screening all the microstructure of the material has led technologists to regard this approach as a merely "theoretical" one and no practical attempt to push such "nanocomposites" in the biomedical marked has been so far attempted.

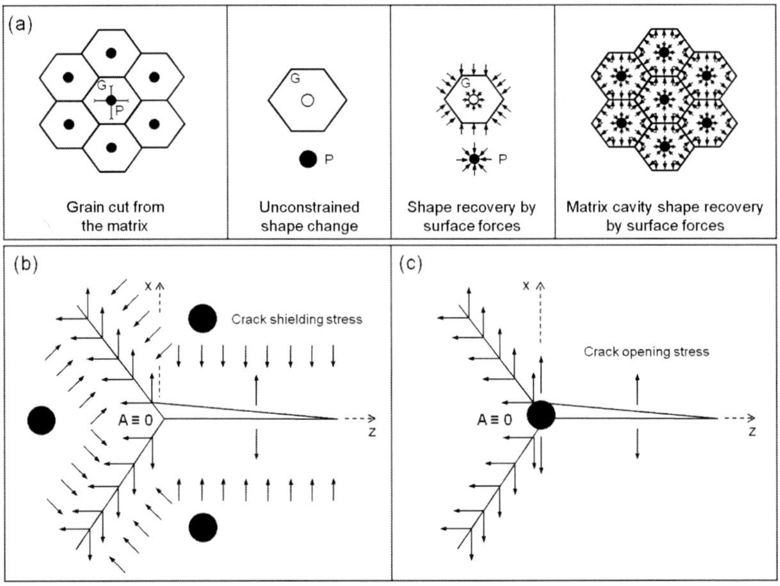

Figure 3.2 (a) Eshelby procedure for visualizing grain-boundary residual stresses due to thermal expansion anisotropy in polycrystalline alumina containing intragranular silicon carbide particles; (b) schematic of the mechanism leading to a shielding action by residual stresses on a grain-boundary microcrack in alumina containing intragranular silicon carbide particles; and, (c) schematic of the mechanism leading to a wedge-opening action by residual stresses on a grain-boundary microcrack in alumina containing intergranular silicon carbide particles.

We have already mentioned that impurities such as Si, Ca, and Na might be present in commercial alumina powders unless strict measures are taken to avoid them [404]. Since these elements show very low solubility limits in alumina, they tend to segregate to grain-boundary regions and to form intergranular glassy films during sintering [405–410]. Bae and Baik [408] determined critical concentrations of silicon, calcium, and related mixtures below which no anisotropic or abnormal grain growth can be observed. Samples doped with Si (>300 ppm) exhibited abnormal grain growth. Doping with only Ca at ≥30 ppm produced the same effect. For co-doping of Si and Ca, intermediate concentration limits were observed. These threshold concentrations approximately correspond to the solubility limits of such impurity elements in alumina, which thus stem as a low-melting intergranular glassy phase. The presence of impurities at the grain boundaries is thus a favorable condition for abnormal grain growth to occur. Segregation of lattice "modifiers" as Ca and Si at the alumina interfaces reduces interface energy at certain specific boundaries and thus favors (abnormal) anisotropic growth of the adjacent grains. Interface energy is found to decrease faster as a function of Na_2O content than as a function of CaO content [411]. From the above considerations, it appears immediately clear how severe must be the chemical control required for raw powders of biomedical alumina grades and how directly their purity impacts on the structural reliability and wear resistance to hip joint components.

The effect of rare-earth elements on the mechanical and wear behavior of polycrystalline alumina yet represents a matter of debate, but certainly constitutes a fascinating and conspicuously unexplored field. We limit here our description to few cases reported in the literature. Segregation of rare earths to grain boundaries was found to alter the room-temperature fracture mode of alumina polycrystals [412]. In pure alumina, it is known that the fracture mode becomes increasingly intragranular as grain size is reduced, a trend that has been explained consistently with thermal expansion anisotropy effects [413, 414]. The addition of rare-earth elements (i.e., Yb, Gd, or La) as dopants to alumina might result in a substantial increase in the proportion of intergranular fracture as compared to a pure material of similar grain size. This can be explained by the significant reduction in the free surface energy that results from rare-earth segregation at grain boundaries, which reduces the work of fracture for intergranular failure. According to our previous statements, this phenomenon should be expected, leading to a reduction in strength. However, one might find that the negative effect is offset by other positive circumstances that the incorporation of a rare-earth dopant can provide to the microstructural network. Some authors [415] have claimed that grain boundaries with more bonds and higher bonding strength should be more resistant to external loading up to high temperatures. As a matter of fact, in their undoped state, grain boundaries of alumina ceramics should have fewer bonds per unit volume than the interior of the grain, which is also why the grain boundaries are mechanically weak points. However, the addition of aliovalent rare-earth elements (i.e., with valence >3) as, for example, yttrium (Y) might eventually provide the boundary regions with additional (stronger) bonds between Y and O ions, which might strengthen the boundaries. A positive stabilization effect of alumina in wet air at high temperature has been also reported for doping by lanthanum (La) [416]. The effect was assigned to the formation of micro-domains of lanthanum aluminate on the alumina surface. Owing to the perovskitic structure of this compound, the Al^{3+} ions in it are stabilized in octahedral coordination.

The above considerations, all related to the performance of polycrystalline alumina as a load-bearing biomaterial, point toward the importance of intrinsically eliminating the weakness of its grain boundaries, namely the most stressed locations of the microstructural array after manufacturing. We shall henceforth assume that any large defect consisting of voids or inclusions of foreign materials (also related to a poor choice of the raw materials or to a flawed manufacturing process) be eliminated either by processing improvement or by proof testing, as already described in Chapter 2. In the clinical practice, alumina heads may be coupled either to polyethylene acetabular sockets or to self-mating alumina liners. The favorable behavior of one type of joint on the other obviously depends upon the intrinsic properties of the manufactured alumina. A "soft" counterpart might conspicuously reduce the risk of fracture and surface damage by interaction of hard asperities. However, when frictionally interacting with polyethylene, the alumina surface should retain extremely high resistance to chemical degradation, especially at grain boundaries. In this context, alumina is known to have a good "chemical" performance in hip joints owing to the ability of its surface to bond hydroxyl groups by chemisorption, which in turn induces a lubricating fluid film at the joint interface.

Biocompatibility, namely the ability of a material to perform with an appropriate host response in the human body [417], is one of the strongest points in favor of the use of alumina in artificial hip joints. Biocompatibility of alumina ceramics addresses all aspects of its interaction with body tissues, as systematically observed both *in vitro* and *in vivo*. From a stoichiometry viewpoint, alumina is a compound in its highest state of oxidation, thus thermodynamically stable with respect to ion extraction in physiologic media. Due to its chemical inertia, alumina is frequently a reference in testing orthopedic biomaterials [418]. Its wettability is higher than that any polymer or metal available to orthopedic implants [419]. *In vitro* tests have demonstrated that water can be adsorbed with high-bond strength. Proteins, even at low concentrations, completely cover the alumina ceramic surfaces with a monolayer [420]. Immediate absorption on the surface of serum proteins is supposed to occur immediately after implantation of alumina ceramics in the human body. This result may also explain the low cellular and tissue reactivity to alumina ceramics [421]. The first clinical case treated with alumina goes back to Boutin [375], followed by Griss and von Adrian-Werburg [422]. Interestingly, experimental data on biocompatibility of alumina using cell culture were mainly published later than its actual clinical use. Fortunately, alumina powder did not induce tumors [422] and direct contact tests proved the absence of toxic effects by alumina powders co-cultured with macrophages and lymphocytes [423]. Alumina is correctly considered a champion material in artificial joint applications for its biocompatibility and high surface wettability. However, recent *in vitro* studies employing analytical tools down to the nanometer scale [71, 101, 424, 425] have suggested that its bioinertness might be lower than what initially believed, especially in presence of additional phases in its microstructural arrangement. The actual impact of a lowered bioinertness, as revealed on the nanometer scale, on the wear properties of alumina will be discussed in some details in a later section of this chapter.

Hard-on-hard alumina bearings have two enormous potential advantages: (i) a very low-wear debris generation; and, (ii) minimum friction among all the available sliding couples. In principle, long-term stability is also expected, because of a significant reduction in third-body wear as compared to metal-on-metal hip implants. However, at least for alumina-on-alumina sliding couples, many details yet need to be precisely addressed in order to actually allow this bearing couple exploiting its best potential value. Details not only concern the already mentioned material quality but also design geometry (i.e., including fixation systems) and surgical implantation. As far as design is concerned, many different designs (and fixation systems) have been explored in the past and new ones are presently being explored. For showing how hard has historically been the path of design improvement, we shall just briefly review how fixation systems have played a major role in clinical outcomes. In early designs, cementless plain alumina sockets (initially with one peg, then changed to two and three pegs) were used. The stem was cemented, and since 1972 it has been made of a titanium alloy. The head-on-cone fixation (32 mm in size) was initially glued and subsequently brazed. However, these two early systems proved leading to a poor performance and produced many failures and fractures. Successively, a design introduced by Mittelmeier included a bulky cementless screw-in-ring alumina socket, a smooth cobalt chromium cementless stem with grooves, and a large head with a Morse taper, which also resulted in many early failures, although not directly related to the employed alumina material, but both to a poor design and to a difficult surgery [426–428]. Higher security levels were finally achieved when technologists improved cone technology in terms of accuracy, tolerance, and roughness, thus enhancing the quality of conical sleeving. Although we will return to design aspects in the next section, a complete description of design issues with alumina-on-alumina implants is clearly beyond the scope of this book. We shall limit henceforth our description mainly focusing on material aspects of the alumina implants.

3.2 Wear Behavior: Wear Patterns on Alumina Hip Joints

As we have already discussed, alumina femoral heads experience the longest history and definitely the most successful performance among ceramics in hip joint prostheses. While this is especially true for alumina heads articulating against acetabular cups made of polyethylene [429, 430], the track record for self-mating alumina joints has shown through the years a more controversial path since its initial development [431]. Nevertheless, the popularity of alumina-on-alumina joints is expected to increase in the near future owing to the achievement of a higher degree of safety, with the substantial elimination from the market of defective joint designs [60, 434], concurrently to the substantial ameliorations of the microstructural design of alumina-based ceramics [3, 435, 436]. Better designs and microstructures enable to minimize the risks of *in vivo* fracture, namely, the most serious concern against the use of (inherently) brittle ceramics as self-mating surfaces in load-bearing hip components. However, from the perspective of alumina-on-alumina hip joints with greater longevity, i.e., to be implanted in younger patients, it is yet essential to accurately understand wear mechanisms as they affect the alumina microstructure on the micro/nanostructural level and, more important, to link them to design aspects of all-ceramic hip implants. Leaving aside the cases of catastrophic liner fracture (as discussed in Chapter 1) unfortunately abundant in joint designs incorporating sandwich-type ceramic liners [60, 434], the challenge remains that of locating the most important factors affecting wear rate of hard-on-hard bearings, thus relating the overall roughness patterns/morphology of *in vivo* worn femoral heads, and the statistical distribution of microscopic surface asperities to specific aspects of joint design. In the field of ceramic-on-ceramic bearings, a study by Nevelos *et al.* [437] has definitely provided a first step forward in the direction of linking microscopic features to macroscopic design aspects, conceptually in line with the above-mentioned perspective. These researchers have pointed out the detrimental effect of edge loading during swinging gait as the mechanism originating the stripe wear phenomenon. This particular wear phenomenon is by far the most severe in terms of abrasive effects on the alumina surface, but systematically appears only in correspondence of a narrow and elongated zone of ellipsoidal shape above the head taper. Being the result of line contact between the femoral heads and the edge of the liner, stripe wear has been attributed to microseparation during gait. Note that due to its peripheral location, stripe wear might not substantially contribute by itself to increase friction in the joint, but it definitely triggers the faster development of high roughness in dome areas of the femoral head through supplying detached alumina grains that act as third bodies between the sliding surfaces. A hip design forgiving some joint laxity has been considered to favor microseparation [438, 439], thus producing a stripe wear zone and adversely affecting the long-term performance of ceramic-on-ceramic hip joints. Jin *et al.* [440] suggested that a smaller radial clearance is better for the fluid film formation between bearing surfaces, which is necessary to minimize frictional resistance and to prevent the severe wear of ceramic joint prostheses by keeping the sliding surfaces apart. However, if the radial clearance is too small, the surfaces will strike due to irregularities or third bodies, potentially leading to high friction [441–444]. On the other hand, a design that substantially eliminates laxity with setting small clearances has been regarded as potentially leading to "high-friction" hip joints [443–445] because of a number of concurrent effects, including liner deformation, equatorial seizing, and scarcity of lubricant access with subsequent entrapment of third-body wear particles between the mating surfaces. Unlike metal-on-metal hip joints, for which elastoplastic deformation (through deflection of the metal liner) is a main concern in quantifying the amount of friction between head and liner [442, 444], ceramics possess quite high stiffness and all the misfit strains arising from physiological loading in presence of third-body particles might directly reflect in a higher friction and thus a higher wear rate in presence of excessively small clearances. In other words, hard-on-hard bearing couples yet entail high risks of reduced lifetime, either due to third-body wear or to high-friction mating, thus calling for prompt studies to isolate the relevant aspects of wear performance as they stem from cup design.

The rationalization of microscopic surface parameters of *in vivo* worn ceramic heads and their link to hip designs with different clearances (i.e., thus with different degrees of laxity) represents an important step. Screening should be systematically made on the entire surface of the available retrievals with microscopic resolution, by means of scanning electron microscopy, thus not only revealing the typical aspect of wear patterns on the microscopic scale, but also assessing the topological boundaries of each wear region on the macroscopic scale of the femoral head. This practice can be shown to provide a rationale for distinguishing typical geometries of wear zones associated to different hip joint designs. In addition, surface topography by atomic force microscopy, performed on ball-head regions worn to different levels, can provide us with precious quantitative information on the statistical characteristics of surface texture and wear mechanisms leading to frictional surface damage.

In the following, a comprehensive surface topology characterization is shown for a group of four retrieved alumina femoral heads, from implants which were all revised after periods comprised between 7.7 and 10.7 years. All retrievals were from alumina-on-alumina hip joints. Clinical data and other characteristics of these femoral heads are summarized in Table 3.1. Cases 1 and 2 in the Table were 28 mm BIOLOX®*forte* (commercialized by Cremascoli Co., Milan, Italy) ceramic femoral heads used against BIOLOX®*forte* liners directly inserted in a metal shell; the other two heads, Cases 4 and 5 were 28 mm BIOCERAM alumina femoral heads (Kyocera Co., Kyoto, Japan) self-mating against acetabular cups of the "sandwich type". This latter type of joint comprised an alumina ceramic liner housed in an ultra-high molecular weight polyethylene liner (ABS liner), which in turn was held in a (titanium alloy) metal shell (AMS HA shell). Schematic drafts comparing the two investigated hip implants are given in Figs. 3.3(a) and (b) for BIOLOX®*forte* and BIOCERAM types, respectively. Besides other geometrical dissimilarities, an important difference between the two types of implant was the joint equatorial clearance. Clearance values were measured by the authors as 15 μm and 32 μm on each side of the head equator for BIOCERAM and BIOLOX®*forte* implants, respectively (cf. drafts in Figs. 3.3(a) and (b)). These data are in agreement with published literature on the same types of implant [446–448]. The nearly half value of clearance in the BIOCERAM implant as compared to the BIOLOX®*forte* one involves this implant possessing, if correctly implanted, significantly higher "rigidity." It should also be noted at the outset that all the four studied hip joints were correctly implanted at the time of primary surgery, as far as the cup orientation was concerned. The change in clearance during implantation was of a negligible amount in all the femoral heads investigated. Widmer *et al.* [449] concluded that the acceptable range of the cup orientation to yield a stable range of motion (ROM) is between 40° and 45° of radiographic inclination (RI), and between 20° and 28° of radiographic anteversion (RA). RI and RA orientations are explicitly

Table 3.1 Classification of implant type and clinical data of the studied self-mating alumina head retrievals.

Case	Age	Gender	Side	Follow-up	Cup radiographic inclination	Cup radiographic anteversion	Wear area [%]	Generation	Acetabular cup	Cause of revision
I	62	Male	Left	7.7 yr	40°	9°	35.4	BIOLOX®*forte*	Alumina liner	Dislocation
II	70	Female	Right	10.7 yr	43°	23°	29.2	BIOLOX®*forte*	Alumina liner	Stem loosening
III	61	Female	Left	8.6 yr	32°	13°	64.2	BIOCERAM	ABS cup system	Cup liner loosening
IV	50	Male	Right	10.1 yr	43°	6°	46.3	BIOCERAM	ABS cup system	Cup liner loosening

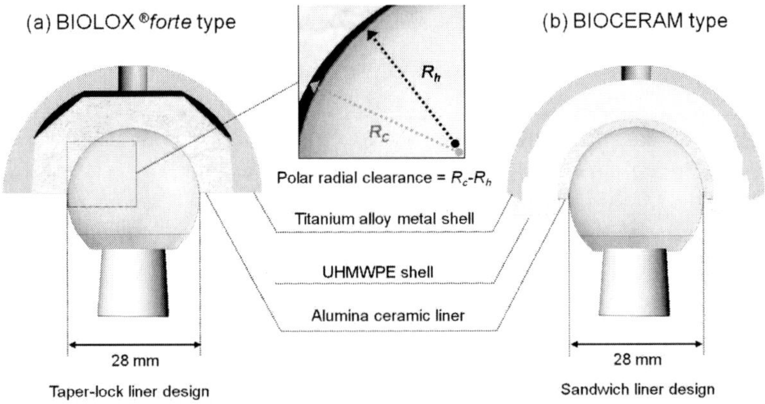

Figure 3.3 Schematic drafts comparing two different types of investigated hip implant; BIOLOX®*forte* and BIOCERAM types in (a) and (b), respectively.

given in Table 3.1 as obtained just after primary surgery, and the positioning error for all the implanted components was minimized within ±10° from the optimal cup orientation suggested by Widmer *et al.* [449]. These angles were determined directly on the plain radiographs centered on the symphysis and showing both hips as proposed by Murray [450]. The causes of revision are also listed in Table 3.1. It is interesting to note that all BIOCERAM implants failed because of problems related to the liner. Such problems have befallen after long-term implantation, while stripe wear was only observed in Case 4, namely (unexpectedly) in an implant that is supposed to possess small laxity at the time of implantation. This body of clinical observation contains interesting aspects to be clarified by a multiscale approach to surface screening from the microscopic level to the macroscopic size of the femoral head. For comparison, two unused femoral heads, one Cremascoli BIOLOX®*forte* and one Kyocera BIOCERAM, which possessed exactly the same manufacturing characteristics of the respective retrieved femoral heads described above, were also investigated. The impurity contents for the unused BIOLOX®*forte* head were: (SiO_2 + CaO + Na_2O) < 0.05 wt.% and MgO < 0.25 wt.%. BIOCERAM alumina had a total impurity content < 0.2 wt.% ((SiO_2 + CaO + Na_2O) < 0.03 wt.% and MgO < 0.01 wt.%.). The average grain size of the two types of investigated femoral head was 1.3 μm and 1.8 μm in BIOCERAM and BIOLOX®*forte*, respectively.

Wear progression on the entire surface of the alumina head has been classified into five levels of increasing wear severity (Grades 1 to 5), based on the scale defined by Shishido *et al.* [451]. However, we reinterpret this wear classification and, particularly, we treat here the wear pattern known as "stripe wear" differently from frictional wear processes related to Grades 1~5, because this distinctive wear pattern is not a consequence of normal sliding during gait, but rather the effect of an "abnormal" microseparation/shock process between head and liner or neck-liner impingement [436, 437, 452]. Here, stripe wear is referred to as "Grade SW," while the as-received surfaces are conventionally classified as "Grade 0." Classification criteria are concisely summarized in Table 3.2 and "standard morphologies" for surfaces worn to different degrees is shown in Figs. 3.4(a)~(f). SEM images

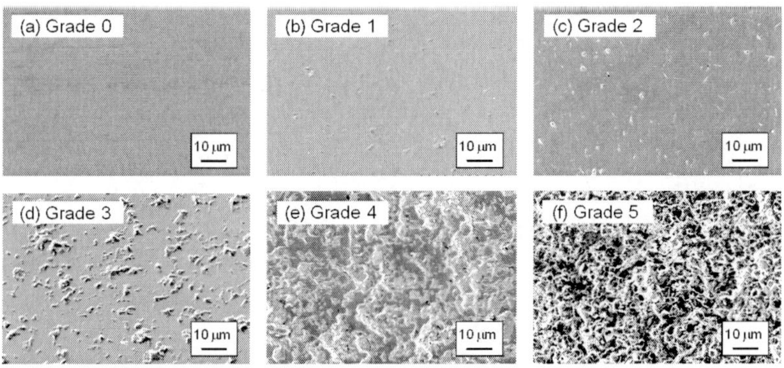

Figure 3.4 Standard morphology of zones of femoral heads worn to different grades (Grades 0 to 5 in (a) to (f), respectively) as visually established according to FEG-SEM micrographs.

were collected along meridian lines with sampling at constant intervals of 500 mm steps while connecting the dome to the edge of each femoral head. Such longitudinal lines were located by taking a (solid) angular step of 15° until covering the total head circumference of 360° (for a total of 1345 SEM images for each investigated head). Wear grades were classified on the head surface on the basis of the qualitative definitions given in Table 3.2. The obtained two-dimensional maps of wear grade on the femoral head were subsequently projected onto stereoscopic images of a femoral head 28 mm in diameter by means of a three-dimensional computer-aided design engineering software. AFM images were systematically recorded on each zone of different wear grade, as preliminary located by SEM inspection on each retrieval surface. Arithmetic mean roughness, R_a, and ten-point mean roughness, R_z, can be obtained from experimental data according to the following equations:

$$R_{\mathrm{a}} = \frac{1}{l}\int_{0}^{l} \left| f(x) dx \right| \tag{3.1}$$

$$R_{\mathrm{z}} = \frac{1}{5}\sum_{j=1}^{5} \left| y_{\mathrm{pj}} + y_{\mathrm{vj}} \right| \tag{3.2}$$

where l is the sampling length, $y = f(x)$ is the profile height relative to the mean line, y_{pj} are height values detected for the five tallest peaks, and y_{vj} are depth values detected for the five lowest valleys of the entire profile. In addition, shape parameters of skewness, R_{sk}, and kurtosis, R_{ku}, for the height histogram can also be mathematically computed from experimentally measured height distribution functions (normalized by the standard deviation of the distribution), according to the following equations:

$$R_{\mathrm{sk}} = \frac{1}{R_{\mathrm{q}}^{3}}\int_{-\infty}^{\infty} f^{3}(x)\, p(x) dx \tag{3.3}$$

$$R_{\mathrm{ku}} = \frac{1}{R_{\mathrm{q}}^{4}}\int_{-\infty}^{\infty} f^{4}(x)\, p(x) dx \tag{3.4}$$

where $p(x)$ is the probability density function given that a profile height occurs between the heights x and $(x + dx)$ [453].

Table 3.2 Classification of worn zones according to qualitative definitions and the related quantitative parametric intervals locating the statistical characteristics of the alumina surface texture on the nanometer scale.

Wear progression	Features	S_f (%)	R_a (nm)	R_z (nm)
Grade 0	As-manufactured smooth surface (with machine marks)	100	<3	<30
Grade 1	Low wear as characterized by small round pits (machine marks are still visible.)	98.7 ± 0.5	4 ~ 9	30 ~ 45
Grade 2	Low wear as characterized by round pits and indistinct machine marks	93.4 ± 1.6	10 ~ 15	45 ~ 60
Grade 3	Mild wear as characterized by polygonal pits and isolated grain pull-out	68.2 ± 4.8	20 ~ 35	295 ~ 430
Grade 4	Severe wear as characterized by total loss of original surface (intergranular erosion followed by grain pull-out)	42.8 ± 3.2	65 ~ 80	655 ~ 740
Grade 5	Disruptive wear as characterized by complete loss of original surface	0	>120	>950

The (root) mean-square roughness, R_q, appearing to the denominator of Eqs. (3.3) and (3.4) is defined as follows:

$$R_q = \sqrt{\frac{1}{l}\int_0^l f^2(x)dx} \qquad (3.5)$$

Figures 3.5(a) and (b) show typical 3D images collected by AFM on the original surface (also referred to as "Grade 0" zone) of unused alumina heads BIOLOX®*forte* and BIOCERAM, respectively. The morphology was conspicuously constant over the entire head surface and quite similar for the two types of head, with common features as machine-scratches and small pits involving similar mean values of arithmetic mean roughness and ten point roughness (R_a = 2.21 nm and R_z = 25.2 nm for BIOLOX®*forte*, and R_a = 2.90 nm and R_z = 27.5 nm for BIOCERAM heads). The maximum and minimum height values in the roughness profiles were R_{max} = 13.2 nm and R_{min} = −16.4 nm for BIOLOX®*forte* head, and R_{max} = 12.0 nm and R_{min} = −15.2 nm for the BIOCERAM head.

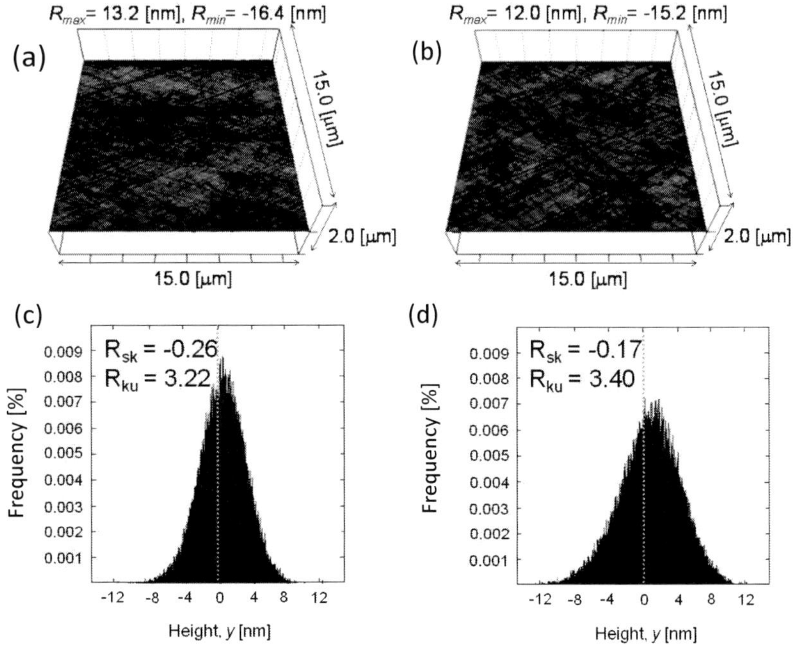

Figure 3.5 AFM images of as-received (grade 0) BIOLOX®*forte* and BIOCERAM types in (a) and (b), respectively; in (c) and (d), their respective surface height histograms are reported (skewness and kurtosis values given in inset).

Slight differences (i.e., arising from different machining procedures) were detected in the recorded height histograms, which are representative of the full sets of statistical data collected on each type of femoral head. Figures 3.5(c) and (d) display such height histograms for BIOLOX®*forte* and BIOCERAM heads, respectively. Both distributions were negatively skewed (R_{sk} = −0.26 and −0.17 for BIOLOX®*forte* and BIOCERAM heads, respectively) and slightly broadened (R_{ku} = 3.22 and 3.40 for BIOLOX®*forte* and BIOCERAM heads, respectively) with respect to a standard Gaussian distribution (i.e., which by definition should experience values of skewness and kurtosis equal to 0 and 3, respectively). It should be noted that the quite low values of roughness in the as-received state (i.e., in the order of the nanometer) is one of the positive aspects of using ceramic materials in hip joint prostheses. Metallic femoral heads in their as-received state might experience, depending on the manufacturer, similar mean roughness values but more than one order of magnitude higher maximum and minimum surface height values as compared with those measured here [454] (eventually also accompanied by sensibly higher (negative) skewness values [455]). Figures 3.6(a)~(d) represent three-dimensional drafts of four retrievals (two BIOLOX®*forte* type and two BIOCERAM type) femoral heads, which emphasize the boundary delineation of zones with different grades of wear. As a general feature, Grade 4 and 5 wear zones were always located at around the superior zone of the femoral head and distributed from posterior to anterior via the superior portion of the head dome. In both types of femoral head, the morphology of the area cumulatively comprising zones of Grades 4 and 5 was always roughly elliptical with preferentially elongating along the direction of primary sliding (i.e., the gait motion) generated at the contact of the joints during *in vivo* loading. However, the cumulative surface area of the zones of Grades 3 to 5 was systematically larger (i.e., more than twice) in the BIOCERAM heads than in the BIOLOX®*forte* heads. This could be attributed to the smaller clearance of the former head type as compared to the latter one. Grade 4 and 5 wear zones, which are characterized by a conspicuous loss of alumina grains from the original surface, are thus also zones producing hard alumina crystallites acting as third-body wear objects. Such pulled-out hard grains, once entrapped between the more tightly adjacent faces of the BIOCERAM implants, might leave the contact area of the joint sliding surfaces with more difficulty as compared to the BIOLOX®*forte* implants with relatively higher laxity. While the optimal clearance to achieve elasto-hydrodynamic lubrication and thus to avoid high friction is still being studied and debated, tribologists recommend the diametral clearance be as small as possible, especially in large-diameter bearings [456]. However, data here clearly show not only that this requirement must be balanced against practical limitations of manufacturing tolerances, but also that in a quite stiff ceramic liner, detached ceramic grains might remain entrapped between the mating surfaces with detrimental effects on friction, on the extension of the wear zone and, ultimately, on a loosening effect on the entire joint.

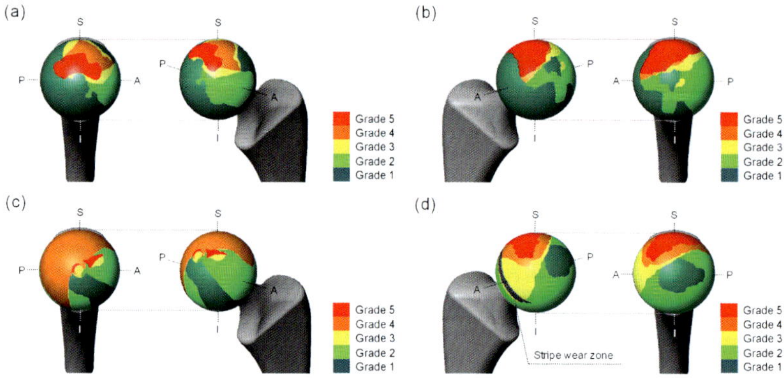

Figure 3.6 Stereoscopic images of the four investigated femoral heads with the related morphology of different wear zones. The heads in (a), (b), (c), and (d) correspond to Cases I, II, III, IV, respectively, as listed in Table 3.1.

The maximum depth of the worn surfaces, arising from grain removal, reached relatively high values in the range 625~916 nm for Grade 5 areas. On the other hand, Grades 3 and 4, which spread peripherally from the zone of Grade 5, could eventually cover significantly large zones of the head (cf., for example, Grade 4 zone in Fig. 3.6(c), which accounts for more than a third of the total surface on the femoral head). In Grade 4 wear zones, most of the original surface was disrupted by the wear phenomenon, with a depth of grain excavation (in the range 506~582 nm) generally shallower than that observed in zones belonging to Grade 5. Some grain pullout and microcracks also occurred in regions of Grade 3, with maximum depth of grain excavation ranging between 222 nm and 318 nm. Histograms of surface heights, from which the full texture characteristics of the worn surfaces can be retrieved, are given for different wear zones of the four head retrievals in Figs. 3.7(a)~(d) (Grade 3 zones), Figs. 3.7(e)~(h) (Grade 4 zones), and Figs. 3.7(i)~(l) (Grade 5 zones). For brevity's sake, data for wear zones belonging to Grades 1 and 2 were not explicitly shown; however, these latter data revealed a gradual alteration from the state of the as-received surfaces to that of worn surfaces belonging to Grade 3. From the obtained height histograms, which are representative of the full set of statistical data collected on five 15 × 15 μm AFM maps for each retrieval, values of skewness

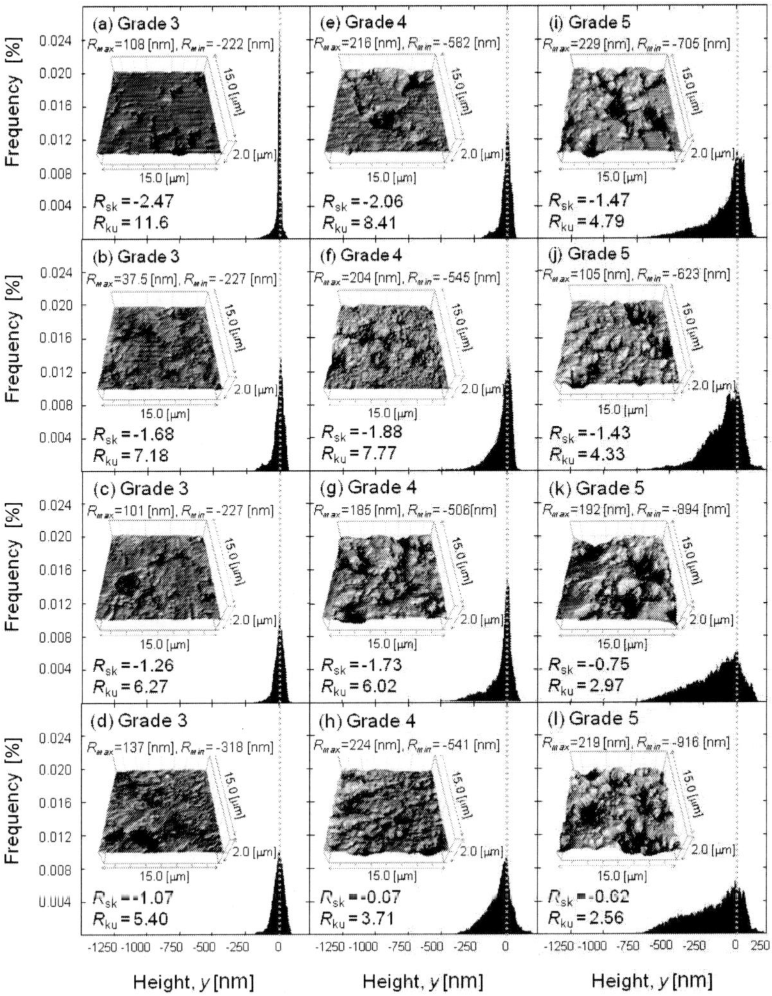

Figure 3.7 Histograms of surface height as obtained from AFM scans on different wear zones of four head retrievals ((a), (e), (i) for Case I; (b), (f), (j) for Case II; (c), (g), (k) for Case III; and (d), (h), (l) for Case IV). Typical AFM images and values of skewness and kurtosis are given in inset to each histogram.

and kurtosis could be calculated as shown in inset to each histogram. The principal features contained in the histograms of Figs. 3.7(a)~(l) (cf. data in inset to the figures) can be discussed as follows:

(i) In all the studied retrievals, the height histograms significantly broadened with proceeding from Grade 3 to Grade 5 wear severity. This is due to the gradual formation of craters as a consequence of grain detachment. Note, however, that if we compare Grade 3 histograms with histograms from unused heads (Grade 0), an inverse (sharpening) process is found for the surface texture. Such effect can be quantified by observing the variation of kurtosis values, which first jump (by at least a twofold increase) from Grade 0 to Grade 3, and then decrease again from Grade 3 to Grade 5 down to values comparable with that of Grade 0. The increase of kurtosis values with increasing wear grade from 0 to 3 might be attributed to an initial process of "reciprocal polishing" of the hard mating surfaces which, losing the artifacts due to the machining procedure, experience sharpened distributions with a width close to that of an ideal Gaussian curve.

(ii) A further finding regarding kurtosis was that independent of wear grade, its values gradually decreased with increasing exposure time *in vivo* of the alumina femoral head. Tayebi and Polycarpou [187] have conducted a useful modeling work on the effect of skewness and kurtosis on the static friction coefficient of rough surfaces. Those researchers predicted that surfaces with high kurtosis, as well as surfaces with positive skewness, exhibit lower static friction coefficient compared to the Gaussian case. However, more important here, they also predicted that for increasing the magnitude of a negative skewness (as observed here in worn surfaces from Grades 3~5), the static friction coefficient increases sharply with decreasing external force. In other words, the static friction coefficient encountered by low torsional forces in even mildly worn areas might be significantly higher (i.e., up to three times) than that occurring in presence of the as-received surfaces.

(iii) Skewness did not generally obey any obvious monotonic trend with increasing the severity of wear loading, but it systematically pointed toward positive values with increasing exposure time *in vivo*. An interesting finding is that all the histograms that were obtained at wear zones of Grades 3~5 were negatively skewed (in the range from −0.62 to −2.47), namely with a number of craters statistically exceeding that of surface protuberances. This gradual transition in the height histogram confirms the preferential occurrence of grain detachment, starting from isolated grain pullout (Grades 1~3) and ending with the total disruption of the original surface (Grade 5) upon wear progression.

(iv) Most of the alumina surface classified into early wear progression (Grade 3) (Figs. 3.7(i)~(l)), conserved portions of the original surface, eventually "re-polished" by the hard-on-hard sliding process but with few locations of grain excavation. As a result, the obtained histograms displayed a sharpened but heavily skewed shape (i.e., with increased static friction coefficient).

Figures 3.8(a)~(c) show a SEM micrograph, a 3D-AFM image, and its corresponding height histogram, respectively, as collected near the center of the edge-loading stripe-wear scar on the surface of Case 4. The latitude of the center of this scar was approximately 10° south of the equator (0°) of the 28 mm femoral head. The long axis of the scar was almost parallel to the equator line. Portions of polished surface were no longer visible in this zone. Interestingly, a large number of convex prominences were observed on the surface of the alumina head and this feature makes the height histogram skewed positively in this region (i.e., an intrinsically different characteristic from that of Grade 5 worn surfaces, despite the apparent roughness similarity). Data for the arithmetic mean roughness, R_a, and ten-point mean roughness, R_z, measured on differently worn surfaces of all retrievals are summarized in Figs. 3.9(a) and (b), respectively. Besides clarifying that roughness values gradually and consistently increased with increasing exposure time *in vivo* within the same grade region, this figure also shows that the highest roughness values were obtained at the center of the stripe wear (R_a = 192 nm; R_z = 1511 nm). In this context, it can also be interesting to note that a stripe wear zone was observed in a hip joint with inherently small clearance, which might be different from the usual simulation of stripe wear arising in joints with initial laxity [457, 458]. The explanation for this experimental observation indeed resides in the high-friction characteristics of the BIOCERAM joint, which ultimately led to loosening of the liner (and laxity) [441, 559], namely to the cause of implant revision in Case 4 and to similar causes for revision in all the other BIOCERAM implants investigated. Finally, according to the above set of statistical data, we have also quantitatively standardized the level of roughness and the values of other statistical parameters of surface texture into quantitative intervals as given in Table 3.2.

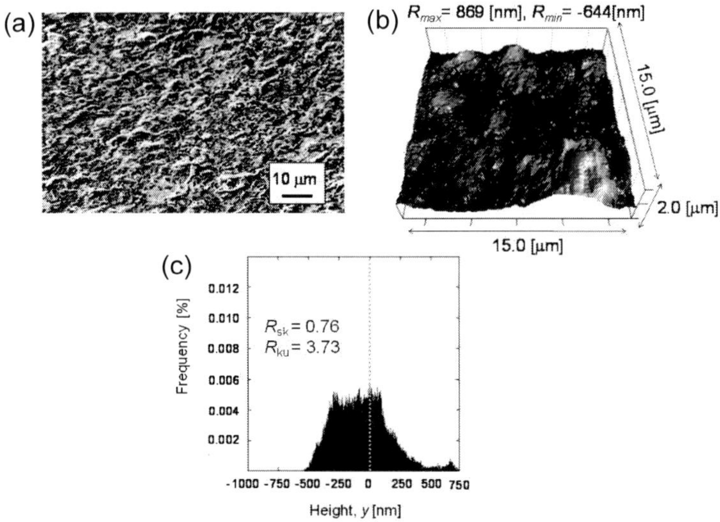

Figure 3.8 FEG-SEM micrograph (a), AFM image (b), and height histogram (c) representative of the stripe wear zone (grade SW) detected in Case IV. Values of skewness and kurtosis are given in inset to (c).

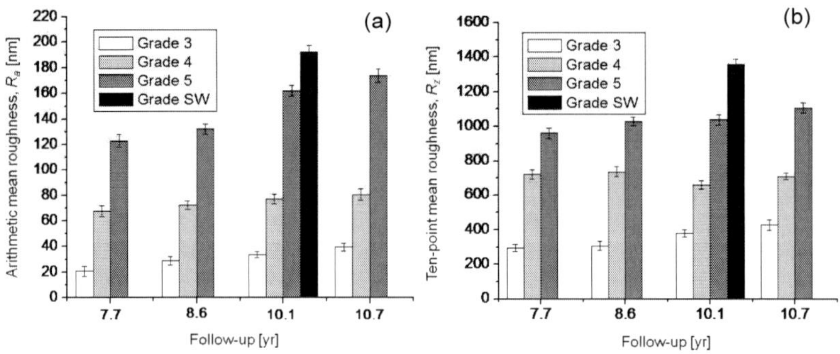

Figure 3.9 Arithmetic mean roughness (a) and 10-point mean roughness (b) in response to wear severity and follow-up time of the head retrievals.

Assessments of long-term *in vivo* exposed alumina femoral head, which uses a composite multiscale procedure involving SEM and AFM morphological examinations, result in an improved view of wear development, which allows one to link nanometer-scale phenomena to the macroscopic characteristics of joint design. The macroscopic morphology of higher-grade wear zones indeed greatly depends on joint design and, in particular, on the equatorial clearance of the femoral head with respect to the liner. Implants with smaller clearance experience larger surfaces for zones heavily worn to Grades 4 and 5, owing to the high friction developed during gait swing and ultimately leading to joint loosening. It has been demonstrated that the microscopic (statistical) features of the surface texture can be rationalized on a quantitative scale with distinguishing among portions of head surface worn to different degrees. Portions of surface worn to different degrees possess surface texture characteristics that lie in common parametric intervals. In particular, the stripe wear zone (produced by repeated contacts/shocks between head and edge of the liner) possesses morphological features which, taken on a statistical base, are significantly different from those of wear zones originated from frictional loading.

3.3 Wear Behavior: The Role of Surface Residual Stresses

The surface damages developed *in vivo* at the bearing surfaces of ceramic hip implants result from repeated fretting contacts between hard surfaces in a highly corrosive environment [460]. Common practices for rationalizing wear processes mainly rely on hip-joint simulators experiments, taking wear rate and roughness evolution (i.e., due to action of local contact loads in simulated reactive environment) as the monitored outputs [373, 461]. According to simulation procedures, ceramic bearings are systematically subjected to cyclic combined actions of sliding and microseparation/shock contacts [373, 462]. Subsequent examinations with respect to weight loss and amplitude of surface roughness profiles in the load-bearing parts are the parameters commonly selected for assessing the quality of a sliding couple. Nowadays, this set of parameters represents a standard for the evaluation of hip joint performance and provides the rationale for predicting joint lifetime *in vivo*. However, from the material physics viewpoint, the outputs of hip simulator experiments appear to be of a purely phenomenological nature. In other words, while simulations provide a phenomeno-logical description of the wear phenomenon in the joint components, they only provide a quite limited physical insight into the nature of surface damage mechanisms. Such a consideration is substantiated by recent spectroscopic studies of ceramic hip joints [99, 100, 117, 120], which have revealed a significant effect by the presence of highly graded residual stress (or permanent strain fields) stored on the bearing surfaces, thus hinting that sound lifetime predictions for *in vivo* exposure need to incorporate the effect of contact-induced residual stresses as well as the occurrence of a stress-assisted grain pullout mechanism at the joint surfaces. We have previously discussed how residual stresses unavoidably exist on the microstructural level in ceramic joint components. Their presence, which originates from the manufacturing process and progresses with bearing history, is acknowledged by those who develop wear and fracture mechanics test methodologies; however, there has always been debate as to how to account for these stresses in hip joints, or even whether they should be accounted for. As a result, not even cautionary notes are being inserted into hip joint test standards.

Residual stresses can enhance or impair the ability of a joint component (especially those made of ceramics) to withstand loading conditions in service, depending on their compressive or tensile nature. The presence of surface residual stresses poses severe problems in lifetime predictions, as they might affect the structural integrity of the whole joint. In addition, the impact of surface stresses on the development of wear damages is of critical importance for manufacturing optimization since it affects component quality and cost. Reliable methods are indeed available for stress measurements in ceramic components. Among the available techniques, in Chapter 2 we have mentioned piezo-spectroscopy, which defines a measurement method for residual or applied stresses in materials using characteristic peak shifts of either vibrational or electronic spectra [463]. The two most common spectroscopic approaches to stress measurement are Raman and fluorescence spectroscopy (in the remainder of this paper, also referred to as photo-stimulated techniques), which both employ a conventional optical microscope to focus the incoming laser and the emitted radiation onto a microscopic volume (i.e., the probe volume). Raman spectroscopy measures vibrational energies, which will slightly change due to the atomic bond in the material getting either more or less "stiff" under stress. The resultant peak shift with stress can be calibrated and used to measure stress. Fluorescence measures the emission of light caused by the excitation and subsequent de-excitation of an electron of a dopant or an impurity ion in a host lattice (e.g., Cr^{3+} in Al_2O_3). In this latter case, the energy of the emission will change under stress due to the crystal field of the lattice altering the energy of the shell electrons of the dopant ion. In both techniques, the probe size is confined to a length scale typically from the single micrometer to the tens of micrometers, according to the combined effects of laser wavelength and the light absorption/diffraction properties of the studied material. An improved, yet less popular, PS method has also been proposed [464–466] that uses an electron beam to excite luminescence from the material and assess residual stresses from the peak shift of such an electro-stimulated spectrum. The main advantage expected in using the electron probe as an excitation source is a substantial improvement in spatial resolution. Relevant to residual stress studies of hip joint surfaces is the minimization of penetration depth (i.e., down to a sub-micrometer scale) along the material sub-surface. In other words, even in the presence of extremely steep stress gradients along the material subsurface, the true magnitude of the surface stress field becomes measurable from PS assessments. In this section, we shall first compare the efficiency of (confocal) laser and electron probes in measuring the actual magnitude of the surface residual stresses piled up *in vivo* on the surface of a hip joint made of monolithic alumina ceramic. An approach adopting the electron beam for high-resolution measurement of surface residual stresses is expected to lead to several orders of magnitude improvement in spatial resolution, with the added benefit of obtaining stress magnitudes less sensitive to gradients along the depth of the sample. It follows that the magnitude of the measured surface stress depends on the probe used to measure it, which is not a favorable circumstance in view of the large dependence of wear rate on surface stress fields. The knowledge of the correct magnitude and of the statistical nature of the residual stress piled up *in vivo* on the surface of alumina femoral heads allows clarifying the nature of wear mechanisms as they develop during *in vivo* service.

An alumina femoral head, which belonged to a left-side implant and was revised after long-term implantation period *in vivo* (≈11 years), is used here as an example. This head was part of a ceramic-on-ceramic total hip prosthesis system that was retrieved because of repeated dislocations. Typical fluorescence and Raman spectra obtained from an alumina femoral head are shown in Figs. 3.10(a) and (b). The fluorescence doublet arises from the presence of an intrinsic Cr^{3+} impurity, substituting for Al^{3+} in the corundum structure of Al_2O_3 [467, 468]. Raman bands belong to the A_g and E_g vibrational modes, namely the Raman active species of the irreducible representation [469, 470]. A typical CL spectrum of the same alumina is shown in Fig. 3.10(c). This latter spectrum, which represents the optical activity of oxygen vacancy sites, consists of the overlap of two sub-bands arising from a single oxygen vacancy trapping one (F^+ centers) or two (F centers) electrons [471, 472].

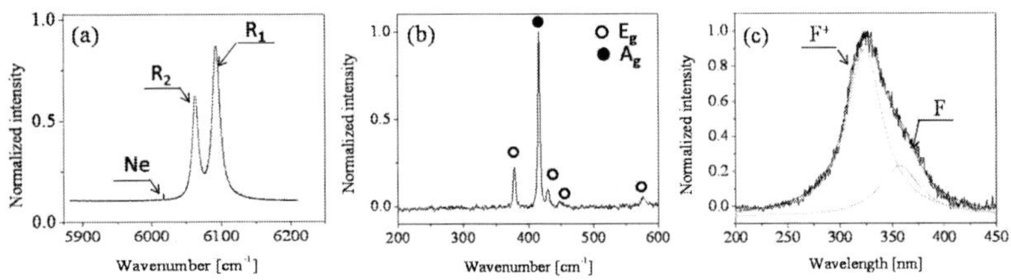

Figure 3.10 (a) Fluorescence (Cr^{3+} doublet) and (b) Raman (A_g and E_g bands) spectra of the investigated alumina femoral head. The band labeled "Ne" in (a) represents the emission from a neon lamp intentionally set in the measurement apparatus for internal calibration. In (c), CL spectrum of the investigated alumina femoral head dominated by the optical activity of oxygen vacancy sites (F^+ and F centers).

The starting point in studying surface stress fields is the observation that the intensity of an optical spectrum emitted from an arbitrary point $P \equiv (x, y, z)$ of the sample depends on the intensity distribution within the probe (i.e., scattered light or electrons) around the irradiation point $P_0 \equiv (x_0, y_0, z_0)$. Such an intensity distribution is usually referred to as the probe response function, $B(z, z_0)$, and it might greatly differ among different probes impinging on the same sample. In the case of surface residual stresses induced by hard-on-hard sliding contacts, the stress gradient along the material subsurface (i.e., along the z-axis) is expected to be particularly steep. Therefore, the morphology of the in-depth probe response function is of main interest in this kind of characterizations. Table 3.3 lists the in-depth probe response functions for confocal fluorescence and Raman probes, and for a CL probe embedded in polycrystalline alumina, together with the numerical values of the related parameters and of probe depth, z^*. This latter parameter is a threshold value for 90% of the intensity emission and it can be assumed as a measure of the probe size along the sample depth. The mathematical character of $B(z, z_0)$ describes both size and morphology of the photo- and electro-stimulated luminescence probes. Probe morphologies are schematically depicted in Fig. 3.11. A full treatment of probe morphology is beyond the scope of this book; however, the interested Readers can find the full details regarding the three-dimensional morphology of the response functions in specialized publications [99, 122, 125, 126, 145, 233]. Briefly here, a common morphology (i.e., but different size) of a truncated cone, whose waist in the focal plane is much smaller than its diameter at the threshold depth, z^*, is found for (confocal) fluorescence and Raman probes; however, these two probes show a clear difference in size, the Raman probe being one third shallower than the fluorescence one (e.g., depth of 36 vs. 50 μm). This phenomenon can be attributed to a difference in the effective absorption coefficients of the compared

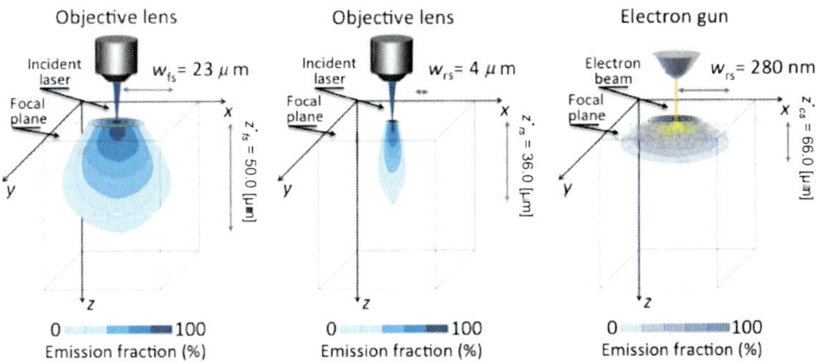

Figure 3.11 Draft comparing both morphology and response functions for laser and electron probes in the studied polycrystalline alumina sample. Probes for the photo-stimulated ruby R_1 and A_g Raman bands (confocal pinhole aperture = 100 μm), and for the electro-stimulated band of F^+ center (electron acceleration voltage, V = 4 kV) are displayed from left to right. The probe widths and depths (for 90% intensity of light emission) are defined by "w" and "z^*," respectively, while their subscripts "fs," "rs," and "cs" refer to fluorescence, Raman, and cathodoluminescence spectroscopy, respectively.

bands (cf. the α_{eff} values reported in Table 3.3). Note that using a confocal probe configuration is known to appreciably reduce the size of photo-stimulated probes; however, the spatial resolution of photo-stimulated spectroscopic assessments in a relatively transparent material as alumina remains unavoidably dictated by a probe volume in the order of at least several thousands of cubic micrometers (i.e., Raman probe). It follows that both photo-stimulated (confocal) probes average the stress information over a large number of alumina grains (i.e., 150 and 5000 for A_g and R_1 bands, respectively) in the depth of the sample, thus washing out the stress magnitude that is expected to reach its maximum value near the surface of the worn sample. Finally, it should be noted that in the case of polycrystalline alumina, the probe size and morphology have been found to strongly depend on grain size. Therefore, the values listed in Table 3.3 are only valid for alumina polycrystals with grain size close to that of the material shown here. The grain size dependence of the response function of laser probes has been explicitly treated in a specific publication [120, 473].

Table 3.3 Probe response function and probe geometry parameters for the three types of investigated probes

Spectral band	p (μm)	α_{eff} (μm^{-1})	w_s (μm)	z_s^* (μm)	V_p (μm^3)	N_g
R_1	75	0.018	23	50	8.4×10^4	$\sim 5 \times 10^3$
A_g	37	0.020	4	36	2.5×10^3	150
F^+		4 kV	0.282	0.066	0.061	<<1
		10 kV	0.416	0.295	0.214	≈1

Note: The probe volume, V_p, and the number of grains, N_g, screened by each probe in a single measurement in the present alumina are explicitly shown. Note that the size of the CL probe can be increased with increasing the acceleration voltage of the electron beam; however, the intensity of the F^+ CL band is strong enough at 4 kV to allow a precise PS measurement of stress on the nanometer scale.

On the other hand, the electro-stimulated probe geometry is that of a semi-ellipsoid (or of a "flattened" onion) whose in-plane semi-axis length is significantly larger than its in-depth axis length, z^*. The most striking feature in Table 3.3 and Fig. 3.11 is that the electron probe is about three orders of magnitude shallower than both photo-stimulated probes. This has a clear effect when a comparison among stress measurements made at the same location by the above three different probes immediately clarifies the strong dependence of the measured stress magnitude on the adopted probe. For each probe, both algorithms and the conversion factors needed for converting spectral shifts to stress magnitudes have been explicitly given in Ref. [122, 226]. It should be noted that the CL probe morphology in polycrystalline alumina differs from that of the typical "onion-like" shape produced by electron scattering in the sample [474, 475], the latter being conspicuously symmetric in shape and less shallow as compared to the former one. It follows that an improved PS method based on low-voltage CL spectroscopy, offers a tangible advantage in terms of spatial resolution and its extreme shallowness is particularly suitable for the characterization of the highly graded stress fields stored onto worn zones of the very surface of alumina hip components. No statistical average among grains can be expected in assessing residual stresses with the electro-stimulated probe, for which both width and depth are smaller than the material grain size. Therefore, in a lack of statistical average over many grains (as in the case of Raman or fluorescence probes), an additional measurement of local crystallographic orientation by EBSD is required, concurrent to CL stress assessments. Such crystallographic information has to be incorporated into the algorithm for the conversion of the observed spectral shift into stress magnitude, as shown in publications specifically devoted to this argument [122, 464]. Finally note that from a spectroscopic point of view, the intensity of electro-stimulated bands arising from the optical activity of oxygen vacancies might also be regarded as a means to monitor the stoichiometric state of the alumina surface after increasing periods of exposure to biological environment. This point will be explicitly treated in the next section dealing with the chemical changes of alumina upon *in vivo* exposure.

Figures 3.12, 3.13, and 3.14 compare mapping experiments conducted at exactly the same area of the investigated alumina hip joint by using fluorescence, Raman, and CL probes, respectively. Two selected areas for spectroscopic measurements were from both wear (worn to Grade 4) and non-wear (worn to Grade 1) zones. No obvious traces of wear or wear scares could be detected in the investigated areas by naked eye or by using conventional optical microscopy inspection. Note also that photo-stimulated intensity maps did not reveal such features as well. This characteristic confirms the appreciable influence of sub-surface contributions for optically stimulated probes. On the other hand, CL intensity maps revealed surface scratches owing to the rather shallow nature of the CL probe. Maps of relative band intensity are given in the (a) and (c) sides (for non-wear and main-wear zones, respectively) of Figs. 3.12~3.14 for the ruby fluorescence, A_g Raman, and F^+ CL bands, respectively. Raman intensity maps revealed the polycrystalline structure of the material slightly better than the fluorescence maps (a relative intensity map for the A_g Raman mode is shown in Fig. 3.13(a)). On the other hand, the electro-stimulated maps of the luminescence intensity from optically active F^+ centers (i.e., Figs. 3.14(a) and (c)) showed a clear pattern of grain-boundary decoration that can be considered to directly relate to the local vacancy concentration in the alumina lattice. PS maps, showing the trace of the local (residual) stress tensor, are given in the sides (b) and (d) (for main-wear and non-wear zones, respectively) of Figs. 3.12~3.14 for the ruby fluorescence, A_g Raman, and F^+ CL bands, respectively. The stress maps were built up according to spectral shift analyses of the respective bands using different PS conversion algorithms, as described in Ref. [122]. A comparison among photo-stimulated spectral maps (cf. Figs. 3.12 and 3.13) shows that the stress maps collected with using the Cr^{3+} fluorescence probe are almost featureless, while a clear resolution improvement is obtained using the Raman probe. This is reflected in a detectable increase of residual stress from nearly zero to a magnitude of the hundredths of MPa. However, as a general trend in photo-stimulated spectroscopy, high spatial resolution on the microstructural scale of the material can be hardly achieved due to the simultaneous collection of out-of-focus light. In alumina, this problem is sharpened by the relatively high transparency of the material to visible irradiation. Note that the use of a confocal pinhole to reduce out-of-focus effects on the detector side does not fully solve the problem (cf. probe sizes listed in Table 3.3), due to a physical limitation on the minimum pinhole aperture needed for providing a detectable emission. As clearly seen from a comparison among Figs. 3.12~3.14, one of the major advantages of using a low-energy electron beam as an excitation source is the possibility of confining the probe to a very shallow volume (i.e., of the order of the tens of nanometer in depth). Furthermore, highly flexible electron scanning can provide finely controlled mapping displacements (i.e., easily in the order of the single nanometer vs. those in the order of the single micron used for building photo-stimulated maps) and, thus, highly resolved stress maps can be collected. As a result of the shallowness of the electron probe, the detected magnitude of surface stress in the femoral head is restored to its actual magnitude (i.e., in the order of the GPa), as shown in Figs. 3.14(b) and (d) for non-wear and main-wear zone, respectively. A comparison between the true magnitude of the residual stress fields stored in the main-wear and in the non-wear zone of the retrieved alumina femoral head also reveals interesting features. Unlike the main-wear zone that is fully embedded in a highly compressive stress field, in the non-wear zone the surface stress field appeared to be of a mixed tensile/compressive nature. However, the maximum stress magnitude is comparable to that recorded in the main-wear zone, although a larger areal fraction of stress-free zones (depicted in green color) is also present. The electro-stimulated PS maps provide us with high-resolution stress measurements on the surface of alumina hip joints, which can be useful to both judge the manufacturing level of the implant and rationalize the progress of its wear behavior. To date, no other stress measurement approach seems to be capable of such a high spatial resolution (i.e., in particular, shallowness) in bulk ceramic materials. The availability of stress measurements at the same location with three probes with different (and known) response functions also gives us a chance for unfolding the "true" subsurface residual stress distribution in the main wear zone of the long-term *in vivo* exposed femoral head. According to the probe characteristics shown in Table 3.3 and data averaged from the maps in part (d) of Figs. 3.12~3.14, it is possible to obtain a deconvoluted profile of average residual stress, $<\bar{\sigma}>$, along the subsurface of the head [99, 122, 233]. A trial function suitable for a sound mathematical deconvolution can be retrieved from published reports on highly graded surface stresses induced by machining in brittle materials [476, 477]. The surface stress field in machined brittle materials is characteZrized by a surface layer under

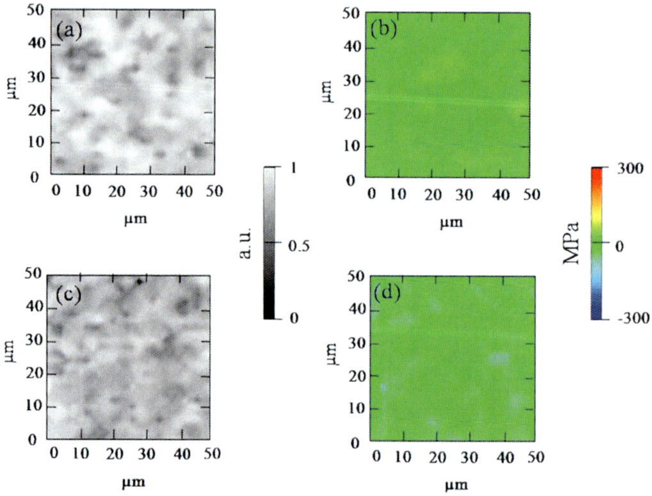

Figure 3.12 Maps of relative band intensity ((a) and (c) for non-wear and main-wear zones, respectively) and residual stress, $<\bar{\sigma}>$, ((b) and (d) for non-wear and main-wear zones, respectively) as measured by applying the PS method to the photo-stimulated R_1 ruby band.

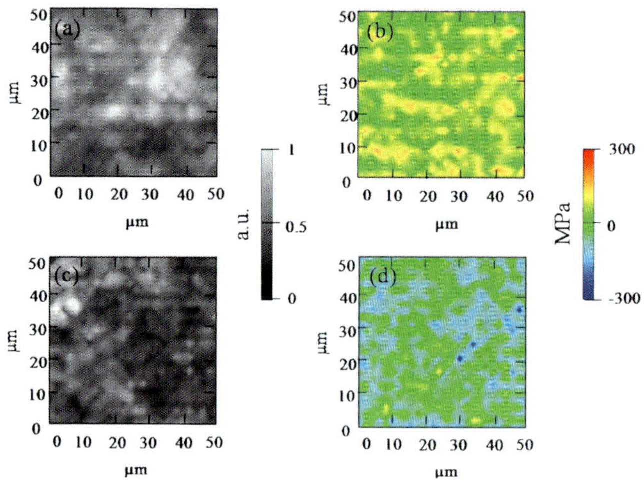

Figure 3.13 Maps of relative band intensity ((a) and (c) for non-wear and main-wear zones, respectively) and residual stress, $<\bar{\sigma}>$, ((b) and (d) for non-wear and main-wear zones, respectively) as measured by applying the PS method to the photo-stimulated A_g Raman band. The maps were collected at exactly the same position as in Fig. 3.12.

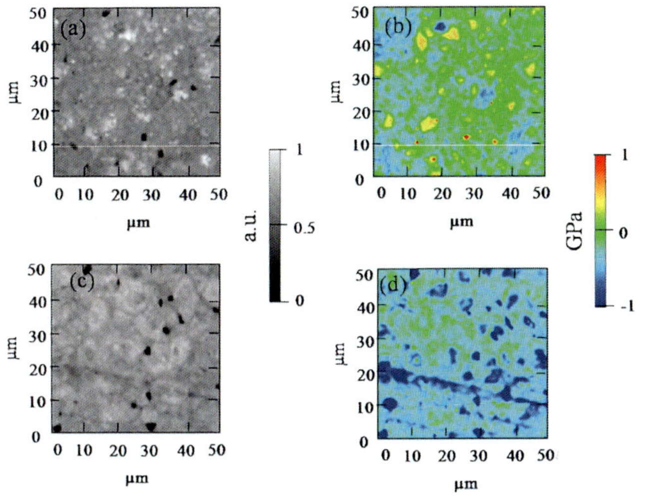

Figure 3.14 Maps of relative band intensity ((a) and (c) for non-wear and main-wear zones, respectively) and residual stress, $<\bar{\sigma}>$, ((b) and (d) for main-wear and non-wear zones, respectively) as measured by applying the PS method to the F^+ CL band. The maps were collected at exactly the same position as in Figs. 3.12 and 3.13.

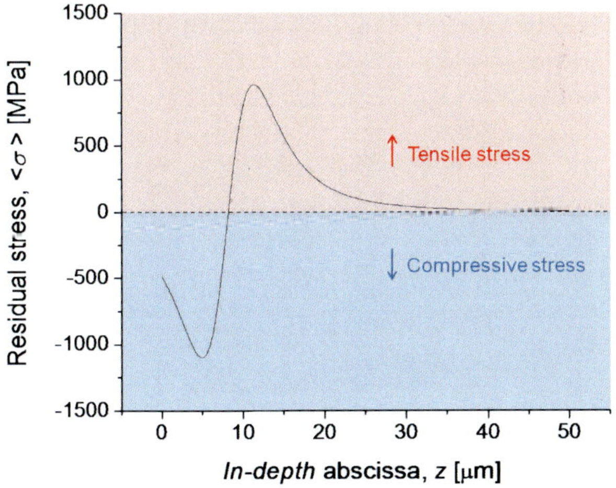

Figure 3.15 Probe-deconvoluted in-depth residual stress profile, $<\sigma>(z)$, as developed in the main-wear zone of a long-term *in vivo* exposed alumina femoral head. Note the steep gradients developed within few microns below the load-bearing surface of the joint.

compression, an abrupt compressive-to-tensile transition, and a deeper-lying region of tension, which ultimately relaxes in the unstressed bulk. The abrupt transition has been attributed to a change from mainly plastic to purely elastic deformation [477], which is also the case of worn alumina surfaces. The deconvoluted profile for the in-depth wear zone of the femoral head retrieval is shown in Fig. 3.15. As seen from the plot, a compressive stress of the GPa order is located within few microns below the worn surface, while the transition point between compressive and tensile residual stresses is located at around a depth of 10 μm. Such steep stress gradient represents an enormous driving force for progressing surface disruption in the wear zone of alumina femoral heads.

Figures 3.16(a)~(f) show histograms of surface (elastic) residual stress fields as measured by CL piezo-spectroscopy on the surface of zones worn to different grades including stripe wear zone, as collected for retrieval Case 4 in Table 3.1. The morphology of the measured stress histograms were quite similar among zones of the same wear grade belonging to different femoral heads, although slight differences in their average magnitudes can be found according to different exposure times *in vivo*. As a general trend for alumina retrievals, the statistical output of CL characterization revealed residual stress histograms slightly shifted toward the tensile side in surfaces worn up to Grade 2, as compared to the as-received surface whose stress histogram is typically centered at zero stress [478, 479]. The residual stress magnitude then progressively turns toward the compressive side with increasing wear grade from Grade 3 up to Grade 5. Stress-free areas could be only observed on worn surfaces up to Grade 3. With further progression of wear grade, the fraction of compressively stressed regions gradually grows, with compressive stress magnitudes in zone of Grades 4 and 5 approaching the GPa level. In these strongly worn zones, the increase in stress magnitude is accompanied by grain detachment, which significantly progresses on the head surface with increasing wear grade. The stripe wear zone experiences the most severe compressive stress magnitude with a significantly different stress histogram as compared to frictionally worn portions of surface (cf. Fig. 3.16(f)). However, the mean stress magnitude in the stripe wear zone is not significantly different from that detected in zones of Grade 5. The mean stress values obtained from the histograms of Fig. 3.16 for each wear region of all the retrievals listed in Table 3.1 are summarized in Fig. 3.17. This latter figure shows that the mean (compressive) stress value is found not only to depend on wear grade, but also to gradually increase with increasing the period of *in vivo* implantation within regions of the same wear grade. Average stress data, $<\bar{\sigma}>$, are re-plotted in Fig. 3.18 as a function of the disrupted surface fraction, S_f, which is expressed in percent of the unit area (also listed in Table 3.2 for each wear grade). A plot of $<\bar{\sigma}>^2$ versus S_f is found to phenomenologically obey a linear trend of linearity, according to the following equation:

$$<\bar{\sigma}>^2 = AS_f \tag{3.6}$$

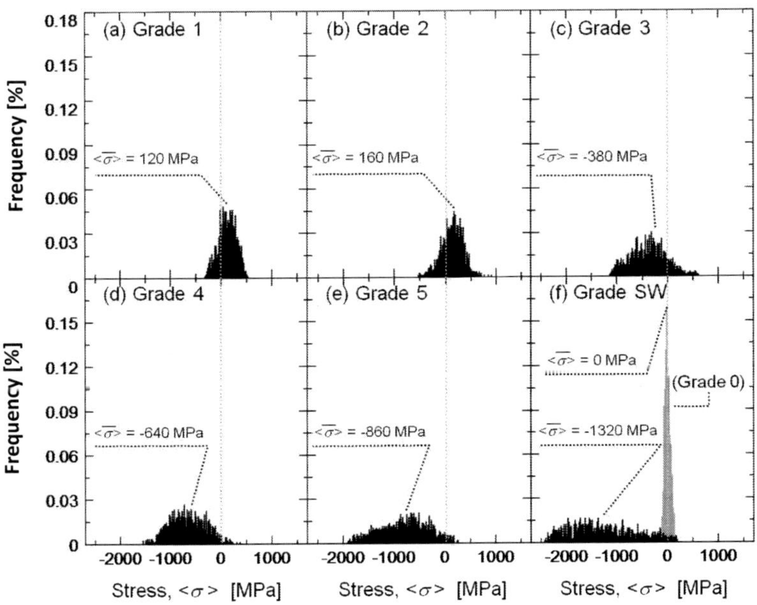

Figure 3.16 Histograms of surface residual stress stored in wear zones worn to different degrees (mean stress values, $<\bar{\sigma}>$, shown in inset) in the retrieval Case IV as compared with the as-received material (Grade 0). Stress magnitudes were measured by means of the F^+-center CL probe.

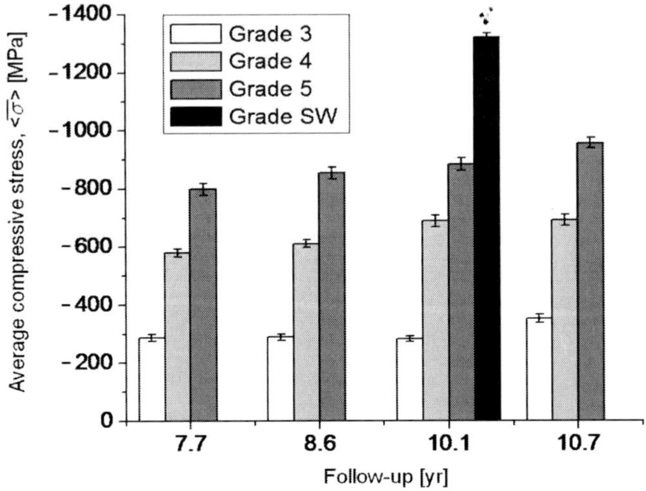

Figure 3.17 Average stress values, $<\bar{\sigma}>$, in response to wear severity and follow-up time of the head retrievals.

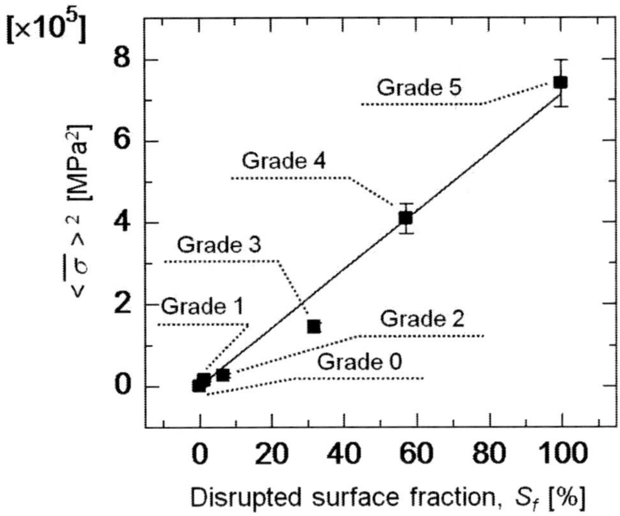

Figure 3.18 Phenomenological plots of average stress data, $<\bar{\sigma}>^2$, as a function of disrupted surface fraction, S_f. The plot obeys the linear relationship given in Eq. (3.6).

where A is the slope coefficient (= 7.13×10^3) of the regression line ($R^2 = 0.98$) plotted in Fig. 3.18, respectively, and S_f is expressed in percent of the total surface for a given wear grade. It should be noted that within the limited interval of exposure time investigated (from 7.7 to 10.7 years) the plot in Fig. 3.18 is found to be independent of exposure time *in vivo*, the slight differences in stress magnitude noticed in Fig. 3.17 being comprised in the error bars of the linear plot (as shown in Fig. 3.18). The presence of surface microcracks, expected to preferentially form at alumina grain boundaries, clearly involves the formation of surface tensile stress fields. On the other hand, it is also known that upon removal of a ceramic grain from the surface, the surrounding (elastic) material attempts to return to its original state (i.e., the shape that it occupied before detachment), producing a self-equilibrating residual stress field. This residual stress is strongly compressive in a narrow annular region adjacent to the hole created on the surface by the detached grains [480–482]. While a compressive stress field can be considered to be useful to avoid further growth of a surface microcrack from the crater location, it also induces tensile stresses in zones of the surface farther away from the crater boundary (i.e., which in turn triggers new cracking and subsequent grain detachment from yet undamaged zones) [481, 483] and in subsurface zones [481], in order to achieve static equilibrium in the material. Such a process of damage accumulation is schematically shown in Fig. 3.19. The plot in Fig. 3.18 and the wear mechanism shown in the draft of Fig. 3.19 elucidate how the fractional increase of surface damage locations is responsible for the evolution of surface texture (as observed in Figs. 3.5(a)~(f)). In conclusion, assessments of long-term *in vivo* exposed alumina femoral head, using a composite procedure involving morphological examinations by SEM and AFM, result in an improved view of wear development, which allows one to link nanometer-scale phenomena to macroscopic joint design. The macroscopic morphology of higher-grade wear zones is found to depend on joint design and, in particular, on the equatorial clearance of the ceramic femoral head with respect to the ceramic liner. Implants with smaller clearance experience larger surfaces for zones heavily worn to Grades 4 and 5, with the high friction developed during gait swing ultimately leading to joint loosening. The microscopic (statistical) features of the surface texture can be rationalized on a quantitative scale among portions of head surface worn to different degrees. A different classification approach should be taken for the stripe wear zone whose

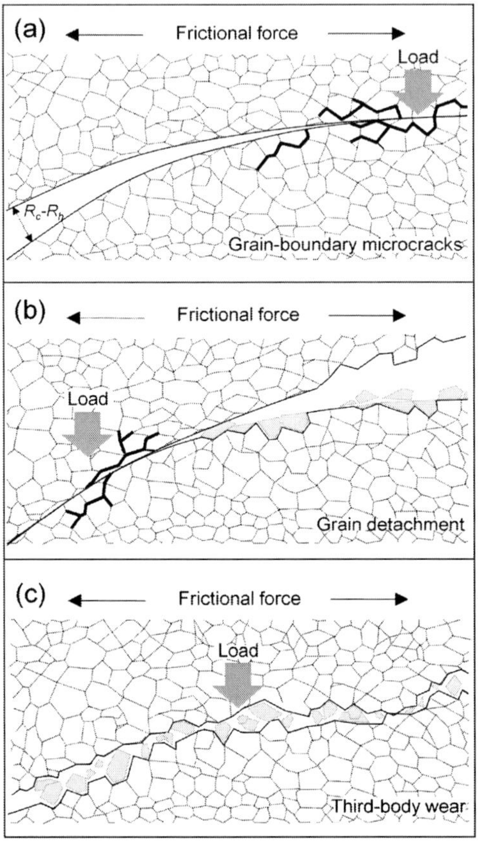

Figure 3.19 Schematic draft of the process of damage accumulation on femoral head surface due to frictional wear processes in alumina-on-alumina hip implants: (a) formation of grain-boundary microcracks, precursor to surface grain detachment, which induces tensile residual stresses; (b) grain detachment with formation of compressive residual stresses on the sliding surface; and, (c) accumulation of wear damage by a third-body wear process.

morphological features, when taken on a statistical base, are significantly different from those of wear zones originated from frictional loading. Surface residual stresses are found to mirror the roughness behavior, their magnitude rising from relatively low tensile values (in wear Grades 1 and 2) into a progressively high compressive regime up to Grade 5, and exceeding the GPa level in the stripe wear zone. A mechanism of damage accumulation, including surface microcracks and grain detachment appears capable of rationalizing the wear resistance of alumina-on-alumina hip joints and only a slight dependence of stress magnitude can be found on follow-up time.

According to the above SEM, AFM, and CL results, we have located the main wear mechanism operative in self-mating alumina hip joints. However, it is widely accepted that the wear resistance of alumina, besides depending on load [484, 485], contact speed [486] and temperature [487, 488], environment [386, 489–491], and grain size [492, 493], might also arise from conspicuously different mechanisms such as chipping due to extension of sub-surface radial and lateral cracks [494, 495], grain dislodgement following grain boundary microcracking [492, 496], plastic ploughing [497, 498], fatigue induced wear [499], and chemical reaction induced wear [489–491, 500]. The combined effect of different mechanisms and their hierarchical importance play a fundamental role in the final wear rate detected for a bearing couple. One might expect that at least in the early stage of wear damage, the main mechanism of surface degradation in self-mating alumina be substantially different from that of alumina operating versus a softer material as polyethylene. While in hard-on-hard surfaces the mechanism of chipping (and grain detachment) by extension of surface cracks (cf. Fig. 3.20) can be regarded, as we have seen, dominant at the early stage of surface damage, in alumina surfaces sliding versus polyethylene, a chemical component is likely to be the main trigger for grain-boundary grooving, which ultimately leads to grain dislodgement on the alumina surface. In the latter case, the formation of grain-boundary microcracks on the alumina surface is thus expected to require a longer time and, therefore, a delay in the process of surface disruption can be generally foreseen as compared to hard-on-hard bearings. Figure 3.21 shows plots of residual stress fields for a series of alumina femoral heads employed against alumina or polyethylene liners. In the curve related to alumina-on-alumina components, data points at the longer *in vivo* exposures refer to the four retrievals listed in Table 3.1. Data belonging to alumina femoral heads mating polyethylene liners were collected on the hip joints, whose clinical data are listed in Table 3.4. The seven retrievals in Table 3.4 were revised after short, medium, or long-term periods of *in vivo* implantation in patients. All the prostheses were retrieved after successful use in patients. However, all the implants underwent aseptic or septic, stem or cup, loosening. Among the seven cases discussed here, only Case 6 refers to a femoral head of the "mushroom-type," the other six balls being of the usual truncated spherical shape, without a ceramic skirt to partially cover the metallic stem. The alumina heads are classified in Table 3.4 as first- to third-generation Al_2O_3, according to the manufacturing year [7, 121]. The most recently fabricated heads were defined as the third generation. The stress magnitudes in Fig. 3.20 refer to those values detected in the main wear zone of alumina femoral heads retrieved after different exposure times *in vivo* (ranging from few months to approximately 19 years). As discussed above, a tensile residual stress on the alumina surface is systematically found at the initial stage of wear and it locates the formation of grain-boundary grooving and/or microcracking, while an increasingly compressive stress field reflects the gradual disruption of the alumina surface. Interestingly, the period of time *in vivo* for which tensile stresses last on the alumina surface is longer for alumina-on-polyethylene than for alumina-on-alumina hip joints. This observation confirms the fact that local asperity collision between hard surfaces (cf. Fig. 3.19) can crack the grain-boundaries at the alumina surface in a shorter service time as compared to the merely chemical attack in presence of a softer counterpart.

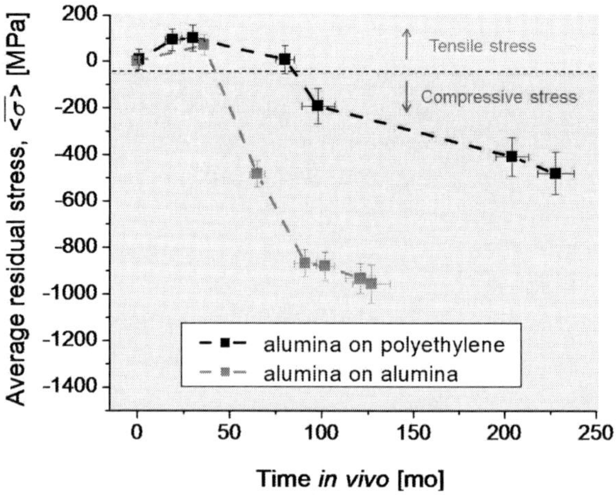

Figure 3.20 Plot of the measured (average) residual stress field, $<\overline{\sigma}>$, in the main wear zone of Al_2O_3 retrieved femoral heads as a function of the elapsed time *in vivo*.

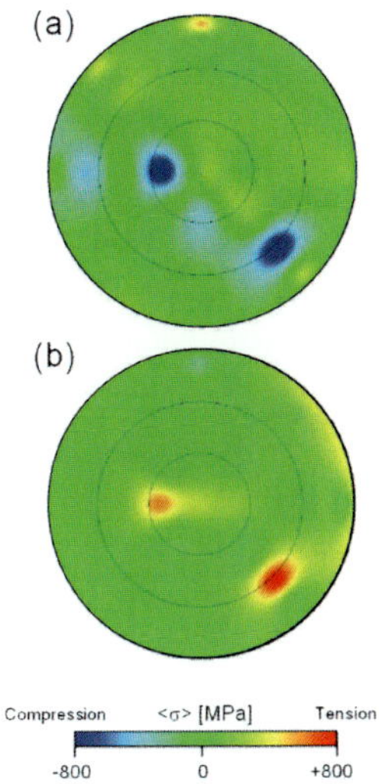

Figure 3.21 Residual stress patterns as collected on an Al_2O_3 femoral head (Case 7 in Table 3.4) after long-term exposure *in vivo*: (A) residual stress on the head surface; and, (B) residual stress state at 30 μm in the sub-surface.

Table 3.4 List of retrieved Al_2O_3 femoral heads, which were used against polyethylene liners, with description of their respective makers, grain sizes and implantation times *in vivo*.

Case	Follow-up	Grain size (μm)	Material type	Generation
1	0.1 yr	1.8	BIOLOX®*forte*	III
2	1.3 yr	1.8	BIOLOX®*forte*	III
3	1.6 yr	4.0	Unknown	II
4	2.5 yr	1.8	BIOLOX®*forte*	III
5	6.7 yr	5.5	Unknown	II
6	17 yr	9.0	Mittelmeyer	I
7	19 yr	2.0	Ceraver	I

An *in toto* statistical collection of residual stress data on the microscopic level for polyethylene-mating alumina femoral heads reveals the loading history *in vivo* and provides an interpretation of the observed wear evolution. Figures 3.21(a) and (b) show the maps of residual stress collected on the entire surface of a first-generation femoral head retrieved after long-term implantation (Case 7 in Table 3.4) by placing the focal plane exactly at the sample surface and 30 μm below the surface, respectively. Two main areas can be recognized, in which mainly compressive stresses were stored on the load-bearing surface of the ball (cf. Fig. 3.21(a)). Note also that the highly stressed zones are quite localized over the entire head dome. However, when the probe was shifted toward the subsurface (cf. Fig. 3.21(b)), residual stresses in the same areas turned to be under stresses tensile in nature. This phenomenon confirms data shown in Fig. 3.15 and can be again explained by considering the static equilibrium that has to be established between sample surface and subsurface. Static equilibrium necessarily requires the development of stress fields with opposite signs in the material subsurface. A significantly different stress trend is found by screening *in toto* second- and third-generation femoral heads retrieved after medium- or short-term implantation in the human body. Figures 3.22(a)~(d) show the evolution of residual stresses on the dome of retrieved alumina heads that served from short- to long-term *in vivo*. On the implant surface, the magnitude of the residual stress field is not only, as expected, lower than that observed in the long-term exposed first-generation femoral heads but also tensile in nature (Figs. 3.22(a) and (b)). As a general trend, the (average) residual stress stored on the wear-zone surface of retrieved heads is increasingly tensile up to 1~2 years exposure *in vivo*, then for implants subjected to medium-term exposure times in the human body residual stress consists of mixed areas of tensile and compressive nature. Note that this composite structure for the stress field conspicuously annihilates the average stress magnitude (cf. Fig. 3.20), but does not lower the maximum value of stress magnitude locally measured. It should be again noted that the topographic location of areas of stress intensification is never the same for all the retrievals. However, this can be considered to be the consequence of different designs of the joints and of the angular set of the acetabular cup at the time of implantation at the time of primary surgery. Thus, the overall morphology of the residual stress distribution on the femoral head arises from different conditions of local loading and impingement that take place during the implantation period. Nevertheless, surface residual stress fields show clear trends whose intrinsic origin should necessarily reside in the mechanical interaction between the surfaces of femoral head and acetabular cup. Based on the present experimental observation of residual stress patterns, we propose that from a phenomenological viewpoint, a similar evolution occurs in both self-mating and polyethylene-mating alumina femoral heads, although through different mechanics, according different time frames, and producing different wear-zone geometries that become involved within the same evolution trend. From a more general perspective, the neat magnitude of the residual stress field can also be considered to represent the loading history stress field. Therefore, piezo-spectroscopy provides a means for screening the concurrent effects of joint design, essential features and peculiarities of the surgery, and material characteristics through the recorded stress patterns on the head surface and subsurface. Finally, it should be noted that a direct comparison between alumina heads belonging to different generations could not prescind from also considering microstructural differences that should originate from different purity of raw powders and other differences in processing parameters during manufacturing.

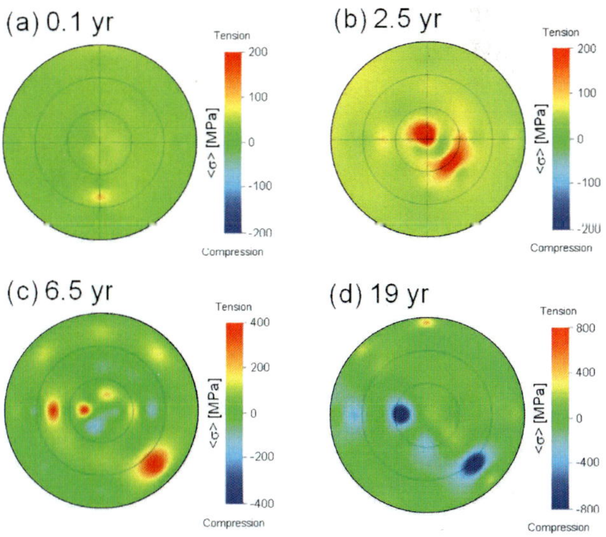

Figure 3.22 Residual stress patterns as collected on the surface of Al_2O_3 femoral heads after different exposure times *in vivo*.

3.4 Wear Behavior: The Role of Chemistry in Wear Damage

Besides conventional morphological features, monitored by AFM, topographic distributions of point defects and lattice strain on the surface of the heads can also be systematically probed by collecting high spatially and spectrally resolved CL spectra from zones of different wear severity. Optically active point-defect sites in alumina ceramics consist of oxygen vacancies, substitutional (aliovalent) cations, and, interstitial aluminum, which in turn can be shown to represent the main defects progressively developed in the alumina lattice during wear loading in human hip joints. In other words, a continuous evolution toward environmentally driven off-stoichiometry is expected with progressing wear. Moreover, as we have partly explained in the previous section, the shallow electro-stimulated optical probe also details the correct magnitude of lattice strain fields (of both elastic and plastic nature) as they develop in the very neighborhood of the bearing surface. CL spectroscopic characterizations thus enable one to substantiate important tribochemical interactions between bearing surface and *in vivo* environment as pivotal parts of progressive events of wear degradation.

We have already mentioned that monolithic alumina is the most widespread ceramic material for bearing parts in hip joints because of its high bioinertness and biocompatibility [421, 501], and a conspicuously low friction coefficient [502]. However, scientists and technologists nowadays believe that its wear resistance could be further improved provided that fundamental aspects of its tribological behavior *in vivo* (i.e., several of them yet unfolded or standing under debate) could be clarified at the nanometer scale. According to basic principles of contact mechanics [503, 504], one could evince that the strong (ionic) lattice bond should ultimately preserve oxide ceramic surfaces from experiencing plastic flow under moderate temperature/stress conditions of low-friction sliding in the human hip joint, with surface asperity contacts being of predominantly elastic nature. This is indeed the regime under which researchers have long tested alumina surfaces *in vitro* in conventional hip simulators [505];

however, the situation *in vivo* can be by far more complex. Not only can be grain-boundary microcracks and grain detachment observed in explanted alumina femoral head that failed due to excessive wear, but also traces of plasticity (i.e., pyramidal slip of dislocations) are already present in mildly worn alumina surfaces [365, 367, 506], which are intrinsically different from those preferentially expected in bulk-crept alumina samples (i.e., prism slip) [507, 370]. In other words, fracture and deformation modes of *in vivo* exposed Al_2O_3 bearings cannot be simply explained in terms of fracture/yield stresses measured in bulk samples, which would result too high to occur in the range of stress and temperature estimated for a hip joint [508]. Systematic microscopy and spectroscopy inspections of a number of long-term *in vivo* exposed alumina surfaces (i.e., with and without a stripe wear zone) lead to believe that the "mechanical" effect of bearing microseparation, although of fundamental importance, represents only one out of several factors exacerbating the degradation of alumina hip surfaces *in vivo*.

The nascent surfaces developed upon wear are proved possessing an extraordinary strong chemical activity, a variety of tribochemical reactions becoming energetically activated there [509, 510]. Hydrothermal environment on the surface of Al_2O_3 crystals is known to lead rather to dissociation than adsorption [511]; this latter phenomenon in turn produces hydroxyl and proton radicals, which promote formation of surface vacancies for maintaining electrical charge neutrality [71, 512]. Under sliding conditions, the continuous formation and frictional removal of hydroxyls should repeatedly create and annihilate a population of different kinds of vacancy site in the outer surface layers of alumina lattice, according to mechanochemically activated processes. The hydrophilic behavior of Al_2O_3 sliding counterparts should in principle minimize surface adsorption of proteins, and thus their consequent denaturation and irreversible unfolding [513–515]. However, a scarcity of synovial fluid lubricant in ceramic-on-ceramic hip joints might indeed create an extremely severe thermomechanical environment [516], in which modifications of the alumina lattice (i.e., especially in correspondence of grain boundaries) might increasingly take place. In this context, one could also hypothesize a role of protein by-products (e.g., hydrocarbons [517]) or released ions (e.g., Ca^{2+}, Mg^{2+}, and Na^{+}) on stoichiometric alterations of the alumina lattice. It is known, for example, that dilution of sodium hyaluronate (with release of Na^{+} ions) takes place in patients affected by rheumatoid arthritis, as systematically detected by Dahl *et al.* [518]. Although the effect of the above tribochemical factors on the wear behavior of alumina bearings has not yet been discussed in details, evidence is shown in the remainder of this section of a clear interaction between body environment and alumina lattice. The ensemble of various tribochemically driven events should give, in the long term, a contribution far from marginal to the lattice structure on alumina bearing surfaces, thus also altering their mechanical resistance of the alumina surface. The challenge is thus to link experimental evidence that clarifies the complex cascade of chemical events (i.e., from the formation of point defects to the occurrence of plastic flow in the lattice) affecting *in vivo* wear behavior of monolithic alumina. The CL probe with its nanometer scale shallowness is capable to resolve both chemical and mechanical features on the very surface of the material, as they develop upon *in vivo* environmental exposure. Drawing upon what has been learned so far about the physical aspects of CL emission in oxide biomaterials, an analysis for retrieved alumina hip surfaces can be attempted. The concentration of point defects (i.e., oxygen vacancies, substitutional impurities, and interstitial aluminum) generated in the very neighborhood of the alumina surface and surface lattice strain can be monitored with a spatial resolution at the nanometer scale. Tribochemical and micromechanical information are thus expected to merge into the common picture of a crystallographic lattice with characteristics of extreme off-stoichiometry and high compressive strain. CL spectroscopy uncovers relevant and so far unexplored connections between the wear resistance of alumina and environmental factors peculiar to the human body.

The CL spectrum of Al_2O_3 contains important information about the oxygen stoichiometry of the lattice [471, 472]. In the ultraviolet (UV) region, a partly overlapping doublet is found consisting of a F^{+}-center band (single oxygen vacancy trapping one electron), located at around 325 nm (3.8 eV), and of a less intense F-center band (single oxygen vacancy trapping two electrons), located at around 415 nm (3.0 eV). The presence of the F^+/F oxygen vacancy doublet was a common feature in the CL spectra recorded from all areas worn to different degrees, for both *in vivo* exposed BIOLOX®*forte* and BIOCERAM alumina materials (shown in Figs. 3.23(a) and (b), respectively). In inset to each figure, spectra are shown after deconvolution into individual Gaussian bands with the F^+ and F bands labeled as (*A*) and (*B*), respectively. Oxygen vacancy centers are Schottky-type defects that act as electric charge compensators; therefore, they should form (or annihilate) on the material surface as a direct consequence of interactions between the sample surface and the environment. In other words, the observed CL intensity in the UV region directly reflects vacancy concentration as it evolves in the Al_2O_3 lattice (e.g., a clear increase in concentration is found here with increasing wear severity).

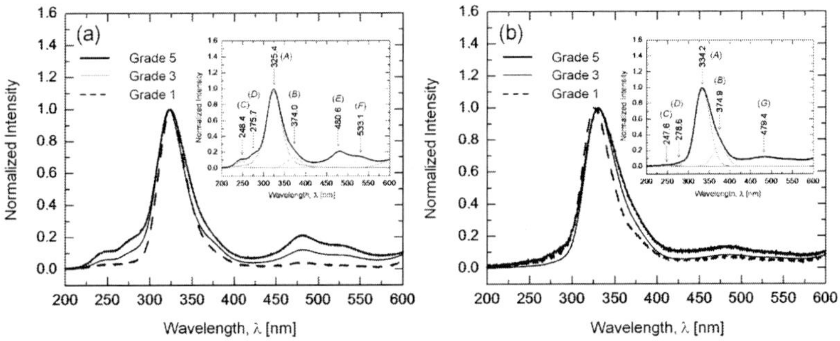

Figure 3.23 CL spectra recorded from areas worn to different degrees for *in vivo* exposed BIOLOX®*forte* and BIOCERAM alumina femoral heads in (a) and (b), respectively. In inset to each figure, spectra are shown after deconvolution into individual Gaussian bands. Intensities are normalized

Unlike virgin femoral heads of both investigated materials, for which the F^+/F doublet was the only CL emission observed, additional CL bands, arising from the presence of aliovalent cations in the Al_2O_3 lattice, were detected in the *in vivo* exposed samples. Relevant to the present study are divalent cations (e.g., Ca^{2+} and Mg^{2+}) that exist as impurities in the raw powders and are also abundantly present in the body environment. Such cations might substitute for Al^{3+} forming a complex F_c-center, namely an F^+-center adjacent to a divalent cation site. F_c-centers of divalent cations emit individual CL bands located in a relatively narrow UV wavelength interval toward 300 nm [519]. An increasingly high presence of such aliovalent cations in the Al_2O_3 lattice, represented by CL bands labeled (*C*) and (*D*) in the deconvoluted spectra in inset to Fig. 3.23, was detected in both materials with increasing wear severity. However, such bands in the retrieved BIOLOX®*forte* material (Fig. 3.23(a)) were stronger than in the retrieved BIOCERAM material (in which mainly band (*D*) was resolved; cf. Fig. 3.23(b)).

Brandt and Mikus [520] have examined the CL emission from worn Al_2O_3 cutting tool surfaces after machining steel. Those researchers observed a double-band emission in the wavelength interval between 450 and 600 nm, which is the same as that we observe here on the worn BIOLOX®*forte* surface (cf. bands labeled as (*E*) and (*F*) in inset to Fig. 3.23(a)). Elemental analyses proved that this emission coincided with Mg-rich areas (Mg being emanated from the workpiece material) and results were substantiated and interpreted with the formation of an $MgAl_2O_4$ spinel phase with higher ductility than Al_2O_3. On the other hand, interstitial aluminum ions in the Al_2O_3 lattice, having the charge of +1 (i.e., Al_i^+-centers), were shown to emit a broad singlet at around 500 nm (2.45 eV) [521, 522]. This emission is similar to what we observed at the same wavelength in CL spectra collected from the worn BIOCERAM surface (cf. band labeled (*G*) in inset to Fig. 3.23(b)). Note also that the MgO content in the initial composition was completely negligible in the BIOCERAM material. Stathopoulos and Pells [523] have clarified by high-resolution electron microscopy the basic mechanism relating the formation of dislocation loops to the presence of intrinsic point defects in the α-alumina. The mechanism was recently reconsidered and refined by Dubinko *et al.* [524]. According to those researchers, Al interstitials aggregate to produce a stoichiometric (although faulted) dislocation loop, while a stoichiometric number of Al and O vacancies remain trapped in the corundum lattice. Note that this circumstance might give us the possibility to (indirectly) judge about the plastic behavior of the alumina lattice on the bearing surface by monitoring the intensity of the CL emission from Al_i^+-centers.

Figures 3.24(a)~(f) show typical SEM pictures of BIOCERAM head surface *in vivo* worn to different grades (i.e., the femoral head displayed in Fig. 3.6(d)). At the same locations, the concentration of oxygen vacancies can also be mapped by collecting the intensity of the CL band centered at 325 m and corresponding to F^+-centers (Figs. 3.24(g)~(l)). Although the absolute CL intensity cannot be directly compared for surfaces with different roughness, the concentration of oxygen lacking sites is found to conspicuously increase with increasing wear severity on the head surface. Exactly the same trend is found for the BIOLOX®*forte* material. Interestingly, locations of high concentration of F^+ centers are also found for bulk grains in mildly worn surfaces (cf. Figs. 3.24(g) and (h)), which confirm the important role of hydroxylation of the bulk grain surface on vacancy formation in the lattice of biomedical Al_2O_3 grades. Note also that the statistical presence of oxygen deficient sites was less frequent in the stripe-wear zone than in the Grade 5 worn zone, confirming that grain removal from the former area was more mechanically than chemically driven as compared to Grade 5 zones.

Another interesting feature in investigating the topology of lattice defects on worn Al_2O_3 surfaces was that bands emitted from divalent impurities labeled (*C*) and (*D*) in the CL spectrum of Fig. 3.23(a), were found to be systematically stronger at grain boundaries than in bulk grains. Figures 3.25(a) and (b) show a SEM picture and a CL (relative) intensity map of band (*C*) from the same area, which belonged to a Grade 3 worn zone in a 7.7 years *in vivo* exposed BIOLOX®*forte* head (cf. Fig. 3.6(a)). In the case of Fig. 3.25(b), all spectra in the CL intensity map were normalized to the intensity of their respective F^+ band, namely the most intense band of the CL spectra. Details of CL spectra taken from selected locations in bulk grains and at intergranular locations (labeled A and B in Fig. 3.25(a), respectively) are shown in Figs. 3.25(c) and (d), respectively. One would expect that cation impurities native to the raw powder mainly segregate to Al_2O_3 grain boundaries after sintering [525, 526]. However, the presence of cation sites in the bulk grains, found in mildly worn surfaces but absent in the virgin material, proves that such sites should have been newly generated upon tribochemical reactions occurred *in vivo*.

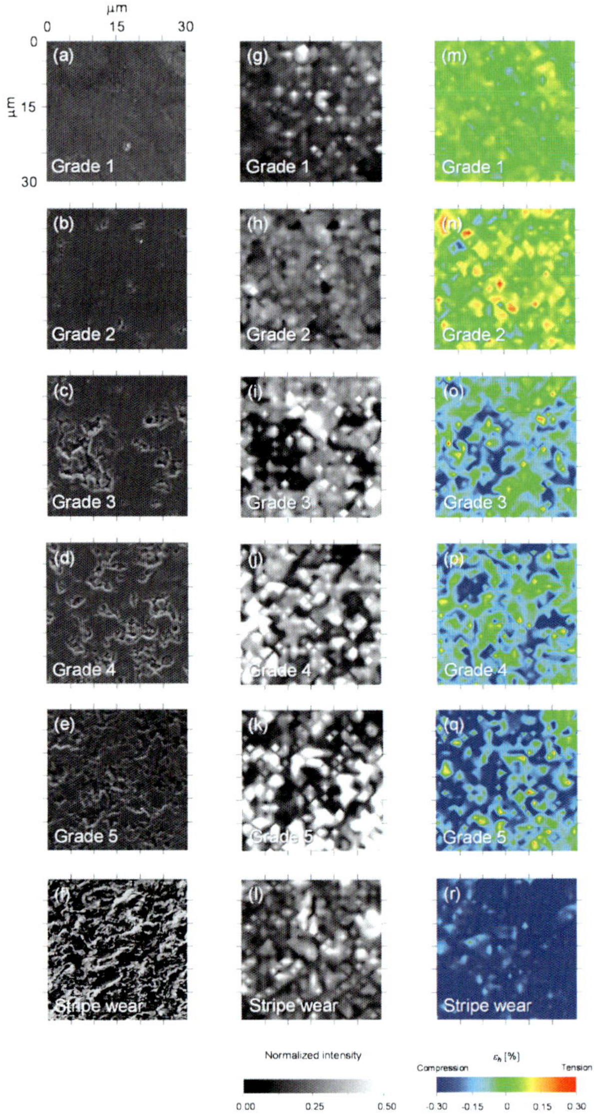

Figure 3.24 SEM micrograph of BIOCERAM head surface (femoral head displayed in Fig. 3.6(d)) *in vivo* worn to different grades ((a)~(f)), the corresponding concentration maps of oxygen vacancies ((g)~(l)) obtained from the intensity of the 325 nm CL band, and the corresponding maps of the trace, ε_h, of the elastic (residual) strain tensor ((m)~(r)) obtained from the spectral shift of the 325 nm CL band.

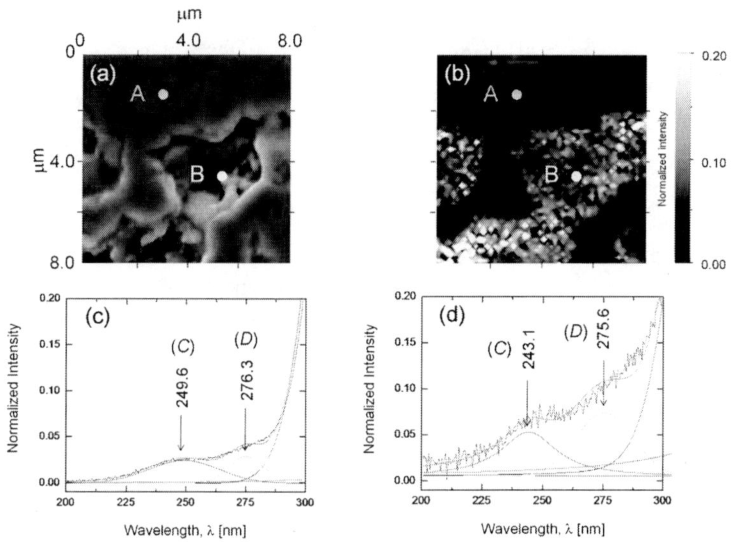

Figure 3.25 (a) SEM micrograph and (b) CL intensity map (b) of band (*C*) from the same area worn to Grade 3 of the BIOLOX®*forte* head in Fig. 3.3(a). Details of CL spectra in the spectral zone between 200 and 300 nm, taken from locations labeled A and B are shown in (c) and (d), respectively.

So far, we have assigned the observed CL emission from *in vivo* exposed Al_2O_3 femoral heads at different wavelengths in the spectral interval between 200 and 600 nm, and mapped the topological evolution on the nanometer scale of intrinsic point defects in the Al_2O_3 lattice upon increasing wear severity. From this body of spectroscopic information, the most relevant items of the CL spectral analysis can be summarized as follows:

(i) The topological concentration of oxygen vacancies on the surface of both types of the investigated alumina material systematically increases with increasing wear severity, namely with successively progressing from Grade 1 toward Grade 5, while the topological frequency of vacancy sites in the stripe-wear zone is lower than that observed in Grade 5 zone.

(ii) Apart from the oxygen vacancy F^+/F doublet, which is similar in both the studied materials, clear differences are noticed in CL bands arising from divalent cations. These latter bands were conspicuously absent in virgin samples, but their relative intensity with respect to the band from F^+ center gradually increases with increasing wear severity after exposure *in vivo*. This can be explained with an increasing presence of "intergranular" areas on the worn surface (i.e., due to grain detachment). However, the increasing presence of divalent cations in the bulk alumina lattice of mildly worn surfaces is interpreted here as a proof of tribochemical interactions between alumina lattice and body environment.

(iii) CL emission from the spectral interval between 450 and 600 nm is also increased with increasing wear severity in both materials. However, while a clear doublet was detected in the worn BIOLOX®*forte* femoral head with maxima at 480 and 530 nm, the spectrum from the BIOCERAM worn femoral head is closer to a broad single band. In both cases, the CL emission can be associated to lattice modifications that ultimately led to plastic deformation. But, the spectroscopic difference is thought here to arise from different mechanisms of wear-induced surface plasticity in the two studied alumina materials: formation of a relatively ductile $MgAl_2O_4$ spinel phase in BIOLOX®*forte* material versus formation of dislocation loops in the Al_2O_3 lattice of the BIOCERAM material.

Finally, it should be noted that the CL spectral zone at >600 nm is of difficult interpretation because it shows a strong overlap between a second order reflection of the F^+ band [527] and an emission from surface hydroxide groups, OH_s, in alumina [528]. The occurrence of both phenomena can be equally related to the formation of surface vacancy sites, which is consistent with the trend observed by monitoring the main F^+ band at 325 nm. However, no additional information could, unfortunately, be obtained at this time in order to improve the above discussion about lattice degradation of Al_2O_3 *in vivo*.

Figures 3.24(m)~(r) show nanometer-scale-resolved maps of elastic lattice strain on the Al_2O_3 surfaces as developed upon *in vivo* wear exposures of increasing severity. These strain maps were collected at exactly the same locations shown in Figs. 3.24(a)~(f) and were built up according to a CL spectral shift analysis of the F^+ band, labeled (*A*) in Fig. 3.23. The shown residual strain magnitudes relate to the very surface of the material and represent the trace (or hydrostatic part) of the strain tensor, ε_h. The main feature found in comparing the strain maps in Fig. 3.24 is an increasing shift toward residual compression in the Al_2O_3 microstructure with increasing wear severity from Grades 3 to 5. Interestingly, the elastic lattice strain detected in surfaces-classified Grades 1 and 2 is increasingly tensile and turns toward the compressive side starting from Grade 3 damage, namely in correspondence of the beginning of grain detachment from the worn surface. The maximum (residual) compressive strain (i.e., $\varepsilon_h \cong 0.3\%$) is found on the surface of the stripe-worn zone. In the previous section, the accumulation of residual tensile stress in head areas worn to different grades has been shown and interpreted in terms of wear mechanism. Data in Fig. 3.24 confirm previous findings, but they also give us a chance for further deepening our understanding of this phenomenon. Figures 3.26(a) and (b) show a high-magnification SEM picture and the related map of elastic strain, respectively, as collected on a Grade 3 worn area in the BIOCERAM femoral head displayed in Fig. 3.6(d). An examination of the topological locations of compressive and tensile (elastic) strains revealed that the former mainly accumulated at locations of detached grains while the latter at partly broken or damaged grain boundaries (cf. arrowed locations in Fig. 3.26). In other words, in an *in vivo* regime of mild wear, grain boundaries are weakened and damaged by the tribochemical attack. Such processes in turn originate localized tensile strain fields at grain boundaries that, upon hard-on-hard bearing contacts, ultimately lead to grain detachment with successive accumulation of residual compressive strain in the material surface.

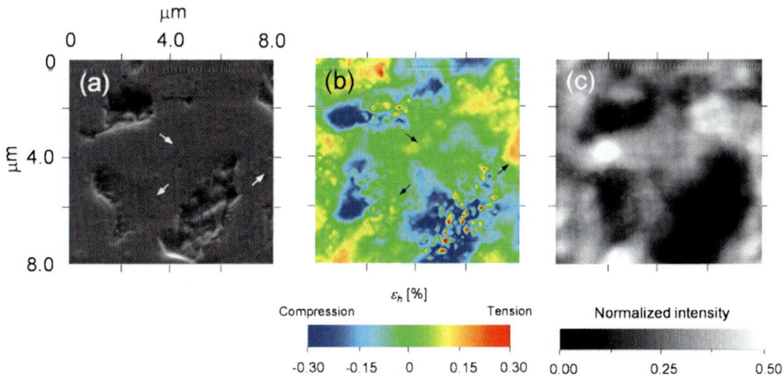

Figure 3.26 SEM micrograph (a), related map of elastic strain, ε_h, (b), and map of relative intensity of band (*G*) (c), as collected on a Grade 3 worn area in the BIOCERAM femoral head displayed in Fig. 3.6(d).

In previous papers, Rainforth [365] and Barceinas-Sanchez and Rainforth [367] have given a discussion about the controversial role of plastic deformation in the wear behavior of ceramic materials. These researchers suggested that surface plasticity in mildly worn alumina is most significantly altered by the adsorption of water. Indeed, environmental effects are long known to strongly affect surface plasticity and fracture in alumina ceramics [101, 529–531]; while it is not possible to get gross surface plasticity, dislocation flow can play a major role, as shown by time dependent effects. For example, Kalin *et al.* [101] showed that in extreme pH environments the main effect controlling wear rate is the dissolution of alumina lattice, with wear rates enhanced by one order of magnitude. Moreover, Castaing *et al.* [530] measured flow stresses in sapphire, which were reduced by a factor of two, due to the presence of water in the lattice, as a result of enhanced dislocation mobility. Concurrently, also grain boundaries in polycrystalline Al_2O_3 were significantly weakened by water. CL studies confirm that all these effects, which obviously involve major changes in lattice stoichiometry (i.e., increase in oxygen vacancies), are important in enhancing surface degradation under regimes of mild wear. In addition, our findings suggest that divalent impurities trapped in the bulk Al_2O_3 lattice might also play a role in enhancing plasticity under mild wear regimes.

Finally, it can be interesting to draw attention to a study of hydrothermally grown sapphire suggesting that "wet" α-Al_2O_3 crystals exhibit enhanced dislocation processes [531]. At the beginning of this section, we have related the broad CL emission centered at around 480 nm to interstitial aluminum sites, Al_i^+, and (indirectly) its intensity to the presence of plastic flow. The relative intensity map of band (*C*), as shown in Fig. 3.26(c), supports this suggestion. As can be seen, the most intense locations of this CL band correspond to bulk grain areas in the SEM picture, which in turn corresponds to regions of very low or no elastic strain, obviously released by the presence of plastic deformation.

Experimental evidence confirms that grain-boundary fracture and bulk quasi-plasticity (i.e., marking the threshold between mild and severe wear transition) of alumina lattice exposed in the human body are affected by both mechanical and chemical factors, especially in regions of mild wear (Grades 1 to 3). CL data appear to bring some new information because they allow us entering upon an updated chapter of hip-joint tribology including the study of *in vivo* tribochemical interactions. CL provides some clear evidence of a conspicuously strong tribochemical interaction between human body environment and alumina lattice. Such interaction can be directly visualized through spectrally resolved CL data, which locates point defects on the worn surfaces with high spatial resolution. Oxygen vacancies abundantly generate in the alumina lattice upon mechanochemical interactions with hydroxyls and aliovalent cations (i.e., Ca^{2+}, Mg^{2+}) from the body fluid. Their successive incorporation into the polycrystalline Al_2O_3 structure should be a consequence of a strong tribologically driven interaction. Such main structural changes lead to both grain-boundary embrittlement and a lowered threshold for bulk lattice plasticity; therefore, microscopic mechanisms pivotal to the observed intergranular microcracks and intragranular dislocation activity are proved to be of a tribochemical nature. Finally, a procedure based on CL spectroscopy seems to be a suitable tool for the systematic search of aliovalent (e.g., with valence >3) dopants enhancing the wear performance of the alumina lattice.

3.5 Fracture Behavior: Intrinsic Brittleness and Strength Fluctuations

Understanding the strength behavior and predicting the reliability of alumina ceramics necessarily involves the rationalization of the effect of the fabrication process on the flaw population present in the material. At the beginning of this chapter, we have described fracture strength as an "extrinsic" property of the material that can be described as arising from the interplay between the size of the largest defect present in the microstructural array and the fracture toughness of the material, namely a local parameter and an average material property, respectively [532–534]. Mechanistic descriptions, which can be considered as physically accurate only for continuum media with isotropic properties, help viewing the fracture phenomenon as a consequence of three combined factors: location of the flaw (e.g., a large pore) with respect to the stress field generated in the component, flaw size and morphology [535, 536]. Thus, in order to gain a deeper understanding on how processing parameters influence the strength of biomedical alumina, one should necessarily trace back the research to the formation and the evolution of flaws as extreme microstructural features. As potential flaw sites mainly develop during material manufacturing, the composite origin of flaws in alumina can be precisely characterized as emerging from three main categories: pores, inclusions, and abnormally grown alumina grains. An efficient non-destructive tool for the direct and systematic detection of flaws in the component is yet conspicuously missing in nowadays-ceramic technology, although a significantly improved accuracy in processing (i.e., which include selection of high-purity raw powders and the use of HIPing) and the introduction of proof testing have led to a conspicuous elimination of large pores and inclusions from biomedical alumina components. Theory teaches us that when large pores are involved with the manufacturing procedure, thermodynamic stability and kinetic evolution during densification dictate the existence of an equilibrium pore size (i.e., determined by grain size, surrounding grain configuration, dihedral angle, and externally applied stress), at which neither shrinking nor growing of the pore can occur [537, 538]. Shrinkage of large pores has only been observed when alumina microstructures were developed under HIPing conditions, owing to plastic deformability at the sintering temperature [538, 539]. A theoretical model by Evans and Hsueh describing the shrinkage of an isolated pore in a dense material supports the need of externally applied hydrostatic pressure for reaching pore closure [540]. In addition, it is also known from experiments that without application of an external pressure, shrinkage of large pores is hardly possible. This phenomenon has only been reported once in the literature, with pores of a starting radius of 50 μm that shrank to about 42 μm [541]. Thus, HIPing becomes a fundamental step in the overall process of alumina bioceramics.

When a fully deterministic control of the microstructure is not feasible, technologists should rely on statistics as the only possible approach in discussing the expected strength values (i.e., in terms of probability of fracture). In such context, it is of fundamental importance to assess which parameters affects strength statistics. Quantitative considerations on the fracture toughness of monolithic alumina have clarified that a rising *R*-curve behavior in this material can only lead to small closure stresses along the crack wake [542]. Such closure stresses are in turn conspicuously ineffective in raising fracture strength [543, 544]. Therefore, a single value of crack-tip toughness (i.e., the critical stress intensity factor at the crack tip, K_{I0}), unfortunately quite low in alumina, fully determines the condition for crack instability when a crack generates from an initial defect [545]. Fracture studies of alumina containing a small volume fraction of artificially controlled pores, including pore evolution during densification (i.e., as measured directly at the fracture origin), have been the object of research by various authors [546, 547]. In this context, evolution of pore size and a computation of the stress intensity factor for semicircular cracks around spherical pores at the condition of crack instability have become the topics specifically placed under deep scrutiny [547]. The most striking outcome of fracture mechanics studies with controlled flaws is that the radius of spherical defects in a size range between 25 and 120 μm has only a small influence on the degradation of fracture strength in alumina, provided that samples possess an average grain size smaller than 1μm. In other words, although we cannot predict *a priori* the size and location of defects belonging to the composite microstructure, we know from systematic experiments that the main strength degradation effect must occur in the presence of defects with size <25 μm. In the absence of significant contributions by closure stresses in the crack wake [542], unstable crack extension might in principle take place under largely scattered stress values and directly lead to the catastrophic failure of the entire joint component.

Biomedical grades of polycrystalline alumina produced in the period between 1965 and 1977, which can be classified as "first generation" alumina materials, possessed an average grain size of ≈4.5 μm. After 1977, additional changes in the manufacturing process were made, which led to the so-called "second generation" alumina grades. These latter materials possessed an average grain size that could be successfully lowered to 3.4 μm. Modern alumina materials ("third generation") are supplied with a grain size conspicuously more homogeneous and slightly closer to the single micrometer as compared to the previous generation. Figures 3.27(a)~(c) show grain size distributions as measured in biomedical alumina grades manufactured before 1977 [391], after 1977, and after 1995. It should be noted that by far more important than the average value of grain size, the right foot of the grain size distribution (i.e., the grain population with the largest sizes observed in the microstructural texture) causes the most detrimental effect on the strength response of the polycrystalline body. In this context, a striking difference in the grain size histograms displayed in Fig. 3.27 appears for the pre-1977 alumina material, in which large grains (from 10 to 18 μm) are present in a cumulative fraction as high as ≈5%. This datum should be compared with the maximum grain size and the fraction of large grains observed in "second" and "third" generation materials. The interesting feature is that one can still find a quite high fraction of grains (i.e., >20%) with size ≥4 μm lying on the right foot of the histogram in materials belonging to the second generation. Such a fraction drops down to ≈2.2% in third-generation materials. Note that the relative density of the materials is quite different according to different generations of manufacturing procedures, with porosity ≈1.7% before 1977, <0.8% after 1977, and <0.1% in modern (HIPed) aluminas. But, for the sake of discussion, let us assume hereafter, in first approximation, that the largest grain population in the microstructural arrangement (or, more precisely, the highly stressed boundaries surrounding such large grains) be the best candidate for becoming the fracture origin.

The strength of a brittle material, σ_f, can be expressed according to the following equation [548]:

$$\sigma_f = \frac{1}{Y}\frac{K_{I0}}{\sqrt{2\pi c}} \tag{3.7}$$

where K_{I0} is the critical stress intensity for crack propagation from a (surface) intrinsic defect of depth, c; and, Y is a shape factor for the defect typically comprised in the interval, $1.1 \leq Y \leq 2$ [549]. The critical crack-tip stress intensity factor, K_{I0}, has been experimentally studied by Seidel and Rödel for alumina materials as a function of grain size [545]. Measurements of crack opening displacement, which were systematically made on crack profiles in the very neighborhood of the crack tip in the SEM, were used to measure crack tip toughness in polycrystalline alumina materials with average grain sizes ranging within the interval 0.9~16 μm. Toughness was confirmed being a material property because no tangible dependence on grain size could be discerned. The K_{I0} value measured in alumina materials with different microstructures was independent of crack geometry, with a mean value of 2.3 MPa × $m^{1/2}$. According to toughness information, we can plot the expected fracture strength for alumina as a function of defect size, as predicted by Eq. (3.7) (Fig. 3.28). In the calculation, we have assumed $Y = 2$, which represents the most conservative assumption for the predicted strength value. Considering now the largest grains in the microstructural populations respectively shown in Figs. 3.27(a)~(c), we can locate different intervals of expected strength for the three generations of alumina by assuming the critical flaw located on the material surface and with depth, c, equal to half the largest grain size observed in the polycrystal (cf. inset in Fig. 3.28). Strength intervals are located on the plot of Fig. 3.28, which were calculated by taking half of the mean grain size and half of the maximum grain size observed in the microstructure as the minimum and the maximum flaw size, respectively. Note that the located strength intervals just represent a "best-expectation" for the strength behavior of the material, namely in absence of any void or impurity inclusion with size larger than the largest alumina grain population.

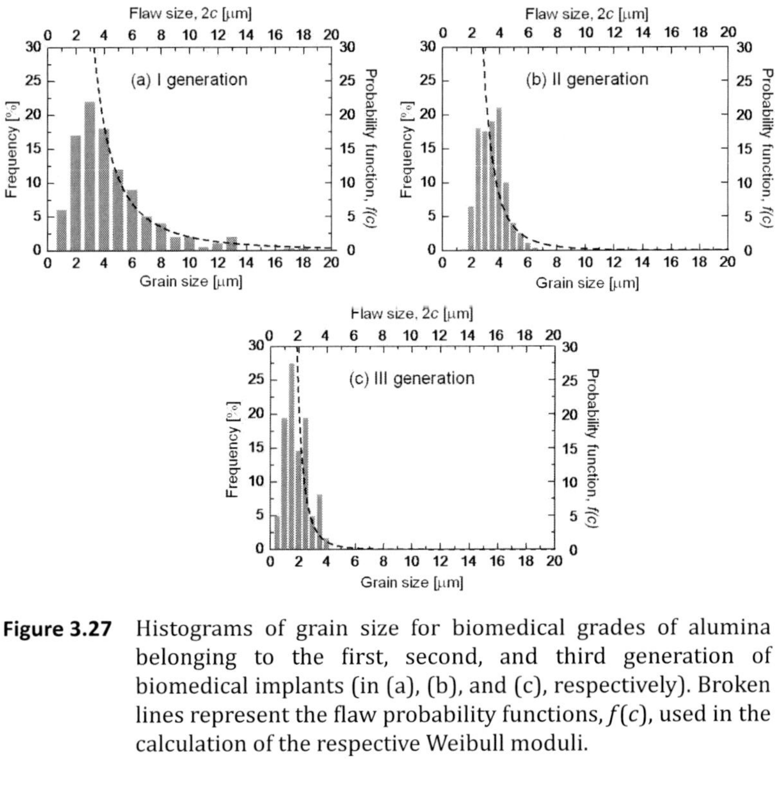

Figure 3.27 Histograms of grain size for biomedical grades of alumina belonging to the first, second, and third generation of biomedical implants (in (a), (b), and (c), respectively). Broken lines represent the flaw probability functions, $f(c)$, used in the calculation of the respective Weibull moduli.

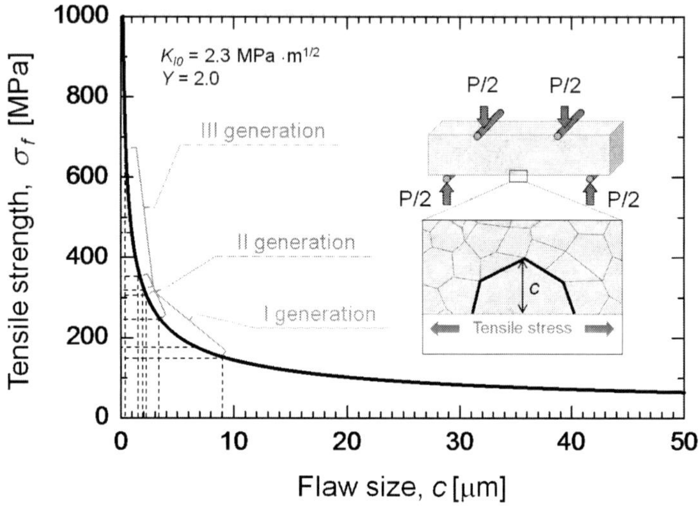

Figure 3.28 Bending strength as calculated for polycrystalline alumina from the crack-tip toughness value through Eq. (3.7). Strength fluctuation intervals predicted for different generations of alumina biomaterials are also shown. In inset, a draft is shown illustrating a bending test with load, *P*, and a microstructural defect, origin of fracture, on the tensile side of the bending bar.

This is a reasonable assumption for biomedical grades of alumina, prepared according to rigorous processing, including hot isostatic pressing. It indeed appears that the conspicuous reduction in grain size, successfully obtained in the most recent alumina components, can lead up to a threefold increase in the expected strength of the polycrystal. In addition, the interval of strength fluctuation, conspicuously reduced from the first to the second generation materials, spans more than a 300 MPa interval in the third generation but systematically remains well above that of the second generation. Nevertheless, the main concept put forward here is that the strength of monolithic alumina is "intrinsically" limited by its own microstructure.

Jayatilaka and Trustram [550, 551] proposed a relationship for directly linking the statistical defect-size distribution to a parameter describing the statistical distribution of strength in a solid, referred to as the Weibull parameter, *m*. The Weibull modulus is a dimensionless number that gives a direct measure of the distribution of flaws, thus also representing the variability in measured strength in a given material. Using a material with a low Weibull modulus will likely lead to products exhibiting greater variation in strength performance and, thus, less reliable. The distribution of defects in the material (or flaw probability function), $f(c)$, obeys a power function of crack size:

$$f(c) = Ac^{-n} \tag{3.8}$$

where A is a numerical constant and the exponent, n, is the rate at which the density of defect probability tends to zero. According to this assumption, the fracture probability, $P_f(\sigma)$, follows a simple equation [550, 552]:

$$P(\sigma_f) \cong 1 - \exp\left[-kN\left(\frac{\pi\sigma_f}{K_{I0}}\right)^{2n-2}\right] \tag{3.9}$$

where k is a constant characteristic of the material, σ_f is the fracture strength of the sample, K_{I0} is the crack-tip (critical) stress intensity factor, and N is the number of defects in the sample. The Weibull modulus, m, is then directly related to the exponent n by the expression [550, 552]:

$$m \approx 2n - 2 \tag{3.10}$$

Interesting for our discussion is that if we assume the population of the largest grains as potential sites for the fracture origin and fit such distributions to Eq. (3.8) (cf. broken lines best-fitting the right foot of the plots in in Figs. 3.27(a)~(c)), we can find a decreasing value of the constant A = 97, 90, and 21 for the first, second and third generation alumina materials, respectively. The n values in the best fitting are 2.4, 3.3, and 4.7 for the plots in Figs. 3.27(a)~(c)), respectively. According to Eq. (3.10), the corresponding m values are 2.8, 4.2, and 7.4, respectively. The majority of Weibull data reported for alumina ceramics (i.e., including biomedical materials) refer to a flexural bending configuration and they indicate values typically comprised in the interval between 6 and 11 [553–555]. In order to compare our predictions for a constant (tensile) stress field with bending strength experiments, a correction factor need to be given, according to Gong [556]:

$$m_b = 0.80 + 0.97m_t \tag{3.11}$$

where the subscripts "b" and "t" refer to bending and tensile loading, respectively. After correcting the values for the different configuration, we find $m \cong 8$ for the latest generation of alumina biomaterials, in good agreement with literature data. In conclusion, we have demonstrated that a low strength and a lack of reliability are intrinsic to alumina ceramics, however good the processing procedure developed and followed by their makers. The mechanical properties of alumina are "locked" to poor values by its own microstructural characteristics. This circumstance calls for an improved approach including the design of composite microstructures, as it will be described in the forthcoming Chapter 5.

Chapter 4

Polycrystalline Zirconia for Joint Replacement

4.1 Zirconia as a Load-Bearing Biomaterial

Since the middle of the 80s, zirconia stabilized with yttrium oxide (Y_2O_3) (also referred to as yttria-stabilized tetragonal zirconia polycrystal, Y-TZP) has been used for producing femoral heads. The main driving force in using this oxide ceramic in load-bearing components for artificial joints has been a reinforcing mechanism induced under tensile stress by a transformation from the tetragonal to the monoclinic polymorph (briefly discussed in Section 2.6 and schematically described in Fig. 2.5). The occurrence of such mechanism on the microstructural scale can be controlled in order to improve the mechanical properties of the bearing components (i.e., toughness and strength significantly improved above those of alumina ceramics). However, in a low-temperature humid atmosphere, a process of surface degradation might also take place, which eventually weakens (and roughens) the Y-TZP bearing surface. This degradation phenomenon just represents a concurrent aspect of the material metastability and another consequence of the aforementioned polymorphic transformation. If uncontrolled, it might potentially increase the roughness of the joint surface with detrimental consequences on the overall joint lifetime. In addition, the high residual stress gradients produced by local phase transformation on the bearing surface might also severely affect

Advanced Materials for Joint Implants
Giuseppe Pezzotti

ISBN 978-981-4316-88-0 (Hardcover), 978-981-4364-39-3 (eBook)
www.panstanford.com

the wear resistance of the material with giving rise to surface microcracks and to the subsequent formation of ceramic debris in the joint. For this reason, hard-on-hard sliding couples made of zirconia ceramics are expected to lead to unreliable wear performances and have not been promoted in the market. Note also that even when a zirconia head is coupled with a polyethylene liner, phase transformation on the zirconia surface may engender malfunction of the joint due to a conspicuous increase of friction with a consequent increase of polyethylene debris dispersed in the human body.

From a physical chemistry viewpoint, the ZrO_2 system has been long and extensively studied since the beginning of the last century [557–559]. Most of the early publications have dealt with structural ceramic materials at various Y_2O_3 contents (mainly below 7 mol.% Y_2O_3), as periodically reviewed by various authors [56, 560, 561]. Nevertheless, it is noteworthy that the unique potential properties of this oxide ceramic were long known, being first studied for its oxygen-ion conductivity by Nernst as early as 1899 [562]. More recently, due to their outstanding mechanical properties (i.e., in particular their high fracture toughness) zirconia ceramics have become a hot topic for materials technologists. With its mechanical properties greatly tunable by varying the yttrium content and with its extremely fine microstructure, Y-TZP has been even regarded as the most outstanding structural ceramic ever manufactured by human hands. Although unstable at room temperature (i.e., in favor of the monoclinic polymorph), the tetragonal form of zirconia (t-ZrO_2) has been deeply studied because of the possibility of (partly) stabilizing it through the addition of dopants sub-valent to Zr^{4+}. The ZrO_2 tetragonal polymorph has accordingly been described as a slightly deformed fluorite-type cell (i.e., a cubic phase that is only stable at elevated temperatures), and Teufer presented the first detailed crystallographic study of the tetragonal cell of zirconia [563]. This researcher described the unit cell of the tetragonal polymorph according to a distorted oxygen sublattice (i.e., with introducing a shift from the original positions of oxygen ions in the cubic unit cell along the c-axis), while the cationic positions of the pseudo-fluorite cell were left unchanged (Teufer-cell). This notion is quite intuitive because the tetragonal phase can indeed be considered a distorted cubic structure including displacements of oxygen ions along the <001> direction (c-axis), which shift the oxygen sub-lattice along this direction and increase the lattice parameter ratio c/a (i.e., referred to as the "tetragonality" of the lattice) from $\sqrt{2}$ to ≈ 1.45 [564]. The fluorite-like (cubic) cell is schematically shown in Fig. 4.1(a). A martensitic-like transformation (i.e., of the shear type) from the tetragonal polymorph t-ZrO_2 (Fig. 4.1(b)) to the monoclinic one, m-ZrO_2 (Fig. 4.1(c)), might spontaneously occur upon cooling from sintering temperature. This transformation temperature is characterized by a large thermal hysteresis between the "martensitic" starting temperature on cooling (i.e., at around 1000°C) and the "austenitic" starting temperature on heating (i.e., at around 1200°C) [565–568]. Note that the terms "martensitic" and "austenitic" are used for a mere analogy with and according to the similarities between the transformation of the ceramic ZrO_2 and the well-known transformation of Fe-based alloys and steel. In ZrO_2, the transformation is described by several steps of successive atomic rearrangements within the unit cell [565, 566, 568] and, as its most striking feature, it is accompanied by a conspicuous increase in volume of the unit cell (for $t \rightarrow m$). Therefore, the volume of each transforming grain in polycrystalline zirconia increases upon cooling and this phenomenon was identified as the main reason for the poor structural consistency (and subsequent rupture) of sintered pieces made of pure ZrO_2 [557]. Depending on heating and cooling rates, the coexistence of t-ZrO_2 and m-ZrO_2 has also been documented by several authors, as summarized by Subbarao *et al.* [569]. Bansal and Heuer have provided systematic studies on the nature of the transformation by transmission electron microscopy, including its salient crystallographic aspects [570, 571], while a comprehensive summary of the $m \leftrightarrow t$ transformation temperatures for Y-TZP and pure ZrO_2 can be found in a publication presented by Chen *et al.* [572]. Garvie reported experimental indications for the occurrence of metastable phases in pure zirconia [573], documenting for the first time the preservation of the tetragonal form down to lower temperatures in fine-grained ZrO_2 polycrystals. An explanation for the experimentally observed grain-size dependent polymorphism was offered in that study with arguing that a smaller size of the crystallites would involve a higher interfacial energy for phase transformation to the monoclinic structure. We shall show in a forthcoming section of this chapter that such size-dependent stabilization plays a key role in the explanation of the outstanding mechanical properties of 3Y-TZP.

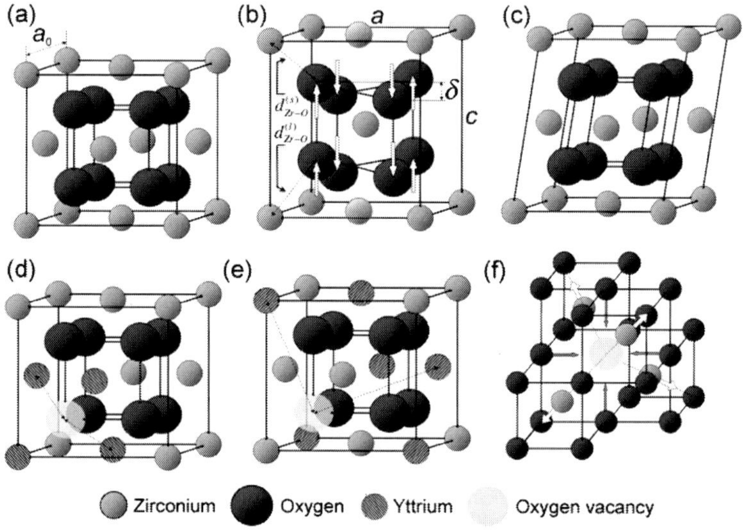

Figure 4.1 (a) Fluorite-like (cubic) lattice cell of ZrO_2; (b) tetragonal ZrO_2 lattice cell; (c) monoclinic ZrO_2 lattice cell; (d) oxygen vacancy in the ZrO_2 cubic cell with Y atoms in the nearest neighbor locations; (e) oxygen vacancy in the ZrO_2 cubic cell with Y atoms in the next nearest neighbor locations; and, (f) crystal relaxation of the atoms neighboring an isolated vacancy in a fluorite lattice (Re-drawn after Fabris *et al.* [246]). White arrows in (b) and (f) represent the displacements of oxygen atoms in a tetragonal ZrO_2 cell without vacancies and after relaxation in a tetragonal ZrO_2 cell including a vacancy. In (d) and (e), broken/arrowed lines represent the distances from nearest-neighbor and next-nearest-neighbor locations, respectively (reported as 0.2195 and 0.4204 nm, respectively [246]).

From the stoichiometry viewpoint and according to current knowledge, stabilization of the tetragonal phase at room temperature in zirconia-based ceramics becomes possible owing to the presence of extrinsic vacancies in the anionic sublattice. Extrinsic vacancies can be induced by doping of ZrO_2, which means by the replacement of Zr^{4+} by cations (e.g., M = Y, Sc, Ca, Mg and others) with lower oxidation states (M^{3+} or M^{2+}) and suitable ionic radii.

Hund first drew the image of a completely filled cationic but deficient anionic sublattice in 1951 [574]. Nowadays, the possibility of alloying ZrO_2 by doping with Y^{3+} ions represents an essential discovery in bioceramic science since ZrO_2 (partly) stabilized by Y_2O_3 is one of the most commonly used ceramic oxides in joint arthroplasty. Through addition of Y_2O_3 to the ZrO_2 structure, oxygen vacancies can form to achieve charge neutrality in the crystal according to the following stoichiometric reaction:

$$Y_2O_3 \rightarrow 2Y'_{Zr} + 3O_O^{x} + V_O^{\bullet\bullet} \tag{4.1}$$

where, Y'_{Zr} represents the Y ions on regular cationic sites (i.e., replacing Zr^{4+} ions) with a relative charge of −1; O_O^{x} stands for oxygen ions on regular anionic sites and $V_O^{\bullet\bullet}$ represents the double positively charged (with respect to the charge of regular oxygen ions) oxygen vacancies. The Kröger–Vink notation for lattice elements and point defects in crystal structures is used here (and will be used throughout the all book) [575], in order to describe the atomistic reactions related to the replacement of Zr^{4+} by Y^{3+}. Note that two dopant Y ions are necessary to introduce a single oxygen vacancy. Accordingly, the concentration of vacancies on the anionic sublattice can be calculated from the concentration of Y ions on the cationic one and might easily reach the range of few percent, as follows:

$$\left[V_O^{\bullet\bullet}\right] = \frac{1}{2}\left[Y'_{Zr}\right] \tag{4.2}$$

The concentration of intrinsic defects thermally induced during sintering is, in contrast, negligible in the usual range of manufacturing temperatures, which explains the full instability of pure zirconia in its tetragonal phase at room temperature. Note that the amount of doping needed for full stabilization is quite substantial (>8 mol.% for various dopants in order to achieve full stabilization [576–578]), thus showing that the electrostatic neutrality of this rather ionic material can only be maintained by large amounts of oxygen vacancies. The simultaneous presence of dopant cations and oxygen vacancies in large concentration also means that the local atomic environments in the stabilized material are very different from the corresponding stoichiometric phases. Unfortunately, there is yet no clear picture of the mechanisms of stabilization on the atomic scale, the most relevant issues concerning the roles of different impurity cations and of oxygen vacancies [579]. In particular, the position of the oxygen vacancy associated with each pair of Y atoms has been the subject of deep discussions. Preliminary experimental data appeared to support the hypothesis that Y is nearest neighbor to the oxygen vacancy (Fig. 4.1(d)) [580–583]; however, the most recent experiments and *ab initio* calculations [584–587] suggest that at low dopant concentrations, Y is instead next near neighbor to the vacancy (Fig. 4.1(e)) and that lattice strain covers a fundamental role in ion diffusional paths. First-principles calculations [588, 589] indeed agree with the latter results, showing that the next-nearest-neighbor position for Y is energetically favored with respect to the nearest-neighbor position. The analyses by Li and coworkers [586, 587] further suggested that the Y atoms have a composition-independent eightfold coordination shell (like in a perfect fluorite structure) in the tetragonal lattice, thus supporting the hypothesis that dopant ions are, on average, at next-nearest-neighbor positions with respect to oxygen vacancies. This peculiar (reciprocal) configuration of oxygen vacancies and sub-valent Y ions has the effect of reducing the average coordination number of the zirconium atoms from 8 (i.e., as in the cubic structure) to values closer to 7 (i.e., similar to the monoclinic phase), thus stabilizing the tetragonal phase at room temperature. Taking these experimental considerations as a guiding light, Fabris *et al.* [246] have recently proposed a theoretical model consistently corroborating a number of experimental studies [590]. In this model, the dopant cations are located in a fluorite-like cation lattice at next-nearest-neighbor sites with respect to the oxygen vacancies and are considered not to take any active part in the stabilization mechanism. Accordingly, stabilization is dominated by the crystal distortions that occur around the oxygen vacancies. When the concentration of vacancies is low, a relatively large volume of crystal is left in the fluorite structure, and it undergoes the tetragonal distortion just as the stoichiometric material. This distortion involves the coordinated motion of all the oxygen sites, so that also the atoms neighboring to the defects are dragged along the tetragonal distortion of the oxygen sublattice by a displacement, δ (Fig. 4.1(b)). When the concentration of defects is high, there is virtually no undistorted cubic region and every oxygen atom is either itself a neighbor of a vacant site or at least four of its six neighboring oxygen atoms are. It follows that there is hardly a region in which the atomic environment could undergo any further distortion. Accordingly, the radial distortions around the vacancies dominate and the resulting atomic structure is cubic only when seen as an average over a large number of atoms, while its short-range atomic arrangement does have tetragonal symmetry (Fig. 4.1(f)). Besides reconciling many different (and apparently contradictory) experimental observations about zirconia stabilization, as offered through the years by many researchers from quite different viewpoints, the model proposed by Fabris *et al.* [246] is intriguing because it suggests that stabilization of the tetragonal zirconia polymorph at room temperature may be achieved, in theory, by "doping" zirconia crystals with oxygen vacancies only, the electronic and structural properties of (partly) stabilized zirconia being mainly controlled by structural disorder and by the local strain stored around the oxygen vacancies rather than by a direct effect of the cation dopant.

Surface structures impart crucially important properties to the performance of a load-bearing biomaterial. Accordingly, experimental techniques and computational modeling have been extensively applied to investigate surface structures and properties of zirconia ceramics. One aspect particularly important here is the difference between surface and bulk stoichiometry. A large body of experimental and computational evidence has proved that Y in stabilized t-ZrO_2 segregates to the surface. From the experimental side, X-ray photoelectron spectroscopy studies by Morterra *et al.* [591] indicated that Y segregation in t-ZrO_2 is favored at low levels of yttria content (~2 mol.% Y_2O_3). Y surface segregation has also been confirmed by low energy ion scattering, which indicated that there is a high enrichment of yttrium on surface monolayers [592, 593]. A study by Bernasik of surface segregation in Y_2O_3-stabilized zirconia shows indeed a Y level at the surface in slight excess of the bulk concentration [594]. Moreover, an upper concentration limit of yttrium at the surface of Y_2O_3-stabilized zirconia has been observed by Zhu *et al.* [595], suggesting that the surface composition is independent of Y concentration in the bulk due to the segregation process. From the computational side, Ballabio *et al.* [596] have confirmed segregation by calculations for the main surfaces (111), (110) and (100) of an Y_2O_3-stabilized crystal. From *ab initio* studies by Eicher and Kresse [597], it is found that the (101) surface of Y_2O_3-stabilized *t*-ZrO_2 becomes more stable if the dopants are located close to the surface, which indicates a driving force for Y surface segregation. In contrast, no significant driving force for Y surface segregation was found for the (001) surface, thus suggesting that stoichiometric oxygen-terminated surfaces are more stable than Zr or O–O terminations. This latter statement might indeed be true independent of the specific orientation of the surface. Since surface orientation is found to cause significant variation in the local concentration of yttrium, all the properties that are a function of defect concentration and distribution (e.g., phase stability) must also be surface dependent. In other words, in polycrystalline materials, surface segregation and, thus, charge compensating oxygen anion vacancies are likely to experience substantial gradients on and below the material surface, with surface chemistry and stoichiometry effects dominating the statistical presence of active sites for the formation of metastable nuclei *in vivo*.

According to the above considerations, it is clear that the stoichiometry of zirconia (especially at its free surface) plays a fundamental role in phase stability and, thus, in the overall performance of the material in bearing components. While this peculiarity has indeed offered wide material design opportunities in many different fields of application, it also forewarns technologists wanting to use zirconia as a structural biomaterial. The human body certainly represents a puzzling chemical environment, in which oxygen vacancies can be easily annihilated and/or cations replaced, especially due to the combined effects of chemical species and high strain gradients at the bearing surfaces. It should be thus very surprising if highly "susceptible" ceramic compounds, as the family of partly stabilized zirconia materials, could preserve unchanged for long time the same stoichiometry given them at the time of material fabrication. In the previous chapter, we have discussed in some detail how even an extremely stable oxide like alumina might undergo substantial stoichiometric changes in the severe tribochemical environment of a human hip joint. We can thus be sure that any (tetragonal) zirconia material embedded in the human body will necessarily change its chemical (and consequently its crystallographic) structure, the change being accelerated by the presence of mechanical stresses and thus preferentially starting from the bearing surfaces. Polymorphic transformation *will* occur; it is just a matter of time.

Pioneering examples of developing Y-TZP as a structural material and of considering it as a suitable alternative to alumina ceramics are presented in early papers by Rieth *et al.* [598] and Christel [599], respectively. A massive industrial development followed since the middle of the 80s, in the attempt of manufacturing femoral heads capable of overcoming the intrinsically limited mechanical properties of alumina ceramics. Explicit evidence of this vast industrial development in Japan remains attested in a paper by Tateishi and Yunoki from the early 90s [600]. Outside Japan, an earliest development focused on magnesia-partially stabilized zirconia materials. However, this material showed a peculiar structure (quite different from Y-TZP), with the tetragonal phase taking the morphology of small acicular precipitates embedded in a matrix of large equiaxed grains of cubic polymorph (i.e., typically 40~50 μm in diameter). As the presence of such a relatively "soft" matrix (i.e., as compared to Y-TZP and to the quite hard alumina biomaterials) was found to negatively influence the wear properties, most of the successive developments were focused on Y-TZP, a ceramic alloy with a more "standard" microstructure. Y-TZP consists of a homogeneous network of equiaxed submicron-sized grains that can be partly stabilized in their tetragonal phase with grain sizes easily confined to <0.4 μm. Since the 90s, Y-TZP (with 3 mol.% Y_2O_3; henceforth, 3Y-TZP) has been considered to be the standard material for clinical applications [601]. Note that using 3Y-TZP indeed relieves several shortcomings related to the use of alumina bioceramics, as discussed in the previous chapter of this book; for example, the higher crystallographic symmetry of the tetragonal structure as compared to the asymmetric hexagonal (corundum) structure of alumina minimizes the grain-boundary residual stresses arising from thermal expansion anisotropy, with direct beneficial aspects for the macroscopic material strength. Furthermore, fully dense 3Y-TZP ceramics can be obtained at sintering temperatures several hundredths of degrees centigrade lower than alumina. It follows, as explicitly shown in a later section, that through introducing a pre-sintering (low-temperature) HIPing cycle in the manufacturing process fully dense samples with a fine and homogeneous microstructure can be promptly obtained. Their grain size is typically in the order of few hundredths of nanometers with a quite sharp grain-diameter histogram, a task that has definitely proved impossible for sintered monolithic aluminas (cf. histograms in Fig. 3.27). However, it should be kept in mind that the fraction of tetragonal phase retained at room temperature will strongly depend on grain size and on the uniformity in concentration of the yttria stabilizing oxide throughout the microstructural network. In other words, the mechanical properties of 3Y-TZP ceramics are strongly affected by manufacturing accuracy and rely on a delicate equilibrium among several microstructural parameters (e.g., dopant dispersion, sintering temperature, etc.). The effect of slight fluctuations in such parameters, as we will see in a forthcoming section of this chapter, can inflict a blow to the ultimate performance of zirconia as a biomaterial, even if fluctuations in processing (and microstructural) parameters are confined to ranges considered to be standard for alumina ceramics. As previously discussed in Section 1.3, the worst (historical) example of ceramic implant failures has certainly been the massive *in vivo* fracture of 3Y-TZP femoral heads in the year 2001. However, even leaving aside such a drastic situation, *in vivo* phase transformation may also involve detrimental effects on the wear behavior of the polyethylene sliding-counterpart. Serious concerns arose in the past on the effect of steam sterilization of 3Y-TZP femoral heads, which was found to have an impact on surface roughness due to the tetragonal-to-monoclinic phase transition. In 1996 [602], in classifying the causes of a number of hip revision surgeries due to osteolysis, surface degradation of retrieved zirconia femoral heads was found to coincide with high wear of UHMWPE sockets. Remarkably, it was found that the femoral heads showing the strongest surface degradation were those very same heads that, although supplied in their sterile status to the hospital, were re-sterilized in steam before implantation. On the positive side, a major discovery the long years of material development has been the effect of a small addition of Al_2O_3 in sintering 3Y-TZP, as comprehensively summarized in recent papers by Guo [603, 604]. There is a double benefit in adding a small amount (typically a fraction of 0.25 wt.%) of Al_2O_3 to 3Y-TZP: (i) an easier densification (i.e., meaning a lower sintering temperature and a finer microstructure [605, 606]); and, (ii) a better environmental resistance in water-vapor environment [607]. However, it might be difficult to solve problems related to the heterogeneity of the small alumina quantities mixed with the 3Y-TZP matrix, due to the strong tendency to agglomeration of raw nanometer-sized powders [608]. It has been then suggested that uniformity in the incorporation of a minor constituent into the matrix can be ameliorated using a coating processing on the raw powder, by means of a colloidal processing or a sol-gel route, a solution coating or a precipitating coating [609, 610]. Although yet not applied to biomedical components, several other methods have also been proposed to avoid low-temperature thermal degradation of 3Y-TZP in hydrothermal environment. Watanabe *et al.* [611] found that below a critical grain size, no polymorphic transformation occurs after ageing in air up to 10^3 h. These researchers estimated the critical grain size being between 0.2 and 0.6 μm for yttria contents between 2 to 5 mol.%. Nitridation [612] has also been proposed as an effective method to enhance the resistance to hydrothermal degradation. In an early study, Hernandez *et al.* [613] observed that bulk-alloying 3Y-TZP with more than 2 mol.% of CeO_2 can significantly increase the hydrothermal resistance. However, such process might lead to a relatively large increase in grain size (i.e., in the order of 2~3 μm), with subsequent reductions in strength and hardness. Sato *et al.* [614] made another interesting discovery as early as 1986. Upon calcining a sintered body of 3Y-TZP on a CeO_2 powder bed at 1400°C for durations up to 10 h, these researchers showed that about 10 mol.% Ce could diffuse deeply into the material. Such heat-treatment greatly enhanced the thermal stability in air of the material, with exposures at 200°C up to 100 h leading to no monoclinic phase formation. Note that this actually was one of the earliest evidence that surface modification can enhance the resistance to hydrothermal degradation of 3Y-TZP without affecting its bulk mechanical properties.

In the remainder of this chapter, we will proceed into the details of the complex behavior of zirconia-based biomaterials, with exploring some physical and mechanical aspects of their structural performances *in vitro* and *in vivo*. From a closer look, we will be able to judge better about the actual potentiality of this intriguing family of materials. While it remains a clear fact that zirconia ceramic implants have gone through a quite controversial history regarding their phase metastability, degradation in water lubricants in simulation studies, and influence on friction and wear phenomena, it is also true that zirconia is a unique ceramic material with its potential for an extremely high toughness. A better correlation between material properties and biological performance appears to definitely be the key to pursue successful designs of improved bioceramics. In this context, it is quite conceivable that some unknown family of zirconia ceramics could be newly discovered, which possess peculiar microstructural features leading to so far unexplored mechanical and chemical properties.

4.2 The Controversial Effects of Polymorphic Transformation

In the previous section, we have discussed about the possibility of obtaining, at room temperature, a zirconia polycrystal in the metastable tetragonal form through the addition to the raw powder of an appropriate fraction of oxides with cations sub-valent to Zr^{4+} (e.g., Y^{3+}, Ce^{3+}, Mg^{2+}, Ca^{2+}, etc.). The obtained t-ZrO_2 alloy will eventually transform into its more thermodynamically stable monoclinic phase under the tensile stress field generated around the tip of a propagating crack. This phenomenon is known as stress-induced transformation toughening (cf. Fig. 2.5(b)). Due to the relatively large volume expansion and shear strain (≈3~5% and ≈7%, respectively) associated to the transformed lattice and the consequent compressive stress field generated upon constraint by the untransformed surrounding material, the local crack tip stress intensity is reduced and so the driving force for crack propagation (i.e., with an apparent increase of the effective toughness of the material). Transformation toughening is thus the result of an extrinsic toughening mechanism associated with the increase in critical stress intensity factor needed for propagating a crack. It is intuitive that effectiveness in polymorphic transformation requires the retention of relatively large fractions of metastable tetragonal phase at room temperature after manufacturing. Therefore, polymorphic transformability is generally regarded as a direct measure of the ability to release a crack-tip stress field [615, 616]. Unlike bone, the majority of synthetic ceramic materials possess

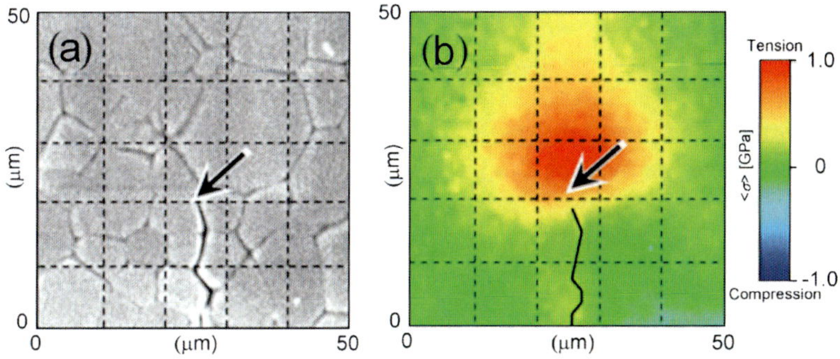

Figure 4.2 (a) SEM micrographs of the crack-tip neighborhood in polycrystalline Al_2O_3 (the arrow locates the location of the crack tip); (b) map of the trace of principal stress tensor collected by Raman piezo-spectroscopy from the same area in (a).

poor resistance to fracture propagation. They thus need to be toughened by extrinsic mechanisms operating both in the crack wake and ahead of the crack tip. Such toughening effects give an assurance of reliability after implantation in the human body. Macroscopic fracture mechanics studies have provided quantitative characterizations of the actual resistance of bone to fracture in terms of critical stress intensity factor and critical strain energy release rate as measured at the onset of crack initiation [617, 618]. This approach has also been coupled with characterizations of toughness as a function of crack length (rising R-curve behavior), which is useful to quantify the toughening contribution arising from microscopic mechanisms occurring behind the advancing crack front [277, 278, 619, 620]. This set of characterizations has allowed scientists for an improved understanding of the fracture phenomenon in biomaterials. The same methods can be used to assess the actual potentiality of transformation toughening mechanisms in zirconia, thus enabling to take one step forward from the viewpoint of developing highly tough synthetic materials. From the perspective of microscopic characterizations, information of the stress patterns developed around the crack path in (metastable) tetragonal zirconia polycrystals leads to a better understanding of the relationships between toughness and polymorphic transformation zone. Microscopic fracture studies employing a Raman microprobe might enable direct investigations on how a macroscopically applied external load engenders transformation at the microscopic level, thus linking the macroscopic toughening effect to microstructural parameters [621, 622]. The stress intensification at the tip of a propagating crack can be also directly measured by the COD method in the electron microscope (cf. Section 3.5) and the partial stress release linked to the occurrence of a crack-shielding mechanism. It should be noted that the use of a confocal probe enables to minimize in-depth averaging of the Raman signal, so that relatively sharp stress maps can be obtained. In crack-tip Raman experiments, the confocal probe can also be shifted below the free surface of the sample (by about 10 μm) in order to minimize disturbing effects arising from surface roughness and stress-releasing effects associated with the presence of the free surface. In this context, it is interesting to compare the crack-tip stress field developed (at the threshold for crack propagation) in a brittle biomaterial as synthetic polycrystalline alumina (cf. scanning electron micrograph and stress map in Figs. 4.2(a) and (b), respectively) with that developed in a toughened biomaterial as partially stabilized zirconia. The stress field in alumina can be visualized by monitoring the stress response (i.e., the so-called piezo-spectroscopic (PS) behavior) of the 418 cm^{-1} Raman band of alumina [623]. In finely grained biomedical alumina, no toughening mechanisms can be found around the crack tip and thus no stress relaxation effect is recorded in the microscopic crack-tip stress map. Under such micromechanical conditions, the crack-tip stress field preserves both magnitude and morphological symmetry characteristics, as expected in linear elastic materials [624]. In other words, no crack-tip toughening effect can be operative in arresting or delaying crack propagation, with the material fracturing with no microstructural "reaction" to the advancing crack. On the other hand, partially stabilized tetragonal zirconia is among the toughest synthetic biomaterials. As already mentioned, the improvement in mechanical properties, including toughness, strength and Weibull modulus, has been theoretically related to stress-induced phase transformation from the tetragonal to the monoclinic polymorph, which takes place in the neighborhood of a propagating crack [615, 616, 625]. Raman spectroscopy can visualize the occurrence of transformation toughening mechanisms through providing quantitative microscopic information on the effect of a polymorphic transformation on crack-tip stress patterns developed ahead of an advancing crack. Figures 4.3(a)~(c) show the monoclinic transformation field in the neighborhood of the crack tip and, in the same zone, the stress field developed in the tetragonal and in the monoclinic phase, respectively. The corresponding equilibrium stress field acting on the crack faces is given in Fig. 4.3(d). This latter stress field, compressive in nature, represents the stress field computed as the average (weighted by the respective volume fractions) of the stress fields respectively stored in the freshly transformed monoclinic phase and in the residual tetragonal phase. Stress fields can be evaluated by exploiting the PS behavior of selected Raman bands of monoclinic and tetragonal zirconia polymorphs [117, 626, 627]. As already mentioned, significant volume expansion of the crystallographic lattice occurs upon stress-induced tetragonal-to-monoclinic transformation, which in turn induces the observed compressive stress field shielding the crack mouth. In other words, partly stabilized zirconia materials are capable to release the tensile crack-tip stress through the development of a self-induced highly compressive stress field arising from polymorphic transformation. Such an intrinsic material "reaction" against fracture propagation can be thoroughly captured on the microscopic scale by Raman microprobe spectroscopy. Besides the importance of a stress visualization procedure from the basic materials science viewpoint, the quantitative knowledge of the exact amount of polymorphic transformation and the related residual stress magnitude is a fundamental step in improving the microstructural design of zirconia ceramics. It also helps materials scientists and technologists in correctly understanding the difference in mechanical properties among zirconia materials designed to achieve different microstructures through different chemical compositions. From this perspective, Raman spectroscopic evaluations can be considered a complementary tool to the set of macroscopic fracture mechanics characterizations, the latter locating the critical stress intensity factor at the onset for crack initiation (as well as the rising *R*-curve behavior), while the former visualizing the physics behind such mechanistic results.

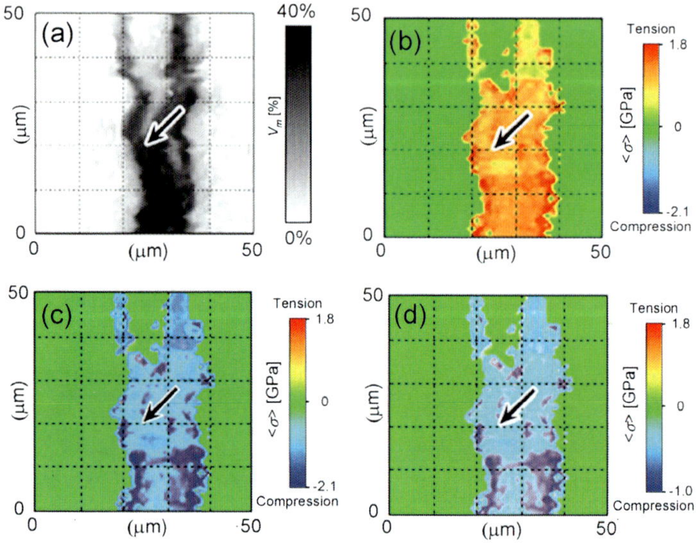

Figure 4.3 (a) Map of the monoclinic volume fraction developed in the neighborhood of the tip of a crack propagated in partly stabilized polycrystalline ZrO_2 (the arrow locates the location of the crack tip); (b) and (c) represent the stress fields developed in the tetragonal and monoclinic phases, respectively; in (d) a map of equilibrium stress is given, which represents the compressive (closure) action developed upon polymorphic transformation on the crack faces.

While transformation toughening definitely represents the most positive aspect of the metastability of zirconia ceramics (i.e., resulting in an unrivaled performance in terms of toughness among polycrystalline ceramics), it is exactly the same metastable behavior that leads to spontaneous transformation and surface degradation at low temperature when the zirconia material is exposed to hydrothermal environment. As the environmentally driven $t \rightarrow m$ transformation progresses from the surface toward the interior of the material, it can ultimately affect the structural integrity of a joint component and definitely compromise its wear resistance. At the present time, a conclusive and comprehensive theory that explains all the aspects of the complex events accompanying low-temperature hydrothermal degradation in zirconia is hard to put forward. However, several researchers have proposed valid models explaining, through different pieces of experimental evidence, the multifaceted and somewhat puzzling aspects of this phenomenon. Sato and Shimada [628] studied the phase change and the microstructure of Y-TZP annealed between 65°C and 120°C and argued that water reacts with the Zr–O–Zr bonds to form Zr–OH. This reaction releases the strain that stabilizes the tetragonal lattice on the material surface and consequently allows local transformation to take place. Similar to water, also non-aqueous solvents with lone-pair electron orbital accelerate the degradation. Yoshimura *et al.* [629] proposed an alternative mechanism based on a four-step model, including: (i) chemical adsorption of water at the sample surface; (ii) formation of Zr–OH and/or Y–OH bonds at stressed sites on the surface; (iii) accumulation of stress by the migration of surface OH^- in the lattice to form nucleating defects; and, (iv) nucleation of monoclinic phase in the tetragonal grains followed by nuclei coalescence. This latter model was supported by infrared absorption experiments and by direct measurements of volumetric and gravimetric changes of the lattice. In particular, the observed increase in weight suggested that about 60% of the oxygen vacancies were occupied by hydroxyls. An additional and more recent model, proposed by Guo [603, 604], consisted of five successive steps: (i) chemical adsorption of water at the zirconia surface; (ii) reaction of water with O^{2-} on the zirconia surface to form hydroxyl ions OH^-; (iii) penetration of OH^- into the inner part through grain boundaries; (iv) filling of surface oxygen vacancies by OH^- ions with subsequent formation of interstitial H^+ proton defects; and, (v) occurrence of $t \rightarrow m$ transformation for oxygen-vacancy concentrations below a threshold value for instability of the tetragonal phase. Note that the mechanism proposed by Guo only requires diffusion of proton defects in the bulk at low temperature (i.e., rather than hydroxyls) and it is supported by X-ray photoelectron spectroscopy results, infrared adsorption spectroscopy and Fourier transform infrared transmission spectrometry data. The oxygen adsorption state on the free surface of zirconia depends on the local defect configuration as well as on surface irregularities, which should accelerate the degradation process. Therefore, a general trend exists with respect to the Zr coordination number, the more strongly reduced oxygen species lying at substrate sites containing lower coordinated Zr ions. The most stable adsorption configuration should then correspond to a redistribution of charge density among the surrounding oxygen ions with a consequent increase in the Zr coordination as in the ground state for ZrO_2. However, despite different charge states for the oxygen species in relation to surface topology and composition, the di-oxygen pair is expected to be more stable than dissociated monoatomic oxygen atoms. In other words, oxygen adsorbed zirconia surfaces can be considered to be consisting of strongly "non-stoichiometric" structures with an excess of oxygen. The Zr coordination number is a criterion for structure stability that suitably applies to such strongly non-stoichiometric surfaces.

An important experimental study from Schmauder and Schubert [630] placed emphasis on the fact that phase transformation starts mainly at grain corners, where residual tensile stresses are amplified, while protruding grains (i.e., relatively stress-free) at the surface of Y-TZP specimens do not transform in humid atmosphere even after long-term exposure times. This model was the first to emphasize the role of surface strain on the environmental degradation of polycrystalline zirconia. Hereafter, we shall experimentally demonstrate the importance of residual stress fields in the progression of phase transformation on the surface of both *in vitro* and *in vivo* exposed zirconia femoral heads.

The long-term performance of zirconia ceramics as a load-bearing material for artificial hip joints has been severely questioned by various research groups [631, 632]. One major concern has been the degradation of the ceramic *in vivo* with transformation of the surface slab of material from the tetragonal into the weaker monoclinic polymorph. Another serious concern has dealt with the frictional heating induced by zirconia femoral heads on their polyethylene liners counterparts during testing in hip simulator [633]. The steady-state temperature of polyethylene under frictional conditions was reported to reach 99~200°C for ZrO_2 heads in comparison to the 45°C reached with alumina heads. Clearly, the enhanced frictional heating may account for long-term degradation by wear in hip joint implants because of structural changes in the bearing surfaces and degradation of the lubricating monolayer proteins. Similar to microscopic studies of fracture mechanisms, Raman spectroscopy may enable prompt and quantitative assessments of phase transformation in zirconia hip joints, either tested *in vitro* under hot/humid atmosphere or retrieved after failure of the hip joint in the human body [117, 634].

As already shown in crack-tip maps, transformed volume fractions can be easily computed from measuring the relative intensity of Raman bands belonging to the monoclinic and to the tetragonal polymorphs [635]. In addition, confocal Raman piezo-spectroscopy proves again suitable in quantitatively assessing the nature and the magnitude of the residual (surface) stresses accompanied with phase transformation. The bearing surface of zirconia hip implants can be thoroughly scrutinized on a microscopic scale by means of the Raman spectroscopic "eye" (i.e., eventually coupled with a computer-aided automatic mapping device), thus providing a great help in understanding the microscopic phenomena laying behind surface deterioration and fracture. Provided that the Raman spectroscopic analysis is performed using a confocal microprobe configuration, a powerful and highly reliable tool becomes available for assessing the biomedical reliability of hip implants produced by different makers or retrieved from different patients. As typical examples of microscopic characterizations, we shall show hereafter two typical applications of the confocal Raman technique in detecting environmental degradation patterns in zirconia materials: (i) phase transformation fractions measured in the early nucleation stage and related residual stresses stored within both tetragonal and monoclinic phases on the surface of an unused ZrO_2 femoral head after *in vitro* soaking in humid environment; and, (ii) tensile stress intensification within the tetragonal phase and its relationship with the $t \rightarrow m$ transformation fraction in a retrieved piece of *in vivo* fractured femoral head. Both studied implants were of the same type and they have been now withdrawn from the market.

An unused ZrO_2 femoral head (St. Gobain Desmarquest, Evreux, France; 28 mm in diameter), containing 3 mol.% Y_2O_3 as a stabilizing agent (i.e., with no Al_2O_3 addition) showed in its as-received state a bearing surface extremely well polished, appearing to the naked eye as a mirror-like surface. Due to a careful machining procedure and successive annealing, no significant residual stress was found to be stored on the surface of the as-received component, as well as no $t \rightarrow m$ transformation could be detected at such stage. The as-received head was kept for 5 h in vapor environment at 394 K, which roughly corresponded to 1 year exposure in the human body. Figure 4.4(a) shows an optical micrograph taken on the surface after this autoclaving cycle. Raman microprobe mapping revealed that the humid atmosphere induced severe surface blistering

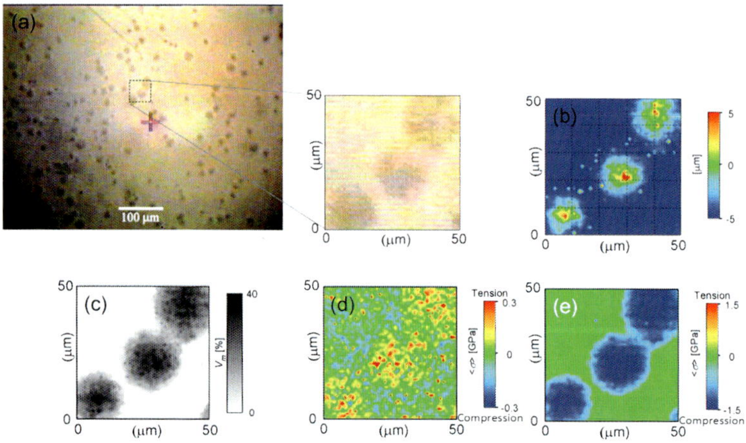

Figure 4.4 (a) Optical micrograph of an 3Y-TZP surface that underwent an initial (nucleation) stage of phase transformation in hydrothermal environment; (b) and (c) are maps of axial elevation and monoclinic phase fraction that were collected from the area depicted in the square inset of (a); (d) and (e) represent maps of the stress fields stored within the tetragonal and the monoclinic phases, respectively. These latter maps were collected from the same area of (b) and (c).

with the formation of monoclinic domains protruding from the surface (cf. three-dimensional laser micrograph in Fig. 4.4(b)). The confocal Raman map was collected with a pinhole confocal aperture corresponding to a laser penetration depth of few microns. The maximum monoclinic content in the surface blisters was found to be as high as 40% (cf. quantitative map of phase transformation in Fig. 4.4(c)). As explained at the beginning of this section, $t \rightarrow m$ transformation occurs with consistent volume expansion, therefore the transformed ZrO_2 crystals are expected to partly protrude out of the (originally) smooth surface. An additional consequence is that the transformed monoclinic phase undergoes significant compressive residual stress with leaving, for the equilibrium, the yet untransformed tetragonal crystal under a strong residual stress of tensile nature. Such tensile stress indeed represents the driving force for further transformation of the residual tetragonal phase. This micromechanical situation is clearly captured at the microscopic level by the Raman microprobe characterization, as summarized in the piezo-spectroscopic stress maps collected on the tetragonal and monoclinic phases (cf. Figs. 4.4(d) and (e), respectively). It is clear that the presence of such large (and hard) protruding monoclinic blisters on the head surface should have an extremely detrimental effect on the wear rate of the softer polyethylene counterpart, with consequent increase of friction and local temperature at the bearing interface, with the final formation of polyethylene debris.

Intensification of surface stress fields in zirconia hip joints may be rather severe because of the overlapping of several factors, including pre-existing defects, surface chemical effects, phase transformation, and machining effects. As seen in the previous Raman assessments, residual stresses are expected to be tensile in the residual tetragonal phase and compressive in the newly formed monoclinic phase. Obviously, the presence in the material of "islands" of tetragonal phase subjected to very high tensile stress weakens the material and makes the implant prone to catastrophic fracture. Figure 4.5(a) shows an *in vivo* broken zirconia femoral head, while (b) shows the largest of its three fractured pieces. The femoral head was from the same maker of that shown in Fig. 4.4 and it was retrieved from the patient after only 5-year implantation. No significant internal transformation was noticed on the fracture surface (with the exception of the fracture origin area), but relatively high fractions of monoclinic phase were systematically found in contact areas, namely both on internal and external surfaces. Raman data strongly suggest that brittle fracture originated somewhere from the inner surface in contact with the metallic stem and propagated toward the inner volume of the head. Given the complex morphology of the fractured pieces, the determination of a single location of fracture origin can be difficult in this case. However, in the machined region in contact with the stem, where the metallic taper-cone impinged on the ball, one site of probable fracture origin could be located (i.e., marked with an asterisk "*" in Fig. 4.5(b)). A confocal Raman analysis at the site of fracture origin revealed that the taper-edge zone underwent evere phase transformation with a maximum fraction up to about 30 vol.% of monoclinic polymorph (Fig. 4.5(c)). Consequently, the residual stresses stored within the tetragonal phase were highly tensile and fracture might have easily found its propagation path within such yet untransformed tetragonal regions (cf. stress map

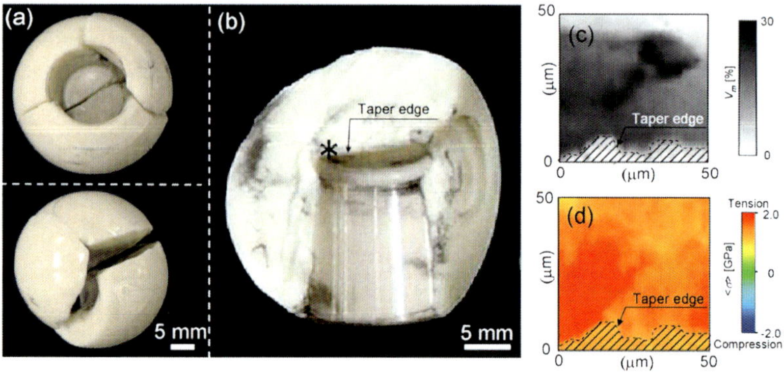

Figure 4.5 (a) An *in vivo* fractured 3Y-TZP femoral head and the fracture surface of its largest fractured piece in (b). The asterisk represents the fracture origin. In (c) and (d), maps of monoclinic volume fractions and residual stresses in the tetragonal phase are shown as collected by Raman spectroscopic assessments in the neighborhood of the fracture origin.

in Fig. 4.5(d)). One of the main parameters influencing the attitude of the material to spontaneously transform at low temperature is its density [636]. Low density involves the presence of open porosity, which in turn provides a free path for water molecules to penetrate in the bulk of the material. This process results in severe aging both on the surface and at internal parts. In such cases, the material rapidly loses its structural integrity, and the load-bearing component might experience a dramatic decrease in mechanical strength. As we have discussed at the beginning of this chapter, zirconia femoral heads have been designed to provide an increased strength performance with respect to alumina heads. However, several hundredths of zirconia head failures were documented since 2000 with cases having been isolated to heads sintered in a "tunnel" furnace introduced in 1998. Similar to the results shown in the above example, the monoclinic composition at the taper surface of fractured and non-fractured heads was significantly elevated (between 21% and 68%) as compared to that of control zirconia heads (<5%) [637]. Microscopic inspections identified fracture features unique to the zirconia heads produced in the tunnel furnace and a common characteristic of slightly lowered density. While one can easily conclude that whatever the manufacturing ability, monoclinic phase transformation following implantation will always and unavoidably remain a potential mechanism for ceramic head failure, it is also clear how delicate is the processing of zirconia biomaterials with extremely amplified effects on potential fracture risks of even apparently insubstantial processing parameters.

Among zirconia materials stabilized by other cation elements, Ca-doped zirconia has been the first transformation-toughening system to be developed [638]. However, little commercial application was predicted for this material because of its high microstructural sensitivity to isothermal tetragonal-to-monoclinic phase transformation at low and room temperature. CeO_2-stabilized zirconia materials might display considerably greater stability in moist environment as compared to 3Y-TZP under similar environmental conditions. However, as we will see in some detail in the last section of this chapter, for similar fracture toughness values, the grain size of the Ce-doped materials is larger than 3Y-TZP and an intrinsic drawback in using this material in hip joints is represented by a hardness value up to 40% lower than that of 3Y-TZP. This characteristic necessarily reflects in a poor wear resistance and thus in an intrinsic unsuitability for the severe tribochemical conditions existing in artificial joints. Roy *et al.* [639] first reported that Mg-doped zirconia polycrystals might possess excellent resistance to environmental degradation, being also resistant to roughening and loss of hardness. Magnesia-stabilized zirconia was proven to be stable and conspicuously free from degradation and roughening both in retrieval series [640] and in *in vitro* aging studies [641]. This positive experimental evidence indeed proves that the properties of polycrystalline zirconia as a biomaterial can span from very positive to very negative trends and should by no means be generalized under the same category. A careful examination of the published literature also shows clear hints that we might yet know too little about the actual potentiality of zirconia as a load-bearing biomaterial for artificial joints.

4.3 Toughening versus Environmental Resistance: The Role of Grain Size

When considering 3Y-TZP as a candidate material for load-bearing joint surfaces, one must take into consideration the two main negative aspects of its phase metastability: (i) the volume expansion that accompanies $t \rightarrow m$ transformation, which might lead to an enhancement of surface roughness; and, (ii) the localized residual stresses stored within the material microstructure upon phase transformation (i.e., highly tensile in the untransformed tetragonal crystals), which can ultimately compromise the structural stability of the component. Enhancement of phase stability in polycrystalline zirconia can be pursued by means of a substantial refinement (and thorough control) down to the nanometer scale of its grain size. To substantiate this concept, experimental evidence can be obtained with the aid of spectroscopic techniques based on quantitative analyses of the Raman and fluorescence bands emitted from 3Y-TZP ceramics and the trace of Al_2O_3 dopant within. A viable approach might thus consist in quantitatively evaluating the phase stability of nanostructured samples made of 3Y-TZP in water vapor environment as a function of time and grain size and in concurrently monitoring the structural modifications of the different phases constituting the 3Y-TZP polycrystals as their microstructures evolve toward a crystalline network of increased grain size.

3Y-TZP powder containing 0.25 wt.% Al_2O_3, was cold isostatically pressed under 300 MPa into small pellets and sintered at nine different temperatures in the range between 1300 and 1500°C, for 2 h in air. The sample sintered at the lowest sintering temperature (i.e., 1300°C) contained large open pores and was thus excluded from further consideration. The remaining eight sintered samples (listed as sample A~H in Table 4.1) were subjected to a HIP cycle at 1350°C for 1 h, after which they all reached full density. Dense samples were then polished by fine diamond paste and evaluated with regard to their phase stability. After quantitatively evaluating their respective grain size distributions, the investigated materials were kept for increasing times (i.e., ranging between 0 and 150 h) into an autoclave operating at 121°C under a vapor pressure of 0.1 MPa, in order to simulate by an accelerating test the effect of environmental aging in the human body [642, 643]. Raman and fluorescence spectra were then collected in order to map phase fractions at room temperature before and after aging in moist environment. A confocal probe was used throughout the spectroscopic experiments in order to keep the penetration depth below the sample surface to few micrometers.

Figures 4.6(a)~(h) are scanning electron micrographs of the fine microstructures (after thermal etching) obtained for 3Y-TZP after sintering at increasing temperatures and after the post-HIPing treatment at 1350°C, which as mentioned above was the same for all materials. In the inset, grain-size histograms are also shown that can provide quantitative insight into the microstructural populations of the investigated samples. The grain-size histogram tended to broaden with increasing sintering temperature. However, independent of sintering conditions, the grain morphology observed on the plane of polish was always equiaxed, with no clear evidence of abnormal grain growth (grain size ≤700 nm under any sintering conditions). The average grain size of the 3Y-TZP materials increased with increasing sintering temperature, with average values typically ranging between 190 and 320 nm. Average grain sizes are also listed in Table 4.1 and a plot as a function of sintering temperature is shown in Fig. 4.7. No detectable contents of monoclinic phase could be found in the samples before testing in autoclave and, independent of sintering temperature, all samples mainly consisted of a tetragonal phases. The results of hydrothermal acceleration tests at 121°C under a vapor pressure of 0.1 MPa are shown in Fig. 4.8 as a function of aging time and sintering temperature. As seen, the 3Y-TZP samples sintered at temperatures below 1370°C showed amounts of $t \rightarrow m$ transformation <1.5 vol.% after exposure times as long as 150 h under any hydrothermal conditions (cf. also data at 121°C in Table 4.1). On the other hand, increasingly larger amounts of phase

Table 4.1 Microstructural, polymorphic transformability and lattice characteristics of eight 3Y-TZP samples prepared from the same raw powder and sintered at different temperatures

	A	B	C	D	E	F	G	H
Sintering temperature [°C]	1326	1339	1352	1362	1383	1401	1452	1485
Average grain size [nm]	192	197	207	198	204	217	272	318
Monoclinic volume fraction, V_m^{max} after 150 h at 121°C [%]	0	0	0	0.7	10.2	67.4	85.6	85.1
Tetragonality, *c*/*a*	1.01518	1.01519	1.01525	1.01534	1.01544	1.01552	1.01575	1.01596

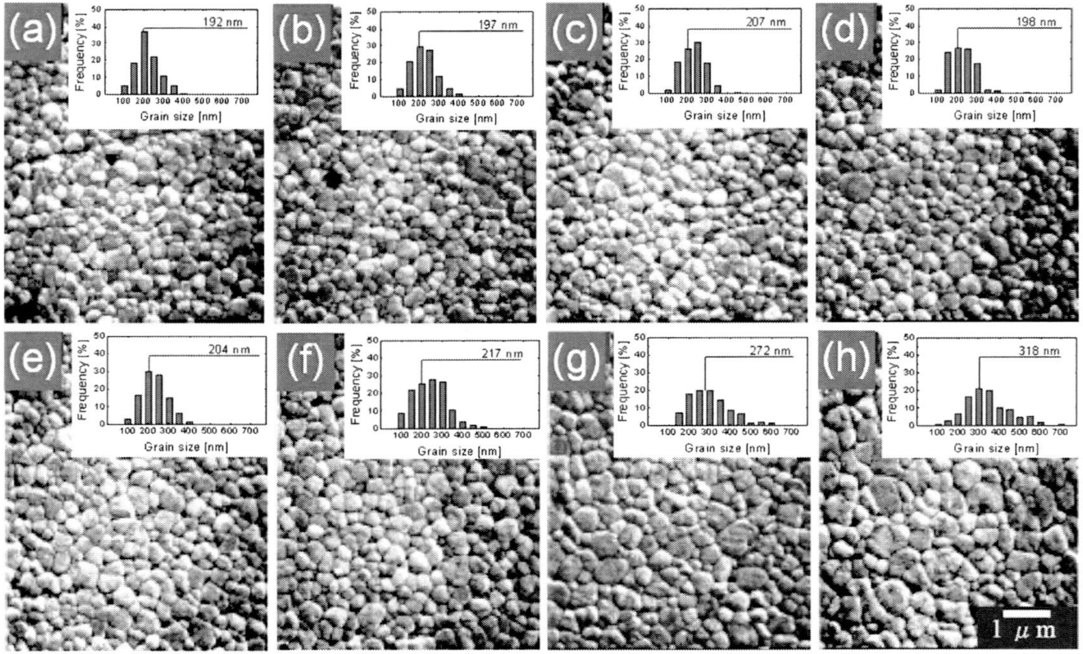

Figure 4.6 Scanning electron micrographs of 3Y-TZP surfaces sintered at: (a) 1326°C; (b) 1339°C; (c) 1352°C; (d) 1367°C; (f) 1401°C; (g) 1452°C; and (h) 1485°C. All samples were sintered for 2 h and then HIPed at 1350°C for 1 h. The micrographs were taken on polished surfaces after thermal etching at 1300°C for 30 min. In inset to each micrograph, grain size histograms and average grain sizes are shown.

transformation could be observed for all samples sintered at temperatures >1370°C, the higher the sintering temperature the steeper the increase of monoclinic volume fraction with exposure time. The data shown in Fig. 4.8 suggest that $t \rightarrow m$ phase transformation in 3Y-TZP can be conspicuously suppressed with lowering sintering temperature below a threshold value of 1370°C (namely, with refining the grain size of the polycrystal down to <200 nm). This finding appears to confirm the estimate of a threshold grain size given by Watanabe *et al.* [611] for 3Y-TZP. However, from a comparison between data in Figs. 4.7 and 4.8, it can also be noticed that the average grain size of 3Y-TZP sintered at temperatures ≤1390°C (samples A~E in Table 4.1) are very similar and, therefore, it is not possible to clearly infer a critical (average) grain size below which phase transformation can be fully inhibited. Figure 4.8 shows that after an initial time of slow increase, the transformed phase fraction, V_m, undergoes a steeper gradient, while a tendency to saturation is observed after relatively long elapsing times in the climate chamber. This trend, which was more pronounced in materials with coarser microstructures, can be rationalized in terms of transformation kinetics parameters by invoking the Mehl–Avrami–Johnson law [644, 645]:

$$V_m = a\left[1 - \exp(bt)^n\right] \tag{4.3}$$

where t is the aging duration, a is a constant that equals 1 when the initial monolithic fraction is zero, b is a parameter that is directly proportional to the $1/n$ power of the nucleation rate of monoclinic nuclei per unit time and area, and n is referred to as the Avrami exponent and ranges between 0.3 and 4 [644]. As previously discussed by other authors [644], exponent values n close to 4 reveal a preponderant contribution to the kinetics of transformation from growth of pre-existing monoclinic nuclei and lead to a sigmoidal dependence of V_m versus t; on the other hand, n values close to 0.3 represent phase-fraction increases fully governed by the process of nuclei formation. Best fitting of experimental data is shown in Fig. 4.8 according to Eq. (4.3). As a result of this best fitting procedure, the obtained n and b^n values are plotted in

Fig. 4.9. As seen, an increase in sintering temperature was accompanied by a decrease of n and an increase of b^n. By translating these findings into a $t \rightarrow m$ transformation model of nucleation and growth [604], it can be deduced that an increase in sintering temperature involves (i) a decreasing preponderance in the contribution of nuclei growth rate (as compared to nuclei formation rate) to the increase of monoclinic phase fraction, as demonstrated by the gradual decrease in the observed exponent value, n and (ii) an increased formation rate of monoclinic nuclei, which is testified by a sharp increase in the parameter b^n. Guo [604] provided an interpretation of this trend by arguing that the cubic phase of 3Y-TZP is extremely resistant to transformation into the monoclinic polymorph. Such high resistance arises from the concentration of oxygen vacancies on a cubic surface being significantly higher than that of tetragonal zirconia. Now, it is conceivable that a higher fraction of cubic grains (i.e., with a lower tetragonality) exists in the microstructural network of materials sintered at lower temperature (i.e., with a finer grain size). Accordingly, a low nucleation rate of monoclinic sites could also be expected. Therefore, the role of the cubic phase fraction in the sintered material on transformation rate should be discussed first based on its quantitative assessment.

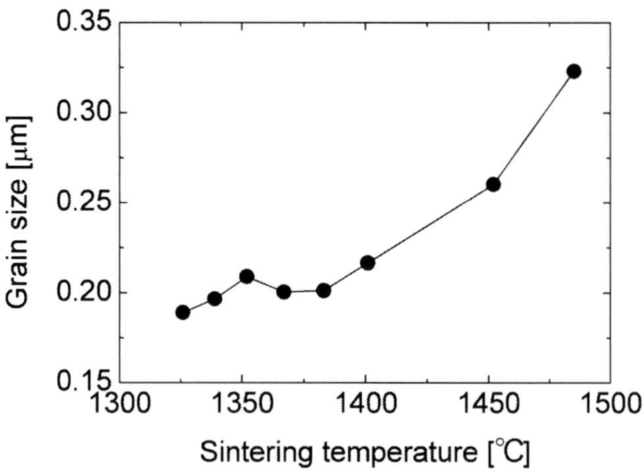

Figure 4.7 Plots of average grain size as a function of sintering temperature for the samples A~H listed in Table 4.1.

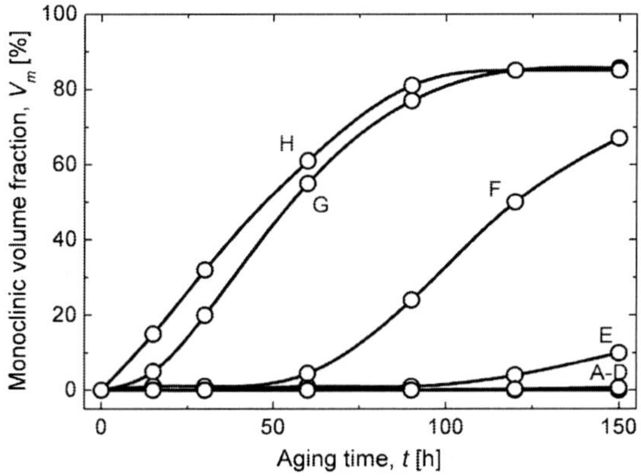

Figure 4.8 Results of hydrothermal acceleration test at 121°C up to 150 h conducted in water vapor environment on the samples A~H listed in Table 4.1. Transformed monoclinic fractions, V_m, are shown as a function of exposure time, t, in autoclave. Best fitting curves were obtained according to a least-square fitting routine to Eq. (4.3).

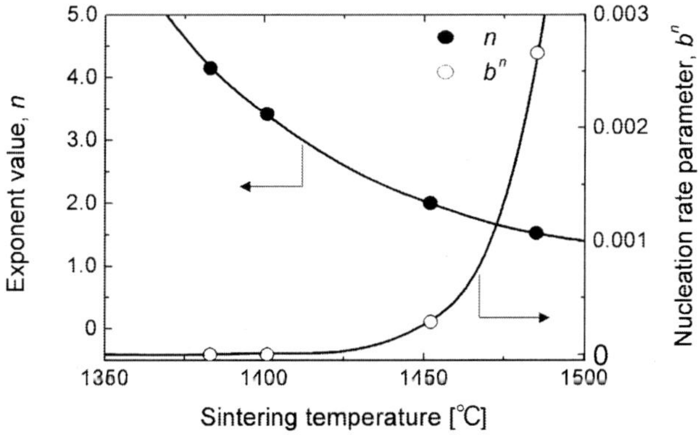

Figure 4.9 Dependence on sintering temperature of the MAJ parameters: exponent value, n, and nucleation rate parameter b^n.

Figure 4.10(a) shows the experimental relationship found between sintering temperature and tetragonality, c/a, of the tetragonal cell, according to a Rietveldt analysis of X-ray diffraction data on the series of eight 3Y-TZP samples listed in Table 4.1 (cf. also c/a values explicitly listed in the table). A comparison between tetragonality data and monoclinic fraction data in Fig. 4.8 indeed indicates that as the tetragonality of the polycrystal

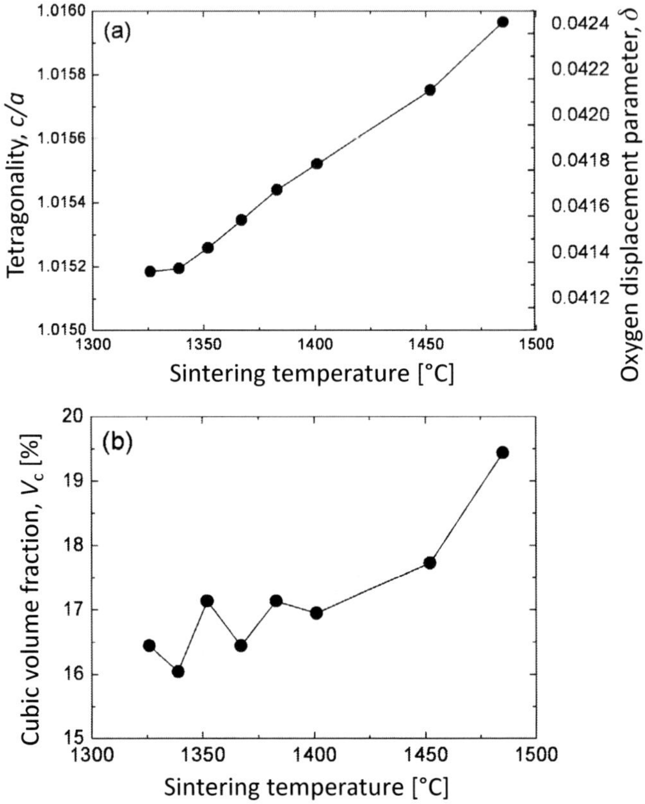

Figure 4.10 (a) Dependence of lattice tetragonality, c/a, and (b) volume fraction of cubic phase, V_c, on sintering temperature; the plot in (a) is rescaled in terms of the oxygen displacement parameter, δ, in the tetragonal lattice cell according to Eq. (4.6).

becomes smaller (i.e., closer to the unity value characteristic of the cubic phase), phase stability in hydrothermal environment increases. In other words, a c/a ratio closer to 1 can actually be interpreted as arising from a larger amount of cubic phase in the crystalline network. In this context, Yashima *et al.* [646] reported that tetragonality approaches unity with increasing the amount of the oxide stabilizer added to the zirconia polycrystal. Moreover, Kim *et al.* [647] reported that small amounts of Nb_2O_5, when added to 3Y-TZP, have a detrimental effect on phase stability due to an increase of grain tetragonality. Data shown here clarify that lowering the sintering temperature and, thus, refining the grain size of a 3Y-TZP polycrystal indeed can effectively bring the tetragonality ratio closer to unity; this phenomenon is accompanied by a consistent improvement in phase stability. Note, however, that when we attempt to translate the observed increases of tetragonality into a volume fraction change of cubic phase, V_c, an increase of few percent units ($\Delta V_c \approx 3.5\%$) is found (Fig. 4.10(b)). Since X-ray diffraction analyses can only read tetragonality values averaged over relatively large surface areas as compared to individual grains, it is not possible to clarify whether the observed increase refers to an increase in number of isolated cubic grains or instead is an average lattice property. Nevertheless, an increase in cubic phase with increasing sintering temperature is commonly found in the literature. Ohmichi *et al.* [648] have reported Rietveld analysis results showing that the amount of cubic phase on the surface in Y-TZP increased and the Y_2O_3 concentration within tetragonal phase decreased as the sintering temperature increased. Matsui *et al.* [649] have inquired into the morphological state of the cubic phase in an otherwise tetragonal grain network according to nanoprobe chemical analyses and proposed a stereological model foreseeing Y-rich cubic phase regions selectively located at grain boundaries and spreading into grain interiors as the sintering temperature increased. Yamashita and Tsukuma [650] indeed substantiated a two-phase tetragonal/cubic microstructural model for 3Y-TZP based on quantitative X-ray analyses. Depending on sintering temperature and duration, cubic grains exhibiting 6~7 mol.% Y_2O_3 could coexist with tetragonal grains containing less than 2 mol.% yttria. In order to fit together a large body of published evidence, Chevalier *et al.* [651] suggested that cubic grains enriched in yttrium lead to a depletion of yttrium in the neighboring tetragonal grains, which in turn act as nucleation sites for tetragonal-to-monoclinic transformation. Even for samples sintered at relatively low temperatures, i.e., 1450°C, the presence of a fraction of cubic phase can be expected from the phase diagram, leading to a significant effect on aging sensitivity. Data shown here confirm that an increase of cubic phase fraction indeed starts from sintering temperatures <1450°C. Nevertheless, in the case of isolated cubic grains, one might wonder how such a small change can alter so dramatically the phase stability of the material. It could, however, be that the measured increase in V_c value, although limited in its absolute value, occurs at fractions close to a stereological percolation threshold on the material surface, thus involving an amplified effect on phase stability. This hypothesis might be particularly realistic in view of the stereological model foreseeing a grain-boundary network for the cubic phase fraction as in the model proposed by Matsui *et al.* [652].

In addition to the crystallographic information provided by X-ray diffraction/Rietveldt analyses, Raman and fluorescence spectroscopy characterizations can also convey chemical, structural and mechanical information, as they all display convoluted in the spectral bands. Spectral band position, intensity, and width provide an interpretable and fairly unique fingerprint for quantitative analyses. A complete spectroscopic analysis of the Raman spectrum of zirconia ceramics used in biomedical applications has been reported in the literature [117]. Here, we focus on the spectroscopic analysis of the 260 cm^{-1} Raman band arising from Zr–O′ bond-stretching (i.e., where O′ is a threefold coordinated oxygen) in the tetragonal polymorph [652]. This band was selected because of its relatively high spectral intensity and because it is fairly isolated from bands arising from zirconia polymorphs other than the tetragonal one. In addition, the Raman band of the tetragonal polymorph located at 640 cm^{-1} (i.e., representing Zr–O bond stretching [652], where O is a fourfold coordinated oxygen) was also monitored. However, this latter band experiences a shoulder located at around 600 cm^{-1}, which arises from splitting of the cumulative 640 cm^{-1} band in the presence of the cubic phase in the polycrystal. Figures 4.11(a) and (b) show typical Raman spectra collected on the 3Y-TZP materials sintered at the two extreme temperatures in the investigated interval of sintering conditions (samples A and H in Table 4.1), respectively. A spectroscopic analysis of the 260 and 640 cm^{-1} bands as a function of sintering temperature revealed that the main morphologic characteristics of these Raman bands (i.e., band intensity and full width at half maximum (FWHM)) were conspicuously independent of sintering temperature; a similar trend was also observed for the band intensity ratio, I_{600}/I_{640} (cf. insets in Figs. 4.11(a) and (b) for samples A and H, respectively), which showed little (if any) variation over the investigated interval of sintering temperature. This latter observation indeed confirms the rather small variation of cubic phase fraction detected with increasing sintering temperature. On the other hand, as a

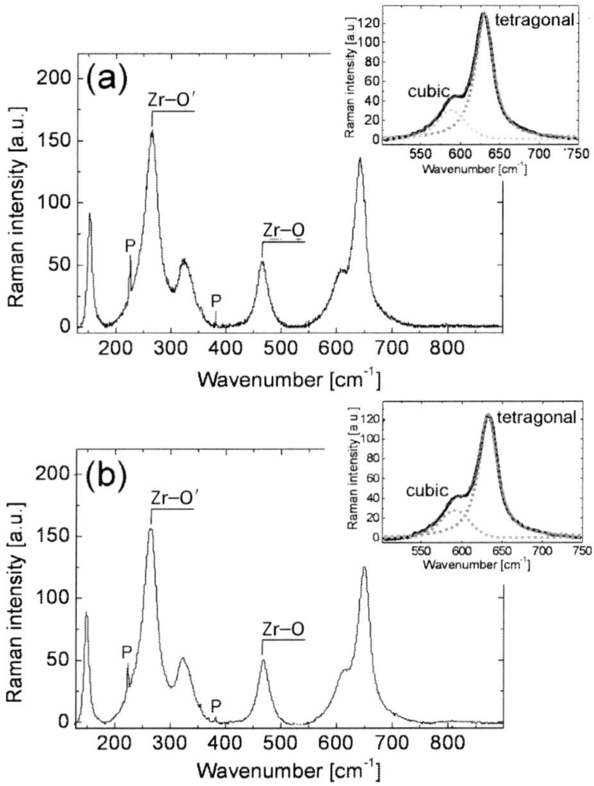

Figure 4.11 Typical Raman spectra collected from: (a) Sample A sintered at 1326°C; and, (b) Sample H sintered at 1485°C. In inset to (a) and (b), enlarged portions of the spectrum are shown that are centered at around 630 cm^{-1}. The letter "P" identifies plasma lines that do not belong to the investigated samples but represent an internal reference to the Raman device.

common characteristic to the three bands located at around 260, 600 and 640 cm^{-1}, band maxima in the sintered samples clearly shifted toward higher wavenumbers with increasing sintering temperature (Fig. 4.12). A similar spectroscopic analysis was performed on the Cr^{3+} fluorescence bands located at around 6089 and 6059 cm^{-1} (these two bands are henceforth referred to as R_1 and R_2, respectively), which could be detected in all the 3Y-TZP sintered samples and arose from the presence of the small amount of alumina added to the mixture of raw powders. Unlike Raman bands, the morphology of the Cr^{3+} fluorescence doublet from the

Al_2O_3 dopant showed clear morphological changes. Figure 4.13 shows the evolution of the Cr^{3+} doublet as a function of sintering temperature. The salient spectroscopic features of the doublet as a function of sintering temperature are summarized in Figs. 4.14(a)~(c) (for band intensity, FWHM and spectral position, respectively). As seen, the Cr^{3+} fluorescence doublet becomes conspicuously more intense, sharper and its spectral position shifts toward higher wavenumbers as the sintering temperature increases. Spectral responses to an applied stress of the Raman bands related to Zr–O′/Zr–O bond stretching in 3Y-TZP were reported to experience shifts toward higher wavenumbers for increasingly tensile stress magnitudes [117]. On the other hand, under increasingly compressive stress magnitudes, the fluorescence bands of Al_2O_3 are known to shift toward higher wavenumbers [224, 479]. Therefore, one can conclude that with increasing sintering temperature, the alumina and the tetragonal zirconia phases undergo increasingly compressive and tensile states of residual stress, respectively.

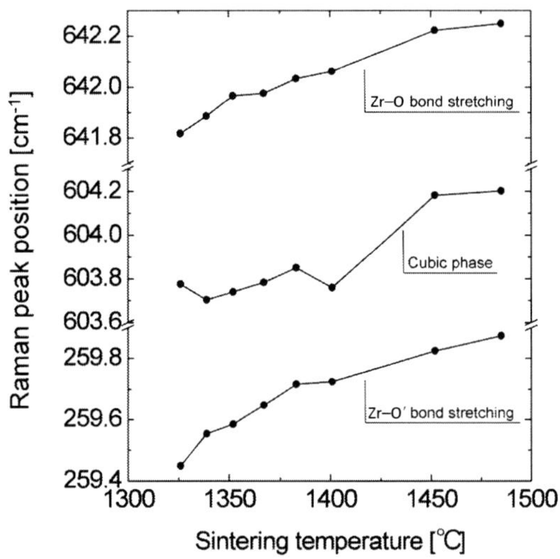

Figure 4.12 Relationships between sintering temperature and Raman spectral position for the bands located at around 260 cm^{-1} (bottom), 604 cm^{-1} (middle), and 640 cm^{-1} (top). Top and bottom plots represent Zr–O and Zr–O′ bond stretching, respectively. The band at 604 cm^{-1} originates from the presence of a fraction of cubic phase in the investigated samples.

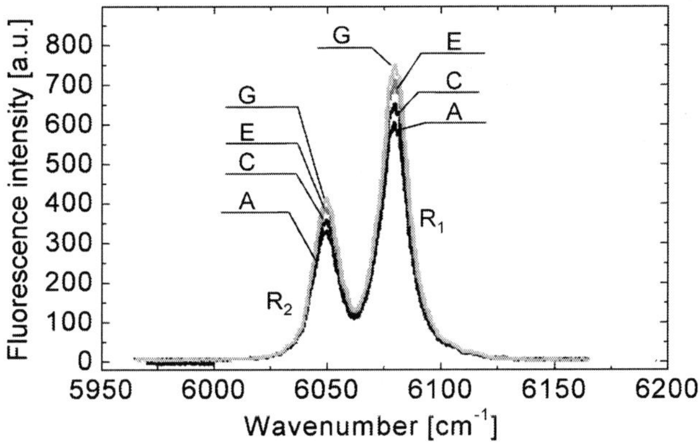

Figure 4.13 Evolution of the Cr^{3+} fluorescence doublet detected from 3Y-TZP samples as a function of sintering temperature (cf. Samples A, C, E, and G as listed in Table 4.1).

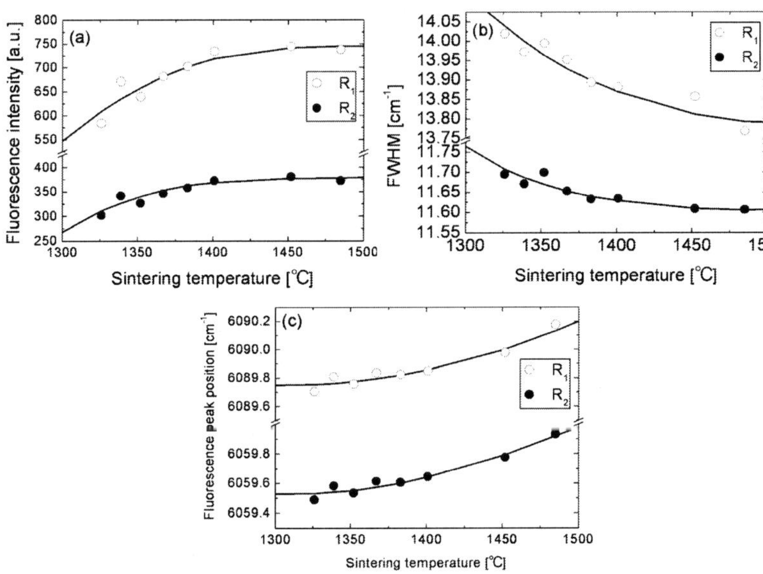

Figure 4.14 Dependences on sintering temperature of the intensity (a), FWHM (b), and spectral position (c) for the chromophoric fluorescence doublet as detected in 3Y-TZP Samples A~H.

As a consequence of tetragonal distortion, the lengths of the short and long Zr–O bonds in the crystal structure of zirconia (cf. Fig. 4.1(b)) can be represented as:

$$d_{\text{Zr-O}}^{(\text{s})} = \sqrt{\frac{a^2}{8} + c^2\left(\frac{1}{4} - \delta\right)^2} \tag{4.4}$$

$$d_{\text{Zr-O}}^{(\text{l})} = \sqrt{\frac{a^2}{8} + c^2\left(\frac{1}{4} + \delta\right)^2} \tag{4.5}$$

in which the subscript Zr–O should be eventually replaced with Y–O at the cation substitutional sites; δ is the oxygen displacement parameter (cf. Fig. 4.1(b)), which represents the O^{2-} ion shifts from the ideal lattice site to moderate the instability arising from distortion of the cubic structure, and can be related to the tetragonality of the polycrystal according to the following equation [653, 654]:

$$\delta = 0.24\sqrt{1 - \left(\frac{a}{c}\right)^2} \tag{4.6}$$

According to Eqs. (4.4)~(4.6), a plot of tetragonality versus sintering temperature (in Fig. 4.10(a)) can be translated into plots of bond length versus sintering temperature (Fig. 4.15) or into a plot of oxygen displacement parameters versus sintering temperature (also plotted in Fig. 4.10(a)). The plots of short ($d_{\text{Zr-O}}^{(\text{s})}$) and long ($d_{\text{Zr-O}}^{(\text{l})}$) Zr–O bond length in Fig. 4.15 show that an increase in sintering temperature involves a decrease and an increase of $d_{\text{Zr-O}}^{(\text{s})}$ and $d_{\text{Zr-O}}^{(\text{l})}$, respectively. This is indeed the same trend as that reported by Howard and Hunter [653] for Y-TZP materials in which an increase in tetragonality was obtained by decreasing the content of Y_2O_3 stabilizer. Raman spectroscopy appears to possess enough sensitivity to reveal subtle variations in the bond length of Zr–O, as demonstrated by studies of aliovalent dopant substitution for Zr^{4+} ions in Y-TZP tetragonal solid solutions [655]. We already mentioned that among the six characteristic Raman modes of a tetragonal crystal, the 260 cm^{-1} line corresponds to the stretching of Zr–O′, while the band located at 640 cm^{-1} relates to that of Zr–O. The frequencies of these stretching modes have been shown to be sensitive to the ionic size, the mass, and the content of dopants. A slight increase in the average bond length as a result of the increased substitution of the dopant for Zr^{4+} decreases the bond strength and,

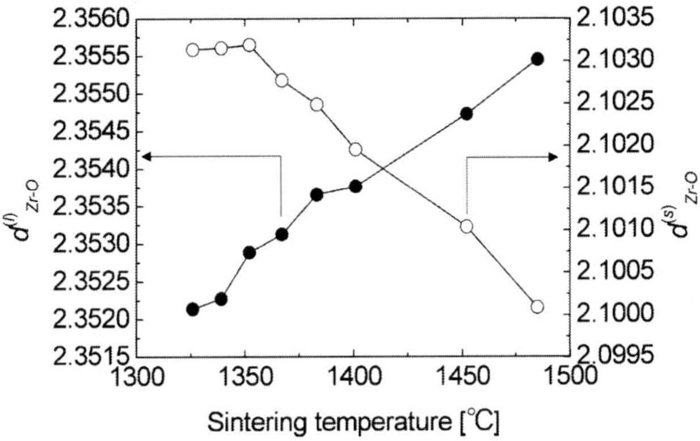

Figure 4.15 Dependence on sintering temperature of the short ($d^{(s)}_{Zr-O}$) and long ($d^{(l)}_{Zr-O}$) Zr–O bond lengths in the 3Y-TZP-lattice cell.

consequently, shifts the Raman modes toward lower frequencies. However, in the case of increasing amounts of Y_2O_3 dopant, the influence of the decreased bond strength on the Raman modes can be partly annihilated by the concurrent increase of oxygen vacancies [656]. Oxygen vacancies are created to achieve electrical neutrality in the lattice when Y^{3+} substitutes for Zr^{4+}, and a decrease in the average coordination number of zirconium ions [657] results in increased bond strength. A proof of this counterbalancing mechanism was given by the observation of a broadening of both the 260 and 640 cm^{-1} Raman bands, which indicates an increased structural disorder with increasing Y_2O_3 concentration [655, 656]. Structurally, the doublet 600/640 cm^{-1} arises from interactions between Zr–O stretching mode and symmetric and asymmetric rocking modes, respectively [657, 658]. The intensity ratio I_{600}/I_{640} increases with increasing the content of Y_2O_3 dopant until a fully stabilized cubic structure only shows a single broad band. Therefore, it has been suggested that the intensity ratio I_{600}/I_{640} represents the degree of distortion of the fluorite ZrO_2 structure [655, 656]. When these notions are applied to the Raman spectroscopy data collected in the present 3Y-TZP material as a function of sintering temperature (cf. Fig. 4.12), we become able to give a sound interpretation to the three following experimental evidence: (i) no reductions (but rather remarkable increases in frequency) were observed with increasing sintering temperature for Raman modes representing both Zr–O and Zr–O′ bond-stretching;

(ii) no changes in FWHM were found for both the above Raman bands with increasing sintering temperature; and, (iii) no tangible increase was found for the intensity ratio, I_{600}/I_{640}. While evidence (i) may just reflect the constant (nominal) content of Y_2O_3 in the present materials, evidence (ii) proves that altering the sintering temperature within the investigated interval induced no change in the amount of substitutional Y^{3+} present in the zirconia lattice. This finding might disprove a previous interpretation of Rietveldt data collected on 3Y-TZP, according to which the reduced tetragonality observed with decreasing grain size was entirely attributed to a change in the fraction of Y_2O_3 in solid solution [659]. The failure in detecting a clear change in the intensity ratio I_{600}/I_{640} as a function of sintering temperature, as already mentioned, supports the finding of a rather low increase in cubic fraction found by Rietveldt characterization. Rather than confirming a direct detrimental effect arising from an increased tetragonality of the 3Y-TZP lattice (i.e., owing to an increase in sintering temperature), the spectroscopic outcomes presented here suggest a role for residual stresses on transformation rate. For the ZrO_2 tetragonal phase, the band located at around 260 cm^{-1} clearly shifted toward higher wavenumbers as the sintering temperature increased. Since no significant morphological change was noticed for this band with varying sintering temperature, the spectral shift can be fully attributed to a pile-up of residual stress (i.e., corresponding to increasingly tensile stresses in the tetragonal ZrO_2 phase). Such stresses are counterbalanced by increasingly compressive stressed in the Al_2O_3 phase, as confirmed by the spectral shifts observed for the R_1 band. It should be noted that compressive residual stresses in the Al_2O_3 phase are conceivable because of its lower thermal expansion coefficient with respect to that of ZrO_2. Furthermore, stress inhomogeneity should cause broadening of the fluorescence lines in polycrystalline alumina [560]. However, we have observed both sharpening and intensity increase for such lines with increasing sintering temperature, which suggest a higher crystallinity and a more homogeneous stress distribution. A schematic model is shown in Fig. 4.16, which shows the evolution of the material microstructure with increasing sintering temperature. In the material sintered at low temperature, a network of fine ZrO_2 grains (the dark lattice in Fig. 4.16) contains a continuously distributed

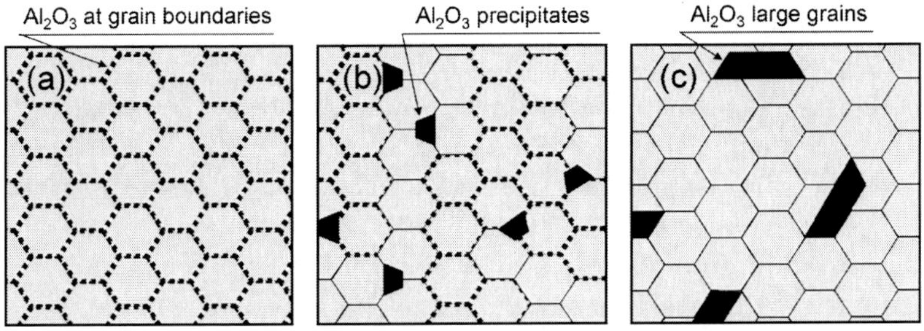

Figure 4.16 Schematic draft of the distribution of the alumina phase in the 3Y-TZP samples as a function of sintering temperature: (a) a sample sintered at low temperature shows the alumina phase homogeneously dispersed at grain boundaries; (b) a sample sintered at intermediate temperatures shows precipitated alumina particles and zones with grain boundaries lacking of alumina; and, (c) a sample sintered at elevated temperature (>1450°C) shows only relatively large alumina grains embedded in the 3Y-TZP network. The dark lattice indicates zirconia grains, while the black spots indicate alumina particles.

network of Al_2O_3 phase at grain boundaries (fine black spots in Fig. 4.16(a)), which is a consequence of the intimate mixing procedure adopted in the preparation of the raw powder mixture. The presence of Al_2O_3 phase at grain boundaries is known to prevent $t \rightarrow m$ phase transformation; therefore, its continuous distribution throughout the microstructural network may impede spreading of transformed areas to neighboring grains. On the other hand, when the material is sintered at higher temperatures, a more substantial diffusional flow may take place at grain boundaries: accordingly, the Al_2O_3 phase might increasingly tend to agglomerate at the triple junctions of the ZrO_2 grains (Fig. 4.16(b)) and, ultimately, to form isolated grains (cf. black grains in Fig. 4.16(c)). If this hypothesis is correct, it is under the combined effects of a higher tensile residual stress field and of the local depletion not only of yttria but also of alumina phase from ZrO_2 grain boundaries that $t \rightarrow m$ transformation may nucleate and spread faster through the polycrystalline ZrO_2 structure. Note that this model might also substantiate the observed decrease in the parameter n of the Mehl–Avrami–Johnson law with increasing sintering temperature. The above data also prove that quite large effects can result from even slight increases in sintering temperature. Furthermore, according to the features observed in the Raman and fluorescence spectra of zirconia and alumina phases with increasing sintering temperature, it appears that residual stresses play a role in the complex cascade of microscopic events leading to environmental phase transformation.

Since biomedical 3Y-TZP has been developed to become an improved alternative to alumina bioceramics, excellent structural characteristics are also required, in addition to biocompatibility. In particular, superior fracture toughness is necessary for guaranteeing high reliability of the joint during its implantation lifetime. Improved fracture toughness characteristics are indeed expected to arise from transformation of the tetragonal polymorph into the monoclinic one during crack propagation. However, we have just discussed above that the suppression of low-temperature degradation is possible but requires a reliable microstructural control that allows one safely confining the grain size of 3Y-TZP to ≤200 nm. Therefore, the next step is to investigate how grain size actually affects fracture toughness in 3Y-TZP, in order to check if a highly tough and environmentally stable bioceramic can be obtained. With this in mind, in the remainder of this section, we shall show an evaluation of the crack-tip fracture toughness of 3Y-TZP by means of microscopic COD assessments and the use of Raman spectroscopy for visualizing the polymorphic phase-transformation zone around the crack path as a function of grain size.

Fracture toughness results by COD analysis are shown in Fig. 4.17 for four 3Y-TZP materials, three materials selected among those listed in Table 4.1 (i.e., Samples A, C, and H) and another material with significantly larger grain size (~700 nm) sintered for comparison at 1600°C (referred to as Sample I, henceforth). As seen, an increase in grain size can produce a substantial increase in the crack-tip fracture toughness of 3Y-TZP and this should be the result of a different width, Δ, of the phase-transformation zone around the crack path. Maps of monoclinic volume fraction as developed along the profile of cracks propagated in the 3Y-TZP samples A, C, H, and I are shown as a function of average grain size in Figs. 4.18(a)~(d), respectively. This latter assessment indeed shows that both the geometrical size of the transformation zone and the maximum amount of monoclinic polymorph fraction contained in the transformation zone are higher in samples with larger grain size (cf. plots in Fig. 4.19). It is thus clear that the

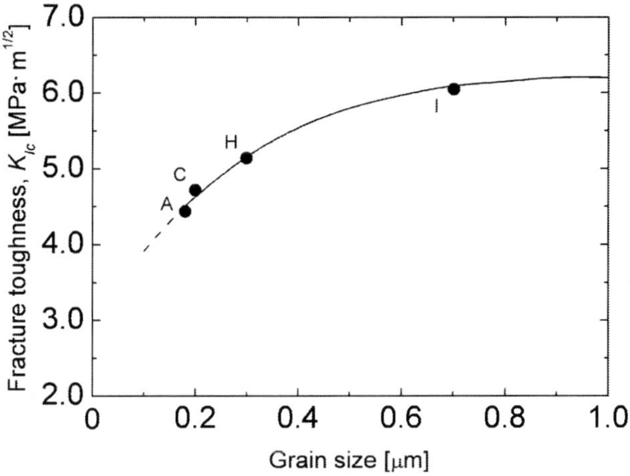

Figure 4.17 Dependence of crack-tip fracture toughness, K_{Ic}, (by the COD method) and grain size in 3Y-TZP polycrystals.

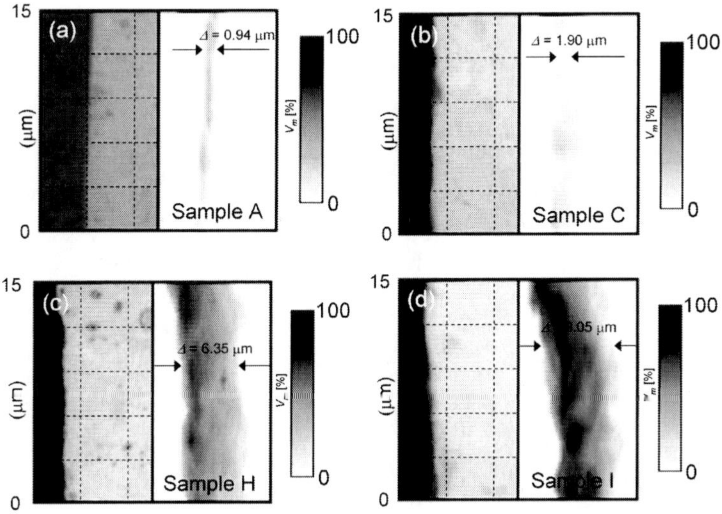

Figure 4.18 Optical micrographs (left side) and maps of monoclinic volume fraction (right side) taken on one side of the profile of a crack propagated in 3Y-TZP samples with different particle sizes. The crack opening displacement is on the right side of the optical micrographs. The Raman maps revealed that Samples A, C, H, and I (in (a), (b), (c), and (d), respectively) with average grain sizes equal to 192 nm, 207 nm, 318 nm, and 700 nm, respectively, experienced substantially different transformation-zone widths, Δ (cf. arrowed zones in insets).

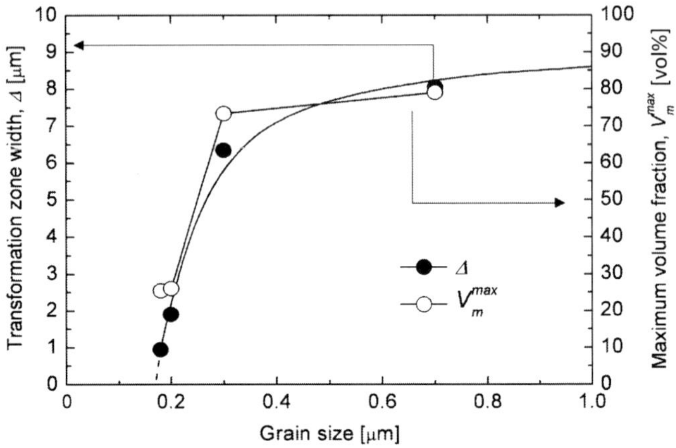

Figure 4.19 Relationships between transformation zone width, Δ, and maximum monolithic fraction in the transformation zone, $V_{\mathrm{m}}^{\mathrm{max}}$, in the neighborhood of the crack path as a function of the average grain size of the 3Y-TZP polycrystal.

tougher 3Y-TZP materials are also those materials more prone to environmental transformation, although the fracture toughness of the most brittle (and most stable) 3Y-TZP material remains about 40% higher than that of fine grained alumina polycrystals (cf. Section 3.5). Figure 4.20 shows the change of fracture toughness as a function of aging time in moist atmosphere. It is clearly observed that fracture toughness always decreases with aging, but the decrease is more substantial in materials with larger grain sizes. This is an obvious result if one thinks that the environmental transformation reduces the fraction of tetragonal polymorph available to the toughening effect during crack propagation within the tetragonal microstructure. Similar to the relationship observed between spontaneous transformation fractions and aging time, fracture toughness decreases more significantly in coarse-grained samples as compared to fine-grained ones. Note that it was not possible to measure fracture toughness by the COD method in Sample I after exposures in moist atmosphere >35 h. This was because of the formation of a cloud of microcracks, which hampered the observation of the main crack paths. The microcracking effect confirms the intrinsic structural weakness of 3Y-TZP surfaces after long-term exposure in water-vapor environment. In conclusion, from the results of aging experiments, it is actually shown the possibility of conspicuously preventing low-temperature degradation in 3Y-TZP by confining its grain size below ≈200 nm. However, this approach seems to be somewhat incompatible with the concurrent achievement of high fracture toughness, which instead requires grain sizes close to the micrometer level. This conclusion is fully conceivable, if one thinks that toughening and environmental degradation just represent different aspects of the same phenomenon of polymorphic instability in 3Y-TZP, the tougher the material the higher its instability in moist environment.

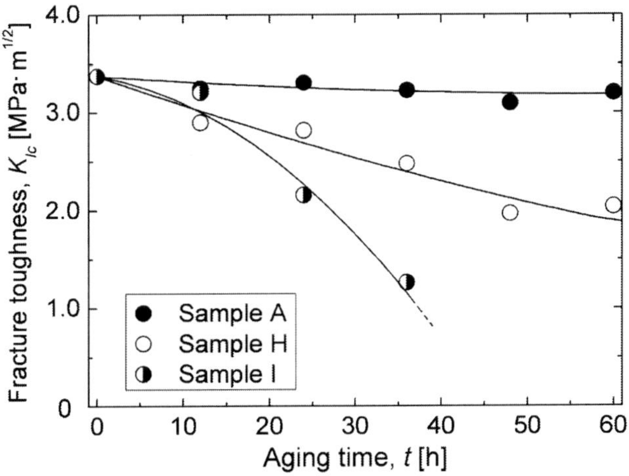

Figure 4.20 Relationship between crack-tip fracture toughness (by the COD method) and aging time, *t*, in hydrothermal environment (121°C) for Samples A, H, and I.

4.4 Environmental Resistance of Zirconia Heads from Different Makers

In Chapter 3, topographic analyses have been shown for the residual stress fields piled up in Al_2O_3 femoral heads. Data by confocal Raman, fluorescence, and cathodoluminescence spectroscopy on retrieved femoral heads have revealed clear changes in residual stress distributions as a function of exposure time *in vivo*. Obviously, these observations can be extrapolated to all ceramic bearings and, from a macroscopic design viewpoint, a possible migration of the polar position of maximum stress can be expected owing to local changes in surface curvature and roughness, especially in the case of a softer (e.g., polyethylene) bearing counterpart to the ceramic femoral head. More important, a drastic change in roughness of the femoral head can have a direct impact on the surface deterioration of the polyethylene liner, with the formation of wear debris, thus increasing the risk of osteolysis. As discussed in the previous sections of this chapter, metastability of 3Y-TZP and its potential effect on surface residual stresses and surface roughening might indeed represent a strong environmental effect affecting the structural performance of a hip joint *in vivo*. We have seen that some aspects of zirconia metastability are useful to improve the bulk fracture toughness of the joint material and, thus, they have been welcomed by joint designers; however, the drawback is a potential embrittlement and a roughening of the bearing surface upon aging *in vivo*. This latter effect, which can be extremely deleterious in the case of 3Y-TZP/polyethylene bearings, strongly depends on the microstructural characteristics of individual materials and on the manufacturing process [564–566]. However, not all types of zirconia materials should be assumed to behave identically with respect to hydrothermal attack from the environment. In this context, it is important to precisely test and to compare the intrinsic stability of their surfaces under hydrothermal conditions. On the one hand, it is somewhat surprising that at the time this book is written manufacturers are still distributing monolithic zirconia ceramic femoral heads (e.g., in Japan), while fundamental information is yet lacking on their characteristics of hydrothermal degradation. In particular, direct comparisons are hardly made among zirconia ceramic heads manufactured by different makers. In this section, we show the results of testing commercially available 3Y-TZP femoral heads with respect to their phase-stability. The roughness responses of their bearing surface to hydrothermal environment are monitored as the output of the study. The purpose here is twofold: (i) to clarify whether or not an actual improvement has been achieved in terms of structural performance with designing 3Y-TZP microstructures instead of adopting monolithic alumina and (ii) to make it available to the scientific community detailed information about the intrinsic material quality of commercially available zirconia femoral heads.

Unused femoral heads of two commercially available types made of monolithic zirconia (22 mm-sized heads by JMM Inc., Osaka, Japan, and 26 mm-sized heads by NGK, Komaki, Japan, both manufactured in 2007) are tested *in vitro* with respect to their surface stability and compared. In the remainder of this section, these samples will simply be referred to as sample "J" and "N," respectively. An additional sample (i.e., sample "ND") is also investigated, which was an unused 26 mm-sized ball manufactured by Norton Desmarquest in 1995 (i.e., the same type that originated several hundredths of head failures since the year 2000 [637]; cf. Figs. 4.5 and 4.6). This latter type of femoral head is now withdrawn from the market. Experimental results of *in vitro* surface phase stability obtained before and after aging tests (conducted in water vapor as a function of exposure time at four different temperatures: 90, 98, 121, and 134°C) are shown in Figs. 4.21(a) and (b) for femoral heads of the types J and N, respectively. Data at similar temperatures are shown in Fig. 4.21(b) for the head of type ND, as redrawn from an early study by Chevalier *et al.* [645]. In the graphs, the fraction of monoclinic zirconia polymorph, V_m, detected by the confocal Raman probe on the surfaces of femoral heads from different makers is plotted in a semi-logarithm scale as a function of exposure time in the autoclave, *t*. All plots can be rationalized according to a MAJ nucleation/growth model [644, 645], as discussed in Section 4.3 (cf. Eq. (4.3)). As foreseen by the MAJ model, the fraction of monoclinic polymorph on the sample surface increases in a relatively slow fashion at the initial stage of aging, according to the time needed for monoclinic nuclei formation; then, the monoclinic fraction experiences an exponential rise after relatively longer time exposures, this stage corresponding to nuclei coalescence and, ultimately, to nuclei extension toward the bulk of the material. The most striking feature in comparing the different plots in Fig. 4.21 is that the increase in monoclinic phase content in both zirconia heads J and N was found to be significantly slower as compared to the zirconia head ND. Polymorphic transformation in sample J was also extremely delayed as compared to sample N, but only at temperatures of hydrothermal aging <121°C. It should be noted that 3Y-TZP in femoral head of types J and N contained the same small fraction of alumina dopant in the raw powder mixture.

However, these two femoral heads were presumably sintered at different temperatures. As a matter of fact, the tangible difference detected in the environmental resistance is the reasonable outcome of the difference in grain size between these two materials (220 nm and 410 nm in heads J and N, respectively) (cf. also data in Figs. 4.7 and 4.8). In addition, alumina was observed as isolated dispersoids in the microstructure of head N, while it was uniformly distributed at grain boundaries (and conspicuously invisible by SEM inspection) in the head J. This microscopic observation, which will be substantiated in a forthcoming paragraph of this section, might confirm the model proposed in Fig. 4.16 for explaining the microstructural development during sintering of nanostructured zirconia polycrystals in the presence of a small fraction of Al_2O_3 dopant. The relatively large (average) grain size of sample ND (i.e., 500 nm) together with a lack of Al_2O_3 dopant can fully justify the relatively speedy transformation behavior in water vapor of this old type of 3Y-TZP femoral head.

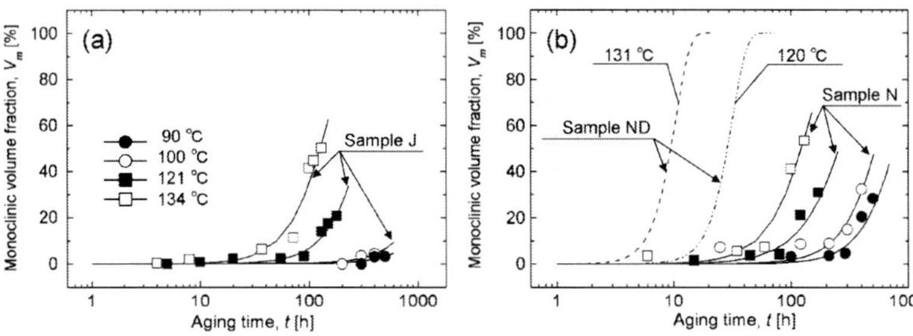

Figure 4.21 Relationship between monoclinic volume fraction, V_m, and aging time, t, in different hydrothermal environments: (a) Sample J, (b) Samples N and ND. Data for Sample ND were re-plotted from Ref. [645].

Best fitting of experimental data in Fig. 4.21 (i.e., according to Eq. (4.3)) leads to the determination of n and b values for each material, as listed in Table 4.2. Furthermore, plots of ln b as a function of the inverse absolute temperature, $1/T$, of hydrothermal exposure can be obtained, whose slope represents the activation energy, Q, for environmentally driven phase transformation (Fig. 4.22). In Al_2O_3-doped samples, the activation energy slightly decreased with decreasing grain size, with values of 140 and 188 kJ/mol in samples J and N, respectively. Both Q values

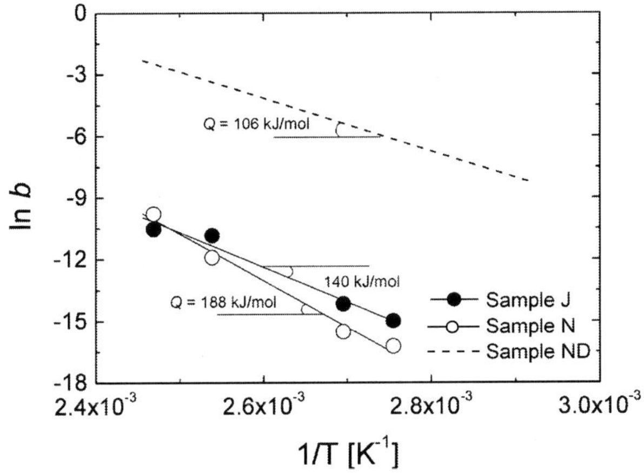

Figure 4.22 Arrhenius plots of the nucleation rate parameter, *b*, for samples J, N, and ND, from whose slopes an activation energy value, *Q*, can be calculated as shown in inset and listed in Table 4.2. The plot for Sample ND was redrawn from Ref. [645].

were detectably higher than the value 106 kJ/mol reported for sample ND lacking in Al_2O_3 dopant [645]. Extrapolations to body temperature suggest that 1 year in the human body invariably corresponds to a few hours in autoclave at 132°C. Therefore, testing in autoclave for times as long as 100 h greatly exceeds the human lifetime. However, it should also be considered that the results of polymorphic transformation upon *in vitro* hydrothermal testing likely represent an underestimation of the actual transformation rate *in vivo*. This is because *in vivo* other factors, e.g., the presence of stress and of chemical elements in the body fluid, might contribute to worsen the material response. As far as the *n* values are concerned, the lowest value found for material J reflects the lowest transformation rate of this femoral head, to be compared with the value of *n* equal to 3.6 ± 0.4 detected for the highly transformable material ND (cf. Table 4.2), which corresponds to a fast nucleation accompanied by a three-dimensional growth process [644]. From the viewpoint of environmental stability, the 3Y-TZP material of femoral head J should be considered the most advanced grade of biomedical zirconia presently available on the market, owing to its optimized sintering schedule and fine (sub-micron scale) grain structure. *In vitro* data indeed confirm the following two main points: (i) intrinsically, superior environmental stability in 3Y-

TZP materials can only be obtained by refining the grain size; and, (ii) 3Y-TZP with poor environmental stability have been released in the past in the hip joint market with negative consequences on the structural reliability of the hip joints, on the wear rate of the polyethylene counterparts, and on the overall image of biomedical ceramic bearings.

Table 4.2 MAJ parameters and thermal activation energies for polymorphic transformation *in vitro* for two commercially available 3Y-TZP (Sample J and Sample N)

	n	T [°C]	b	Q [kJ/mol]
Sample J	2.10 ± 0.5	98	1.82×10^{-7}	140
		121	3.78×10^{-6}	
		134	3.21×10^{-5}	
Sample N	2.17 ± 0.2	98	7.10×10^{-7}	188
		121	1.99×10^{-5}	
		134	2.17×10^{-5}	
Sample ND	3.6 ± 0.4	100	5.73×10^{-2}	106
		120	8.76×10^{-4}	
		131	2.70×10^{-4}	

Source: Data for Sample ND, now out of the market, were obtained from Ref. [645].

Figures 4.23(a)~(d) and 4.24(a)~(d) show a comparison between typical AFM images (i.e., displaying the height distribution on the surface), which were recorded on the surfaces of the femoral heads of type J and N, respectively. In both figures, AFM micrographs in parts (a), (b), (c), and (d) were taken after 0, 10, 50, and 100 h exposure in autoclave at 134°C, respectively. The topographic details of the maps recorded on unexposed heads made of monolithic zirconia indeed confirmed a considerable difference in grain size, finer in the femoral head J as compared to N. Both 3Y-TZP surfaces revealed morphological changes with increasing exposure time. A closer examination of the AFM maps shows distinct isolated asperities for the surface of the femoral head J as compared to the craters found on the more transformed surface of the femoral head N. Interestingly, the AFM images capture an important difference between the rates of both formation and coalescence of transformation sites on the surfaces of the two different monolithic zirconia heads, type J showing only sporadic transformation sites after 30 h exposure in autoclave, as compared to an advanced state of coalescence in the transformed surface of type N after the same exposure time. Figures 4.25(a)~(d) and 4.26(a)~(d) show histograms of surface depth asperities as statistically detected on the surface of the femoral heads J and N, respectively (samples unexposed and after autoclave exposures of 0, 10, 50, and 100 h are displayed in (a), (b), (c), and (d), respectively). The statistical height distributions for the two 3Y-TZP materials showed marked morphologic variations and large differences among different exposure times. Both head types experienced an increasing tendency to bimodality with increasing autoclaving time. In type J, a shoulder located between 10 and 30 nm tended to increase with increasing the exposure time in autoclave. On the other hand, autoclave exposure induced more complex and prominent changes in the symmetry of the histogram recorded for type N, including not only symmetry changes but also successive appearance and disappearance of shoulders both at positive and negative heights.

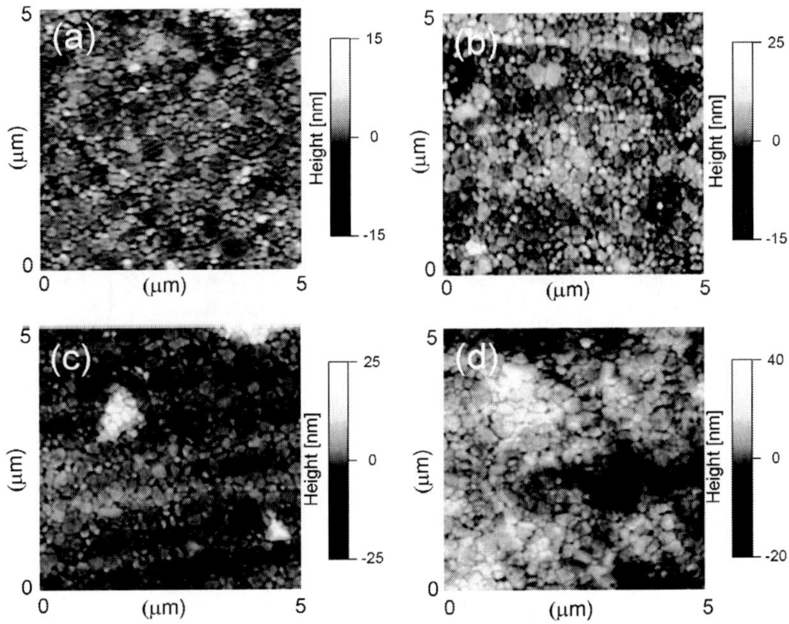

Figure 4.23 AFM micrographs of sample J after hydrothermal aging tests at: (a) 0 h, (b) 10 h, (c) 50 h, and (d) 100 h.

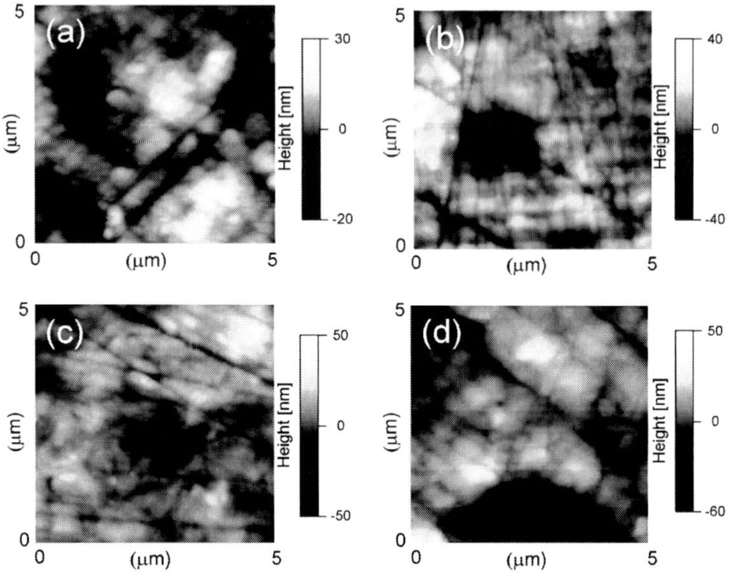

Figure 4.24 AFM micrographs of sample N after hydrothermal aging tests at: (a) 0 h, (b) 10 h, (c) 50 h, and (d) 100 h.

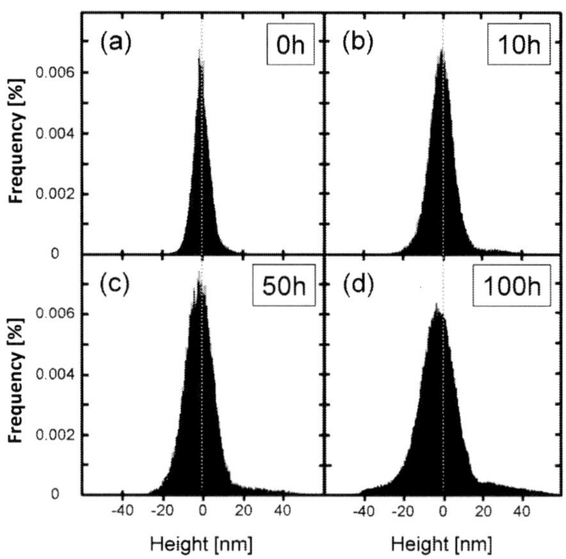

Figure 4.25 Frequency height histogram measured on the surface of sample J after hydrothermal aging tests at: (a) 0 h, (b) 10 h, (c) 50 h, and (d) 100 h.

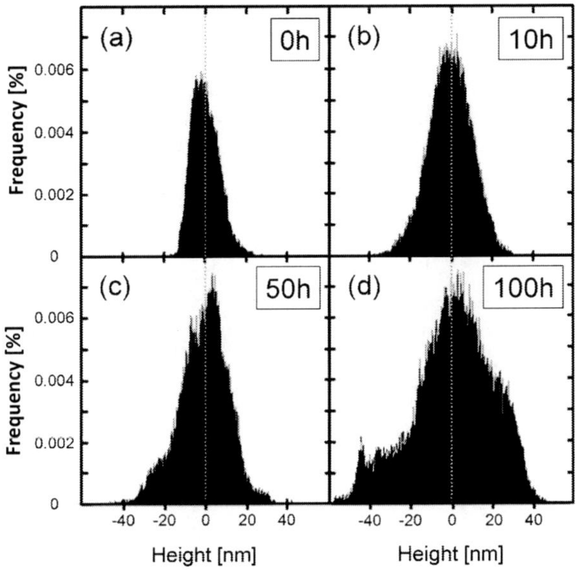

Figure 4.26 Frequency height histogram measured on the surface of sample N after hydrothermal aging tests at: (a) 0 h, (b) 10 h, (c) 50 h, and (d) 100 h.

A quantitative statistical analysis of topological features also captured important differences among the two 3Y-TZP femoral heads in terms of both intensity and morphology of their height frequency distributions. Such different characteristics are summarized for all measurement conditions in Figs. 4.27(a) and (b), in terms of arithmetic mean roughness, R_a, and 10-point mean roughness, R_z, respectively. As discussed in Chapter 3, the 10-point mean roughness is the average difference in height between the five highest peaks and five lowest valleys found on the surface. It should be emphasized here that surface roughness is a useful single-value parameter for comparing surfaces, but it might be largely insufficient for completely describing the surface topology, thus potentially leading to draw erroneous conclusions. For example, it can occur that similar surface roughness values are obtained for surfaces that have completely different global or local topology. Therefore, in order to provide a more meaningful description of the surface, it is important to examine the complete surface height histogram from the AFM images (as given in Figs. 4.25 and 4.26). In other words, the height histograms of the

AFM image represent a superset of the data contained in a surface roughness value. Regarding the present 3Y-TZP femoral heads, we indeed deal with strongly non-Gaussian distributions of surface elevations. A meaningful parameter for characterizing these types of distribution is the skewness, R_{sk}, which measures the asymmetry of the data around their mean value and thus the dissimilarity relative to a Gaussian distribution. As an additional parameter, the kurtosis, R_k, qualifies the flatness of the height distribution and is a measure of the extent to which the surface height variance is due to infrequent extreme deviations. Figures 4.28 and 4.29 show plots of skewness and kurtosis of the statistical height distributions. The surface of the sample N shows skewness values that become increasingly negative with increasing exposure time in autoclave. On the other hand, the surface of the type J shows a clear exponential rise in skewness with increasing exposure time in autoclave. Interestingly, this latter zirconia femoral head was also the only sample showing a significant increase in kurtosis with increasing aging time in autoclave. There are small differences between the contents of SiO_2 and cubic ZrO_2 phases between the two 3Y-TZP investigated materials. However, the slightly larger amounts of both phases present in the femoral head N should be beneficial in delaying phase transformation [661], which does not appear to be the case here (more details on this point will be given in a forthcoming paragraph by means of CL data). Therefore, the grain size refinement should be considered the dominant effect in explaining the higher hydrothermal resistance of femoral head J. Nevertheless, in type J, statistical data of skewness and kurtosis showed quite high values. These parameters quantify the symmetry of the height distribution and the frequency of maxima and minima in it, respectively. The high (positive) skewness of the surface of the femoral head J locates a surface with a number of peaks on an otherwise flat surface plane. Its high (positive) kurtosis coefficient, which is a statistical measure of the divergence of the experimental distribution from a Gaussian one, (i.e., characteristic of a perfectly random distribution of peak heights and valley depths) also confirms that peaks prevail over valleys or pores. It is conceivable that the isolated surface uplifts found in the femoral head J correspond to initial agglomerations of the ZrO_2 raw powder that are poor in Al_2O_3 contents. In considering how polymorphic transformation affects wear, isolated elevations emerging from a relatively flat surface appear to represent the worst scenario in the process of wear debris formation when the zirconia femoral head slides against an acetabular cup made of polyethylene. However, investigation of surface stability in autoclave can only partly represent the actual exposure in the human body, in which high surface stresses at the bearing surfaces might accelerate degradation [56, 662]. Therefore, we can only conclude here that femoral heads of the type J experience an intrinsically slower environmental resistance as compared to those of type N, but analysis of surface stability are necessarily needed of retrieved implants for an ultimate evaluations of phase stability (as shown in the last paragraph of this section).

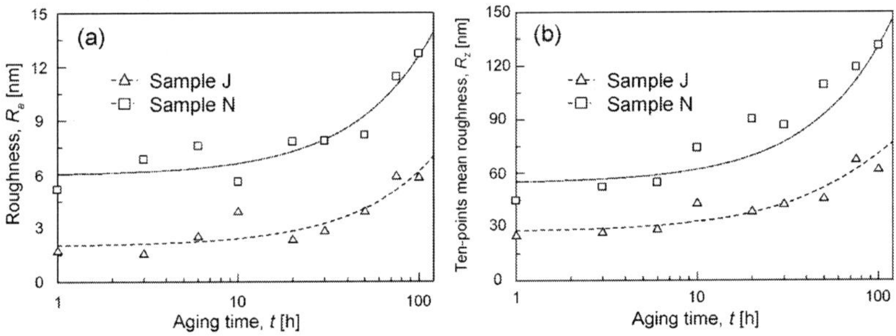

Figure 4.27 Relationship between aging time in hydrothermal environment and: (a) roughness, R_a, and (b) 10-point mean roughness, R_z, for the surfaces of samples J and N.

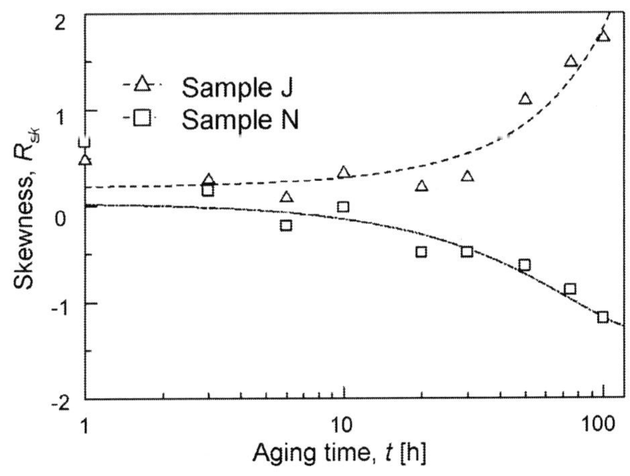

Figure 4.28 Relationship between aging time in hydrothermal environment and the skewness, R_{sk}, of the surfaces of samples J and N.

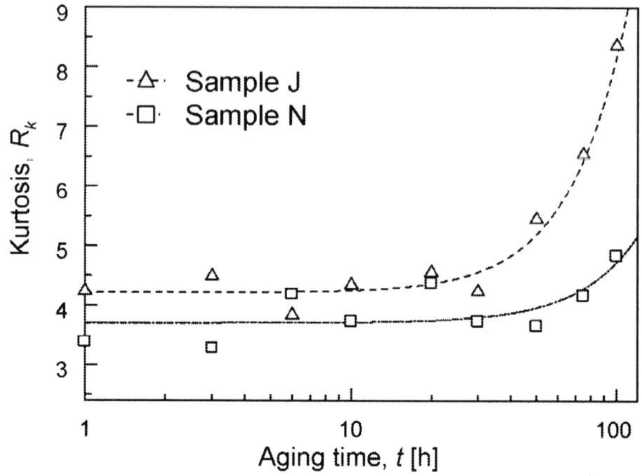

Figure 4.29 Relationship between aging time in hydrothermal environment and the kurtosis, R_k, of the surfaces of samples J and N.

Lu *et al.* [663] studied the effect of oxygen vacancies on the stability of 3Y-TZP phase structures and related it to polymorphic transformation at low temperature by means of an electrochemical technique. This pioneering study provided straightforward experimental evidence that a decrease in oxygen vacancy concentration decreases the stability of metastable tetragonal zirconia and thus promotes its transformation into the monoclinic phase. On the other hand, as already discussed, an increase in concentration of substitutional Y^{3+} to replace Zr^{4+} increases Zr–O bond length (i.e., decreases bond strength) [655, 656]. It is thus from the delicate balance between the level of bond strain in the tetragonal network and vacancy concentration in it that the polymorphic stability of the 3Y-TZP surface is decided. In this context, it is also clear that a residual stress field of tensile nature "destabilizes" the 3Y-TZP lattices. Raman experiments have revealed fundamental differences between the hydrothermal stability of femoral heads J and N. A systematic study has also shown (cf. Fig. 4.15) that 3Y-TZP materials can experience relatively high bond-stretching variations when their sintering temperature is altered. In addition to Raman spectroscopy, CL experiments can provide complementary evidence to substantiate some inherent differences between femoral heads of type J and N in their stoichiometric structure. Figures 4.30(a) and (b) show SEM micrographs of the surfaces of femoral heads J and N, respectively, after exposure for

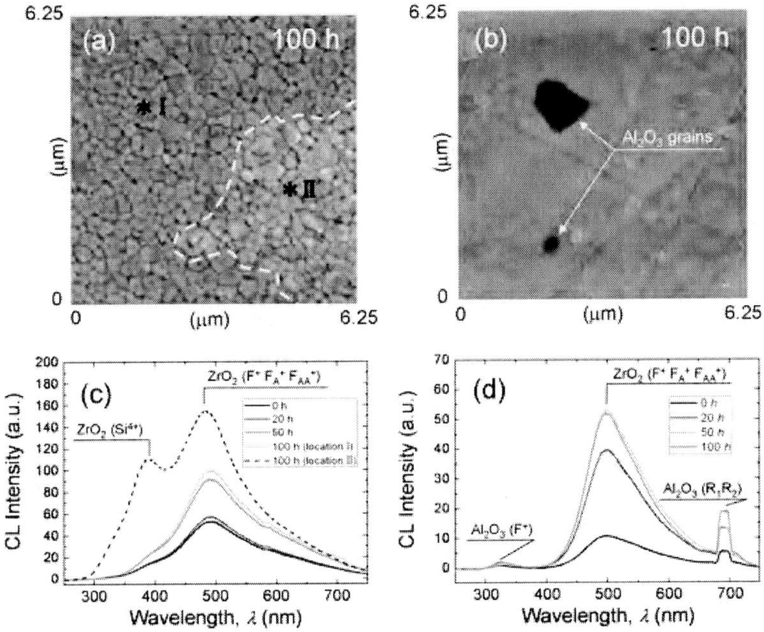

Figure 4.30 SEM micrographs of the surface of Samples J and N after 100 h exposure in autoclave at 121°C (in (a) and (b), respectively). The broken line in (a) locates a nucleus of polymorphic transformation in Sample J. The dark particles in (b) are Al_2O_3 grains. In (c) and (d), CL spectra collected on Samples J and N, respectively, after increasing periods of exposure in hydrothermal environment. Bands are labeled according to their respective physical origins.

100 h to hydrothermal environment 121°C. CL spectra are given in Figs. (c) and (d) for samples A and B, respectively, which were collected before and after exposure in autoclave for increasing times up to 100 h at 121°C. Striking differences are found in the morphology of the Al_2O_3 phase (cf. large grains only visible in Sample N (Fig. 4.30(b)) and in the complete absence of CL bands belonging to Al_2O_3 in Sample J (cf. Fig. 4.30(c)) as compared to Sample N (cf. F^+ and R_1R_2 bands located at around 330 and 695 nm in the CL spectra of Fig. 4.30(d)). In other words, unlike Sample N, which contains relatively large Al_2O_3 grains, Sample J, sintered at lower temperature, contains Al_2O_3 homogeneously dispersed at grain boundaries in the form of such small precipitates that they can conceivably be considered as existing in the amorphous state

(i.e., with quite low CL emission efficiency). These observations confirm the effect of sintering temperature on the stereological distribution and the crystallinity of the dispersed Al_2O_3 phase, as discussed in the previous section and depicted in the model of Fig. 4.16. As far as CL emission from the ZrO_2 lattice is concerned, the CL spectra recorded in the two types of femoral head show a common feature in a main broad band, which represents the sum of three distinct emissions from oxygen-related defects of different structure [664]. The broad band (peaking at around 500 nm) has been reported to consist of three distinct sub-bands of Gaussian nature located at 460 nm (2.69 eV), 550 nm (2.25 eV), and 600 nm (2.07 eV). The emission at 460 nm (commonly referred to as the F^+-center of ZrO_2) was at tributed to singly occupied anion vacancies, thus involving the presence of an intrinsic defect where all Zr^{4+} ions are nearest neighbors to the vacancy [665]. The two extrinsic bands located at 550 and 600 nm (i.e., referred to as F_A^+ and F_{AA}^+ centers, respectively) were associated to electron transfer from the valence band to local mid-gap states. Their structures show one and two Y^{3+} ions as nearest neighbors to the vacancy, respectively [664, 666]. The intensity of the CL emission is related to the presence of vacancy sites in the ZrO_2 lattice, their annihilation leading to an increase in CL intensity. The intensity increase arises from the fact that oxygen vacancy annihilation involves additional Zr–O bond stretching, which enables a more efficient emission as compared to oxygen vacancy sites themselves. CL data on both Samples J and N thus consistently confirm that annihilation of oxygen vacancies on the surface of the sample accompanies polymorphic transformation. In addition to CL emission due to Zr–O bond stretching, which is a consequence of vacancy annihilation, the presence of Si impurity in the ZrO_2 lattice might involve the presence of an additional band in the blue region of the CL spectrum (i.e., here corresponding to the shoulder observed at around 390 nm (3.18 eV) in Sample J), as demonstrated by Gholinia and Leach [667]. This shoulder-band was only observed in highly transformed monoclinic nuclei on the surface of the femoral head J (cf. SEM picture and photomultiplier CL map centered at 390 nm in Figs. 4.31(a) and (b), respectively). This observation is consistent with the detrimental effect reported for Si impurities on the hydrothermal resistance of finely

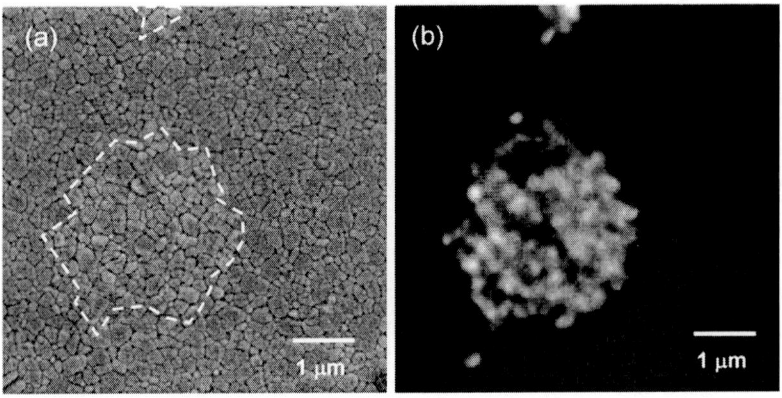

Figure 4.31 (a) SEM micrograph of a monoclinic nucleus in Sample J; and, (b) photomultiplier CL image at the wavelength of 390 nm taken at the same location of (a).

grained 3Y-TZP [668]. Indeed, the content of SiO_2 in Sample J is six times larger than that in Sample N (i.e., the respective makers declare maximum values of silica contents of 60 and 10 ppm, respectively). Furthermore, as another consequence of the relatively low sintering temperature (and thus greatly lowered grain-boundary diffusion), the presence of SiO_2 in the microstructure of Sample J might be strongly localized. In other words, CL experiments have revealed that Si-rich areas on the surface of Sample J become preferential sites for phase transformation in an otherwise extremely resistant microstructure to hydrothermal transformation. Figure 4.32 summarizes the average intensity variations of the cumulative CL band centered at around 500 nm as a function of exposure time in autoclave. Since the two compared samples were set on the same stage and CL spectra measured during the same experimental session, the CL intensity can be compared. Despite averaging over a large area (300 μm^2), the comparison systematically shows a slightly higher CL emission from Sample J as compared to N, due to the exceptionally strong off-stoichiometry effect experienced in the transformation nuclei. However, the relative increase of CL intensity (i.e., the progressive amount of oxygen vacancy annihilation) over aging time was nearly the same for the two investigated microstructures. From this set of SEM and CL data, we can conclude the following:

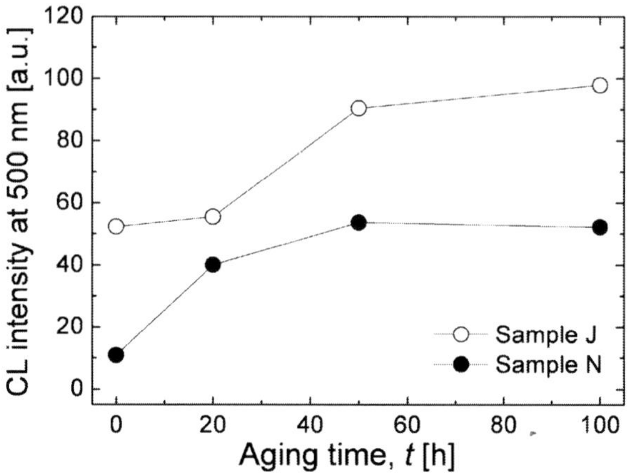

Figure 4.32 Intensity of the cumulative CL band at 500 nm as a function of aging time in hydrothermal environment for both Samples J and N.

(i) The femoral head Sample N, sintered at higher temperature and possessing a grain size larger than Sample J, shows a highly localized presence of Al_2O_3 with high crystallinity. The presence of Al_2O_3 phase is observed as large dark grains in the SEM micrograph of Fig. 4.30(b) and it is substantiated by the presence of relatively strong CL bands emitted from Al_2O_3 point-defect sites (Fig. 4.30(d)). On the other hand, Al_2O_3 bands are conspicuously lacking in the CL spectra detected from Sample J (Fig. 4.30(c)). A lack of homogeneity in the distribution of the Al_2O_3 phase involves its lesser efficacy (i.e., for the same added fraction) in impeding transformed areas to spread over the material surface (cf. model in Fig. 4.16). The higher sintering temperature of sample N could also have promoted abnormal grain growth in the zirconia grain texture. Large grains, rich in Y-content, are associated to of Y-depletion from the grain bulk as depicted in the model by Matsui *et al.* [649], thus creating an increased number of preferential locations for transformation nuclei in the material microstructure.

(ii) The femoral head Sample J, for which less amount of diffusional flow occurred at grain boundaries during sintering (i.e., as a consequence of a low sintering temperature) in comparison with femoral head Sample N, appears to sporadically contain zones rich in Si impurity. Such zones, which might exist in the material since agglomerations of the raw powder mixture, are shown to become the nuclei from which polymorphic transformation originates. The process of Y-depletion from the grain bulk should not be substantial in Sample J, given its relatively low sintering temperature. Consequently, polymorphic transformation spreads over the sample surface from the sporadic locations of SiO_2-rich material.

(iii) The presence of monoclinic domains (under a compressive residual stress field) on the surface of the femoral head Sample J involves, for static equilibrium, high tensile stresses in the residual tetragonal phase as compared to untransformed zones (cf. Fig. 4.4). Such tensile stresses represent the driving force for spreading the polymorphic transformation throughout the microstructural network.

These characteristics fit well with both transformation kinetics and AFM analyses performed on the two types of femoral heads, showing a larger number of nuclei and a higher propagation rate on the surface of femoral head Sample N as compared to Sample J. In conclusion, it appears that lowering sintering temperature helps minimizing grain size, which in turn reduces nuclei formation rate (i.e., according to a lower tetragonality of the lattice and to a lower content of Y-rich cubic phase, in addition to limiting the coalescence of the dispersed Al_2O_3 additive into large grains). All these factors produce a positive effect in delaying polymorphic transformation. However, the presence of SiO_2 impurity in the ZrO_2 raw powder is found to originate transformation nuclei in the sintered material. The main practical consequence of SiO_2-rich agglomerations resides in a degraded morphology of the head surface after hydrothermal exposure. This, in turn, leads to high skewness values of positive sign, which form rather quickly after the polymorphic transformation starts to take place.

To clarify the response of 3Y-TZP femoral heads *in vivo*, we shall show hereafter results for two retrievals, as follows: (i) an implant used for only one year by a 65-year-old woman with osteoarthritis (right hip surgery in 2001). In this case, a 26-mm diameter head made of 3Y-TZP manufactured by NGK (the same material as Sample N above) was used against a polyethylene liner. This implant, which is henceforth simply referred to as the "short-term retrieval," was retrieved due to repeated dislocations; and, (ii) another implant containing a 28-mm-diameter 3Y-TZP femoral head (also in this case manufactured by NGK, i.e., the same as Sample B above) that belonged to a 56-years-old woman who underwent total (right) hip arthroplasty in 1998 due to osteoarthritis. This latter implant was a bipolar system for which revision surgery was performed after 10 years and 2 months because of central head migration. This sample is simply referred to as the "long-term retrieval," henceforth. Figures 4.33(a) and (b) show the results of polar line maps along the hemisphere of the short- and long-term retrievals, respectively. In Fig. 4.33(b), the transformation profile show local values of monoclinic fraction as high as ≈19% in the long-term implanted retrieval, while the maximum amount of phase transformation in the short-term retrieval (Fig. 4.33(a)) was V_m = 13.6%. In the long-term retrieval, the transformed fractions were similar on both sides of the head (i.e., the right side of the plot here corresponds in both cases to the side of the main wear zone of the femoral head). According to activation energy arguments, 1 h of autoclave exposure under the above standard conditions corresponds to few years' exposure *in vivo* [669]. However, Raman maps collected on the surface of the retrievals clearly show areas with monoclinic fractions higher than those predicted according to *in vitro* experiments (cf. Fig. 4.21(b)). This evidence strongly suggests that, *in vivo*, additional causes of mechanical and/or chemical nature (e.g., tribochemical and stress effects) may overlap to accelerate phase transformation with respect to *in vitro* conditions. Being non-conservative, data collected *in vitro* can thus only represent fairly optimistic predictions of *in vivo* transformation lifetime.

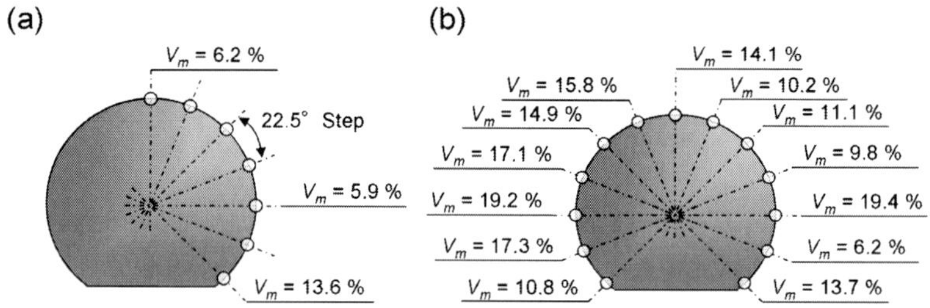

Figure 4.33 Results of polar line maps along the hemisphere of the short- and long-term 3Y-TZP retrievals (in (a) and (b), respectively). In (a), locations without V_m labeling showed monoclinic contents $V_m \approx 0$.

With the purpose of clarifying and comparing the surgical performances of alumina and zirconia femoral heads when employed against polyethylene liners, Liang *et al.* [670] used a computer-aided technique to measure polyethylene wear radiologically in 46 hips with alumina heads and 58 hips with zirconia heads. Sampling was quite homogeneous with the preoperative diagnosis in all cases being osteoarthritis. The mean linear wear rate of polyethylene sockets against zirconia heads was 0.133 mm/year, significantly larger than the mean linear wear rate against alumina heads (0.078 mm/year). Mean volumetric wear rates were 24.1 and 39.8 mm^3/year in alumina and zirconia femoral heads, respectively. These researchers also found that age at operation, patient body weight, height and thickness of polyethylene, and socket abduction angle did not significantly influence the wear rates. They, thus, attributed the excessive polyethylene wear to the occurrence of phase transformation on the surface of zirconia heads, leading to an increase of surface roughness. However, besides the reported poor wear performance of 3Y-TZP heads against polyethylene liners, another important difference between alumina ceramics and 3Y-TZP resides in their different thermal conductivity. It has been reported that the thermal conductivity of 3Y-TZP is more than 15 times lower than that of alumina [671], which not only might accelerate the $t \rightarrow m$ phase transformation of the 3Y-TZP surface *in vivo* [672], but also increase the contact temperature during frictional sliding with detrimental consequences for the molecular structure of the polyethylene counterpart. In conclusion, besides a clear unfeasibility of hard-on-hard zirconia bearings [58], the reported clinical data also fail to substantiate a clear improvement in wear performance for 3Y-TZP femoral heads (i.e., with respect to the alumina ones) even when the sliding counterpart is polyethylene.

4.5 Open Issues and Yet Unexplored Possibilities for Zirconia Biomaterials

In the 80s, technologists turned their strategy to zirconia ceramics because they believed in the possibility of overcoming the structural limitations (i.e., low strength, low fracture toughness and unsatisfactory Weibull modulus) encountered with polycrystalline alumina microstructures when manufacturing artificial joint components. Development and subsequent commercialization of 3Y-TZP femoral heads later demonstrated that overcoming such difficulties is indeed possible by means of a strict control of the manufacturing procedure, which enabled to obtain fine and homogeneous microstructures and, thus, of joint components with high strength (i.e., about twice that of monolithic alumina) and improved Weibull modulus [673]. In the previous section, we have also shown that toughness at least 40% higher than that of alumina can be obtained even in 3Y-TZP materials with an average grain size as fine as ≈200 nm. However, a strict control of the manufacturing process has been found to be an extremely delicate task for nanocrystalline 3Y-TZP, with fluctuations in local stoichiometry potentially leading to extremely amplified consequences (of a detrimental nature) on the structural and environmental efficiency of the artificial joint implants. All this premised, we emphasize here that 3Y-TZP is only one, although the most popular, among the zirconia materials that can potentially be used for manufacturing biomedical joint components. In other words, the unique capacity of the zirconia lattice of being alloyed with large fractions of sub- or super-valent ions and the consequent possibility of modulating its lattice stoichiometry is a unique and intriguing property among bioceramics. From the viewpoint of materials design, this property should be regarded as an additional degree of freedom in engineering a biomaterial microstructure with suitable desired properties.

Similar to 3Y-TZP, although less popular than it, various other classes of materials based on binary ZrO_2 systems have been proposed as potential material candidates for joint prostheses. For example, the ZrO_2–CeO_2 system has been long known for its high fracture toughness and moderate strength and hardness [274, 674]. Therefore, this system has been somewhat regarded as the natural counterpart of the Y-TZP system, which instead possesses relatively low toughness but high strength and hardness. It is thus quite conceivable to speculate that a suitable composition based on the ternary system ZrO_2–Y_2O_3–CeO_2 could be tailored with designing their microstructures for concurrently achieving high strength, high hardness and improved fracture toughness. Hence, one could in principle follow two different paths in approaching the design of a microstructure with improved structural properties, namely: searching for a hardening mechanism in the CeO_2-doped material system or developing a toughening mechanism in the Y_2O_3-doped counterpart. Materials technologists have nowadays focused on advanced processing procedures that have led to the development of a new generation of Y-TZP–Al_2O_3 composites, also referred to as zirconia-toughened alumina (ZTA) materials, which will be extensively described in the next chapter. On the other hand, the search for hardening in highly tough (but softer) zirconia alloys lies yet conspicuously unexplored in the field of joint arthroplasty. On the tortuous path of rationalization for this new branch of research, a major unresolved issue resides in identifying the underlying mechanism by which Ce-TZP can resist so strongly to moisture attack. An improved understanding is indeed relevant to the future of ceramic biomaterials because a clarification (and the subsequent control) of the stoichiometric details leading to the substantially reduced hydrothermal susceptibility of Ce-TZP could definitely open the path to advanced designs of zirconia microstructures.

Figures 4.34(a) and (b) show SEM pictures of the microstructures of 3Y-TZP and 12Ce-TZP, respectively, sintered according to the same thermal cycle (1400°C for 2 h). The difference in the microstructural network is striking, with the latter material showing a significantly larger grain size (explicitly indicated in inset) with a broader histogram as compared to the former material (cf. histograms of grain size in inset). The transformability responses of the two materials to surface loading are also quite different. Figures 4.35(a) and (b) show optical micrographs of Vickers indentation prints produced with the same load on the surface of 3Y-TZP and 12Ce-TZP, respectively. The larger print detected in the latter material clearly reveals its lower hardness. However, Raman maps of $t \rightarrow m$ transformation fractions (Figs. 4.35(c) and (d) for 3Y-TZP and 12Ce-TZP, respectively) also reveal a stronger transformation response in the 12Ce-TZP material, with local values of maximum monoclinic fractions as high as 50% (vs. the maximum fraction of ≈23% found in 3Y-TZP). The magnitude of internal stresses was also found to be quite different in the two materials. Figures 4.35(e)/(g) and 4.35(f)/(h) show maps of residual stresses around the indentation print, as collected for the monoclinic/tetragonal phase of 3Y-TZP and 12Ce-TZP, respectively. As seen, in the monoclinic phase, for similar residual stress magnitudes (in the order of the GPa), the 12Ce-TZP material shows a considerably larger extension of the stressed zone, consistent with the observation of a larger indentation print. On the other hand, the tensile stress intensification in the residual tetragonal phase appears, despite the similar stress field morphologies, more pronounced in the 12Ce-TZP material as compared to 3Y-TZP. This is a consequence of the lower fraction of tetragonal phase left untransformed in the 12Ce-TZP material after indentation, as noticed in comparing Figs. 4.35(c) and (d). The stress maps vividly visualize the higher propensity to phase transformation of the "softer" 12Ce-TZP material as compared to 3Y-TZP. Equilibrium stress maps (i.e., calculated as explained in Section 4.2) were also calculated, as shown in Figs. 4.35(i) and (j) for 3Y-TZP and 12Ce-TZP, respectively. A comparison between these two latter maps again visualizes a stronger compressive effect on the surface of the 12Ce-TZP, thus confirming its better propensity to react against external loading with polymorphically transforming under stress.

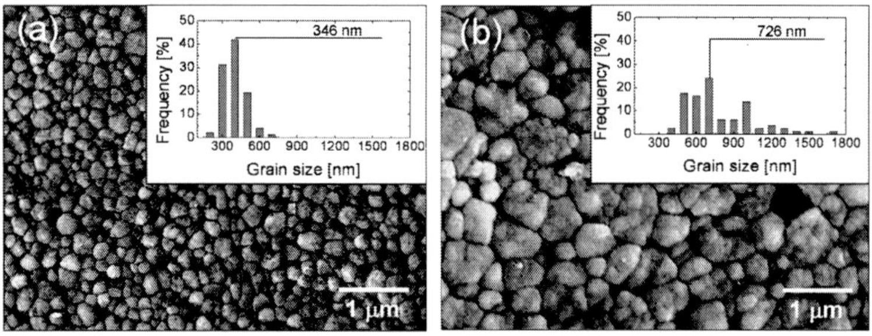

Figure 4.34 SEM pictures of the microstructures of 3Y-TZP and 12Ce-TZP (in (a) and (b), respectively). Both materials were sintered at 1400°C for 2 h.

We already mentioned that the 260 cm^{-1} Raman line of tetragonal zirconia corresponds to the stretching of the Zr–O′ bond in its lattice. The band frequency of this stretching mode has been reported to be rather sensitive to the content of dopant, a slight increase in bond length as a result of a larger substitution of the dopant for Zr^{4+} decreasing the bond strength and, consequently, shifting the Raman mode frequency. For reaching mechanical and electrical equilibrium a concurrent increase of oxygen vacancies occurs [656], with a consequent decrease in the average coordination number of zirconium ions [657]. A semi-quantitative evaluation of bond-stretching mechanisms can be thus obtained by monitoring the shift of the 260 cm^{-1} Raman band before and after exposure in water-vapor atmosphere. One can then assume that the spectral shift of such band be related to the two possible reasons leading to bond stretching, namely, the development of internal lattice stresses and the evolution of oxygen off-stoichiometry in the tetragonal lattice. Figure 4.36(a) shows an optical micrograph taken on the surface of a coarse-grained 12Ce-TZP material (i.e., sintered at 1600°C). As already mentioned, this material, unlike Y-TZP, was found to be conspicuously insensitive to low-temperature degradation. Polarized/confocal intensity maps of the tetragonal Raman bands located at approximately 260 (A_{1g} vibrational mode) and 145 cm^{-1} (E_g vibrational mode) are shown for the same area in Figs. 4.36(b) and (c), respectively. According to a quantitative analysis based on Raman selection rules for the tetragonal lattice (i.e., as described in a recently published specialized literature [675]), these latter two maps can be converted into an angular orientation map of the *c*-axis of the tetragonal cell with respect to the plane of polish (i.e., referred to as angle, θ, in Fig. 4.36(d)). Figure 4.36(e) then represents a map from the same area of spectral shift of the tetragonal band located at 260 cm^{-1}. However, it is hard to attribute the entire amount of spectral shift observed for this band to the presence of residual stresses developed upon sintering in the microstructural network. As a matter of fact, one should consider that thermal expansion anisotropy in the ZrO_2 tetragonal cell is significantly less pronounced than that discussed for the hexagonal cell of alumina. Accordingly, the relatively large spectral shifts detected here can be conceivably interpreted as mainly arising from the effect of local variations in oxygen off-stoichiometry on the tetragonal surface of 12Ce-TZP, which in turn represents the origin of the valence switch of cerium ions solved in this ceramic alloy. An experimental confirmation of this assertion can be given according to the stress map shown in Fig. 4.36(f), which was retrieved from the same area by means of the tetragonal Raman band located at around 145 cm^{-1} and shows, as expected, quite moderate residual stress values. Note that unlike the 260 cm^{-1} band directly related to bond stretching, the 145 cm^{-1} Raman band arises from a coupling mode related to Zr–O–Zr and O–Zr–O bending vibrations and, thus, it is conspicuously less affected by both Zr–O and Zr–O′ bond lengths [652, 676]. Furthermore, entirely attributing the shifts observed for the 260 cm^{-1} band to residual stress fields would lead to unacceptably high stress magnitudes, in contrast with the values shown in Fig. 4.36(f).

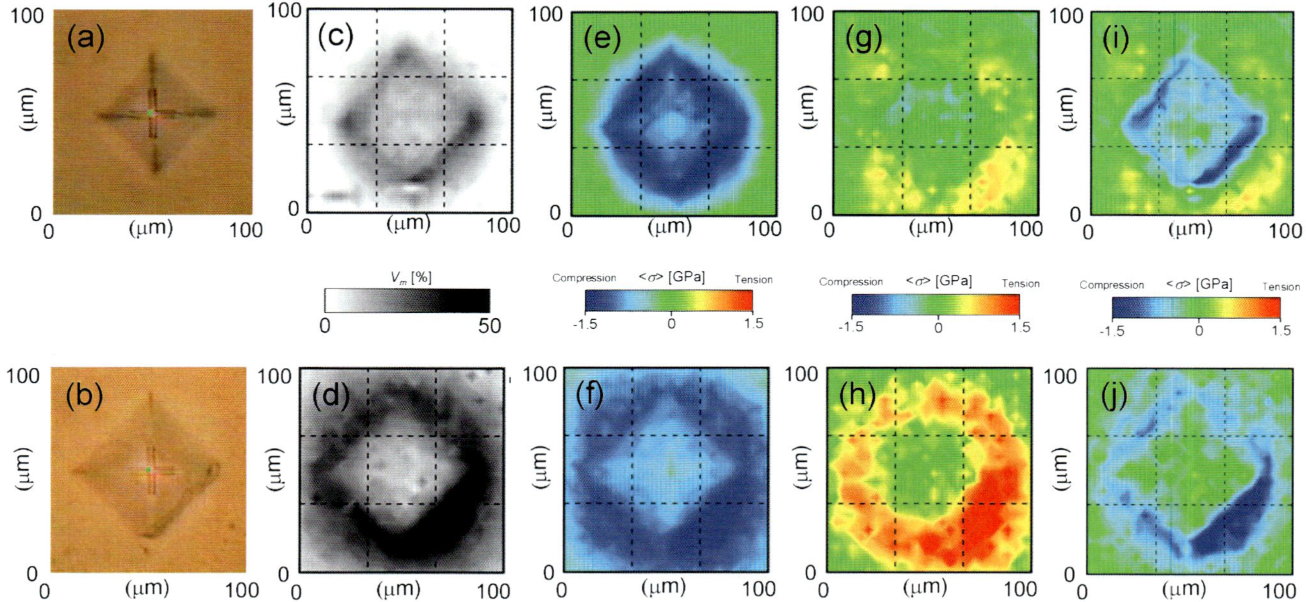

Figure 4.35 In (a) and (b), optical micrographs of Vickers indentation prints produced on the surfaces of 3Y-TZP and 12Ce-TZP, respectively. Raman maps of $t \rightarrow m$ transformation fractions are shown (c) and (d) for 3Y-TZP and 12Ce-TZP, respectively. In (e)/(g) and (f)/(h), maps are shown of residual stresses around the indentation print, as collected for the monoclinic/tetragonal phase of 3Y-TZP and 12Ce-TZP, respectively. In (i) and (j), maps of equilibrium stress are shown, which visualize the hydrostatic stress state around the indentation print under the hypothesis of an idealized material with phase homogeneity and continuum characteristics.

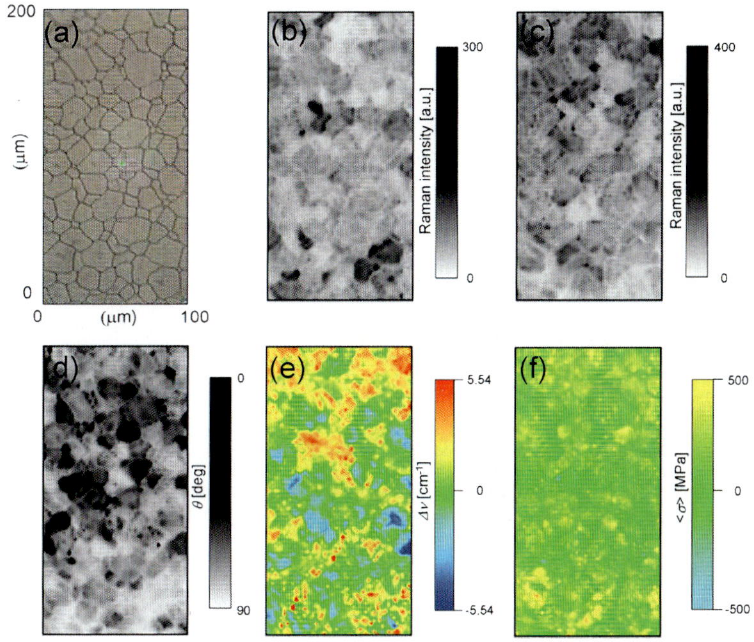

Figure 4.36 (a): Optical micrograph taken on the surface of a coarse-grained 12Ce-TZP material; (b) and (c): polarized/confocal Raman intensity maps (from the same area of (a)) of the tetragonal bands located at approximately 260 cm^{-1} (A_{1g} vibrational mode) and 145 cm^{-1} (E_g vibrational mode), respectively; (d) angular orientation map of the angle θ between the *c*-axis of the tetragonal cell and the plane of polish (θ = 0° and 90° for *c*-axis perpendicular and parallel to the plane of polish, respectively); (e) map of frequency shift, $\Delta\nu$, of the 260 cm^{-1} Raman band; and, (f): residual stress map obtained from the 145 cm^{-1} Raman band.

It is well known that oxygen mobility in zirconia is higher than in pure zirconia, when stabilization is made with cerium ions [677]. This property arises from a possible valence change of the cerium ions from 3+ to 4+ and vice versa. Accordingly, a large modulation effect in the "storage" capacity of oxygen from the environment becomes possible. The effective ionic radii of Ce^{4+} and Ce^{3+} are equal to 0.097 and 0.114, respectively (i.e., both larger than the 0.084 nm of Zr^{4+}). Upon oxygen storage in the lattice from hydrothermal environment, the volume of the compound increases in proportion to the change in cerium oxidation state. Accordingly, lattice bond stretching increasingly generates from volume expansion, which would restrict further valence change in the Ce ion. We have now located a Raman band (at 260 cm^{-1}), which appears to possess enough sensitivity for directly visualizing the material stoichiometry according to its frequency shift (cf. Fig. 4.36(e)). Pushkarev *et al.* [678] have published a similar study, although based on a different *in situ* Raman spectroscopic approach. According to Kim *et al.* [655], the frequencies of Raman modes associated with Zr–O′ bond-stretching decrease as the amount of (oversized) Ce^{4+} cations incorporated in the lattice increases. In analogy, one could expect higher positive shifts in Raman frequencies for higher vacancy contents (i.e., Ce^{3+}-rich) areas as compared to a neutral situation in which only Ce^{4+} are present in the lattice. This chemically driven Raman shift should indeed be the key for interpreting the meaning of the map shown in Fig. 4.36(e).

Ce-TZP intrinsically differs from Y-TZP because no vacancies are required for charge compensation of the stabilizer in the Ce^{4+} state. We have previously shown according to CL data and discussed that the mechanism for low-temperature degradation arises from annihilation of oxygen vacancies upon diffusion toward the material sub-surface of OH^- ions. While the lack of oxygen vacancies in Ce-TZP can indeed represent a valid argument for interpreting its high resistance to degradation, this argument fails to answer the question as to why Ce-TZP partly, although quite slowly, transforms. There are two possible hypotheses for explaining low-temperature degradation in the absence of charge compensating vacancies [679]: (i) native oxygen vacancies, namely those vacancies present for thermodynamic equilibrium at the sintering temperature, are retained at room temperature and are responsible for mediating the inward diffusion of moisture species; and, (ii) there exists a finite concentration of Ce^{3+} ions in the alloyed zirconia lattice. In the case (i), it is conceivable that the concentration of native vacancies be significantly lower than that of charge compensating vacancies in zirconia stabilized by sub-valent ions. Despite possible structural differences in the vacancy sites (partly discussed at the beginning of this chapter for the case of oversized dopants), sevenfold coordinated oxygen ions around the Zr cation are an invariable feature to different lattice configurations and, thus, the different availability of oxygen vacancies to Zr^{4+} should be responsible for a more effective stabilization effect by oversized trivalent dopants. From this viewpoint, it is quite conceivable that doping by trivalent Y^{3+} cations is much more efficient in relieving oxygen overcrowding (via both oxygen vacancies generation and dilatation of the cation network) than doping by tetravalent Ce^{4+} cations. For example, this provides a sound conceptual explanation for the fact that 1.5 mol.% of Y_2O_3 is as effective as 10 mol.% of CeO_2 in stabilizing tetragonal zirconia at room temperature. The Raman data in Fig. 4.36(e) might provide new physical insight that seems to support the above hypothesis (ii) and, in addition, add evidence that an extremely various stoichiometric population exists on the surface of Ce-TZP. Interestingly, a closer comparison between maps in Figs. 4.36(d) and (e) reveals that large variations in Raman shift toward higher wavenumbers were often associated with the presence of grains oriented with their *c*-axis nearly parallel to the plane of polish (i.e., $\theta \rightarrow 90°$). In other words, the surfaces of these grains are proved to be the richest in Ce^{3+} cations and thus they represent the only planes that can potentially interact with hydroxyls through a process of vacancy annihilation.

It is interesting to mention, at this point, the results of an *ab initio* study by Eichler [680] demonstrating that oxygen diffusion in tetragonal zirconia doped by large trivalent ions can only occur perpendicular to the (001) (*c*-)axis. Diffusion along the (001) direction is limited by a huge potential barrier since the oxygen ion has to pass between two dopant ions with ionic radius bigger than that of Zr^{4+}, so that the gap between the two ions is small, and hence the barrier high. On the other hand, diffusion along the (110) direction is activated by a lower energy arising from the energy difference between the most and less favorable vacancy position along the pathway plus the diffusion barrier of an oxygen vacancy along the (110) direction. Experimentally determined values for the diffusion barrier were indeed in good agreement with the theoretical estimate by Eichler [680] and by other authors [681–683]. Data in Fig. 4.36 point to grain surfaces corresponding to crystallographic planes nearly perpendicular to the *c*-axis of the tetragonal cell as Ce^{3+}-rich areas and, thus, as preferential sites for oxygen off-stoichiometry. On the other hand, such planes are also those for which inward oxygen diffusion is strongly hampered by a huge potential barrier. It is thus suggested that the competition between favorable stoichiometric conditions and unfavorable OH^- diffusion paths represents the origin of the strong environmental resistance of Ce-TZP. From a more general perspective, Raman spectroscopy provides both direct confirmation of local off-stoichiometry processes in 12Ce-TZP and insight into their local development on the material surface.

In the stream of early reports by Hernandez *et al.* [613] and Sato *et al.* [614], Marro *et al.* [684] recently employed a procedure of uniaxial compaction of CeO_2 powder on a sintered 3Y-TZP sample followed by a post-sintering heat-treatment. This practice induced diffusion of a small concentration of cerium ions in 3Y-TZP (through a surface layer few microns in thickness, which totally prevented the formation of monoclinic phase during hydrothermal exposures as long as 30 h at 131°C. Surface modification by Ce ions produced grain growth close to the sample surface, but no degradation in hardness or elastic modulus could be found on the surface layer. This study clearly shows the possibility of producing zirconia materials with significantly improved properties by selecting a suitable blend of cation dopants. Zirconia doped or co-doped with multiple cations may provide stronger and safer alternatives to materials presently available on the market. The target is clear: to achieve the highest phase transformation effect under stress but the lowest transformation driving force in hydrothermal environment. Understanding the role of oxygen vacancies and the way they supply a diffusion path for hydroxyls from the environment is definitely the key for a successful microstructural design of advanced zirconia ceramics.

Chapter 5

Alumina–Zirconia Composites for Joint Replacement

5.1 Alumina–Zirconia Composites: A Natural Choice

Alumina–zirconia composites represent the latest development in ceramic biomaterials technology and, from the viewpoint of material design, the most natural extension of monolithic alumina or zirconia bioceramic microstructures. Such composites were originally developed in the search for an improved biomaterial that could not only preserve both biocompatibility and stability of monolithic alumina in the human body, but also display an enhanced toughness and strength performance through the exploitation of the polymorphic transformation toughening mechanism peculiarly experienced by monolithic zirconia. It was indeed long known that materials with broadly different microstructures could be achieved in the alumina–zirconia system, as reported in an early review by Claussen [685]. Originally, zirconia-toughened aluminas (henceforth simply referred to as ZTA materials) were investigated in France, Italy and Spain [686–688] in view of advanced load-bearing applications in orthopedics. One selected material obtained full qualification as a joint biomaterial and reached the orthopedic market of hip joint components in Europe in 2000 owing to the pioneering efforts of German scientists

Advanced Materials for Joint Implants
Giuseppe Pezzotti

ISBN 978-981-4316-88-0 (Hardcover), 978-981-4364-39-3 (eBook)
www.panstanford.com

[689, 690]. The selected composite was an Al_2O_3-matrix whose reinforcing phase consisted of a low-Y_2O_3-containing ZrO_2 phase and other minor fractions of oxides including chromia. This material was concurrently shown to be suitable for biomedical applications by a number of studies from different researchers [691–695]. ZTA materials are expected to combine the outstanding properties of alumina (i.e., high hardness, chemical inertness, biocompatibility, and wear resistance) with an improved fracture resistance. Similar materials have also been long and extensively used in different applications as, for example, in the field of machining and cutting tools [696, 697]. Similar to the phenomenon that we have described for monolithic zirconia polycrystals in Chapter 4, transformation of tetragonal zirconia into its monoclinic polymorph under the tensile stress field induced by a propagating crack is unanimously assumed as being the main toughening mechanism in ZTA materials. Additionally, a compressive state of residual stress developed in the alumina matrix due to a thermal expansion mismatch between the tetragonal zirconia and the alumina phases has also been suggested to contribute toughening and strengthening ZTA composites [698]. A substantial size refinement of the alumina microstructure, due to the presence of the zirconia particles, can instead be considered as being partly responsible for the significantly improved strength observed in ZTA composites above that of monolithic alumina. From a micromechanical viewpoint, internal (residual) stresses in ceramic composites pile up upon cooling from fabrication temperature, owing to thermo-elastic mismatches between their constituent phases [698, 699]. Stresses of substantial magnitude might locally generate in an alumina matrix that includes partially stabilized (tetragonal) zirconia second-phase particles, since the linear thermal expansion coefficient of the alumina matrix (i.e., $8.50 \times 10^{-6}{}^{\circ}C^{-1}$) [700] is consistently smaller that of the tetragonal zirconia particles (i.e., $10.6 \times 10^{-6}{}^{\circ}C^{-1}$) [701]. When the ZTA composite is cooled down from sintering temperature, the zirconia reinforcement contracts more than the alumina matrix, such physical circumstance resulting in a tensile stress in the particles and a compressive stress in the matrix. Although the mean residual field stress can be considered in first approximation hydrostatic, its local components might be highly anisotropic with compressive tangential stresses coexisting with tensile radial stresses at the interface between matrix and reinforcement [702, 703]. The residual stress fields developed in a ZTA microstructure upon cooling strongly affect the stress field generated ahead of a propagating crack. Tensile residual stresses in metastable zirconia particles can improve both the volume fraction and the size of transformation zone around the crack path. Moreover, when hydrostatic stresses compressive in nature pile up in the matrix phase, they can also lead to an increase of material resistance to crack propagation upon crack extension. Another interesting feature in using zirconia second-phase particles as reinforcement in analumina matrix arises from the fact that unlike the tetragonal phase, the thermal expansion coefficient of the monoclinic phase is smaller (i.e., 7.50×10^{-6}°C^{-1}) than that of alumina. This circumstance thus leads to an opposite micromechanical situation compared with the presence of tetragonal dispersoids, in which the matrix alumina and the monoclinic zirconia particles are, after sintering, under a tensile and a compressive residual stress state, respectively. Spontaneous transformation of ZrO_2 particles upon cooling was reported by Garvie and Goss to occur at $T_{st} = 1447 \pm 6$°C [704], while Sergo *et al.* [705] reported a stress-free temperature value (i.e., a threshold temperature for which residual stresses start to pile up within the constituent phases upon cooling) for ZTA materials of $T_{sf} \approx 1180$°C. Therefore, being $T_{st} > T_{sf}$, polymorphic transformation upon cooling from manufacturing temperature should be completed before thermal stresses start to pile up in the microstructure. Accordingly, even if a fraction of monoclinic phase forms upon cooling from sintering temperature in the ZTA material, one could still interpret the bulk residual stress magnitude as arising from the mismatch in thermal expansion coefficients between the Al_2O_3 matrix and the ZrO_2 dispersoids. Spontaneous transformation upon cooling of the zirconia particles from the tetragonal (t-ZrO_2, henceforth) to the monoclinic (m-ZrO_2, henceforth) polymorph can be controlled by the amount of Y_2O_3 phase incorporated in solid solution in the ZrO_2 lattice. It follows that one could in principle be able to control the fraction of monoclinic phase developed in the sintered body (and thus the "average" thermal expansion coefficient of the second-phase dispersion) through finely modulating the amount of Y_2O_3 additive. By doing so, for example, one might obtain a three-phase composite (i.e., $Al_2O_3/t\text{-}ZrO_2/m\text{-}ZrO_2$) in which the alumina matrix is, in the average, residual stress-free. In this context, however, it should also be clear that larger ZrO_2 particles transform more easily upon cooling. Therefore, controlling both average size and breadth of the ZrO_2 particle size distribution in the composite represents a crucial issue. The particle size distribution of the ZrO_2 dispersoids usually ranges between two limit values: a lower boundary, d_L, namely the size below which polymorphic transformation is completely hindered by size effects, and an upper boundary, d_U, above which spontaneous transformation fully occurs upon cooling from sintering temperature. Lower and upper boundaries for particle size, which were also found to depend on the total amount of ZrO_2 in the composite, were reported by Heuer *et al.* [706] to be 0.1~0.4 and 0.6~2 μm, respectively. The strict necessity to keep as fine as possible the grain size of biomedical ceramics, as discussed in Chapters 3 and 4, represents a further boundary condition for microstructural design of the composite. In other words, increasing the ZrO_2 grain size is usually not given consideration as a viable approach to control the fraction of monoclinic polymorph in the final ZTA microstructure, and only the amount of stabilizing Y_2O_3 phase is used as a design parameter.

In order to clarify residual stress-related concepts in a ZTA microstructure, we shall show hereafter a theoretical estimate of the average hydrostatic stress stored in the alumina matrix in the case of ZrO_2 particles with size, d, comprised within the range $d_L < d < d_U$. Computations are shown as a function of the fraction of monoclinic phase (i.e., the fraction comprised within a fixed amount of added second-phase ZrO_2 particles) that spontaneously transform during cooling from sintering temperature due either to a particle size effect or to a reduced amount of stabilizer dopant. If one consider in first approximation the misfit strain induced by thermal expansion mismatch as simply dilatational, thus neglecting any anisotropy and grain shape factors for both dispersoid and matrix phases, the average hydrostatic stress fields in the matrix, $\langle\sigma\rangle_m$, and in the dispersed particles, $\langle\sigma\rangle_p$, can be expressed as [698, 707]:

$$\langle\sigma\rangle_m = -E_m \frac{2V_{fp}\beta\alpha^*}{A} \tag{5.1}$$

$$<\sigma>_p = E_p \frac{2(1-V_{fp})\beta\alpha^*}{A}. \qquad (5.2)$$

where V_{fp} is the volume fraction of the ZrO_2 particles, E_m and E_p are the Young's modulus of the Al_2O_3 matrix and of the ZrO_2 particles, respectively; the parameters $A, \beta,$ and α^* are given by

$$A = (1 - V_{fp})(\beta + 2)(1 + \nu_m) + 3\beta V_{fp}(1 - \nu_m) \qquad (5.3)$$

$$\beta = \frac{(1+\nu_m)E_p}{(1+2\nu_p)E_m} \qquad (5.4)$$

$$\alpha^* = (\alpha_p - \alpha_m)\Delta T \qquad (5.5)$$

where ν and α are the Poisson's ratio and the thermal expansion coefficient, respectively (the subscripts "p" and "m" refer to ZrO_2 and Al_2O_3 phases, respectively); $\Delta T = T_{sf} - T_0$ refers to the temperature interval between the stress-free temperature and room temperature (i.e., ΔT = 1160°C, as discussed above, with taking T_0 = 20°C). Note that the volume fraction, V_{fp} refers to the overall fraction of ZrO_2 particles embedded in the Al_2O_3 matrix, and thus it might include both fractions of tetragonal, V_{fp}^T, and monoclinic, V_{fp}^M, phases. According to the rule of mixture, the thermal expansion coefficient of the ZrO_2 phase can be then expressed as

$$\alpha_p = \alpha_p^M V_{fp}^M + \alpha_p^T V_{fp}^T \qquad (5.6)$$

where α_p^M and α_p^T are the thermal expansion coefficients of the monoclinic and tetragonal ZrO_2 polymorph, respectively. The bulk residual stresses in the alumina matrix, and in the tetragonal and monoclinic phases should in turn obey static equilibrium, as follows:

$$<\sigma>_{eq} = V_{fm}<\sigma>_m + V_{fp}^M<\sigma>_p^M + V_{fp}^T<\sigma>_p^T = 0 \qquad (5.7)$$

where, $<\sigma>_{eq}$ is the net (hydrostatic) stress field (simply referred to as "equilibrium stress," henceforth) stored in the bulk of the material; and, $V_{fm} + V_{fp} = 1$, with $V_{fp} = V_{fp}^M + V_{fp}^T$. Assuming common values for the elastic constants of the two ZrO_2 polymorphs [701] and introducing the parameters in Eqs. (5.1)~(5.5) as listed in Table 5.1 [701,708], it is possible to obtain an estimate of the average (hydrostatic) residual stress fields stored in the Al_2O_3 matrix (as shown in Fig. 5.1) and in the tetragonal or monoclinic ZrO_2 particles. Experimental data collected by Akiniwa *et al.* [700] are plotted, which reasonably support the theoretical estimates. As seen from Fig. 5.1, for $V_{fp}^{M} = 0$, a compressive hydrostatic stress is predicted (and experimentally confirmed) in the Al_2O_3 matrix, whose magnitude increased with increasing the volume fraction of ZrO_2. On the other hand, for $V_{fp}^{T} = 0$, a tensile hydrostatic stress is predicted in the Al_2O_3 matrix, whose magnitude increases with increasing the volume fraction of ZrO_2. For intermediate ratios, $0 < V_{fp}^{M} < 1 - V_{fm}$, the residual stress in the matrix is gradually lowered in magnitude and a matrix stress-free can be found for a fraction $V_{fp}^{M} \approx 0.55V_{fp}$. The residual stress in the tetragonal zirconia particles, which is also of some interest in the following discussions, can be shown to become strongly tensile and compressive for $V_{fp} = V_{fp}^{T}$ and $V_{fp} = V_{fp}^{M}$, respectively. In both cases, the stress magnitude is in the order of 700~800 MPa and varies only slightly with varying the fraction covered by the monoclinic polymorph within a fixed value of V_{fp}. Note that below a given threshold value for spontaneous transformation during cooling from sintering temperature, a tensile residual stress field stored in the tetragonal ZrO_2 phase actually represents a "driving force" for polymorphic transformation to take place under the stress field of a propagating crack. It can thus increase the effectiveness of the transformation toughening mechanism through increasing both the fraction of transformed phase around the crack tip and the extension to which transformation occurs. This physical circumstance is well expressed by the concept of "intensity of the transformation," which was first put forward by Budiansky *et al.* [709] and later quantified by Amazigo and Budiansky [710] as a function of transformation strain and volume fraction of transformed material. A material showing a small value of transformed volume fraction under stress is a "weak transformer", as the case of a strongly stabilized tetragonal phase of ZrO_2. A strong stabilization, thus, requires a large critical stress for conspicuously activating the crack-tip transformation mechanism; otherwise, only a toughened effect of lowered "intensity" can be obtained in the ZTA composite. In summary, the

Table 5.1 Values of elastic constants and thermal expansion coefficients for the Al_2O_3 matrix and two ZrO_2 polymorphs [701]

Phase	Thermal expansion coefficient α [°C^{-1}]	Young's modulus *E* [GPa]	Poisson's ratio ν
Al_2O_3	8.5×10^{-6}	406	0.231
m-ZrO_2	6.6×10^{-6}	243	0.310
t-ZrO_2	10.9×10^{-6}	214	0.310

Note: The values were used in calculations made by Eqs. (5.1)~(5.5).

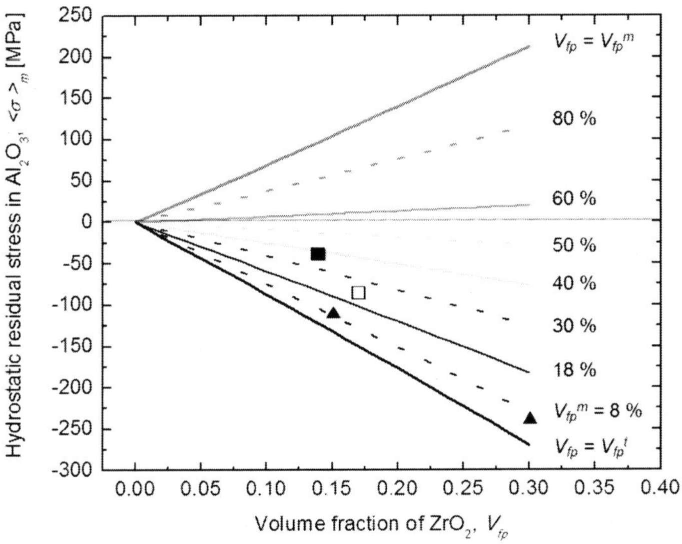

Figure 5.1 Theoretical estimate of the average (hydrostatic) residual stress fields stored in the bulk Al_2O_3 matrix, as arising from thermal expansion mismatch, in a three-phase composite made of alumina, monoclinic and tetragonal zirconia in various fractions. Experimental data are also shown, which refer to data published by Akiniwa *et al.* [700] (closed triangles), and to composites A and B (open and close squares, respectively), as discussed in the remainder of this chapter.

above considerations and (simplified) calculations provide clear vectors for design considerations and instruct us about the complexity of the microstructural design of a three-phase ZTA biomedical composite. We attempt here to summarize the possible design concepts according to three rules of thumb, as follows:

(i) Residual stresses in the Al_2O_3 matrix are compressive in nature when ZrO_2 dispersoids are retained in their tetragonal phase (e.g., through Y_2O_3 addition) at room temperature. Strong compressive stresses in the matrix material can lead to an increase in crack-propagation resistance with increasing crack extension. Such toughening mechanism is additive to, but probably less effective than, the toughening effect produced by polymorphic transformation of the tetragonal ZrO_2 dispersoids.

(ii) Increasing fractions of monoclinic ZrO_2 phase in the ZTA composite (e.g., as obtained by "destabilizing" the ZrO_2 dispersoids through limited or null addition of Y_2O_3) increasingly push the residual hydrostatic stress field in the Al_2O_3 matrix toward the tensile side. The residual stress state in the Al_2O_3 matrix phase can conceivably be set at nearly zero magnitude by suitably balancing the ratio of tetragonal to monoclinic fraction.

(iii) An increasing presence of monoclinic fraction in the ZTA composite after sintering obviously reduces the amount of ZrO_2 potentially available for crack-tip transformation (and toughening), but it also enhances the magnitude of the tensile residual stress stored in the tetragonal phase after sintering. Therefore, a reduced fraction of stabilizing agent and, thus, an enhanced tensile residual stress, might make the residual tetragonal phase more prone to transformation during crack propagation. Such micromechanical circumstance might improve the "efficiency" of the transformation toughening effect by promoting a more "intense," although less extensive, shielding effect around a propagating crack.

A literature search brings about a very large number of papers aimed at empirically optimizing the microstructure of ZTA composites by using as variable parameters the grain size of the ZrO_2 starting powder and/or the amount of stabilizing element(s) contained in it (e.g., [711–714]). An instructive study by Szutkowska [715] investigated in detail the role of either fully unstabilized or Y_2O_3 partially stabilized ZrO_2 particles on the fracture toughness of ZTA composites. It was demonstrated that the two materials experienced a completely different fracture behavior, with the best results in terms of fracture toughness being achieved with the presence of unstabilized ZrO_2 particles. These results also seemed to provide an experimental confirmation about the importance of the transformation "efficiency" concept mentioned in the above point (iii). An experimental work by Shin *et al.* [716] also provides further confirmation of the thesis expressed in the above point (iii). Those researchers indeed demonstrated that the enhancement in fracture toughness due to $t \rightarrow m$ transformation depends on the fraction of monoclinic phase freshly transformed at the crack tip and around the crack path. Such fraction proved higher in the presence of fully unstabilized ZrO_2 particles. In an extensive review on transformation toughening mechanisms, Hannink *et al.* [274] stated that for significant transformation toughening to occur, the microstructure in the transformed zone must contain a component of net residual (shear) strain. As theoretical models of transformation toughening have been refined in the past, they have mainly been progressed from only considering the dilatational component of the transformation strain to increasingly recognizing the importance of a deviatoric component of strain. While a proof of this concept must await the development of an analytical tool capable of distinguishing hydrostatic and shear stress components, it is now experimentally clarified and widely accepted that it is necessary to consider a variation in the degree of transformation within the transformation zone in order to explain the different toughening behaviors found in zirconia-containing materials. As far as ZTA composites are concerned, we have shown here that even simple arguments related to thermal expansion mismatches between the (three) constituent phases and to purely hydrostatic residual stress fields can be helpful in discussing the "intensity" of the crack-tip transformation and thus of the variable toughening effect observed in different ZTA materials.

In addition to the structural performance in terms of strength and toughness, the design of a ZTA microstructure to be employed as load-bearing components in artificial joints should also fulfill additional main issues as bioinertness (i.e., particularly surface phase-stability with respect to both morphological and mechanical effects on the joint surface) and wear resistance. Based on the concepts described above, a number of design approaches become conceivable. However, it immediately appears that some combinations should be *a priori* discarded. For example, a ZTA composite in which the alumina matrix is under a strong tensile stress field would definitively prove unsuitable in terms of strength and wear-resistance performance, especially in hard-on-hard bearings. As we previously discussed in Chapter 3, in polycrystalline alumina a microscopic residual stress field piles up upon cooling as a consequence of the pronounced thermal expansion anisotropy of the corundum structure. Such thermal stress field can locally be strongly tensile and thus weaken a fraction of Al_2O_3 grain boundaries. This will in turn hinders the macroscopic material strength and lowers the wear resistance of the material. It is straightforward that an additional residual stress component of tensile nature, induced in the Al_2O_3 matrix by dispersed (monoclinic) ZrO_2 particles could exacerbate the effect of the residual stress field due to thermal expansion anisotropy, with deleterious effects on the strength and the wear resistance of the composite. Therefore, only the lower part of the plot in Fig. 5.1 is usually considered for a sound microstructural design. Owing to the above considerations, two design approaches can be conceived and have so far been followed, which in turn led to the commercialization of two different ZTA materials: (i) the ZTA so-called BIOLOX®*delta*, a material manufactured by CeramTec GmbH with about ten years of clinical records in hip replacements all over the world); and, (ii) a new ZTA material, commercialized under the brand name KM AZ209, manufactured by Japan Medical Materials Corporation (now Kyocera Medical) with so far no published clinical records. These two materials (i.e., whose microstructures are shown in Figs. 5.2(a) and (b)) will henceforth be simply referred to as composites A and B, respectively. Both ZTA materials contain a similar fraction of fine ZrO_2 particles (cf. Al_2O_3 and ZrO_2 particle-size histograms in insets to Figs. 5.2(a) and (b)) and minor fractions of oxide additives (≈3 vol.%). Composite B appears to possess a finer microstructure than composite A, with respect to both the Al_2O_3-matrix and the ZrO_2-dispersoid grains. Table 5.2 lists the compositional characteristics of the two ZTA materials. Both materials can be classified as finely structured ceramics and were reported to achieve flexural strength values well above 1 GPa [717,718]. An important difference between the two ZTA microstructures resides in the amount of stabilizing Y_2O_3-agent present in the raw ZrO_2 powder, namely 2 mol.% and zero fraction in composites A and B, respectively. This different choice in turn reflects in a different amount of monoclinic phase in the ZTA final microstructure, as developed after cooling from sintering temperature. Clearly, different criteria were followed for designing the microstructures of the two composites. However, both designs commonly hint that a reduction of Y_2O_3 content (i.e., compared with the standard monolithic 3Y-TZP material) in the ZrO_2 phase of a ZTA composite is a desirable approach in order to achieve a more tangible toughening effect. The results in Fig. 5.1 also show that owing to a different phase composition in the final microstructure, the micromechanical equilibrium between the constituent phases in terms of residual stresses could be quite different in the two ZTA materials. Predictions will be compared with experimentally measured values and the effect of the residual stress fields on toughness clarified in the following sections. Another important aspect of the microstructural design of a ZTA composite resides in the dualism between the "positive" toughening effect of $t \rightarrow m$ transformation under stress during crack propagation and its "negative" counterpart, leading to a spontaneous process of surface transformation during exposure in a hydrothermally activated environment (e.g., in the human body). We have seen in the previous chapter that both the above effects are indeed aspects of the same physical phenomenon, namely the room-temperature metastability of the tetragonal ZrO_2 polymorph. While the substantial volume expansion associated to $t \rightarrow m$ phase transformation can shield an advancing crack, it might also alter the surface topology of the joint upon *in vivo* hydrothermal attack with producing a roughening effect (cf. Sections 4.2. and 4.4). Conceivably, the monoclinic fraction of ZrO_2 formed upon cooling from manufacturing temperature would not contribute to the roughening effect, and the fraction of potential asperity sites formed by hydrothermal attack could be lower than that of materials retaining a preponderant fraction of tetragonal polymorph after sintering. Nevertheless, the actual output of different design criteria needs to be experimentally verified on a case-by-case base. In the meanwhile, it is clear at the outset that the microstructural design criterion adopted for composite A focuses on maximizing the toughening effect while keeping phase stability of the material surface within acceptable limits. On the other hand, the design criterion behind composite B mainly foresees a tendency to maximize surface phase stability while keeping the fracture toughness of the material above an acceptable value. The effectiveness of these two different approaches will be discussed and judged in some detail in the following sections of this chapter.

Table 5.2 Compositional characteristics of the investigated composites A and B

Composition	Composite A		Composite B	
Al_2O_3 [vol.%]	82.0		84.0	
ZrO_2 [vol.%]	17.0		14.0	
Other oxides [vol.%]	Cr_xO_{19}	0.5	SrO	2.0
	$SrAl_{12-x}$	0.5	TiO_2	
			MgO	
			SiO_2	

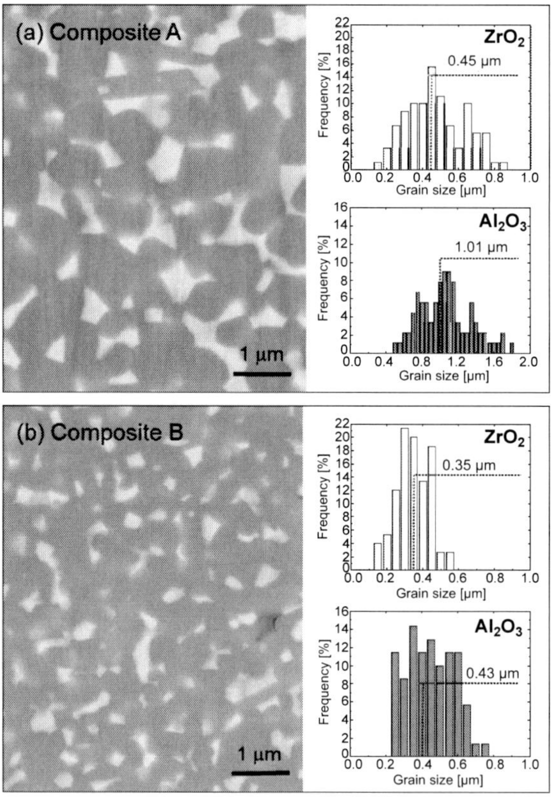

Figure 5.2 The microstructures of composites A and B are shown in (a) and (b)), respectively. Al_2O_3 and ZrO_2 grains display in the micrographs as dark and bright features, respectively. For both materials, histograms and average values of Al_2O_3 and ZrO_2 particle size are given alongside the respective SEM micrographs.

5.2 Stability, Residual Stresses and Surface Morphology Evolution in ZTA

Given the profound impact of surface phase stability on the reliability of ceramics components for artificial hip joints, as previously discussed in Chapter 4, a thorough scrutiny needs to be preliminary performed according to *in vitro* experiments, in the attempt to quantitatively estimate their actual lifetime *in vivo*. In this context, wear testing procedures conducted in hip-joint simulators have been continuously improved to better reproduce conditions the closest possible to the actual wear solicitation of the joints in the human body. The addition of realistic features to wear simulation tests is also ongoing and it certainly represents a fundamental step in properly assessing the reliability of the hip joint on the macroscopic scale. However, any substantial improvement in microstructural design of hip joints must also rely on a more profound physical understanding of the microscopic mechanisms behind wear degradation of the joint surfaces, which is the specific target of the investigations reported in this chapter. From this latter point of view, major concerns are related to the physical modifications of the ceramic joint surface as they arise from the combined effects of biological environment and wear under the unavoidable presence (and continuous evolution during exposure in the human body) of residual stress fields. Deeper understanding from the material physics standpoint is a particularly urgent requirement especially when hard-on-hard bearings are considered, because of the extreme severity of surface loading and, thus, wear damage in such circumstances. The availability of advanced spectroscopic analytical tools, capable of quantitatively scrutinize the joint surface not only on wide areas but also with high spatial resolution leads to fundamental advantages in research and development. In the previous chapters, we have already shown and discussed how confocal Raman and fluorescence spectroscopies are powerful and versatile methods for promptly analyzing the presence of different polymorphs and residual mechanical stress in ceramic materials with a high spatial resolution. In this chapter, similar to what was done in Chapters 3 and 4 for monolithic materials, we apply the Raman and fluorescence spectroscopic techniques to the quantitative evaluation of both physical and mechanical modifications of ZTA composite hip-joint surfaces, as they arise from aging in a vapor moist atmosphere. Through this spectroscopic study, a comparison is carried out between the two most advanced ceramic hip prostheses available at this time available in the biomedical market, namely those made of composites A and B, as we have introduced them in the previous section. Target of the spectroscopic investigations here is the clarification of the $t \rightarrow m$ polymorphic transformation as a function of exposure time in hydrothermal environment and its overall impact on the joint lifetime. In the following, while confirming the suitability of confocal spectroscopy as an advanced evaluation tool for artificial joint surfaces (and sub-surfaces), physical insight into understanding the possible lifetime limitations of advanced ceramic materials is also obtained, including a direct visualization of transformation and stress patterns of the joint surface under the effect of hydrothermal attack.

Figures 5.3 (a) and (b) show typical Raman spectra collected in confocal probe configuration on the surface of as-received femoral heads (in the polar region) of composites A and B, respectively. The size of the confocal probe was typically in the order of 5~8 μm in depth. Both spectra are commonly dominated by the intense Raman emission of the ZrO_2 phase versus the weaker Raman bands of Al_2O_3; among the latter ones, only the strongest band located at around 435 cm^{-1} is visible in both spectra of Fig. 5.3. However, some difference between the spectra of the two composite materials can be found in the relative intensity of bands belonging to different polymorphs of the ZrO_2 phase, which in turn represents the presence of different volume fractions in their composite microstructures. A partly transformed structure could be clearly resolved in both the as-received composites A and B, as shown by the presence of Raman bands belonging to the monoclinic polymorph (cf. bands labeled "*m*" in Figs. 5.3(a) and (b)). On the other hand, a slightly higher intensity of Raman bands belonging to the monoclinic polymorph (i.e., compared with tetragonal bands, labeled "*t*") was observed in composite B, which reveals a somewhat larger fraction of monoclinic phase already present since the manufacturing process. Figure 5.4(a) shows the evolution of the monoclinic volume fraction in the microstructure of composites A and B, respectively, as a function of aging time in a climate test chamber operating in water vapor (0.1 MPa) at 121°C. The autoclave exposure was extended up to very long duration times (i.e., up to 300 h) in order to observe the final response of the material to hydrothermal environment. As seen, composite A experienced a continuous increase of the monoclinic fraction (with a relatively high statistical scatter) from an initially low amount (i.e., in the order of few percent of the overall material) up to ≈70 vol.% of the added ZrO_2 fraction (i.e., approximately corresponding to 12 vol.% of the overall material).

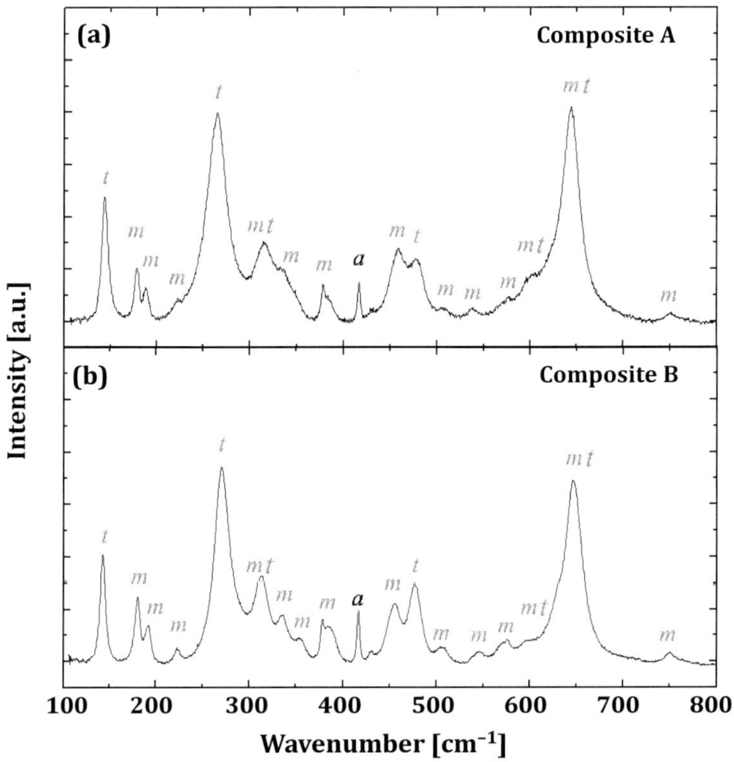

Figure 5.3 Typical Raman spectra collected in confocal probe configuration on the surface of as-received femoral heads (in the polar region) of composites A and B (in (a) and (b), respectively). The size of the confocal probe was typically in the order of 5~8 μm in depth. Bands from the alumina phase, and from the tetragonal and monoclinic polymorphs are labeled "*a*," "*t*," and "*m*," respectively.

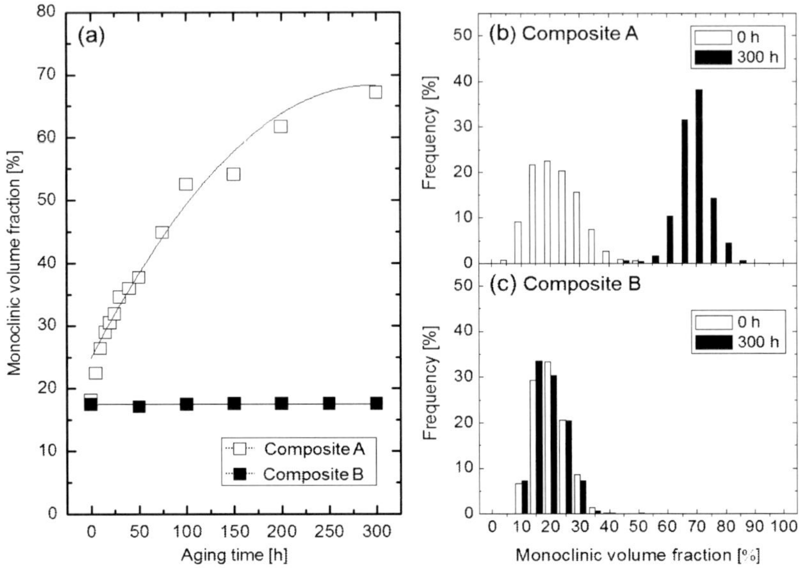

Figure 5.4 (a) Volume fraction evolution of the ZrO_2 monoclinic polymorph in the microstructure of composites A and B as a function of aging time in climate test chamber operating at 121°C in water vapor. Histograms of monoclinic phase fractions detected by the confocal Raman probe on the surface of the two studied bioceramics in the as-received state and after 300 h exposure in autoclave are given in (b) and (c) for composites A and B, respectively.

On the other hand, composite B possessed an initial volume fraction of monoclinic phase in the order of 30% of the overall ZrO_2 phase, which remained conspicuously unaltered up to 300 h exposure in autoclave. Histograms of phase fractions detected on the surface of the two bioceramics are given in Figs. 5.4(b) and (c) for composites A and B, respectively. These different phase-stability characteristics are a direct consequence of the different contents of stabilizing agents added to the raw powder mixtures of the two materials (i.e., 2 mol.% and null in composites A and B, respectively). In other words, the microstructural design of composite B enables to control the initial amount of monoclinic phase in the material and ensuring surface stability when embedded in hydrothermal environment. Such characteristics should be related on both stoichiometry and residual stress equilibrium of the material surface during exposure *in vivo*. As previously discussed in Chapter 4, there are potential drawbacks for spontaneous phase transformation in biological environment as, for example, surface roughening with subsequent acceleration of surface degradation of the conjugated acetabular cup, increased formation of fine debris, etc. The modification of the residual stress state on the surface of the joint, which accompanies the polymorphic transformation of zirconia, might also have an impact on the strength of the component and on the wear resistance of the its bearing surface. This eventuality requires precise experimental investigations, as shown in the forthcoming section 5.3. It is also conceivable that wear degradation processes are related to the presence of residual stresses in the material microstructure. Figures 5.5(a) and (b) show the evolution with aging time at 121°C (under 0.1 MPa) in water vapor atmosphere of the hydrostatic stress field stored in the main constituent phases (i.e., tetragonal and monoclinic zirconia polymorphs, and alumina phase) of composites A and B, respectively. The shown data represent stress values averaged over the femoral heads surfaces of the as-received and autoclaved samples at a large number of microscopic locations (>1000) randomly selected on the polar region of each joint. In both materials, the tetragonal zirconia phase in the as-received femoral heads was found to be under a severe tensile stress state of similar magnitude (i.e., ≈1 GPa), but the tensile hydrostatic stress revealed in the tetragonal ZrO_2 phase of composite A experienced a magnitude approximately double that of composite B. The monoclinic ZrO_2 phase underwent stresses with magnitudes in the order of 1 GPa in both the as-sintered composites. The Al_2O_3 matrices of both the as-received composites experienced stress values in line with the predictions shown in Fig. 5.1, namely both compressive in nature but of lower magnitude in composite B than in composite A. Unlike composite B, whose residual stress state was conspicuously independent of autoclave exposure, the stress fields stored in various phases of composite A changed with increasing time exposure in autoclave, as a consequence of the evolution of the environmentally driven polymorphic transformation of the ZrO_2 phase. The residual stress field related to polymorphic transformation is additive to that arising from thermal expansion mismatch upon cooling from manufacturing temperature and, in partially stabilized materials, is a consequence of the higher specific volume of the ZrO_2 monoclinic phase compared with its tetragonal counterpart. With elapsing exposure time in moist atmosphere (i.e., with progressing phase transformation), the tensile residual stress field stored in the tetragonal zirconia phase of composite A decreased significantly. On the other hand, the magnitude of the compressive residual stress stored within the monoclinic phase decreased less abruptly, retaining a considerably high magnitude even after an autoclave exposure of 300 h. The residual stress in the Al_2O_3 matrix phase gradually increased toward the tensile side with increasing aging time until reaching a magnitude of 200 MPa after 300 h aging. It is clear from the surface residual stress analysis shown in Figs. 5.5(a) and (b) that environmentally loading hip joints made of composite A promotes phase transformation and produces a significant rearrangement of the residual stress fields and of the overall mechanical equilibrium among the constituent phases of the composite. Conversely, hydrothermal attack had almost no effect on hip joints made of composite B. The residual stress values that we observed on the material surface are the result of thermomechanical interactions between the constituent phases of the composite. It should be noted that although the laser beam was focused on the surface of the joints, the laser also penetrated along the material subsurface, introducing spectral contributions from bulk regions of the sample. In such probe configuration, surface stress fields were partly counterbalanced by the residual stress fields stored within the material sub-surface. According to a procedure similar to that shown in Chapter 3 for femoral heads made of monolithic alumina, confocal stress assessments on the composite A femoral head were also performed with translating the focal plane of the laser probe toward the head subsurface. This procedure confirmed a lower amount of monoclinic phase in the material subsurface, as we will show at the end of this section. We anticipate here that the amount of monoclinic transformation in the material selectively occurs on the material surface and that the depth probed in confocal Raman experiments is comparable with the depth of the transformation zone but its emission intensity is highly graded in it. For this reason, the Raman probe is only capable to provide values of both volume fraction and stress magnitude averaged over a finite length in depth. It follows that the balance of the residual stress fields probed on the surface in the different phases might become $<\sigma>_{eq} \neq 0$. In other words, the condition of static equilibrium can only be achieved with taking into account less- or non-transformed sub-surface regions that undergo a residual stress field of opposite sign counterbalancing that stored on the material surface. Translating this notion into a static equilibrium equation among the magnitudes of the hydrostatic stress fields stored within the constituent phases leads to a modified version of Eq. (5.7), in which $<\sigma>_{eq} \neq 0$ (i.e., a zero value for equilibrium stress can only be reached when the probe fully scans the graded stress fields stored in both surface and sub-surface of the material). While bearing this important distinction in mind, Eq. (5.7) can be applied to the data shown in Fig. 5.5 in order to calculate the evolution of the equilibrium stress field piled up in the joint materials versus time elapsed while the joints are placed in the moist atmosphere. The results of this calculation are also plotted in Fig. 5.5. For the femoral head made of composite A, they show an initial moderate decrease and then a gradual increase of $<\sigma>_{eq}$ toward the tensile side with increasing aging time in hydrothermal environment. The magnitude of $<\sigma>_{eq}$ was always relatively low, in

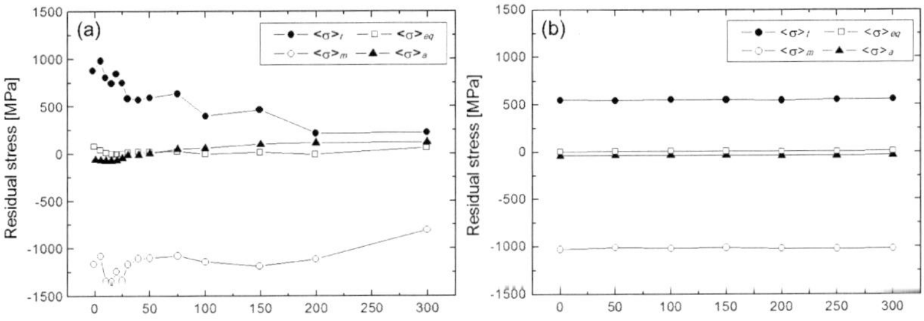

Figure 5.5 Evolution with aging time at 121°C (under 0.1 MPa) in water vapor atmosphere of the bulk hydrostatic stress field stored in the main constituent phases (i.e., tetragonal and monoclinic zirconia polymorphs, and alumina phase) of composites A and B (in (a) and (b), respectively). Each data plot represents an average over ≥1000 locations randomly selected on the polar region of each joint. Average stress magnitudes in the Al_2O_3 matrix, the tetragonal and the monoclinic ZrO_2 phases, and the equilibrium stress are indicated as $\langle\sigma\rangle_a$, $\langle\sigma\rangle_t$, $\langle\sigma\rangle_m$, and $\langle\sigma\rangle_{eq}$, respectively.

the order of the tens of MPa. On the other hand, $<\sigma>_{eq}$ was constantly zero in composite B, whatever extended is the exposure in hydrothermal environment, thus again demonstrating the microstructural phase stability of this material. While average stress data clearly demonstrate the micromechanical consequences of long-term progression of polymorphic transformation by environmental aging, the knowledge of the statistical details of both phase fractions and equilibrium stress distribution may greatly help in understanding the actual origin of the degradation phenomena observed on the joint surface. In such context, spatially resolved maps of such parameters are useful to visualize the gradients developed on the microstructural scale. Exploiting the microscopic spatial resolution of the laser probe, maps of phase fractions and equilibrium (residual) stresses stored on the surface of the composite materials can also be collected. Equilibrium stress maps can be built up by applying Eq. (5.7) to the stress magnitudes retrieved for each constituent phase at each microscopic location probed by laser. Figure 5.6 shows a comparison between phase transformation and equilibrium stress patterns (in (a), (c), (e), (g), (i) and (b), (d), (f), (h), (j), respectively) as detected in composite A as a function of increasing exposure time in autoclave at 121°C under 0.1 MPa. All maps refer to exactly the same location on the femoral head surface and thus clarify the local evolution of the physical and micromechanical state of the surface upon hydrothermal attack. As can be seen, in the as-received material (Figs. 5.6(a) and (b)), the equilibrium stress field on the joint surface is weakly tensile, while a clear intensification of residual stress can be noticed exactly in correspondence of areas where the fraction of monoclinic zirconia is smaller. A trend toward the release of tensile stresses in favor of compressive stresses was observed in areas containing an increasing fraction of monoclinic polymorph, up to about 100 h of aging time in the autoclave. Figures 5.6(c)~(f) show the pattern evolutions of both monoclinic volume fraction and equilibrium stress with increasing periods of aging up to 100 h. Interestingly, although the average equilibrium stress was found to conspicuously release in its magnitude with progressing polymorphic transformation in the ZrO_2 phase, the locations of residual tetragonal phase became "hot spots" of highly localized tensile stresses with increasing magnitude for

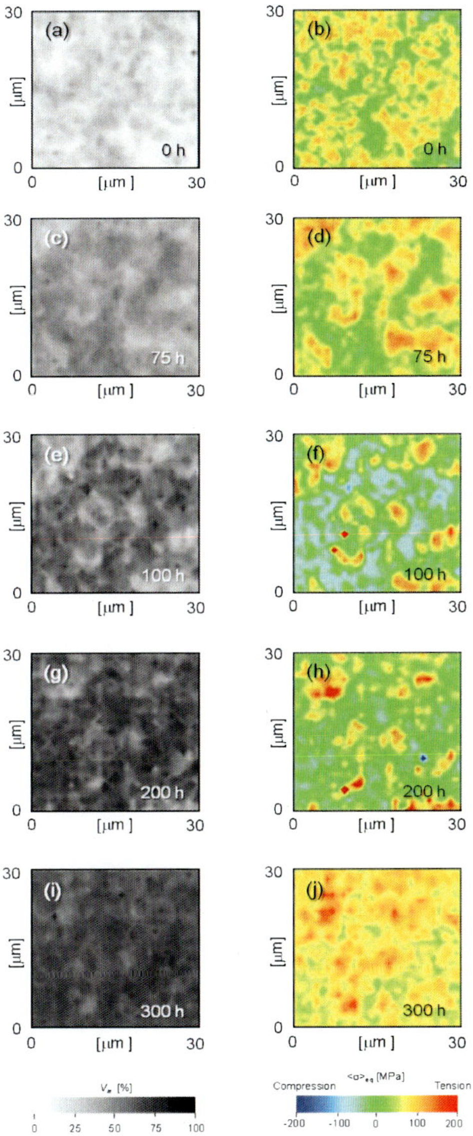

Figure 5.6 Comparison between phase transformation and equilibrium stress patterns (in (a),(c),(e),(g),(i) and (b),(d),(f),(h),(j), respectively) as mapped on the surface in composite A as a function of increasing exposure time (given in inset) in autoclave at 121°C under 0.1 MPa. All maps monitor exactly the same location on the femoral head surface at increasing exposure times in autoclave.

exposure times >100 h (cf. Figs. 5.6(g) and (h)). Beyond 200 h exposure in autoclave, the ZrO_2 phase was almost fully monoclinic over the entire joint surface and this let to the concurrent disappearance of both compressive and stress-free regions in favor of a more homogeneous tensile stress field of higher magnitude. This latter evolution is documented in Figs. 5.6(i) and (j), which both refer to 300 h exposure in hydrothermal environment. Plots showing the equilibrium stress histograms as they evolved upon hydrothermal aging are given in Figs. 5.7(a), (b), and (c) for exposures of 0, 100, and 300 h, respectively. These plots basically give the same information as the stress maps shown in Fig. 5.6, but they also help visualizing in a quantitative fashion the variation of the surface stress field upon aging. Significant broadening of the stress histogram was observed after 100 h exposure (Fig. 5.6(b)) compared with the as-received material (Fig. 5.6(a)), with the average stress magnitude being almost completely released. As a general feature, it should be noted that the edge tensile stresses of

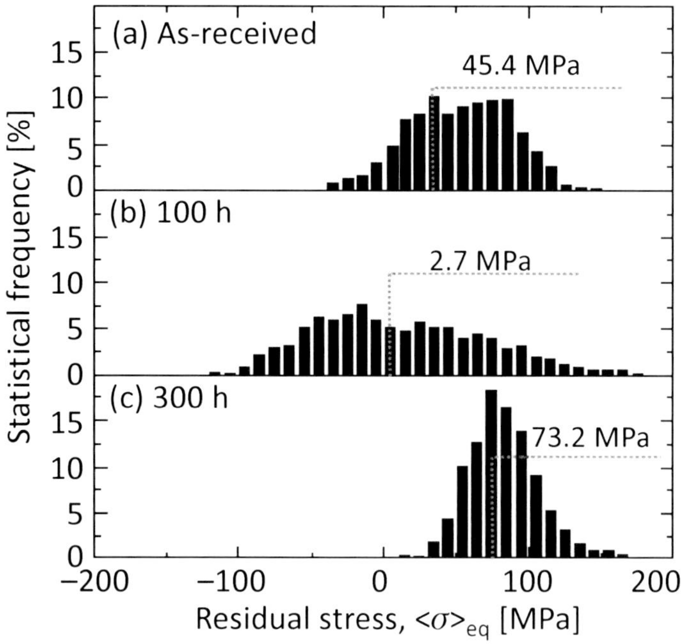

Figure 5.7 Equilibrium stress histograms as they evolved on the surface of composite A upon hydrothermal aging for 0, 100, and 300 h (in (a), (b), and (c), respectively).

the statistical distributions in Fig. 5.6, namely the hot spots observed in the spectroscopic maps collected after medium-term exposure to moist environment, are locations of possible grain detachment, thus involving a potential risk for debris formation during wear, especially under hard-on-hard wear regimes. A similar spectroscopic analysis was carried out on the surface of composite B, for which, however, no appreciable changes could be found up to exposures in autoclave as long as 300 h. Figure 5.8 shows a comparison between phase transformation and equilibrium stress patterns (in (a), (c) and (b), (d), respectively) as detected in composite B in its as-received state and after 300 h

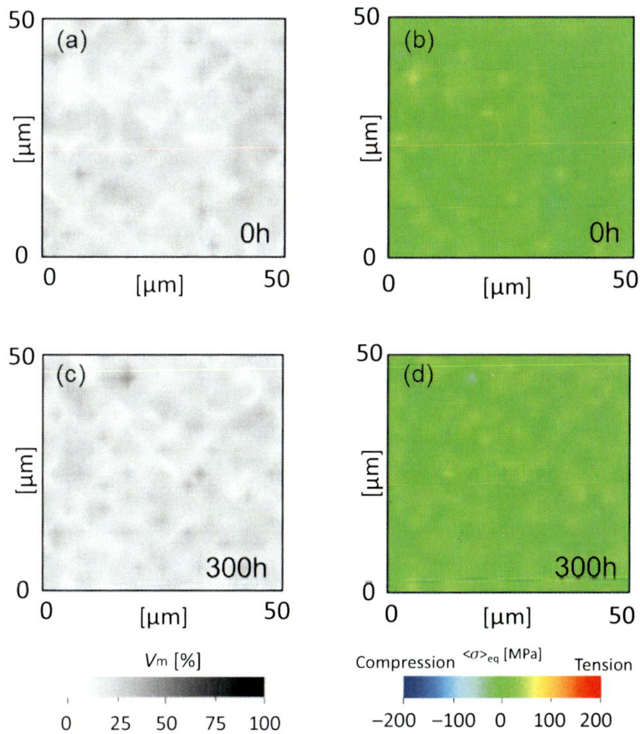

Figure 5.8 Phase transformation and equilibrium stress patterns (in (a),(c) and (b),(d), respectively) as detected on the surface of composite B in its as-received state and after 300 h exposure time in autoclave at 121°C under 0.1 MPa. Maps should be compared with those shown in Fig. 5.6 for composite A. No detectable changes were found, thus confirming that composite B is stable in hydrothermal environment.

exposure time in autoclave at 121°C under 0.1 MPa. As anticipated above, no detectable changes were found, thus confirming that composite B is stable in hydrothermal environment. Histograms of monoclinic fractions and equilibrium stresses (Figs. 5.9(a) and (b), respectively) collected on the surface of composite B confirm this conclusion, both displaying conspicuously unchanged patterns after long-term exposure in autoclave.

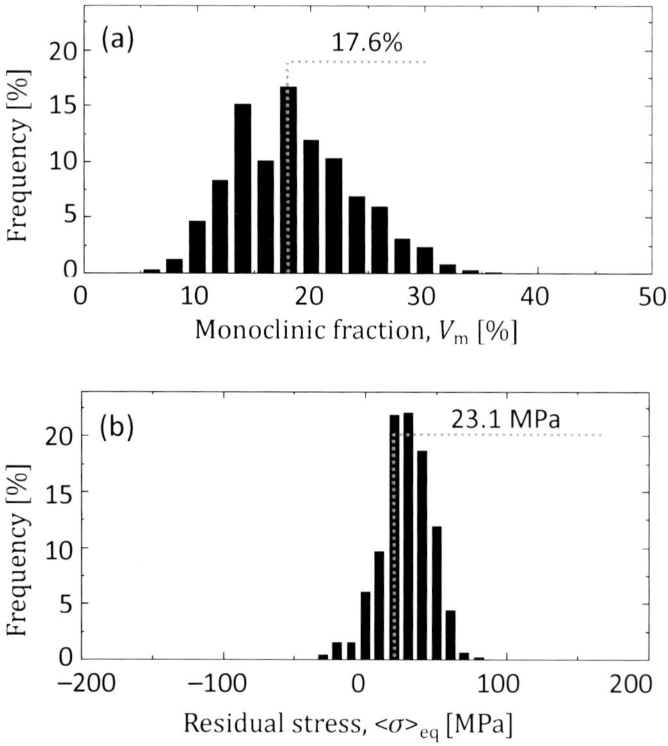

Figure 5.9 Histograms of monoclinic fractions and equilibrium stresses (in (a) and (b), respectively) collected in the neighborhood of the surface of composite B and displaying no change even after long-term exposure in autoclave. The stress histogram in (b) should be compared to those shown in Fig. 5.7 for composite A.

Now, one might wonder what could be the effect of phase instability or, from a different viewpoint, what could be the price to pay in terms of internal stresses in order to suppress it. By means of autoclave experiments, we have environmentally loaded both ZTA composites in the attempt to explore their very ultimate resistance. Thus, we can judge about the mechanisms of surface deterioration. As far as a partially stabilized tetragonal ZrO_2 phase is concerned, Sergo *et al.* [719–721] examined the effect of the residual stress fields arising from room-temperature aging of ZTA composites. These researchers found that aging of zirconia occurred spontaneously at room temperature and even under low humidity levels only when the pristine tetragonal zirconia was subjected to tensile stresses larger than ≈400 MPa. Raman experiments revealed that the residual stress level stored in the pristine tetragonal zirconia phase of composite A is by far higher than the threshold stress value reported by Sergo and Clarke [719] (cf. Fig. 5.5(a)), thus suggesting that the composite A material will necessarily undergo spontaneous transformation and local stress intensification when exposed for a sufficiently long time to the human body environment. On the other hand, phase stability in composite B could be achieved through the balancing action of strongly compressed monoclinic ZrO_2 particles entrapped in the as-sintered microstructure. This balancing effect proved effective in "stabilizing" the material response to hydrothermal environment. In the first section of Chapter 3, we have shown how the presence of second-phase particles with a lower thermal expansion coefficient at grain boundaries of the alumina matrix grains might operate a wedge-like opening effect. We additionally argue here that such wedge-like action might also promote grain pullout under wear regime. Tightly compressed particles will definitely pop out of the surface as soon as the grain boundary surrounding the mismatched particle will fracture. Indeed, zones with a relatively high density of popped out ZrO_2 grains could be extensively observed by SEM even on the surface of as-received femoral heads made of composite B. This pop-out phenomenon became significantly exacerbated when impinging on the surface of composite B with a Vickers (pyramidal) diamond indenter (Figs. 5.10(a) and (b)). Raman assessments of residual stress leave open the reason why such spontaneous ZrO_2-grain pullout phenomenon could not be found in composite A, which showed the same magnitude of compressive residual stress in the monoclinic ZrO_2 phase. The answer resides in the relatively large volume along the sub-surface screened by the Raman probe, as will be clarified in the forthcoming Section 5.4. In summary, our

Raman scrutiny suggests that no microstructural design can be perfect and, apparently, two different phenomena can ultimately take place on the surface of a ZTA composite, depending on the selected microstructural design criterion, namely: (i) the formation of isolated spots of highly tensile stress in correspondence of residual tetragonal ZrO_2 dispersoids after long-term hydrothermal loading; or, (ii) the pristine (and undesired) presence of highly compressive stress spots at the grain boundaries where the monoclinic ZrO_2 dispersoids are located, which will lead to their popping out as soon as hard-on-hard wear contact will occur.

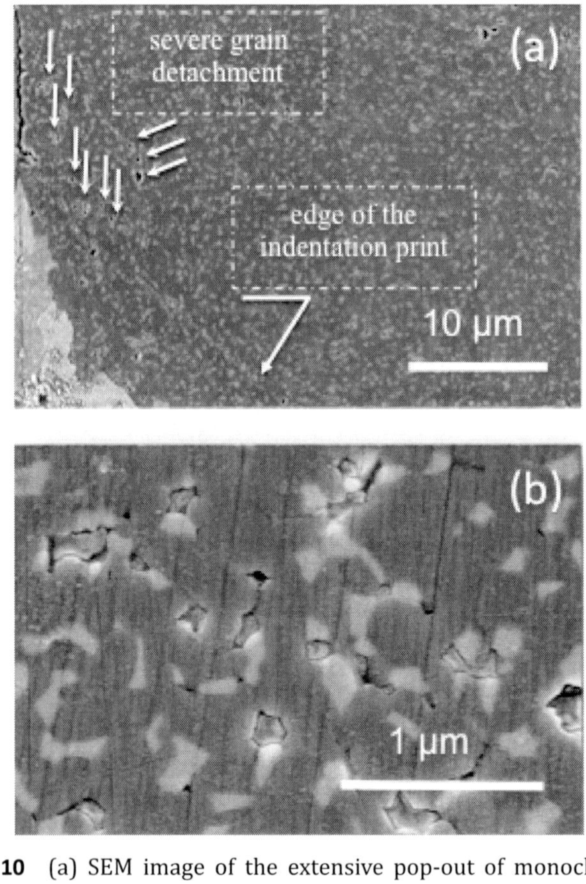

Figure 5.10 (a) SEM image of the extensive pop-out of monoclinic ZrO_2 grains observed near the edge of a Vickers indentation print in composite B; (b) higher magnification SEM micrograph of the area depicted in (a).

In the previous chapter, we have seen that for a given ZrO_2-based material, the long-term aging (in years) at the relatively low temperature of the human body can be reasonably predicted under the assumption that both formation and successive growth of monoclinic nuclei on the material surface are thermally activated. Subjecting metastable zirconia polycrystals to systematic variations of temperature for increasing periods of time has enabled us to assess a value of thermal activation energy in a controlled hydrothermal environment. The output of such experiment is represented by the measurement of monoclinic phase fraction as a function of temperature and time of environmental exposure. With the experimental knowledge of a value of activation energy, extrapolations can be made to reasonably predict the increase of monoclinic fractions *in vivo* as a function of time, although such predictions might not be conservative, because they refer to an environmental loading in the absence of external stress fields. In other words, they can only give an upper (i.e., non-conservative) limit for material stability. The theoretical background lying behind lifetime predictions for surface stability is based on the MAJ theory [644, 645], which was already applied to monolithic zirconia materials in Chapter 4. According to such theory, for example, it was found that for zirconia 3Y-TZP materials 1 hour exposure at 134°C, under 2 bar water steam is equivalent to several years exposure *in vivo*. It is emphasized again that the MAJ theory does not represent a universal law for zirconia containing materials, but it just provides a tool for rationalizing the individual environmental behavior of each particular ceramic composition and microstructure. However, provided that the activation energy is calculated from experimental kinetics measured down to sufficiently low temperatures [645], the application of the MAJ theory to different materials possess both physical meaning and useful comparative significance. The MAJ equation can be applied to composite materials in the following modified form:

$$V_M = V_0 + (V_{max} - V_0)\{1 - \exp[-(bt)^n]\} \tag{5.8}$$

where V_M is the monoclinic phase content for a given test duration, t; V_0 is the initial monoclinic phase content prior to the test, and V_{max} is an apparent upper boundary (or saturation value) for the monoclinic phase after long-term autoclave exposure. The exponent, n, is the time exponent of the MAJ equation, and b is a factor that describes the temperature dependence of the aging effect. This latter factor can be derived from fitting the experimental data according to the following Arrhenius type equation:

$$b = b_0 \exp\left(-\frac{Q}{RT}\right) \tag{5.9}$$

where b_0 is a material constant, Q is the activation energy for phase transformation during environmental aging, R the universal gas constant, and T the absolute temperature. Since composite B showed no phase transformation, we will hereafter apply the MAJ theory only to composite A. In Fig. 5.11, the experimental results of aging tests on composite A are plotted in a logarithmic time scale for different aging temperatures and best-fitted using Eq. (5.8) as a trial function. Fitting was successful over the entire interval of time investigated only for low temperatures, while aging at high temperature involved a sigmoidal shape for the MAJ plots that could not be represented by means of Eq. (5.8). Therefore, the MAJ curves plotted for temperatures >105°C are only valid for exposure times <100 h. By means of the b values obtained by such fitting procedure, an Arrhenius plot can be obtained according to Eq. (5.9) (Fig. 5.12), whose slope reveals a value of activation energy; i.e., Q = 108 kJ/mol. This represents a significantly higher value as compared with a similar composite material, for which activation energy of 78 kJ/mol was reported [722]. Such large variation shows that it is not possible to generalize values of activation energy for different ZTA materials, which thus necessarily require individual characterizations against hydrothermal attack. Figures 5.11 and 5.12 represent plots that are conceptually the same as those previously shown for monolithic ZrO_2 in Figs. 4.21 and 4.22, respectively. Hydrothermal degradation in composite A appears to be extremely slow, although still comparable to the best monolithic ZrO_2 material (i.e., sample J) investigated in Chapter 4 (cf. data in Fig. 4.21(a)). The lower Q value found for composite A compared with monolithic ZrO_2 materials (cf. Samples J and N in Fig. 4.22) is a reasonable consequence of the lower amount of the Y_2O_3 stabilizing agent used in the former material. Upon introducing the experimentally determined Q value in Eq. (5.9), substituting for the factor b in Eq. (5.8), and using a value of the exponent n obtained from the best-fitting of the experimental data ($n = 0.78$), an extrapolation of the hydrothermal aging effect under *in vivo* conditions (37°C) can be obtained from accelerated hydrothermal aging tests. For the composite A with $Q = 108$ kJ/mol, 1 h at 134°C is equivalent to 4 years *in vivo*. According to the newly proposed ISO standard 6474-2 [303], hydrothermal aging should be simulated under autoclaving conditions at 134°C for 10 hours. These conditions result to be equivalent to 40 years *in vivo* for the composite A, which seems to be a realistic upper bound for the expected life time of an artificial hip joint.

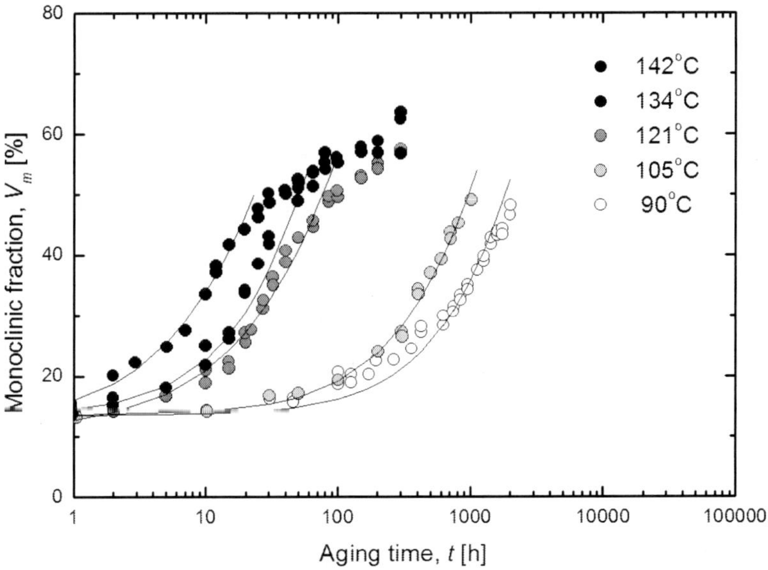

Figure 5.11 Experimental results of aging tests on composite A plotted in a logarithmic time scale for different aging temperatures and best-fitted using Eq. (5.8) as a trial function. Best fitting at $T > 105$°C was made with only including data collected at $t < 100$ h.

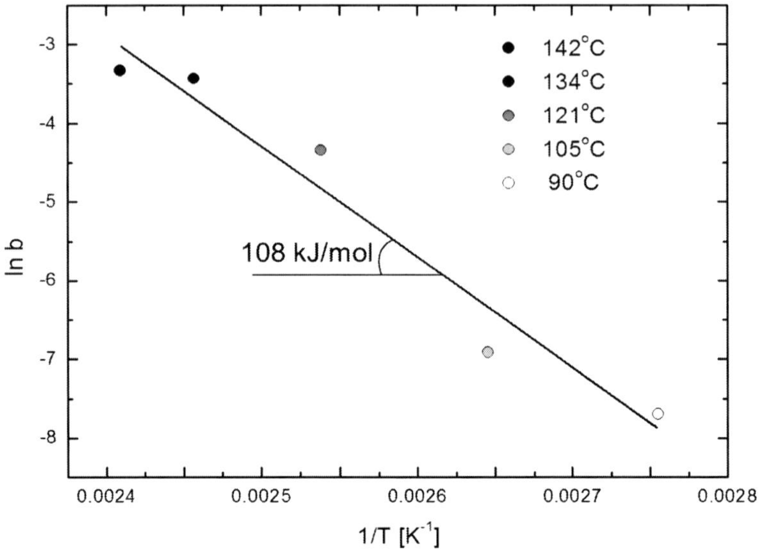

Figure 5.12 Arrhenius plot obtained according to Eq. (5.9). The slope of the plot reveals an activation energy of Q = 108 kJ/mol for surface polymorphic transformation in composite A, when exposed to hydrothermal environment.

In Chapter 1, we have already discussed how the wear debris produced by the articulation of hard-bearing femoral heads against polyethylene sockets in total hip implants can become the main cause of osteolysis [9, 17] and how this disease represents one of the most detrimental factors in the reported failure statistics of hip implants [5]. Besides improving the wear performance of the polyethylene sliding counterpart, a possibility that we will explore in detail in the next chapter, potential solutions to obtain volumetric debris reduction reside in minimizing the surface roughness of the hard bearing counterpart or in employing hard bearing surface combinations (i.e., ceramic-on-ceramic prostheses). As far as morphological characteristics are concerned, standard specifications [723] cover the design and dimensional requirements for metallic, ceramic, and polymeric mating bearing surfaces used in total hip joint prostheses. However, these specifications deal with sphericity, surface finish requirements, and dimensional tolerances, but do not address the tolerance match between the mating bearing surfaces. Concerning this latter point, time-dependent *in vivo* modifications of the microscopic surface structure (i.e., involving significant changes in friction) should be considered, and the surface roughness adequately characterized. Therefore, it is important to monitor and, ultimately, to predict through *in vitro* experiments how the morphology of the joint bearing surface will develop upon long-term exposure to biological environment. Validation of *in vitro* data remains a necessary step before proceeding with implantation in the human body but, as already discussed, it cannot represent the ultimate output of the biomaterial performance. Since composite A was introduced in 2000 in the international market, few retrieval studies have been published on the *in vivo* performance of implants made of this novel ceramic. Waiting for a chance to validate *in vitro* predictions with the analysis of retrieved implants, we aim here at clarifying the actual surface roughening effect associated to the hydrothermally activated polymorphic transformation. Obviously, in the actual *in vivo* performance of prosthetic implants, additional causes of degradation might additively occur (e.g., impingement, stripe wear, and third body wear); thus, a validation of the present data using *in vivo* exposed implants should be necessarily performed as soon as retrievals become available. Nevertheless, the experiments shown in this section represent a necessary step for providing surgeons and technologists with additional information about the actual clinical potential of femoral heads made of composite A. From a practical viewpoint, the ultimate output of an *in vitro* evaluation of hydrothermal resistance should be a predictive plot of surface roughness as a function of extrapolated exposure time in body environment. In Fig. 5.13, the results of in-depth confocal Raman spectroscopy are plotted to clarify non-destructively the impact of the phase-transformation phenomenon along the composite A joint subsurface. A comparison is carried out with the monolithic ZrO_2 femoral head ND shown in Section 4.4. The environmental response refers to aging tests of increasing time, t_{vt}, conducted in water vapor at 134°C as shown in Fig. 5.11. In the plot of Fig. 5.13(a), the thickness of monoclinic phase fraction, T^*, was defined as the distance along the joint subsurface over which the volume fraction of the monoclinic polymorph, perturbed by environmental loading, recovered to the value originally recorded on the surface of the as-received head. The plot was re-scaled in its abscissa to predict equivalent periods of time *in vivo*, t_{vv}, according to activation energy data. As seen, the thickness of material affected by an enhanced amount of monoclinic phase increased with time in both types of femoral head and, in an initial range of exposure time (t_{vt} < 10 h), its in-depth extension in the composite head was comparable to that measured in the monolithic zirconia head. In an intermediate range of time (10 < t_{vt} < 50 h), T^* appeared to be slightly larger in the composite than in the monolithic ZrO_2 material. But, after long-term exposure in hydrothermal environment (t_{vt} > 50 h), the transformation thickness in the composite head saturated at a value about a half that of the monolithic one. In the composite femoral head, the transformed subsurface thickness, T^*, remained confined to < 10 μm (with monoclinic volume fractions <10%) after *in vitro* exposures equivalent to several average human lifetimes. Although both monolithic and composite materials contain fine zirconia grains, a significantly lower fraction of zirconia dispersoids is present in the microstructure of a composite. In addition, in monolithic ZrO_2 materials, polymorphic transformation can easily spread from one grain to its neighbors, thus leading to a fast growth rate both in plane and in depth. However, in the case of a ZTA composite, such a spreading process is hindered by the main presence of alumina grains in the microstructural arrangement. Therefore, dilatational displacements do not easily pile up along the in-depth direction and the composite surface cannot undergo large surface uplifts, as in the case of femoral heads made of monolithic zirconia. This different behavior is clearly seen in comparing plots of surface roughness as a function of autoclave aging time, t_{vt} (and extrapolated to *in vivo* exposures, t_{vv}, through activation energy values) (Fig. 5.13(b)). The surface roughness in the monolithic zirconia femoral head piled up exponentially with increasing hydrothermal exposure times, while it showed only a rather small increase in composite A, despite the increase found in its surface monoclinic content (cf. Fig. 5.11).

The set of experimental data shown above addresses with a relatively high spatial resolution and statistical reliability the morphological changes that occur near the surface of femoral heads made of composite A upon quite severe exposures to a moist water environment. The results, which are relevant to wear-related and joint lifetime issues, unequivocally show that the impact of $t \rightarrow m$ transformation on the surface morphology is minimal in the composite even after very long exposures to environmental loading. Specifically, surface deterioration appears to be appreciably lower than in the case of femoral heads made of monolithic zirconia. We conclude that in the case of composite A, attack by the biological environment *per se* does not appear capable of producing any serious surface deterioration or appreciable roughening effects. It can be concluded that the observed instability in the ZrO_2 phase fraction not only can occur over quite long exposure times (i.e., when extrapolated to *in vivo* conditions), but also does not involve severe enough structural consequences to affect wear debris formation upon articulation against polyethylene sockets.

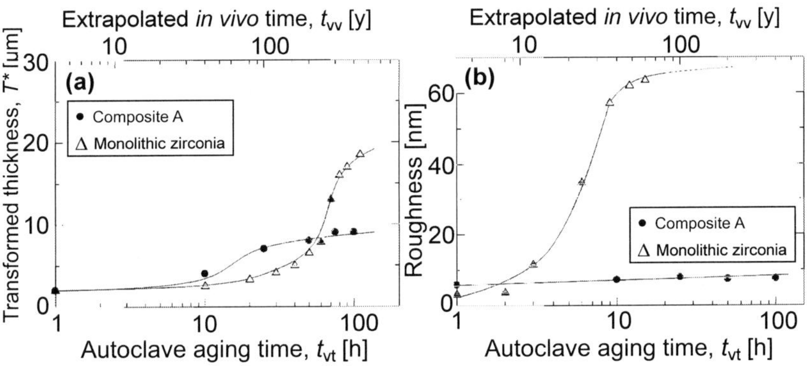

Figure 5.13 Results of in-depth confocal Raman spectroscopy along the composite A joint subsurface in comparison to the monolithic ZrO_2 femoral head ND shown in Section 4.4. Plots are given of transformed thickness (a) and surface roughness (b) as a function of hydrothermal exposure time. The environmental response refers to aging tests of increasing time *in vitro*, t_{vt} (conducted in water vapor at 134°C, as shown in Fig. 5.11) and extrapolated to *in vivo* exposures, t_{vv}, through activation energy assessments.

5.3 Toughness of ZTA Materials and Related Environmental Effects

We have previously discussed that the main advantage in adopting a ceramic-on-ceramic hip prosthesis is the reduced probability of contamination by polymeric debris (leading to osteolysis and eventually to revision surgery) as wear sub-products from polyethylene-made acetabular cups. However, if the softer polyethylene counterpart is eliminated from the joint articulation and the ceramic femoral head directly impinges on an equally hard acetabular cup, superior fracture resistance/reliability requirements become more stringent for the selected ceramic. This is particularly true when joint micro-separation processes occur in heavy-weighted patients [724], as well as in Asian patients, whose squatting and sitting attitudes require a prosthesis design with high joint deflection [62]. Furthermore, such a superior fracture behavior should be retained for long lifetimes, as expected in young patients, who are likely to select ceramic-on-ceramic joints for obtaining an enhanced motion activity. In this scenario, much expectation is placed on the development of new ceramic materials, especially ZTA composites [6,308,725,726], whose fracture behavior and reliability could be significantly improved above those of monolithic ceramics. Polycrystalline alumina indeed possesses a very low coefficient of friction, negligible wear rate and extreme chemical inertness in physiological environment, and has thus emerged as a very suitable bearing material for ceramic orthopedic joints. However, serious concerns arise from its brittleness and, thus, vulnerability to fracture, especially during unexpected loading situations. In order to counteract brittleness, a dispersion of zirconia particles is introduced in the alumina matrix to obtain a ZTA composite, whose fracture resistance can be greatly enhanced by the effect of a phase-transformation process occurring in the zirconia dispersoids [727,728]. It is the main object of this section to evaluate the effectiveness of such a toughening mechanism in ZTA composites, namely the newest generation of ceramic materials for hip joints, and to quantitatively evaluate to which extent toughening can be retained after exposing the material to long-term aging in hydrothermal environment. In particular, we examine here the fracture behavior of composite A with emphasis placed on the effect of environmental surface degradation in water vapor. Samples are taken from femoral heads exposed to accelerate aging tests (i.e., up to 300 h in autoclave operating at 121°C), which, as already discussed, represent quite severe environmental testing conditions. Besides conventional fracture mechanics characterizations, including different types of fracture toughness test, microscopic insight into the effect of environmental surface degradation on toughness are obtained according to Raman and fluorescence microprobe spectroscopy. Comparisons are also systematically carried out with composite B and monolithic alumina.

Near-tip COD assessments, as explained in section 2.6, were used for measuring the surface fracture toughness of the composite material before and after hydrothermal exposure to autoclave. Six to ten COD profiles were analyzed for each aging condition. For comparison, toughness measurements were also made from indentation crack length, according to a standard method [288]. In both types of toughness measurement on indentation cracks, indentation prints were obtained on finely polished portions of surface (i.e., as obtained from femoral heads manufacturers) with a load of 98 N. The bulk toughness of the material was assessed with fracturing bending bars, which contained a controlled flaw. Specimens for fracture mechanics testing were rectangular bending bars 3 × 4 × 20 mm in dimension. A sharp V-shaped notch with a relative length, $a/W \approx 0.4$, was introduced at their center to obtain a SEVNB configuration for fracture mechanics assessments. In order to achieve stable fracture initiation in bending geometry, the crack stabilizer designed by Nojima and Nakai for a three-point bending geometry was employed [729]. The span of the flexure jig was 16 mm and the crosshead speed was 0.005 mm/min. In low crosshead speed fracture experiments, the fracture toughness value relative to crack propagation from the notch root can be calculated according to the equation given by Srawley [730]. For comparison, bending bar samples containing a notch with the same geometry were also unstably fractured at the relatively fast speed of 0.5 mm/min and the K_{IC} value calculated from the recorded fracture load. In all fracture tests in bending, the notch configuration comprised a root radius sharpened down to 5.8 μm. All fracture data shown hereafter represent the average value of seven tested samples per each testing conditions. Both types of fracture test, by indentation and SEVNB methods, were performed on the as-received material and on the same material after long-term aging in autoclave. The impact of environmentally driven phase transformation on the material (surface) toughness can indeed be quantitatively discussed by systematically recording and comparing COD profiles from indentation cracks introduced in the material before and after environmental aging test. Indentation cracks can be considered to be near-surface equilibrium cracks, which thus are stably arrested at about their threshold stress intensity value for crack propagation, K_{IC}. Systematic COD measurements of such cracks give direct access to the inherent toughness of the near-surface portion of the material. In addition, such a toughness value may represent the crack-tip toughness of the material, namely the critical stress intensity factor for crack initiation. The K_{IC} value can be retrieved from the slope of a plot of COD vs. $8b^{1/2}F(a,x)/(\pi E')$, where $E' = E/(1 - \nu^2)$ is the plane strain elastic modulus; x, a, and b are an abscissa along the crack path (behind the crack tip and with origin at the tip), the distance between the crack tip and the geometrical center of the indentation print, and the half diagonal of the indentation print, respectively. $F(a,x)$ is a weight-function for the median surface crack configuration, as first given by Fett *et al.* [298], and recently applied and validated by Kruzic and Ritchie [731]. Figure 5.14(a) shows a SEM image of the main indentation crack path in a zone of relatively high COD values, while Fig. 5.14(b) displays a microscopically branched area in the very neighborhood of the crack tip. Both micrographs refer to composite A in its as-received state. Similar SEM pictures were used for composite B and throughout the investigation of COD assessments in the autoclave-aged materials. In Fig. 5.15, COD plots are shown as collected on typical indentation cracks introduced in composite A in the as-received state, after 10 and 300 h aging in moist atmosphere. From best-fit slopes of the plots, K_{IC} values equal to 3.2, 3.1, and 2.2 MPa × $m^{1/2}$ were found for the as-received, 10 h and the 300 h autoclaved material, respectively. The COD assessments show that nearly no effect occurs on surface toughness after 10 h aging, but also suggest that ultimately, a reduction in toughness by about 1/3 of its initial value will occur after very long-term exposure in autoclave. The reduction in toughness observed in these experiments may also represent the actual contribution of phase transformation to toughening in the as-received material. Table 5.3 shows a comparison between K_{IC} values obtained from COD measurements and those calculated according to the standard indentation method. From a comparison between the two methods, it is clear that K_{IC} values obtained from indentation crack-length measurements were systematically larger than those obtained from COD measurements. An explanation of this discrepancy will be given in a later discussion. However, it is important to note here that despite the observed discrepancy in the absolute values of toughness, a similar reduction in toughness upon autoclaving was found after both COD and indentation-crack-length measurement methods. In Table 5.3 and Fig. 5.15, a comparison is also given with monolithic alumina, which showed a surface toughness value similar to that of composite A after very long-term exposure in moist environment. In Table 5.3, the results of fracture mechanics tests performed as a function of stable crack extension from a sharp notch root are also shown. In such low cross-head speed fracture experiments, the critical stress intensity factor for crack initiation from the notch root was K_{IC} = 3.0 ± 0.24, 2.9 ± 0.20, and 2.8 ± 0.18 MPa × $m^{1/2}$, for the composite A sample as-received and aged in autoclave for 10 and 300 h, respectively. A detectably higher fracture resistance was noticed when notched samples were fractured at high crosshead speed (cf. data listed in Table 5.3). However, unlike surface toughness values, no significant difference in the toughness value could be found before and after autoclaving composite A. In other words, even very long-term autoclaving did not significantly affect the bulk toughness of the composite. In fracturing notched bars at relatively fast crosshead speed, the observed K_{IC} value was almost twice that measured at low crosshead speed. A qualitative explanation for this difference will be given in a later discussion. In this context, it is important to note that as far as the bulk toughness value is concerned, composite A remains at least as tough as monolithic alumina even after very long-term exposures in moist environment.

Table 5.3 Comparison between K_{IC} values in the as-received and autoclaved composite A, as obtained from COD measurements, standard indentation method, and SEVNB at two different crosshead speeds

	K_{IC} [MPa·$m^{1/2}$]					
			SEVNB			
Material	**IFCL**	**COD**	**0.005 mm/min**	**0.5 mm/min**	***c/a***	***E/H***
As-received	6.5 ± 0.6	3.2 ± 0.2	3.0 ± 0.24	5.7 ± 0.6	3.4	0.2
Aged for 10 h	6.5 ± 0.7	3.1 ± 0.1	2.9 ± 0.20	—	3.4	0.2
Aged for 300 h	4.7 ± 0.5	2.2 ± 0.2	2.8 ± 0.18	5.6 ± 0.4	3.8	0.2
Monolithic alumina	3.4 ± 0.8	2.2 ± 0.2	2.2 ± 0.30	—	4.8	0.3

Note: Data collected on biomedical grade monolithic alumina are also shown for comparison.

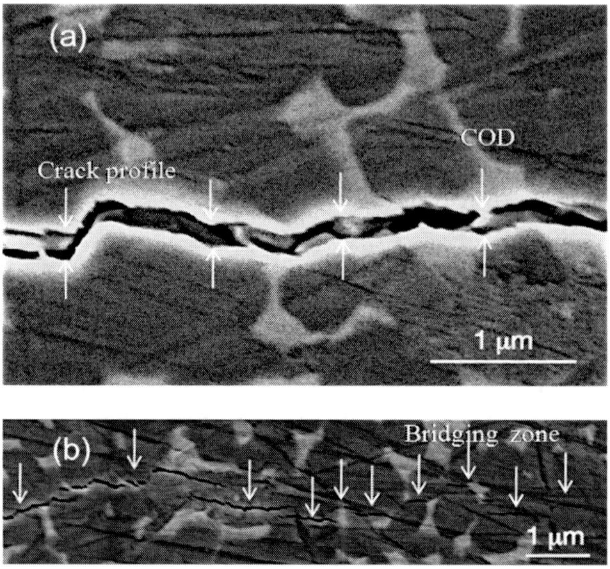

Fgure 5.14 (a) SEM image of the path of an indentation crack propagated in composite A in a zone of relatively high COD values; (b) microscopic branched area in the very neighborhood of the crack tip of the crack in (a). Both micrographs refer to composite A in its as-received state.

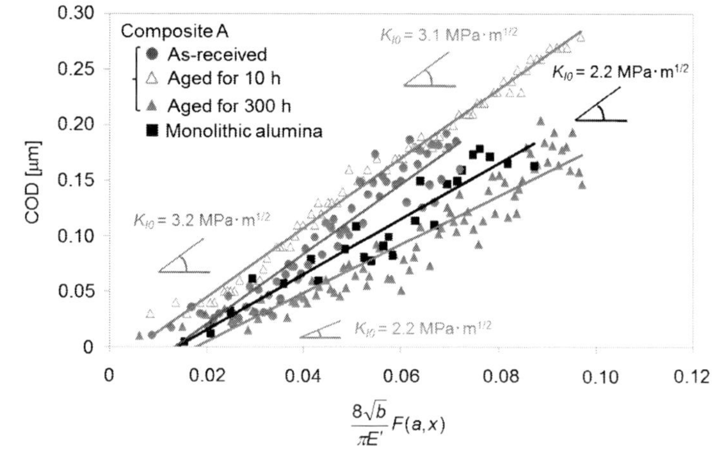

Figure 5.15 Typical COD plots collected on typical indentation cracks introduced in composite A in the as-received state, after 10 and 300 h aging in moist atmosphere. Data are compared with a profile collected on a biomedical grade monolithic Al_2O_3.

In the examination of toughness data collected on composite A by different testing methods (as listed in Table 5.3), large differences among absolute K_{IC} values (i.e., related not only to different testing methods but also to different testing conditions) can be noticed. While this observation might stress the importance of a clear specification of the testing procedure adopted before comparing toughness data from different materials, it also calls for a clarification of the physical reasons behind the observed discrepancies in measuring the toughness value. An attempt to interpret the reasons behind the observed differences in the toughness value is offered in the following.

Experimental practice has shown us that the main difficulty in measuring toughness by indentation-related methods resides in the difficulty of precisely assessing the location of the crack tip in the studied composite. As can be seen from the SEM image shown in Fig. 5.14(b), the location of the tip on crack profile in composite A typically ended with a branched morphology (cf. arrows in Fig. 5.14(b)). The linear extension of this branched portion of crack profile, which in some cases was found to be as large as 10 μm, involves a significant difference in the calculated toughness value. Excluding the branching zone from the considered crack length may lead to an overestimation of the toughness value up to about 15~20%. Toughness assessments by COD in the SEM are more reliable, but also involve a problem in using a weight function for a (branched) crack with a greatly altered geometry, compared with a standard median crack configuration. This problem is visualized in Fig. 5.16, in which the same COD profile, as collected in the as-received composite A, can be routinely best-fitted by the same weight function but selecting different crack-tip locations. The K_{IC} values obtained for different crack-tip locations are also shown in inset to Fig. 5.16. As seen, if we incorporate the branching zone in the COD profile, the computational routine leads to a poor fit to the experimental data in the neighborhood of the selected crack tip location; in addition, a lower K_{IC} value is found as compared with a fitting in which the crack tip location is selected by excluding the crack-tip branched portion from the overall crack length. The toughness value calculated by this latter approach is thus closer to the value calculated by crack-length assessment. An additional consideration about the relatively low value of fracture toughness detected by the COD method can also be stated according to the relatively long period of time (at least several hours) that elapsed until COD experiments were made in the SEM since the indentation was printed. Under such experimental conditions, a K_{I0} (rather than a K_{IC}) value is likely to be measured (i.e., $K_{I0}/K_{IC} = 0.5\sim0.6$) [271,732,733]. The difference in toughness values by SEVNB methods adopting stable and unstable crack propagation can be mainly inferred to the significant difference in crosshead speed between the two testing procedures. It has been already reported in the literature [734] that in partially stabilized zirconia ceramics, the toughness value in notched bars increased with increasing loading speed (i.e., in the same interval of the present testing procedures). This phenomenon has been explained with invoking a sub-critical formation of a shielded (pop-in) crack zone ahead of the notch root in semi-brittle materials [735]. The so-called "rule" of $K_{I0}/K_{IC} = 0.5\sim0.6$ can be invoked to empirically explain the different results [271,732,733]: in SEVNB testing conducted at fast loading speed K_{IC} is measured, while K_{I0} is likely the output of testing at slow loading speed, thus involving the detrimental effect of slow crack growth on the material crack resistance. As far as a comparison between composite A and composite B is concerned, Figs. 5.17(a) and (b) show surface K_{I0} data

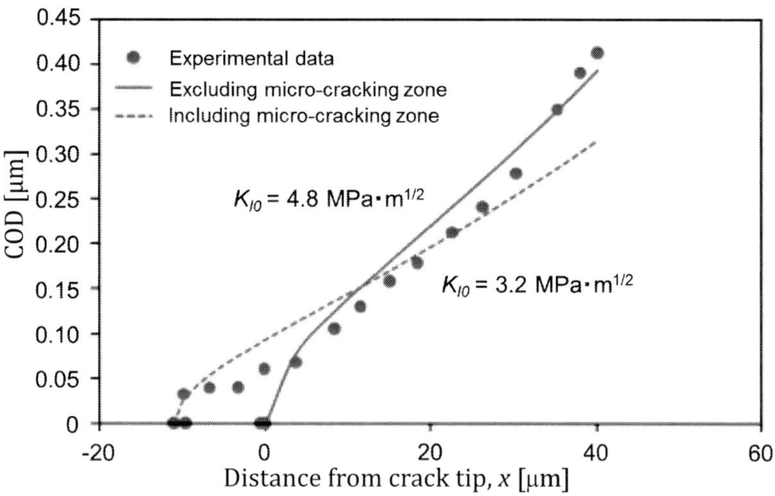

Figure 5.16 A COD profile, as collected in the as-received composite A, was best fitted by the same weight function but selecting different crack-tip locations. The different K_{I0} valuesobtained by selecting different crack-tip locations are given in inset.

collected by the COD method for the as-received and 100 h-autoclaved samples. The two composites experience a similar level of surface toughness in the as-manufactured state (cf. data shown in inset to the figures). However, while composite A experiences a reduction of about 30%, the surface toughness of composite B is almost unchanged after 100 h exposure in autoclave. This is obviously a positive consequence of the high phase stability of composite B in hydrothermal environment.

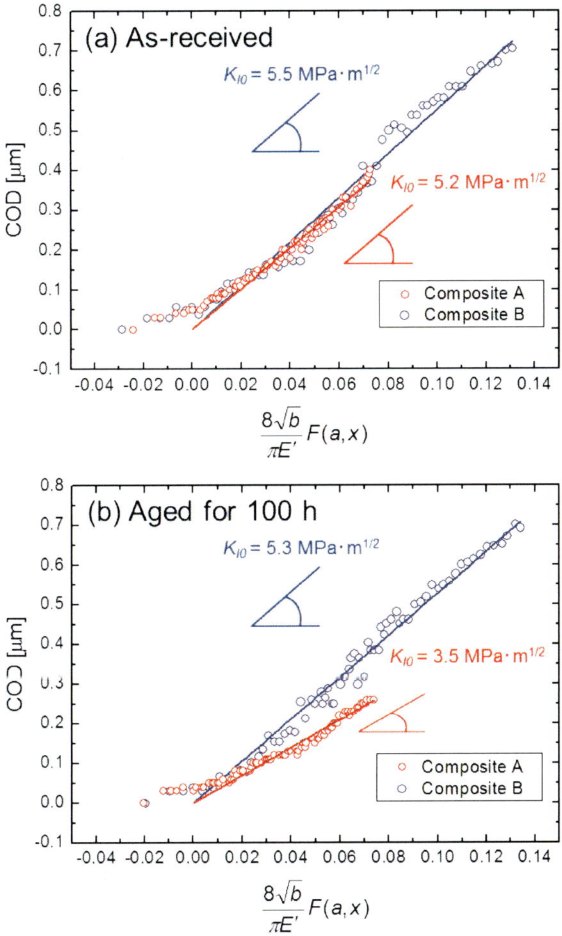

Figure 5.17 Examples of surface K_{I0} data collected in composites A and B by the COD method for as-received (a) and 100 h-autoclaved (b) samples.

Raman maps of monoclinic phase fraction are shown in Figs. 5.18(a) and (b), which were collected in the neighborhood of indentation cracks propagated in the as-received and 300 h-autoclaved composite A, respectively. From a comparison between these two maps, it can be seen that a clear phase transformation zone formed around the crack path in the as-received sample, while in the aged sample the surface crack run in a fully transformed area, with almost no possibility of newly creating a zone of additional transformation in its neighborhood. In Figs. 5.18(c) and (d), the corresponding maps of equilibrium stress are shown for samples tested before and after autoclaving, respectively. Some features in these two additional maps may support the difference found in the measured K_{IC} values before and after autoclaving process. A broader zone of stress intensification is noticed at the tip of the equilibrium crack propagated in the autoclaved material as compared with that propagated in the as-received material (thus reflecting a difference in the K-field to which the crack is embedded). Although the absolute magnitude of the measured stresses can be affected (i.e., underestimated) by the micrometer size of the laser probe, it appears that crack-tip stress intensification presumably spreads towards a larger area as compared with the as-received material, as a consequence of overlapping between the crack-tip stress field and the tensile residual stress field stored in the material surface after long-term aging in autoclave. By comparing the Raman spectroscopic maps in Fig. 5.18 and the surface toughness data in Table 5.3, it can be concluded that in composite A, the main toughening effect (i.e., about 30% increase in toughness with respect to monolithic alumina) may arise from the formation of a phase transformation zone in the neighborhood of the crack path. Note that in composite A, a contribution to toughness arising from bridging effects by platelet-like grains has also been suggested [6]. The present data instead prove that the preponderant toughening effect arises from polymorphic phase transformation, which is also supported by the rather small fraction of platelet-like grains present in the material (cf. microstructure in Fig. 5.2(a)). Similar Raman characterizations are shown in Figs. 5.19(a)~(d) for composite B. A complete lack of influence is again found for a long-term treatment in hydrothermal environment on the monoclinic fraction present of the composite, while a zone of higher transformation fractions in the neighborhood of the crack path again suggests a toughening contribution by phase transformation (cf. Figs. 5.19(a) and (b)). The crack-tip (equilibrium) stress field was also quite similar for composite B samples observed before and after aging (cf. Figs. 5.19(c) and (d)), although some stress release could be observed after aging. Such partial stress release could be associated to the same process of pulling out of monoclinic grains that was displayed in Fig. 5.10(b).

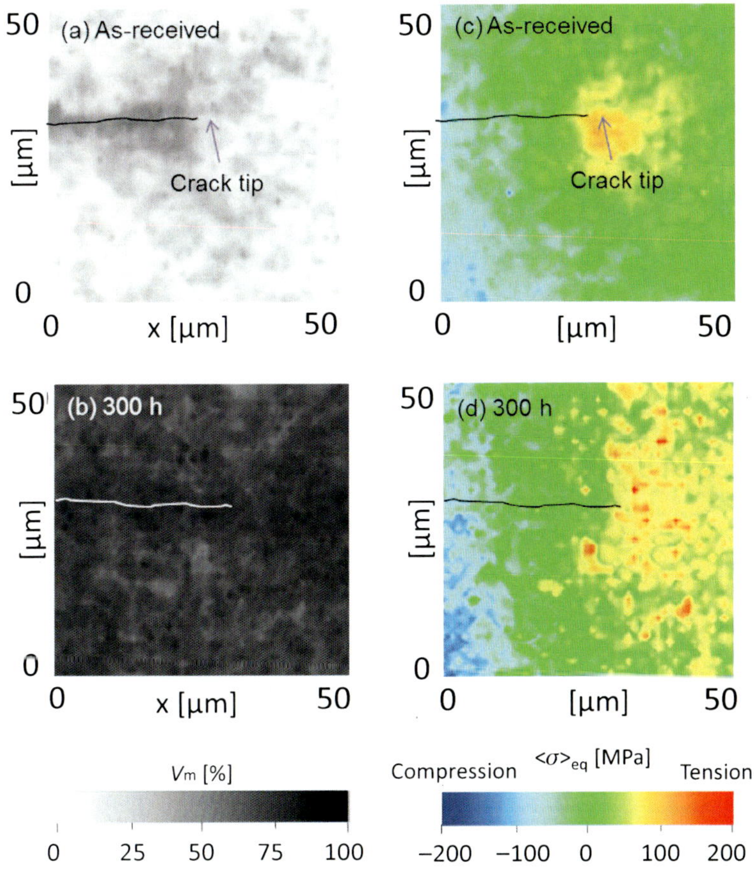

Figure 5.18 Raman maps of monoclinic phase fraction collected in the neighborhood of indentation cracks propagated in the as-received (a) and 300 h-autoclaved (b) composite A. In (c) and (d), the corresponding maps of equilibrium stress are shown for samples tested before and after autoclaving, respectively.

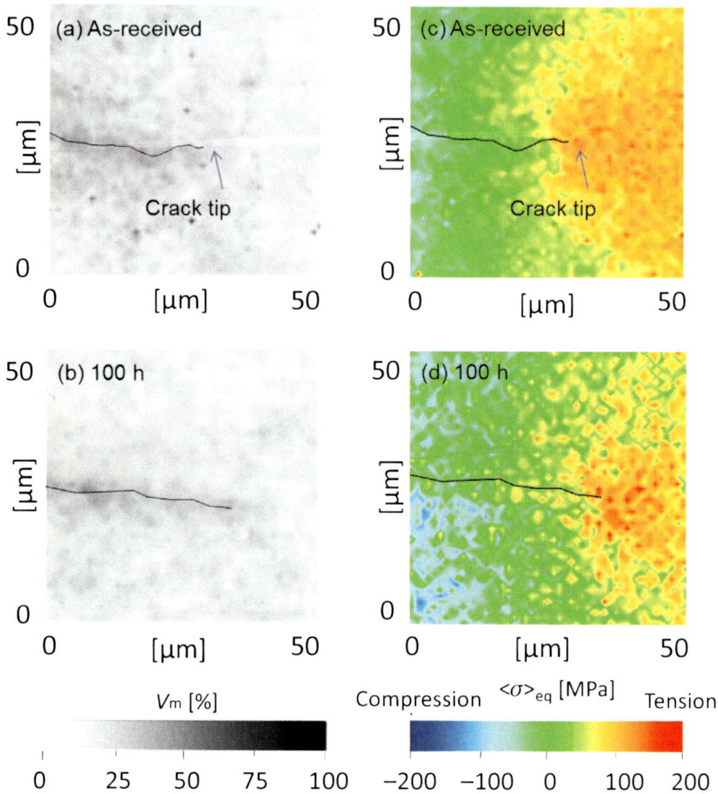

Figure 5.19 Monoclinic transformed fractions in the neighborhood of cracks propagated in composite B before and after aging of 100 h in hydrothermal environment (in (a) and (b), respectively). The corresponding crack-tip (equilibrium) stress field before and after hydrothermal aging is shown in (c) and (d), respectively.

In environmentally assisted phase-transformation processes, polymorphic changes are maximized at the sample surface and vary quite steeply with position along the *in-depth* axis. On the other hand, the Raman probe is of a finite diameter and depth, and thus the spectrum collected at each location represents an averaged (and Gaussian-weighted) Raman emission over the entire probe volume [98, 120]. The main consequence of the finite size of the probe is that even if the phase-fraction data are collected with a highly confocal microprobe configuration, they need to be treated by a mathematical deconvolution procedure to retrieve the actual *in-depth* transformation profile. The experimental profiles of monoclinic phase fraction, $V_m(z_0)$, which were collected with an *in-depth* confocal scanning along the subsurface of samples of composite A in the as-received condition and autoclaved for 100 and 300 h, are shown in Fig. 5.20. In this plot, z_0 corresponds to the *in-depth* abscissa, which locates the probe focal plane, with origin at the material surface. A positive z_0 value refers here to a translation of the focal plane below the free surface of the sample. The plot, $V_m = V_m(z_0)$, can be translated into a plot, $V_m = V_m(z)$, with z being the abscissa of the actual phase fraction distribution along the *in-depth* direction, defined similarly to z_0. In such a probe deconvolution process, the experimental profile of phase fraction is "cleaned up" from probe averaging effects [70]. The results of a mathematical deconvolution procedure are plotted in Fig. 5.20 together with the raw experimental data collected by the confocal Raman probe. The deconvoluted monoclinic fraction profile is compared with the monoclinic fraction profile typically found in the as-received material. This latter profile remained almost unaltered after 10 h exposure in moist environment. On the other hand, after exposures in autoclave as long as 300 h, the thickness of material affected by an enhanced amount of monoclinic phase increased. This particular output of the in-depth spectroscopic assessment may be invoked to explain the reason why the bulk toughness value was almost independent of autoclaving exposure time. In fact, whatever steep is the variance in the transformed near-surface portion of material, it clearly remained confined to the level of a few tens of microns even after very long-term exposure in autoclave. The actual in-depth extension of the transformation layer represents important information because it might severely affect the residual stress fields developed on the bearing surface and, thus, the wear behavior of the material. It has been reported [736] that a compressive residual stress on the bearing surface contributes to reduce both amounts of wear and friction in alumina materials. The residual stress trend found in composite A showed relatively high compressive stresses in the as-received state, and an initial moderate magnitude decrease to reach few tens of MPa in compression after about 20 h exposure (transformation thickness of about 6 μm) and then a further gradual increase of the residual stress to reach zero magnitude after about 45 h and toward the tensile side (with aging time >45 h). The detainment of a compressive stress even after relatively long exposures to hydrothermal environment might be one of the causes that makes the alumina matrix in the ZTA composite A intrinsically more wear resistant than monolithic alumina. Additional details about the surface conditions of composites A and B in comparison with monolithic Al_2O_3 will be given in the following Section 5.4, in which spectroscopic data collected with an extremely shallow CL probe will provide further insight into the physical, chemical and mechanical state of the hip joints in the very neighborhood of their bearing surfaces.

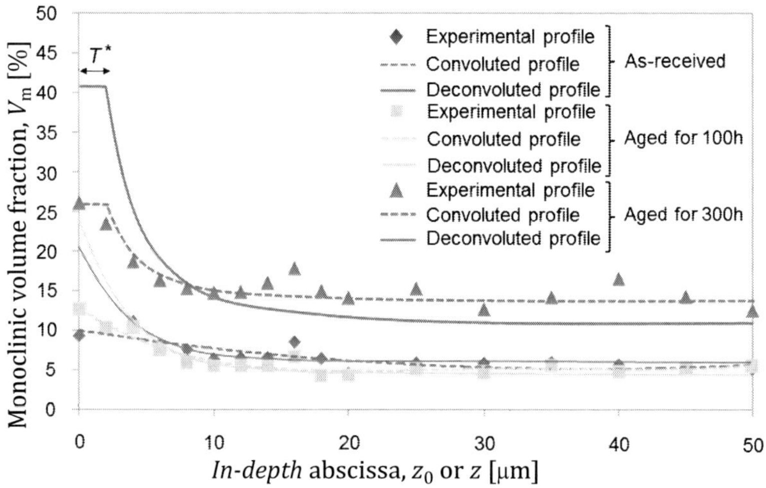

Figure 5.20 Experimental profiles of monoclinic phase fraction as collected along the *in-depth* direction by confocal scanning of composite A in the as-received condition and autoclaved for 100 and 300 h. Results of mathematical deconvolution procedures are also plotted as full lines. The *in-depth* spectroscopic assessments provide a rationale for the conspicuous invariance of bulk toughness with respect to increasing autoclaving exposure times (cf. SEVNB data in Table 5.3).

5.4 Surface Stoichiometry, Surface Stresses and Their Evolution in Hydrothermal Environment

The physicochemical processes governing surface stability in hydrothermal environment of composites A and B, namely the two leading ZTA biomaterials available in the modern market of hip-joint applications, can be investigated at the molecular scale by means of spatially and spectrally resolved CL spectroscopy. Principles of CL spectroscopy have been introduced in Chapter 2. CL characterizations are conceptually similar to those already shown for monolithic Al_2O_3 and ZrO_2 in Chapters 3 and 4, respectively. As far as composite biomaterials are concerned, we have already mentioned that the microstructures of composites A and B were designed according to completely different microstructural concepts. Quantitative CL analyses are then expected to convey different outputs, thus providing additional experimental evidence for judging about the validity of the two different design criteria. CL assessments allow concurrently monitoring oxygen sub-lattice stoichiometry and stress alterations on the surface of the joints, as they continuously evolve under the effect of hydrothermal environment. Oxygen stoichiometry and residual stresses can be tracked down at increasing times of *in vitro* environmental exposure in both Al_2O_3 and ZrO_2 phases, and the intimate relationship between the (surface) oxygen activity in the two phases clarified. It is anticipated that significantly different trends could be found between the two investigated composites, especially with respect to the delicate issues related to surface stability of the tetragonal ZrO_2 polymorph. Similar to the case of monolithic biomaterials, the off-stoichiometry characteristics of both Al_2O_3 and ZrO_2 oxygen sub-lattices play a pivotal role in the environmental behavior of hip joints made of ZTA ceramics. In addition, the presence of a minor fraction of different doping elements might induce significant differences in the hydrothermal behavior of the composites.

The CL spectra of composites A and B before and after increasingly longer exposures in autoclave are shown in Fig. 5.21. They can be analyzed according to the spectroscopic notions already stated in Chapters 3 and 4. Three characteristic spectral zones were studied in detail: (i) the interval 275~425 nm (Figs. 5.21(a) and (b)), which is dominated by the emission from F^+ centers (peaking at around 325 nm) in the Al_2O_3 lattice; namely, oxygen vacancy sites trapping one electron [471, 527]; (ii) the interval 425~575 nm (Figs. 5.21(c) and (d)), which mainly encompasses emissions from F^+ and F_A^+ centers (peaking at ≈460 and 550 nm, respectively) contained in the ZrO_2 lattice; namely, the defective sites associated to singly occupied oxygen vacancies and to oxygen vacancies embedded in complexes with Y^{3+} stabilizing ions (or other dopant/impurity elements), respectively [664, 737]; and, (iii) the interval 600~800 nm (Figs. 5.21(e) and (f)), which includes a second-order reflection of the F^{+} band of Al_2O_3 [527] and/or complex optical emissions from hydroxide groups present on its surface [528] (both types of emission are located in the same spectral interval at 600~650 nm). In both composites, the spectral region at >650 nm is dominated by emissions related to the main solute element present in the Al_2O_3 lattice (i.e., Cr and Ti for composite A

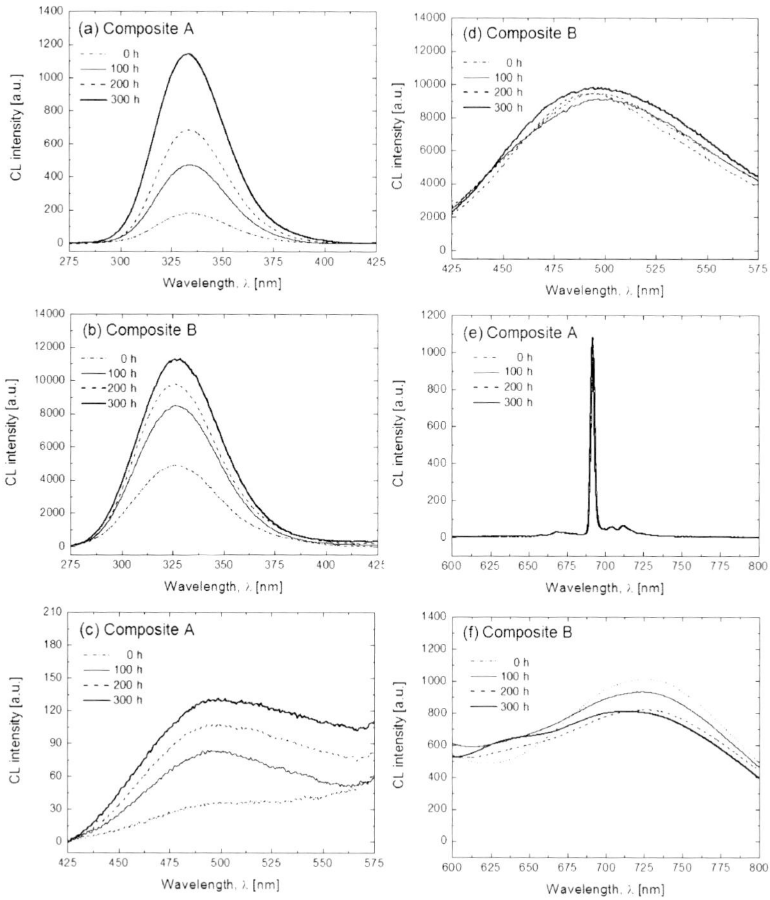

Figure 5.21 The CL spectra of the two studied composites before and after increasingly longer exposures in autoclave. Three characteristic spectral zones are shown, as explained in the text, which were relevant to the present investigations.

and B, respectively). Two spectrally close lines (the ruby doublet at 692 and 694 nm, but seen as a singlet in Fig. 5.21(e)), which relate to non-phonon radiative transitions from the first excited state ^2E to the ground state $4A^2$ of substitutional Cr^{3+} ions in the alumina lattice [738], dominate the red zone in the spectrum of composite A. On the other hand, near-infrared emission from the $^2E \rightarrow {}^2T_2$ radiative transition of Ti^{3+} ions at around 725 nm [739] is a peculiar characteristic of the CL spectrum of the Al_2O_3 lattice in composite B (Fig. 5.21(f)). Regarding the spectrum of composite B displayed in Fig. 5.21(b), the presence of a CL emission component at around 290 nm, which is lacking in the spectrum of composite A (cf. Fig. 5.21(a)) and arises from excitons localized at Ti in solid solution [739], confirms the presence of Ti ions in the Al_2O_3 lattice. In the absence of Y^{3+} or other triply charged cations, the cumulative emission at 550 nm from the ZrO_2 phase of composite B should merely arise from F_A^+ centers that are related to the intrinsic concentration of oxygen vacancies in the tetragonal ZrO_2 lattice. No CL emissions could be obviously observed from other dopants (e.g., Si^{4+} ions which, despite being a common trace element present in the structure of corundum [740], do not directly alter the oxygen sub-lattice and are optically traceless).

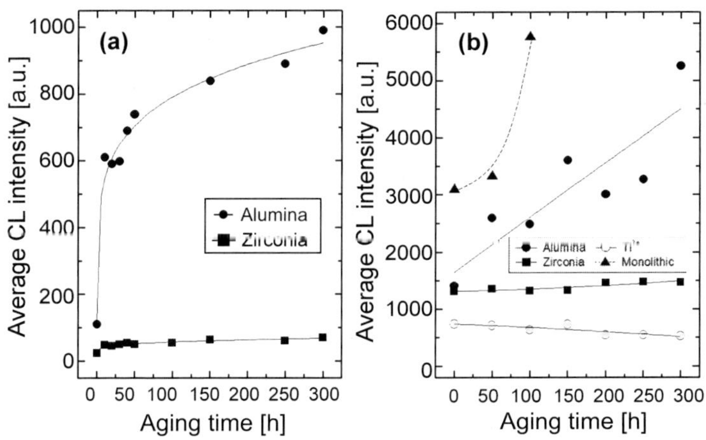

Figure 5.22 Trends found for the CL intensity of various bands as a function of exposure time in autoclave. Plots in (a) and (b) refer to composite A and B, respectively. Close circles and close squares (labeled in inset as "alumina" and "zirconia," respectively) represent F^+ centers in Al_2O_3 F^+ and F_A^+ and centers in ZrO_2, respectively. In (b), the CL behavior of monolithic alumina is also shown for comparison (close triangles labeled "monolithic" in inset).

After having categorized individual emission bands with attaching them to specific stoichiometric features, we are now ready to properly discuss the differences between lattice defect populations in the two studied composites and to interpret their structural modifications upon aging in hydrothermal environment. The trends found for CL intensity of various bands as a function of exposure time in autoclave are summarized in Figs. 5.22(a) and (b) for composite A and B, respectively. Data were rigorously collected under the same experimental conditions and can thus be compared. Relevant features and main spectral alterations related to the effect of environmental exposure can be listed as follows:

(i) The intensity of the F^+-center emission (at 325 nm) from the Al_2O_3 lattice was quite low in the as-sintered composite A compared with composite B, although it consistently increased in both composites with increasing exposure time in autoclave. This means that oxygen vacancies were increasingly created on the surface of the alumina matrix of both composites by the effect of hydrothermal treatment, but such increase started from quite different initial concentrations (i.e., significantly lower in composite A).

(ii) Emission at around 720 nm, whose intensity represents the concentration of Ti^{3+} ions in solid solution in the Al_2O_3 lattice of composite B, appreciably decreased with increasing autoclaving time, thus proving the progressive extinction of such defective sites upon autoclaving.

(iii) The cumulative intensity of the CL emission from F^+ and F_A centers (at around 460 and 550 nm, respectively), representative of oxygen vacancies in the ZrO_2 lattice, strongly increased upon autoclaving composite A but remained almost constant (at high intensity) in composite B up to 300 h exposure. Since a distorted lattice configuration leads to a more efficient CL emission compared with oxygen vacancy sites themselves [737], the intense green emission found in composite B is a consequence of the highly strained (intrinsic) oxygen-vacancy sites in its unstabilized ZrO_2 phase. Conversely, the ZrO_2 structure of composite A, relaxed by the presence of a relatively high concentration of Y^{3+}-induced oxygen vacancies, emitted a CL spectrum of rather low intensity compared with that of composite B.

The increasing trend for the F^+ emission from the Al_2O_3 lattice is the obvious consequence of a process of water-vapor dissociation producing hydroxyls and proton radicals on the Al_2O_3 surface with successive formation of oxygen vacancies for maintaining electrical equilibrium on the material surface [512] (cf. also data on monolithic Al_2O_3 in Fig. 5.22(b)). However, owing to the presence of different dopants, there are fundamental differences between the processes of vacancy formation occurring in the Al_2O_3 matrices of the two studied composites. The very low initial amount of oxygen vacancies in the Al_2O_3 phase of composite A (cf. CL intensity at 0 h in Fig. 5.22(a)) can be explained by considering that Cr^{3+} isovalent cations behave as a luminescent protection against oxygen defect formation [741]. On the other hand, Ti^{3+} ions do not possess such property, besides their incorporation in the Al_2O_3 lattice being possible without alteration of its native oxygen sub-lattice [742]. This leads to an initial concentration of oxygen vacancies in composite B in the same order as that of undoped Al_2O_3 (i.e., reported for comparison as a broken line in Fig. 5.22(b)). Despite the steep vacancy-formation rate in the first 50 h of autoclave exposure, the CL emission from F^+ centers in composite A remains always distinctly below that recorded in composite B. This indicates a systematically higher oxygen vacancy concentration in the latter biomaterial. Regarding the optical activity at around 600 nm, independent of whether it arises from oxygen vacancy or from surface hydroxide groups, it should follow the same trend as the F^+ emission at 325 nm, which is in fact what we observe in the present data (cf. Figs. 5.21(e) and (f)). Concurrent to oxygen vacancy formation, a mild decrease (with a constant gradient) in the concentration of Ti^{3+} sites is also observed in the Al_2O_3 lattice of composite B (cf. Fig. 5.22(b)). Being a donor-type dopant, Ti^{3+} sites should tend to annihilate through enhancing the incorporation of oxygen excess in the crystal lattice (i.e., with providing the electrons that are required for trapping O^{2-} from the environment). The progress of this phenomenon is indeed observed in composite B through a gradual and moderate intensity decrease of the CL band located at 725 nm (cf. Figs. 5.21(f) and 5.22(b)). However, the water-dissociative process leading to the formation of oxygen vacancies appears to be preponderant on that of oxygen incorporation as shown by the substantial increase of the intensity of the F^+ band (at 325 nm). Oxygen vacancies might then gain the outer electron of Ti^{3+} sites creating (Ti^{4+}-F^+) spatially correlated complexes in the Al_2O_3 lattice. A comparison between data in Figs. 5.4 and 5.22 suggests that a high concentration of oxygen vacancies in the Al_2O_3 lattice (i.e., a high initial content and/or their successive formation under hydrothermal attack) is a positive factor for increasing the stability of the tetragonal ZrO_2 polymorph.

As far as the information available from the CL emission of ZrO_2 is concerned, the rather high intensity of the 500 nm band from composite B reflects a strong bond straining at intrinsic vacancy sites (conspicuously unaffected by hydrothermal attack), while the weak CL emission from the ZrO_2 phase of composite A is symptomatic of a relaxed tetragonal lattice with a high initial concentration of oxygen vacancies (as expected, due to the incorporation of Y^{3+}). However, Y^{3+}-related oxygen vacancies annihilate at a significantly fast rate in hydrothermal environment (cf. Figs. 5.22(a)), and their annihilation directly triggers polymorphic transformation into the monoclinic polymorph [679, 743]. Therefore, it is confirmed that polymorphic transformation occurs as a consequence of vacancy annihilation in the tetragonal ZrO_2 lattice and it is also demonstrated that the oxygen stoichiometry data represented in Fig. 5.22 exactly reflects the different phase-stability behaviors of the two studied composites, as depicted in Fig. 5.4.

Figure 5.23(a) shows the evolution of the residual stress magnitude on the surface (values averaged over depths of about 70 nm) of the Al_2O_3 matrix phase of composites A and B as a function of aging time in a climate test chamber operating at 121°C in water vapor (i.e., the values for monolithic Al_2O_3 tested under the same conditions are also plotted for comparison as a broken line). As seen, both the recorded stress values in the as-sintered status and the successive stress evolutions are markedly different for the two composites. The Al_2O_3 phase in composite A was found undergoing a strongly compressive residual stress in its as-received state, then it experienced a steep increase toward a stress-free state (i.e., up to 50 h exposure in hydrothermal environment), and finally endured tensile stresses for further elongated autoclave exposures. Even after very long-term exposures in autoclave, the surface residual stress in composite A remained confined to a magnitude below 500 MPa. In composite B, exposures to autoclave up to 300 h produced only a mild increase on the average residual stress stored in the surface of its Al_2O_3-matrix. However, the recorded stress magnitudes, always tensile in nature, were close to 1 GPa level. Histograms of residual stress magnitudes, collected with nanometer-scale spatial resolution on the surface of the two Al_2O_3 matrices, are plotted in Figs. 5.23(b) and (c) for composites A and B, respectively. This statistical set of data differs from what was shown by Raman assessments in Section 5.2 because the CL probe screens within an extremely shallow volume below the material surface (i.e., in the nanometer scale), thus locating mechanical and chemical characteristics that can unquestionably be defined as peculiar to the material surface. Surface stress magnitudes on the material surface indeed prove being quite different from those stored in the bulk composite microstructures. One would expect that bulk residual stresses (i.e., as measured by Raman spectroscopy) mainly determine the strength level of the composite, while surface stresses (i.e., as measured by CL spectroscopy) are critical for the wear behavior of the material. In other words, the remarkably high tensile stresses found stored on the surface of the Al_2O_3 matrix in composite B, should have no significant role on the burst strength of the femoral head, but they could significantly affect the wear behavior of the components when employed in hard-on-hard joint configurations. Similar to Raman data, CL characterizations show a shift toward tensile magnitudes in the surface stress distribution stored in the Al_2O_3 matrix of composite A after hydrothermal exposure (cf. Figs. 5.5(a) and 5.23(b)). The histogram in Fig. 5.23(c), representative of composite B, confirms a mild increase of the average tensile stress magnitude upon autoclaving with no tangible broadening of its distribution even after long-term exposure in autoclave. It should also be considered that in order to achieve static equilibrium, a tensile stress state in the Al_2O_3 matrix should involve compressive stress in the ZrO_2 grains. Compressive stresses have a stabilizing effect on the tetragonal ZrO_2 polymorph [744]. However, a residual stress field of compressive nature should also be established in the immediate Al_2O_3 subsurface in order to counterbalance the tensile stress field stored on the surface. In other words, a quite steep stress gradient becomes established within a depth interval in the order of about 10 μm, which might be expected to somehow weaken the wear resistance of the material [745]. CL analyses prove, from a general viewpoint, that the residual stress state on the material surface is exacerbated with respect to the stress state in the bulk. Furthermore, a clear residual stress contribution in enhancing the environmental resistance of composite B against polymorphic ZrO_2

transformation could be achieved, but the main drawback of such phase stabilization is a strong alteration of the residual stress state of the Al_2O_3 matrix on the materials surface and, consequently, of the mechanical equilibrium between surface and sub-surface.

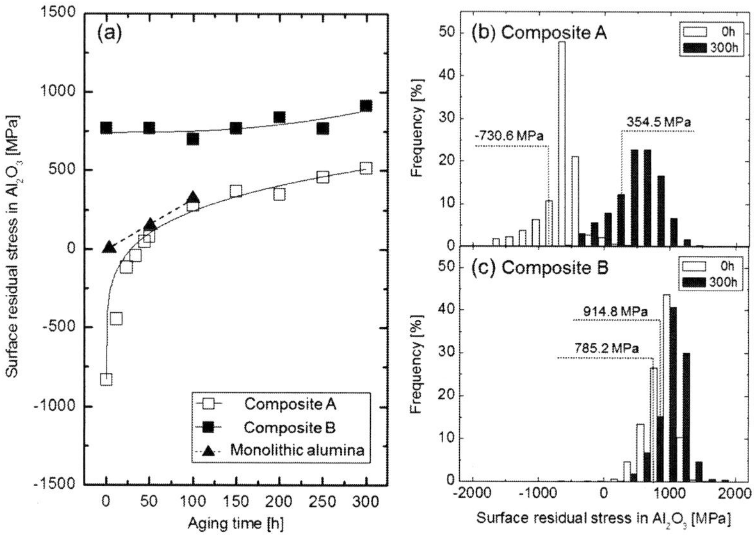

Figure 5.23 (a) Evolution of the residual stress magnitude on the surface (values averaged over depths ≤70 nm) of the Al_2O_3 matrix phase of composites A and B as a function of aging time in a climate test chamber operating at 121°C in water vapor. Surface stresses found in monolithic alumina are also shown for comparison. Histograms of residual stress magnitudes, collected with nanometer-scale spatial resolution on the surface of the two Al_2O_3 matrices, are plotted in (b) and (c) for composites A and B, respectively.

A brief review of the main causes of residual stress in Al_2O_3/ZrO_2 composites might help clarifying the origin of the different hydrothermal behaviors of the two studied composites. Contributions of different nature can affect the final stress state on the material surface: (k) thermal residual stresses, which arise from cooling from the manufacturing temperature and are caused by a mismatch in thermal expansion between the constituent phases; (kk) phase-transformation-induced residual stresses, which stem from the volume expansion that accompanies polymorphic transformation of the ZrO_2 lattice; and, (kkk) compositional (or chemical) residual stresses peculiar to the material surface, which might become significant when a strong oxygen off-stoichiometry is accumulated in the material surface (i.e., upon dopant addition combined with interactions with the environment). Thermal stresses in the Al_2O_3 matrix are expected to be of a compressive nature when the ZrO_2 phase in the composite is predominantly tetragonal, owing to the lower thermal expansion coefficient of Al_2O_3 compared with tetragonal ZrO_2 [746]. On the other hand, a stress component of tensile nature might gradually pile up in the Al_2O_3 phase in order to counterbalance the compressive stress field created in the constrained ZrO_2 grains upon their transformation into the monoclinic polymorph (i.e., accompanied by lattice expansion) [746, 747]. The lattice contraction associated with the formation of oxygen vacancies, which would lead to volume shrinkage in the absence of any constraint, instead originates a tensile stress field of chemical origin on the very surface of the Al_2O_3 phase due to the resistance operated by the (stoichiometrically unaltered) sub-surface [748]. These notions might help in rationalizing the surface stress behavior of the two composites.

As far as composite A is concerned, in a conspicuous lack of oxygen vacancies (due to the "protective" effect of the solute Cr^{3+} ions) in the Al_2O_3 matrix of the as-manufactured material and owing to the presence of only a minor fraction of monoclinic ZrO_2, the Al_2O_3 phase mainly displays the compressive thermal stress field expected from its lower thermal expansion coefficient compared with tetragonal ZrO_2. Note, however, that the compressive stress field measured on the material surface is more than one order of magnitude larger than that measured in the material bulk by Raman or fluorescence spectroscopy [749]. This latter magnitude indeed mainly reflects the effect of thermal expansion mismatch between the constituent phases (as predicted in Fig. 5.1). Additional compression stress might have piled up in the Al_2O_3 lattice of the material surface as a consequence of chemical effects (i.e., the formation of a high concentration of oxygen vacancies) peculiarly occurring in the ZrO_2 phase on the material surface during sintering. Autoclave exposure for increasingly longer periods of time then progressively introduced stress components associated to both phase-transformation and environmentally driven chemical alterations of the surface. Both these components pushed the overall residual stress field stored in the Al_2O_3 matrix toward the tensile side (cf. Fig. 5.23) until static equilibrium between surface and sub-surface could be achieved. In other words, the gradual stress increase toward the tensile side observed in composite A upon increasing autoclave exposure should be attributed to the cumulative effect of both phase-transformation and variation of surface vacancy concentrations. Bulk stress contributions only arising from transformed ZrO_2 grains lead to a linear stress increase with a significantly lower slope than what we observed here [747]. Note also that the similarity of the trends in Figs. 5.4(a) and 5.23(a) again suggests that the process of polymorphic transformation in ZrO_2 and that of vacancy formation in Al_2O_3 are related to each other. As explained above, both processes enhance the magnitude of the compressive stress stored in the residual tetragonal ZrO_2, and this explains the fact that the transformation behavior tends to saturate after long-term hydrothermal exposures. In the case of composite B, surface chemistry effects dominate the residual stress field, because neither thermal expansion mismatch nor phase-transformation-related stresses can give rise to the remarkably high tensile stress magnitude recorded in the as-received material.

A straightforward visualization of the relationship between vacancy concentration and tensile stress could be obtained by collecting CL maps at a fixed location on the surface of both composites A and B, before and after long-term exposure in autoclave. Figure 5.24 shows the evolution of oxygen vacancy population in Al_2O_3 ((a)~(e)) and ZrO_2 ((f)~(j) lattices of composite A. The corresponding evolution of surface stress field in the Al_2O_3 lattice is given in (k)~(o). Data were obtained from CL maps collected at exactly the same location on the composite surface after increasing exposure to autoclave for periods of time of 0 ((a), (f), and (k)), 10 ((b), (g), and (l)), 60 ((c), (h), and (m)), 160 ((d), (i), and (n)), and 300 h ((e), (j), and (o)). Increase and decrease of vacancy population in the Al_2O_3 and ZrO_2 lattices, respectively, are clearly envisaged by the respective increases of CL intensity. Note also the difference in CL intensity by a factor ten in the scales of the (arbitrary) intensity maps, which documents the stronger CL emission from Al_2O_3 compared with ZrO_2. The tensile stress piled up on the Al_2O_3 surface appears to exacerbate with progressing off-stoichiometry evolution in the oxygen sub-lattices of the constituent phases. Figures 5.25(a) and (b) show CL intensity maps of the F^+-center band in the Al_2O_3 lattice of composite B, in as-received and

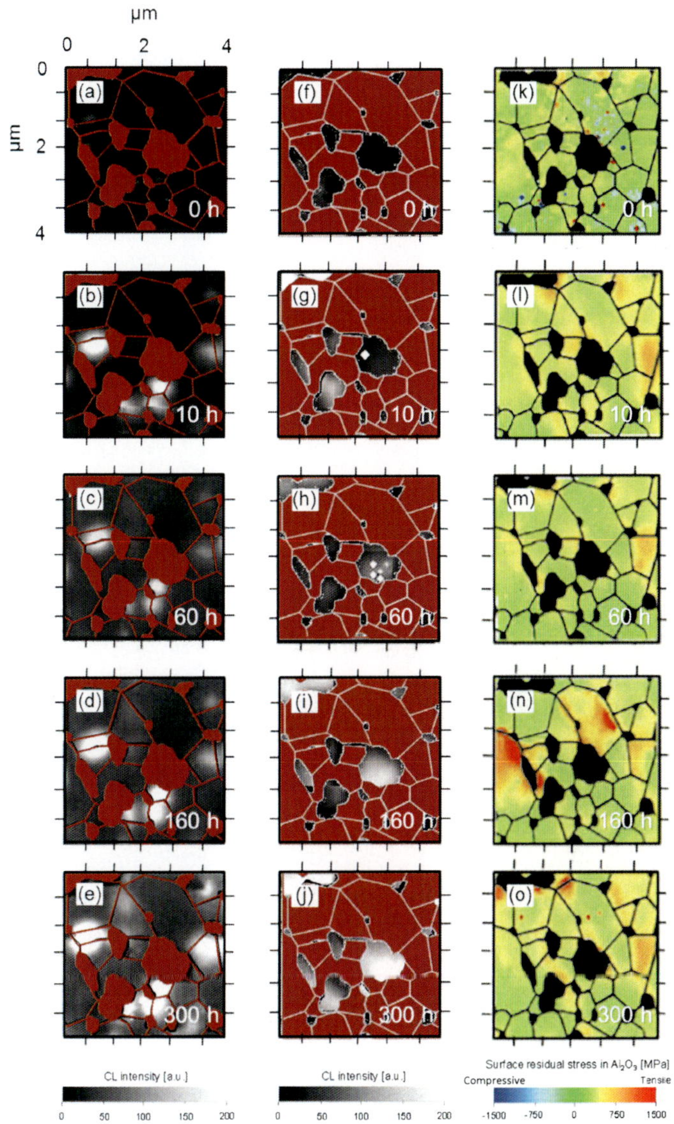

Figure 5.24 Evolution of oxygen vacancy population in Al_2O_3 (a)~(e) and ZrO_2 (f)~(j) lattices on the surface of composite A. The corresponding evolution of surface stress field in the Al_2O_3 lattice is given in (k)~(o). Data were obtained from CL maps collected at exactly the same location on the composite surface after increasing exposure to autoclave for periods of time as given in insets.

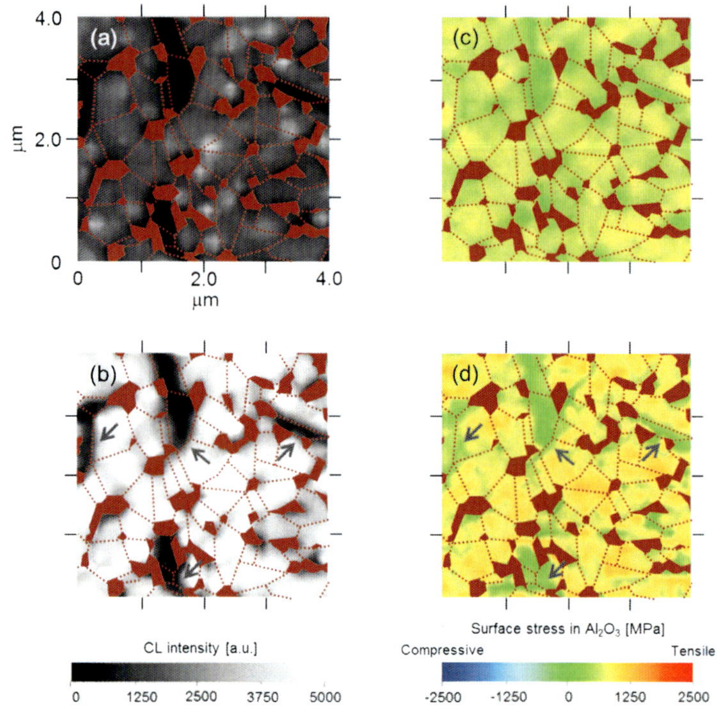

Figure 5.25 In (a) and (b), CL intensity maps of the F^+-center band (i.e., directly related to oxygen vacancy concentration in the Al_2O_3 lattice), in as-received and 300 h-autoclaved samples, respectively. The corresponding stress maps are given in (c) and (d) for as-received and 300 h-annealed samples, respectively. Arrows locate regions with low vacancy concentration, which systematically experienced low tensile stress levels.

samples, respectively) reveals that regions with low vacancy concentration systematically experienced low (or null) tensile stress 300 h-autoclaved samples, respectively. A comparison with the corresponding stress maps (Figs. 5.25(c) and (d) for as-received and 300 h-annealed levels (cf. arrow labels in Figs. 5.25(b) and (d)). Such regions, seen as dark spots in the CL intensity maps, were found by EBSD analyses to systematically correspond to Al-terminated (0001) Al_2O_3 surfaces, which are known to be stoichiometrically and energetically more stable [750]. On the other hand, areas of tensile stress intensification corresponded to highly vacancy-populated regions. Therefore, it is proved that the strong tensile stress field stored on the surface of composite B is a direct consequence of the presence of a high concentration of oxygen vacancies in the Al_2O_3 matrix. Such surface stress field induces, for maintaining static equilibrium, a strong compressive stress in the ZrO_2 grains, which in turn has the effect of completely "freezing" any environmentally driven phase-transformation effect on the surface of the material, as proved by data in Fig. 5.4(a).

In conclusion, the pivotal role of oxygen off-stoichiometry in the Al_2O_3 and ZrO_2 lattices on surface phase stability of ZTA composites for hip joint applications has been proved by means of CL analyses. The hydrothermal responses of the two leading composites presently available in the world market revealed environmentally driven modifications, both of chemical and mechanical nature, hierarchically occurring at the molecular scale on the material surface. The obtained results uncovered the behaviors of two quite different composite biomaterials with rather antithetic mechanochemical evolutions in hydrothermal environment: Composite A (containing Cr^{3+} dopant) underwent polymorphic transformation in its ZrO_2 phase upon hydrothermal exposure and experienced a compressive residual stress state in the Al_2O_3-matrix phase on its surface in the as-manufactured state, while the counterpart composite B (containing Ti^{3+} dopant) was completely stable with respect to ZrO_2 polymorphic transformation but, for gaining such phase stability, incorporated quite strong residual tensile stresses (i.e., in the GPa order) in the surface of its Al_2O_3-matrix phase. Such high tensile stresses slightly worsened upon hydrothermal exposure. While confirming the impact of lattice strain on the environmental stability of ZTA biomaterials, the present data also unfold its relationship with the oxygen sub-lattice characteristics at the molecular scale, in particular with respect to the role of the selected dopant. Through monitoring the antithetical effects of Cr and Ti ions, we could also learn about the possibility of tailoring the surface properties of ZTA materials through doping with selected elements. A tensile residual stress stored on the free surface of the material (e.g., in the case of Ti-dopant) might have serious repercussions on the wear behavior of a hip joint sliding couple, especially in the case of hard-on-hard bearings. In this context, the fact that high phase stability was achieved at the expenses of the mechanical equilibrium of the material surface and, thus, in extreme mechanical conditions of the load-bearing surface, might represent a major drawback to the lifetime of implanted hip components made of composite B in the case it being employed in hard-on-hard bearings.

5.5 Wear Resistance of ZTA vs. Monolithic Al_2O_3 Investigated by *in situ* Raman and Fluorescence Spectroscopy

Despite the large amount of investigations conducted in the past years regarding wear and frictional sliding in artificial hip joints, no attempt has been yet made to investigate the behavior of ceramic femoral heads *in situ* during wear tests. The literature on tribological assessments of artificial hip joints has been quite successful in establishing phenomenological correlations between joint composition, size, and specific wear rates, but has conspicuously ignored the physical aspects behind the occurrence of degradation mechanisms of friction and wear. In actuality, surface degradation in artificial joints occurs because of local increases in temperature and exacerbation of contact stresses at surface asperities during moving contact, as a consequence of physical and chemical modifications of the sliding surfaces. *In situ* assessments appear to be an ideal choice, besides being the only viable procedure, for obtaining physical insight into wear degradation effects. This section describes the collection of experimental data obtained by a newly developed photo-stimulated-spectroscopy-assisted tribometer that enables to investigate wear processes using *in situ* Raman and fluorescence techniques. This innovative tribometer (amply presented in Section 2.7) enables to investigate abrasive wear during frictional sliding of a rotating femoral head, which is employed, without any manipulation, as-received from the maker, against a non-rotating pin made from a sectional cut of a separate femoral head of the same type as the rotating head. The sliding geometry is specially designed to bring about not only the usual conventional outputs of tribological parameters according to international standards, but also *in situ* quantitative information of temperature, stress and phase transformation in the tested femoral heads. One main advantage, as already mentioned, is that the femoral head component can be directly tested as-received from the maker, thus avoiding any manipulation that could alter the nature of the hard-on-hard sliding counterparts. Raman and fluorescence spectra at the point of sliding contact are concurrently recorded during reciprocating hard-on-hard sliding tests. Results collected on two different types of commercially available ceramic-on-ceramic hip joints made of monolithic alumina and alumina–zirconia composites, are shown and interpreted here. The comparison is useful to judge about the obtainment of eventual improvements in the intrinsic resistance to abrasive wear, as targeted by adopting a composite ceramic microstructure rather than a monolithic one. *In situ* collected data could also be compared with the outputs of *ex situ* analyses, in order to elucidate further the nature of surface degradation processes.

The investigated sliding couples were obtained from two kinds of commercially available ceramic femoral heads, widely employed worldwide in artificial hip joints: BIOLOX®*delta* and BIOLOX®*forte* (both manufactured by CeramTec, Plochingen, Germany). BIOLOX®*delta* is the same material referred to as composite A in the previous sections of this chapter. The BIOLOX®*forte* material was made of monolithic (high-purity) polycrystalline alumina and was already introduced and characterized in Chapter 3. Composite and monolithic self-mating biomaterials are henceforth simply referred to as *delta*-on-*delta* and *forte*-on-*forte* sliding couples, respectively. All the analyzed femoral heads were 32 mm in diameter and, as already explained, were self-worn against pins made of the same material and with the same surface curvature of the femoral head. Before wear testing, both femoral head and pin were washed ultrasonically in high purity acetone for 0.5 h, then immediately rinsed with high purity ethanol and dried for additional 0.5 h at room temperature. Before clamping the sliding parts to their respective holders, their weight was accurately measured. After mounting both pin and femoral head in the tribometer machine, the eccentricity of the rotating ball was checked using a profilometer and adjusted using a bolt to reach a tolerance better than 10 μm. The pin and the attached weight system were then rotated to obtain the desired contact angle between pin and ball head (i.e., 45° in the present case). The tribometer machine was finally allocated into the Raman spectrometer equipment and the incoming laser beam (the blue line of an Ar ion laser with wavelength 488 nm) focused through a long-focus objective lens at the contact point between pin and ball. Throughout all wear tests described in this section, a load of 10 N was applied to the lever-arm device and a sliding velocity, v = 0.1 m/s, set on the tribometer controller. Tests were always divided into two steps: (i) a pre-testing step lasting about 30 minutes, in which sample positioning and various other adjustments were performed in order to allow all test parameters reaching stability; and, (ii) the main tribological test that lasted for about 6 h, which was intentionally terminated when the sliding distance reached the value of 2×10^3 m, as recommended by international standards. All wear tests were performed on self-mating couples and were carried out at room temperature under dry sliding conditions. The dynamical conditions selected for the present pin-on-ball wear testing configuration were also fixed in order to obtain a precise correspondence with the recommendations given by international standard for the pin-on-disk wear testing configuration (i.e., ASTM G99/G95, DIN 50324 and ISO/FDIS 20808:2003(E)). The interaction between laser beam and sliding couple has been explicitly analyzed in preliminary technical studies, in which a description of the complex optical interaction between laser and sliding couple at the contact point was given, together with the analytical configuration of a probe response function. Such computational procedures enable to correctly compute local values of the measured parameters at the contact point with correcting the averaging effects arising from the finite size of the spectroscopic probe [751].

At the end of the wear test, both femoral head and pin samples were ultrasonically cleaned to remove ceramic and metal debris formed at the taper joint. Then, after drying, the weights of the worn pin and ball were again measured and subtracted from the respective pristine weights recorded before wear testing. In addition, the worn surfaces were observed by optical microscopy to visualize the elliptical scar on the pin and the longitudinal scar on the femoral head, as created by the dry sliding process. Optical inspections served for a quantitative evaluation of the length of the elliptical axes of the pin scar and of the average width of the longitudinal scar on the femoral head. A profilometer stylus was also used to measure the depth in the cross sectional area of the latter scar. These geometrical parameters enabled to quantify the average volume loss and calculating the specific wear rates. The worn-out volumes of the pin, V_p, and of the femoral head, V_h, could also be calculated according to the following equations:

$$V_p = \frac{\pi a^3 b}{64R} \tag{5.10}$$

$$V_h = 2\pi r S \tag{5.11}$$

where, a and b are the lengths of the short and long axes of the elliptical pin scar, respectively; R is the radius of curvature of the pin; r is the radius of the diametral trajectory of the wear scar on the head sample, and S is its average cross sectional area. Note that Eq. (5.10) can only be used in the case of $b < 1.5a$, otherwise the wear volume must be calculated by accurately profiling the wear scar with a profilometer. The specific wear rates for the pin, W_p, and for the head, W_h, could then be calculated according to the respectively measured worn volumes, as follows:

$$W_{p(h)} = \frac{V_{p(h)}}{FL} \tag{5.12}$$

where, F is the applied force (i.e., 10 N) and L is the sliding distance applied in the wear test. The coefficient of friction, μ, a function of sliding distance, could be calculated as the ratio of the measured frictional force to the axial force component. In the characterizations described in this section, we will present both the coefficient of friction in the transient period of initial sliding and its value as successively reached at the steady state of the wear process.

During wear testing, part of the kinetic energy is converted into frictional heat, which develops from the contact zone and might result in a considerable temperature increase at the contact point between pin and ball. The outputs of a theoretical analysis can provide a solution for the heat-propagation equation from a hot-spot source of appropriate shape (i.e., in the present case, frictional heat generation from the contact Hertzian zone and transfer through the bulk in the absence of lubricant). Heat transfer can be then described by a partial differential equation, which locates the distribution of heat (or variation in temperature) in a given region over time. The final output of the theoretical analysis is to locate a temperature function at and in the neighborhood of the contact point, which in turn depends on three spatial variables and the time variable [751]. Heat conduction in a stationary medium in the case of a time dependent point source arises from the effect of heat inputs at different times, which can be considered as directly additive since heat is not a vectorial quantity. Therefore, the temperature distribution at any time can be set as the integration over time of a sequence of instantaneous sources of heat at each unit of sliding contact time. In the case of a rotating head, the contact time is given by the ratio between the diameter of the contact area between head and pin, and the rotation speed of the head. As far as the spectroscopic sensor of contact temperature is concerned, it is known that the width of the fluorescence bands of Cr^{3+} in Al_2O_3 obeys a linear dependence on temperature (0.108 and 0.077 $cm^{-1}/°C$ for the bands R_1 and R_2 of the chromophoric doublet, respectively [224, 752]). Therefore, temperature variations at the contact point can be monitored *in situ* by focusing the confocal probe at the contact point and detecting the broadening of fluorescence bands during wear testing. Note that bandwidth can also be affected by stress gradients, but such broadening is negligible in comparison with that arising from temperature increases [479]. During wear testing in the tribometer, two stress components of different nature are concurrently generated at the contact point between pin and ball: a shear stress generated by friction, and a uniaxial pressure created by the two parts in contact under load. The uniaxial pressure applied at the contact between pin and ball in turn splits into two variable stress components parallel and perpendicular to the sliding surface at the contact point, henceforth referred to as σ_{xx} and σ_{zz}, which can be theoretically expressed according to principles of Hertzian contact mechanics [753, 754]. The stress field stored on the surface around the contact point can also be determined by means of fluorescence piezo-spectroscopy, taking again advantage of the characteristic spectral shifts of the strong fluorescence bands produced by Cr^{3+} impurities in Al_2O_3. In the case of untextured polycrystalline samples, the observed spectral shift of a selected fluorescence line will depend on the magnitude (or, in the general case, on the trace) of the applied (principal) stress tensor, which is thus the *in situ* measurable quantity. The shift/stress correlation factor for the most intense chromophoric band of the fluorescence emission doublet in Al_2O_3 was experimentally determined by a preliminary *ex situ* calibration procedure in bending geometry as -2.53 cm^{-1}/GPa and -3.02 cm^{-1}/GPa, for *delta* and *forte* materials, respectively. Contact stress magnitudes can thus be retrieved from fluorescence spectra recorded *in situ* at the contact point as a function of sliding distance. However, in this case, one complication arises from the fact that fluorescence band shifts are concurrently affected by stress and temperature. Therefore, an additional computational step is needed, according to which the spectral shift components arising from stress and temperature are separated (i.e., spectral shifts computed from the known temperature field at each sliding distance were preliminary subtracted from the observed overall shifts [751]).

Monoclinic zirconia volume fractions, V_m, were quantitatively evaluated *in situ* from the relative intensities of selected Raman bands belonging to the tetragonal (145 cm^{-1}) and to the monoclinic (178 cm^{-1} and 189 cm^{-1}) polymorphs of the ZrO_2 phase. The following equation was used, according to Katagiri *et al.* [635]:

$$V_m = \frac{0.5(I_{189}^{(m)} + I_{178}^{(m)})}{0.5(I_{189}^{(m)} + I_{178}^{(m)}) + 2.2I_{145}^{(t)}} \tag{5.13}$$

where, I is the intensity of a Raman band belonging to the polymorph indicated by the superscript in brackets ((m) and (t) for monoclinic and tetragonal polymorph, respectively) and spectrally located at the frequency given in the subscript. *Ex situ* assessments of monoclinic fractions and elastic residual stresses stored on the surface of the worn samples were also made after the end of the tribological test by means of the above Eq. (5.13). In a similar way, a piezo-spectroscopic approach using the frequency shift of the chromophoric fluorescence bands emitted from the alumina phase [19,479,660] was employed to obtain an *ex situ* spatial profile of surface residual stress across the wear scar on both monolithic and composite femoral heads.

The outputs of wear tests on the two different self-mating ceramic-on-ceramic couples, namely the monolithic *forte*-on-*forte* and the composite *delta*-on-*delta* couples, are summarized and compared hereafter. Figures 5.26(a) and (b) show micrographs of the damaged zone and the related length measurements on the head side for the *forte*-on-*forte* and *delta*-on-*delta* couple, respectively. The observation refers to the worn samples at the end of the respective wear tests conducted over a sliding distance of 2×10^3 m. In the same figure, micrographs of wear scars, as observed after wear tests on the pin side, are also shown for both monolithic and composite couples (in Figs. 5.26(c) and (d), respectively). According to length measurements done on the micrographs (summarized in Table 5.4) and weight loss measurements, the specific wear rates on ball and pin could be calculated as listed in Table 5.4. Interestingly, the composite couple showed slightly wider but significantly shallower (i.e., in the order of the single micron) scar damage on the head side compared with the monolithic one. On the other hand, the damage on the pin side was detectably smaller in the composite than in the monolithic material. Accordingly, the specific wear rate of the composite sample was about 2.63 and 4.48 times lower than that of the monolithic sample for the head and the pin, respectively. The friction coefficients were also distinctly different between the two investigated couples (cf. Table 5.4), consistently showing values higher by about 12 and 20% in the *delta*-on-*delta* couple for initial and regime conditions, respectively. This difference is conceivably a consequence of the intrinsically higher coefficient of friction of zirconia compared with alumina. Figures 5.27(a) and (b) show SEM micrographs taken in the damage scar region of the *forte*-on-*forte* and *delta*-on-*delta* couple, respectively. The micrographs reveal a quite high level of surface damage in the monolithic material, with significant grain detachment. On the other hand, the damage on the surface of the composite material was limited to micro-scratches and sporadic/partial detachments, while only sporadically zirconia grains were pulled out from the worn surface (none is indeed seen in the shown micrograph). In summarizing the comparison of the tribological characteristics of the tested monolithic and composite hard-on-hard couples, it could be said that despite the conspicuously larger friction coefficient measured for the composite couple, this couple was by far more resistant to grain detachment and wore at a significantly lower rate compared with the monolithic couple.

Table 5.4 Topological, tribological, physical and mechanical outputs of wear tests performed in the newly developed spectroscopy-assisted tribometer

Parameter	BIOLOX® *forte*	BIOLOX® *delta*
Scar width (pin side) [μm]	$a = 232$, $b = 325$	$a = 240$, $b = 255$
Scar width (head side), d [μm]	366	388
Specific wear rate (pin), W_p [m^2/N]	1.02×10^{-16}	2.23×10^{-17}
Specific wear rate (pin), W_h [m^2/N]	9.67×10^{-14}	3.67×10^{-14}
Friction Coefficient, μ (initial)	0.38	0.43
Friction Coefficient, μ (regime)	0.41	0.52
Contact temperature, T_{max} [°C]	48	134
Contact frictional stress, $\sigma_{xx,max}$ [GPa]	−1.72	−2.41
Contact pressure, $\sigma_{zz,max}$ [GPa]	−1.25	−1.74

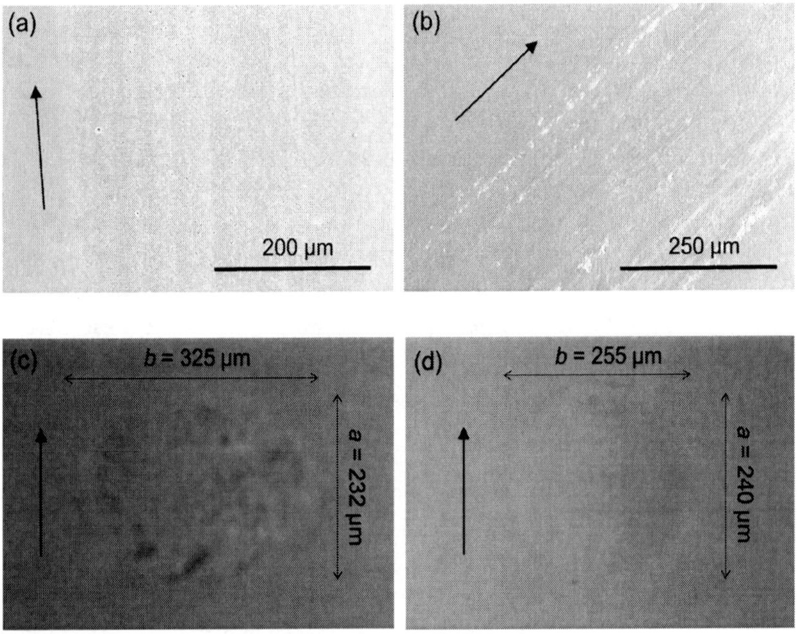

Figure 5.26 In (a) and (b), optical micrographs of the damaged zone and related length measurements on the ball side for the *forte*-on-*forte* and *delta*-on-*delta* couple, respectively, as observed at the end of the respective wear tests conducted for a sliding distance of 2×10^3 m. In (c) and (d), micrographs of wear scars, as observed after wear tests on the pin side for the monolithic and the composite couples, respectively. Arrows indicate the sliding direction.

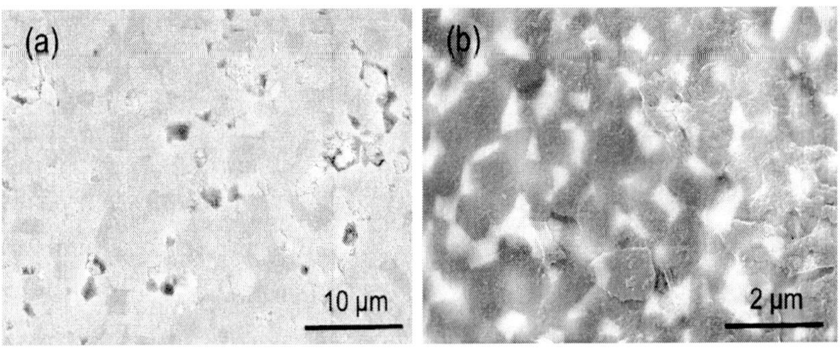

Figure 5.27 In (a) and (b), SEM micrographs taken in the damage scar region of the femoral head in *forte*-on-*forte* and *delta*-on-*delta* couples, respectively.

As mentioned above, temperature variations can be determined from the variation of time-dependent line width of fluorescence spectra *in situ* recorded at the contact point during running a wear test on the ceramic couples. Figures 5.28(a) and (b) show the variation of contact temperature, ΔT, as obtained from broadening of a selected fluorescence band for *delta*-on-*delta* and *forte*-on-*forte* sliding couples, respectively. Data are plotted as a function of sliding distance after deconvolutive correction for laser probe broadening in the sample [751]. A rapid increase and then a saturation (at sliding regime) of the local temperature recorded at the contact point were commonly found, as a consequence of the friction generated between the sliding components. A significantly lower contact temperature was found at sliding regime in the *forte*-on-*forte* couple compared with the *delta*-on-*delta* one (i.e., 48°C vs. 134°C), which could be considered as being the cumulative consequence of the lower friction coefficient measured in the former couple (i.e., μ = 0.41 vs. 0.52) and of the lower thermal conductivity of the zirconia polymorphs compared with alumina. The steep temperature gradients generated at sliding regime in the neighborhood of the contact point from the pin side could also be plotted as a function of distance in depth from the contact point, *r*, according to the solution for the heat-propagation equation from the additive effect of a series of instantaneously generated hot-spot sources [751]. The plots are shown in Fig. 5.29. A comparison between the curves obtained for the two investigated couples shows similar trends but quite different temperature ranges, with significantly higher temperatures in the composite couple consistent with the plots in Fig. 5.28. In both cases, the temperature field rapidly decayed below the contact surface, within a range of few microns. A similar estimation of temperature gradients was also made from the ball side. However, unlike the pin that was subjected to a continuous frictional load, the time needed for the ball to complete one-round rotation at the rotation speed selected in this study, namely about 0.32 s, was by far longer than the time needed for heat diffusing away from the contact point on the ball side. Therefore, only insignificant changes in local temperature (<1°C) could be detected on the femoral head side.

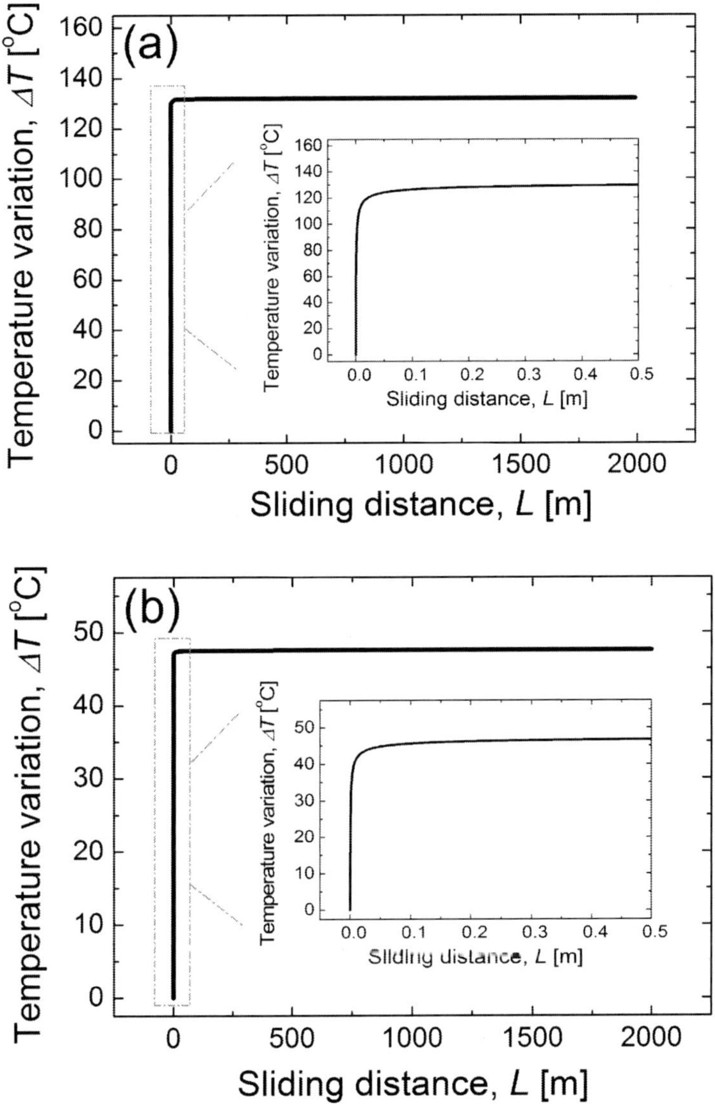

Figure 5.28 Variation of temperature at the contact point between pin and ball as a function of sliding distance for *delta*-on-*delta* and *forte*-on-*forte* sliding couples (in (a) and (b), respectively). Enlargements of the transient zones to regime are shown for better clarity in insets.

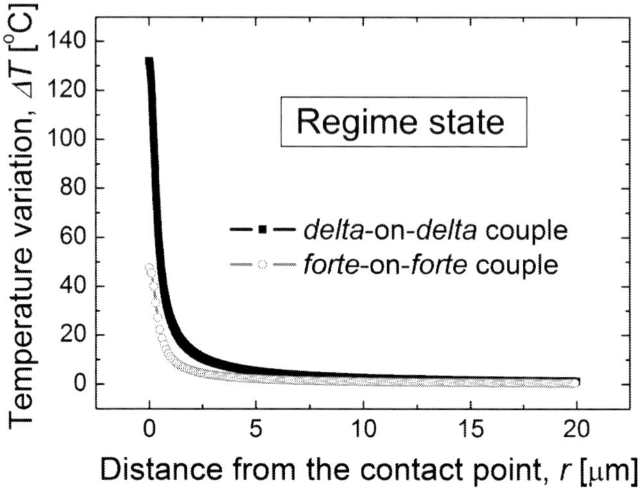

Figure 5.29 Comparison between gradients of deconvoluted regime temperature as a function of distance from the contact point along the radial direction, r, as recorded for *delta*-on-*delta* and *forte*-on-*forte* sliding couples.

The magnitude of the stress field developed around the contact point is given in Fig. 5.30(a), which shows the deconvoluted stress variation at the contact point as a function of sliding distance for both cases of *delta*-on-*delta* and *forte*-on-*forte* sliding couples. Rather high compressive stresses were found at the contact point, which slightly increased in magnitude with increasing sliding distance. This variation could be ascribed to the generation of scars on both ball and pin, with consequent increase of friction in the contact area between the sliding counterparts. On the other hand, the stress magnitude at sliding regime rapidly decreased with increasing the in-depth distance away from the contact point towards the center of the ball (or pin) (cf. Fig. 5.30(b)). A significantly lower stress magnitude was found for the *forte*-on-*forte* sliding couple compared with the *delta*-on-*delta* one (cf. Table 5.4). The bi-axial load cell of the tribometer also recorded a similar difference in maximum contact forces. Such large difference in stress magnitude might again be related to the higher friction coefficient of the *delta*-on-*delta* sliding couple, but it could also be related to the strong initial state of residual stress stored on the surface of the composite material (cf. Section 5.4). However, also contributions related to polymorphic transformation in the zirconia phase, which was found in the *delta* material by spectroscopic analyses of the scars at the end of the test, cannot be ruled out, as discussed in the following part of this section. The stress results, complementing the temperature assessments shown in the previous section, reveal that the composite couple behaves in a more "dissipative" way compared with the monolithic one. However, the intriguing feature if this behavior is that the composite couple was also found to experience a lower specific wear rate by a factor 2.63 and 4.48 on the head and pin side, respectively, compared with the monolithic one (3.67×10^{-14} vs. 9.67×10^{-14} m^2/N at the ball side, and 2.23×10^{-17} vs. 1.02×10^{-16} m^2/N at the pin side).

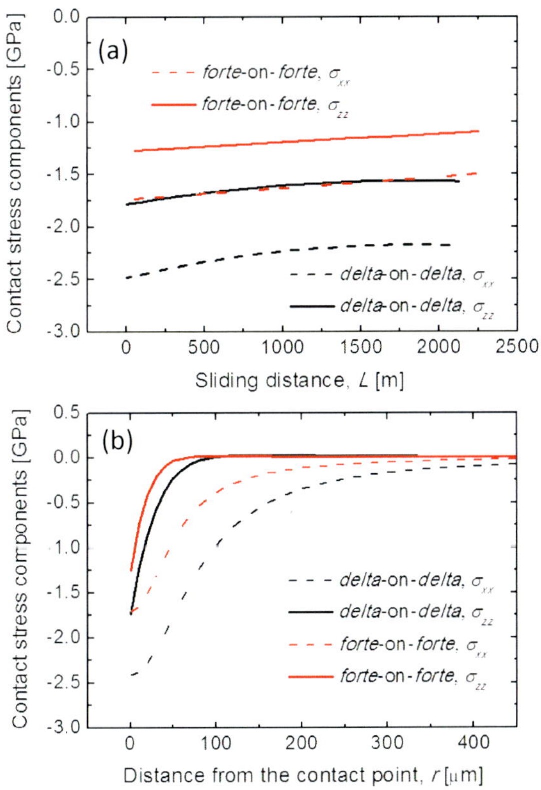

Figure 5.30 Variation of deconvoluted contact stress magnitudes as detected at the contact points for *delta*-on-*delta* and *forte*-on-*forte* sliding couples as a function of: (a) sliding distance; and, (b) radial direction from the center of the pin at sliding regime.

Figure 5.31(a) shows a typical confocal Raman spectrum collected *in situ* from the contact point of the sliding composite couple. In the spectrum, tetragonal and monoclinic bands are labeled and, from their intensities, the volume fraction of monoclinic phase, V_m, could be calculated according to Eq. (5.13). Similar spectra were collected as a function of sliding distance, L, thus obtaining a plot, $V_m(L)$, as shown in Fig. 5.31(b). Plots are given for two different configurations of the Raman probe, namely a confocal configuration (i.e., 100 μm pinhole aperture) and a configuration with the full aperture of the confocal pinhole (referred to as "through focus" in the label). The two different optical configurations lead to different laser penetration depths in Raman assessments, in the order of few microns and few tens of microns for the cases of confocal and through-focus assessments, respectively. The plot collected with a confocal probe indeed shows a clear increase (in the order of 35%) of monoclinic content after $L = 2 \times 10^3$ m, above the initial content of monoclinic polymorph, $V_m^{(0)} \approx 15\%$, in the pristine material. The values recorded by the through-focus configuration are conspicuously lower, showing a monoclinic volume fraction increase from about 5% in the pristine composite to 7.5% at the end of the test (i.e., increase also in the order of 33%). The locally occurred polymorphic transformation is obviously a consequence of the stress and temperature increases at the contact point during dry sliding. However, the extent of transformation along the depth of the sample appears confined to a quite shallow region, because, unlike the confocal probe, the through-focus probe conspicuously fails in locating the actual amount of monoclinic fraction on the sample surface. Since the polymorphic transformation occurs with substantial volume increase, it is conceivable to believe that it can be one additional reason for the higher coefficient of friction measured in the composite couple (cf. Table 5.4). The plot in Fig. 5.31(b) should be compared with a plot of monoclinic fraction across the scar on the ball head, as performed *ex situ* after the end of the tribological test on the worn sample. This plot is given in Fig. 5.32(a) for both confocal and through-focus probe configurations. The two different probe configurations again show different values when recorded at the same locations due to the different probe depths, but the values of monoclinic phase found *ex situ* for both confocal and through-focus plots at the center of the scar were very close to those measured *in-situ* during tribological tests. This can be considered as a confirmation of the spectroscopic assessments obtained *in situ*. An intriguing finding was that a relatively high content (up to about 32%) of monoclinic phase was found at a distance of about 300 μm from the center of the scar, namely quite far from the distance of the developed gradient of temperature. The lower value measured at the center of the scar cannot either be explained as being simply due to pullout of zirconia grains during tribological test, because we have found the occurrence of such phenomenon to be only sporadic in the present test. The agreement between *in situ* and *ex situ* monoclinic volume fraction measurements at the center of the scar also confirms that negligible further transformation occurred during cooling from the sliding regime temperature after the interruption of the tribological test. Therefore, the spatial gradient in monoclinic phase transformation found on the head scar should rather be attributed to the high stress gradients developed on the material surface during sliding than to temperature effects, the higher the gradient toward tensile stresses, the higher the transformed fraction. From a general viewpoint, the trend found for monoclinic phase transformation during tribological test on the *delta*-on-*delta* couple could be interpreted as indicating high stability for the tetragonal zirconia dispersed in the alumina matrix of the composite. However, for ceramics used in joint arthroplasty, the *in vivo* performance of load-bearing surfaces depends on the combined effects of both structural and environmental loading. The dry-sliding results presented in this paper can be considered to be very severe from a micromechanical viewpoint, but the effect induced by the exposure to biological environment is missing. Therefore, additional studies are needed with running the tribometer under wet conditions, namely in an environment that could reproduce as close as possible the real operative conditions encountered by the femoral head in the human body.

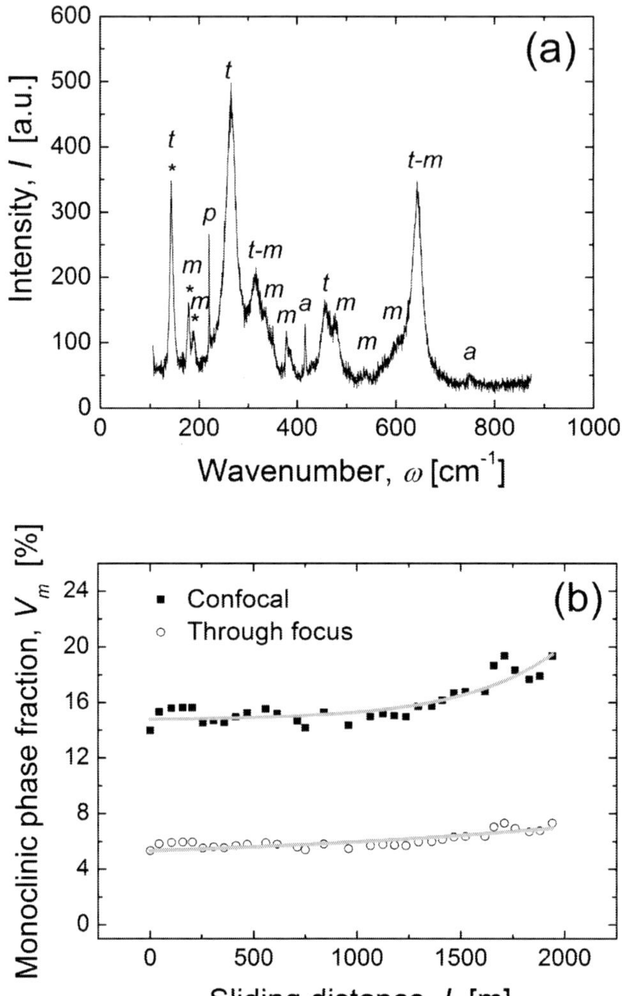

Figure 5.31 (a) Typical Raman spectrum collected *in situ* from the contact point of the sliding composite couple. In the spectrum, tetragonal and monoclinic bands are labeled *t* and *m*, respectively (overlapping bands show both labels). The bands labeled with an asterisk were used for the computation of the monoclinic volume fraction, V_m, according to Eq. (5.13). The label *a* refers to alumina bands, while the label *p* locates a selected plasma line from the laser emission, which was used as an internal standard for spectroscopic calibrations. In (b), a plot of V_m is given as a function of sliding distance.

In Fig. 5.32(b), *ex situ* measured residual stresses, σ, are plotted as measured by collecting the fluorescence spectral shifts of the chromophoric doublet of the alumina phase in the worn monolithic and composite heads. Spectral shifts, which represent the local differences in peak position with respect to the peak average position recorded before wear testing, were translated into hydrostatic stress magnitudes by means of the piezo-spectroscopic coefficients published in Refs. [19, 479, 660]. The region investigated was the same as in the case of the scan shown in Fig. 5.32(a). Two distinct bands, R1 and R2, belonging to the chromophoric doublet provided consistent results, which showed a shift towards compressive values (i.e., with respect to the unworn material) in a region near the center of the scar (abscissa $0 \leq x \leq 100$ μm), and a subsequent gradual stress release starting from $x = 100$ μm to 300 μm. The observed residual stress field in the alumina phase belonging to the wear zone can be interpreted as the superposition of two components, although the fluorescence technique does not allow one to separately assess different stress tensor components. One component of compressive nature arises from the hard-on-hard pressure contact during sliding [745], and another component of tensile nature is induced by the volume expansion associated with the polymorphic transformation of the zirconia phase [747]. The effects of these two stress components are thus competitive with respect to the cumulative spectral shift recorded. Moreover, the high compressive stress component developed at the center of the scar seems to have induced a delaying effect on tetragonal-to-monoclinic phase transformation. The results of *ex situ* experiments shown in Fig. 5.32(a) have indeed shown that polymorphic transformation preponderantly takes place at distances relatively far from the contact point, namely in regions at which the contact compressive stress is significantly released. A similar characterization of *ex situ* residual stresses in the monolithic alumina *forte*-on-*forte* couple (also shown for comparison in Fig. 5.32(b)) revealed stresses of negligible magnitude, as a consequence of the occurrence of significant grain pullout and surface disruption, which released the frictional contact stress, in addition to the absence of a transforming phase.

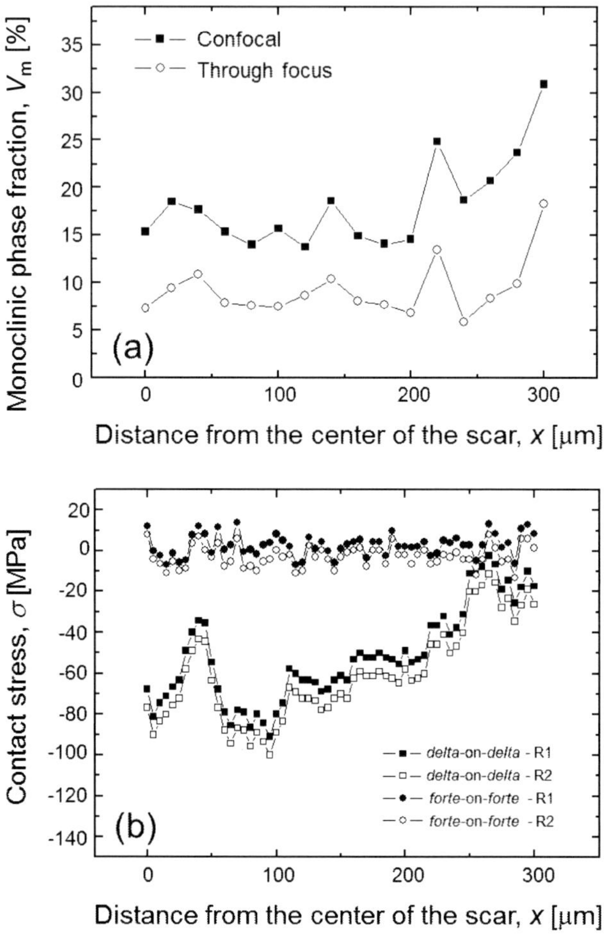

Figure 5.32 (a) Plot of monoclinic fraction across the scar on the ball head, as performed *ex situ* after the end of the tribological test on the worn sample. In (b), *ex situ* measured residual stresses are plotted as measured by collecting the fluorescence spectral shifts of the chromophoric doublet of the alumina phase in the worn monolithic and composite heads.

In conclusion, both *ex situ* and *in situ* characterizations have been presented, which led to different outputs of a comparative tribological analysis of commercially available artificial hip biomedical implants. The *in situ* characterizations were carried out in a newly developed tribometer device, which enabled not only wear testing under standard wear conditions, but also the concurrent collection of Raman and fluorescence spectra at the contact point. From *in situ* collected spectra, information about contact temperature, stress, and polymorphic phase transformation could be retrieved. The intrinsic tribological behaviors of two commercially available hard-on-hard sliding couples, namely a monolithic and a composite ceramic couple, were characterized and compared. The main outcomes of these characterizations can be summarized as follows:

(i) An almost threefold higher temperature (in the order of 134°C) was locally found at the contact point of the composite couple compared with the monolithic one. Such significantly higher contact temperature was a consequence of both a lowered thermal conductivity (i.e., due to the presence of a fraction of ZrO_2 phase) and of the higher friction coefficient developed during sliding of the composite couple. Both materials commonly showed a high magnitude of compressive stress at the contact point, but substantially lower stress magnitudes could be found in the monolithic couple.

(ii) Polymorphic phase transformation occurred *in situ* under conditions of dry sliding in the composite couple. The lattice expansion associated with polymorphic transformation was considered as one of the causes of the higher friction coefficient measured in the composite couple compared with the monolithic one.

(iii) The monolithic couple, which experienced significantly deeper scars and grain pullout after testing compared with the composite couple, wore at three to fourfold higher specific wear rates.

(iv) The degree of damage observed in the monolithic couple was quite high after sliding for 2×10^3 m, with severe pull out and partial disruption of the material surface. Some pullout of the zirconia grain was sporadically observed in the composite sample, but the overall damage on the surface was clearly by far less pronounced than that found on the surface of the monolithic femoral head. In other words, despite its more "dissipative" behavior (i.e., higher friction and higher contact temperature), the composite material was significantly more wear resistant than the monolithic one under dry sliding conditions.

In this section, for brevity's sake, we have not explicitly shown *in situ*-collected tribological data for the ZTA composite B discussed in the previous sections of this chapter. We only mention here the output of hard-on-hard tribological experiments conducted on this composite with the same procedure as that just described for the couples *forte*-on-*forte* and *delta*-on-*delta* (i.e., ZTA composite A). In agreement with the discussion given at the end of Section 5.4, the wear resistance in hard-on-hard (dry) sliding conditions was quite lowered as compared to that of composite A under the same testing conditions. For example, the dimension of the scar width on the pin side (a circle of diameter ~440 μm) was even larger than that of the monolithic *forte*-on-*forte* couple, while significant disruption of the surface with grain detachment was noticed in the scar on the head side. On the other hand, the contact temperature at sliding regime was slightly larger (~161°C) but yet comparable with that measured for composite A, thus supporting the argument that the higher contact temperature in ZTA composites as compared to monolithic alumina mainly arises from the presence of the zirconia particles and, in particular, to their lower thermal conductivity as compared to the alumina matrix. Clarke *et al.* [755] have published a comparative study, which reported about hip-simulator wear testing of *forte*-on-*forte* and *delta*-on-*delta* sliding couples in severe testing modes, including microseparation. Tests were run up to duration of 5 million cycles. The study, which was shown to provide outputs comparable to wear rates measured on *in vivo* worn retrievals, reported a sixfold higher wear resistance for the composite couple compared with the monolithic one. Microstructural observation and Raman spectroscopic analyses, performed *ex situ* at the end of the tests, revealed detachment of the zirconia grains in the composite (only sporadically near the pole of the head and continuously increasing down to the dome of the head) and considerable amounts of phase transformation, with the monoclinic phase present on the material surface in amounts comparable to what we have measured in this study in regions at a distance about 300 μm away from the center of the scar. Despite the completely different way to test the wear resistance of the material between the hip-simulator study and the present study, the wear data obtained in our tribometer could similarly resolve the difference in wear resistance between monolithic and composite couples and can thus be considered comparatively consistent with those collected in wear simulator. Accordingly, at the end of the presented *in situ* tribological characterizations, one might wonder about what we actually could learn in addition to finding the composite material significantly more resistant to abrasive wear and more damage tolerant than the monolithic one under dry sliding conditions, which is actually the same phenomenological output that one could find by conventional hip-simulator experiments [755]. The simple answer is that now we know much more about the physics underlying the wear degradation and, through such information, could get important hints on how to improve the composite microstructure in order to obtain a better wear response. We detected both a more dissipative character and friction-enhanced phase instability in the composite hard-on-hard couple compared with the monolithic one, which in turn arose from the lowered thermal conductivity and from the attitude of the metastable Y-stabilized zirconia phase to undergo polymorphic transformation. On the other hand, recalling the CL spectroscopic findings reported in Section 5.4, one might also better recognize the importance of the peculiar surface characteristics of the *delta* composite, namely its quite low initial oxygen-vacancy concentration, the strong resistance to vacancy formation during environmental loading, and the highly compressive residual stresses stored in the Al_2O_3 matrix after manufacturing. Such characteristics could be successfully induced on the surface of the *delta* composite through the concurrent fortunate choices of Cr^{3+} doping in the Al_2O_3 phase and of a lower amount of stabilizing Y_2O_3 additive (compared with the standard 3 mol.%) to obtain a suitably metastable ZrO_2 phase. Our *in situ* spectroscopic studies of wear mechanism showed that these were key-factors in minimizing wear damage. Therefore, the obtained spectroscopic characterizations are actually giving us hints on how to design more wear-resistant ceramic microstructures based on quantitative and rigorously ontological, rather than phenomenological, arguments. From a more general viewpoint, we have demonstrated in this section that *in situ* tribological tests combined with Raman and fluorescence microprobe spectroscopy have a potential for fully satisfying all the requirements for effective *in situ* and *ex situ* wear evaluations. Such innovative testing procedure enables one not only to measure the intrinsic wear characteristics but also to unfold exactly which physical circumstances might become decisive for further enhancing the wear resistance of ceramic-on-ceramic hip joints.

Chapter 6

Ultra-High Molecular Weight Polyethylene for Joint Replacement

6.1 Polyethylene Hip Components and Their Recent Manufacturing Trends

In the general introduction given in Chapter 1, we have emphasized several main issues related to the use of polyethylene components in artificial joints. The most striking issue found in revisiting the performance of polyethylene acetabular cups was the occurrence of aseptic loosening, the main consequence of osteolytic bone loss. Aseptic loosening has been by far the most common reason for hip implant failure (cf. Fig. 1.4). The *in vivo* generation of polyethylene wear debris actually represents a quite serious problem in modern hip replacements [756]. Polyethylene particle debris, generated upon wear of the cup liner, become attacked by the body immune system, this process ultimately leading to partial bone destruction in and around the joint implant. The associated bone tissue degradation then leads to loosening. Wear-debris-induced osteolysis is thus a consequence of adverse cellular reactions against wear particles in the body. The mechanism leading to osteolysis is complex and consists of a sequential cascade of events including [757,758]: (a) the dispersion of wear debris generated in the joint into the surrounding fluids and tissues; (b) their phagocytosis by

Advanced Materials for Joint Implants
Giuseppe Pezzotti

ISBN 978-981-4316-88-0 (Hardcover), 978-981-4364-39-3 (eBook)
www.panstanford.com

macrophages; (c) the release of cytokines (e.g., tumor necrosis factor TNF-α and prostaglandin PGE2) by the activated macrophages; and, (d) the action of the released cytokines upon osteoblasts and osteoclasts to cause inflammation and osteoclastic bone resorption. The macrophage activation is dependent on both volumetric concentration and size of wear debris, particles in the size range 0.3~10 μm being the most active biologically [758]. Efforts in reducing the generation of polyethylene wear debris have been spent in two distinct directions. From the one side, ceramic femoral heads have gradually been employed versus polyethylene liners to replace metallic heads. Perhaps the earliest proof in support of such innovative surgical policy resides in the original work published in the late 1970s by Semlitsch and coworkers [759]. Those researchers were the first to demonstrate a 20:1 reduction in volumetric wear in a wear simulator with alumina ceramic heads sliding on polyethylene compared with the a sliding couple consisting of chrome cobalt heads on polyethylene liners. Since then, the use of alumina ceramic vs. polyethylene couples in total hip replacement became quite popular all over the world [391]. The reasons for the wear resistance improvement with ceramic heads are manifold and include their better surface finishing (i.e., compared with metal heads) in the as-manufactured state, their superior lubricating properties, as arising from a better wettability compared with metals, their low coefficient of friction at the bearing surface, and less susceptibility to third body wear and scratching of the surface. From the other side, the microstructure of the polyethylene liner has been gradually engineered to more and more sophisticated levels, including the control during manufacturing of both the degree of crystallinity and the molecular chain orientation in three dimensions. *In vitro* hip simulator studies [760–762] as well as clinical studies [763–765] have clearly shown that a robust cross-linking of polymeric chains can alleviate most effectively adhesive/abrasive wear of UHMWPE acetabular cups. Cross-linking, which is mainly achieved in the amorphous regions of the polyethylene structure [762, 766], occurs as the main effect of ionizing irradiation in an inert atmosphere, the optimal γ-radiation dose being individuated as being at around 100 kGy in the case of liners for hip prostheses [762]. Such threshold value for radiation dose stems from the experimental findings that fatigue crack propagation resistance, ultimate tensile strength, and elongation at the break might abruptly decrease with further increasing radiation dose and cross-link density. These negative effects originate on the microscopic scale and are due to a loss of chain mobility (i.e., the residually strained chains, under microstructural constraint, rather crack than deform), which in turn reflects, on the macroscopic scale, in a diminished material ductility [767,768]. A key-factor in the performance of biomedical UHMWPE is the selection of a post-irradiation heat treatment, namely either a remelting or an annealing cycle, which is commonly conducted to eliminate the excess free radicals created during irradiation and leading to premature oxidative degradation *in vivo*. The processing step after γ-ray irradiation is quite delicate because the post-irradiation treatment directly contributes to the microstructural development of the final product with either ameliorating or worsening the physical properties of the liner. In this context, it should be noted that a post-irradiation remelting process (i.e., a thermal cycle involving heating up to above the melting temperature (>135°C)) can most effectively eliminate all the free radicals (and thus annihilate the extra oxidation probability that they potentially introduce), but it might also irreversibly alter the polyethylene microstructure with conspicuously decreasing its crystallinity level with respect to that achieved during irradiation. On the other hand, a post-irradiation annealing cycle conducted below the melting temperature preserves the pristine (i.e., the irradiated) microstructure (or even increases crystallinity), but unavoidably allows for an uncertain amount of residual free radicals remaining trapped in the final product. As a consequence of the complexity of such microstructural issue, the choice between different heating treatments is still argument of controversy among implant makers. However, it should be noted at the outset that in spite of the importance of (and deep controversy on) the choice of an optimal manufacturing process for UHMWPE liners, very few evidences have been so far shown to clarify the actual structure of differently treated UHMWPE liners on the molecular scale, especially with respect to their three-dimensional textures. In other words, evaluation procedures so far presented in the literature commonly discuss microstructural features of the liners that are hard to explicitly visualize and quantify in terms of three-dimensional molecular assembly of the polymeric structure. As a result of such lack of microstructural knowledge on the molecular scale, quantitative structural comparisons among commercially available liners are conspicuously missing in the available literature and the optimum molecular microstructure for UHMWPE liners has not yet been individuated.

The impact of γ-irradiation on retrieved liners was first discussed in an early paper by Eyerer and Ke [769], in which a density increase was found for a large number of explanted UHMWPE liners. This phenomenon was explained by invoking the occurrence of a post-crystallization process as a result of oxidative chain scission. The phenomenon led to a reduction in average molecular weight of the polyethylene material and to an increased extractability of its constituents. These microstructural changes are nowadays generally recognized as the main reason for aging (and failing) of γ-irradiated UHMWPE liners. An increase of crystallinity during the mechanical and chemical loading of the liner *in vivo* can be thus seen as a clear symptom of the presence of residual free radicals in the pristine material and, thus, of the associated occurrence of a time-dependent oxidation process. In this context, a recent study by Fouad [770] investigated the effects of natural aging up to 6 years in air on the thermal, mechanical, and viscoelastic properties of a UHMWPE used in total joint replacement. The results show that the lamellar thickness and degree of crystallinity of UHMWPE specimens increase by 38% and 12% due to aging, with clear indications that the formation of new crystalline fractions occurs within their amorphous region. The tensile properties also show a significant decrease in the elastic modulus, yield, fracture stresses, and strain to failure due to aging. The key to interpret these negative results can be found in a recent study by Oral *et al.* [771]. Those researchers hypothesized and proved that an increased cross-link density might hinder crystallization during processing due to decreased chain mobility. There are two main consequences to the decrease of chain mobility: (i) the fraction of "inhibited" crystallinity during processing can be considered as a measure of the expected *in vivo* instability of the polymeric structure; and, (ii) when crystallization forcedly occurs (e.g., by *in vivo* loading) under conditions of a lack of chain mobility, the result is an embrittlement of the material. In order to circumvent the problem and to achieve high crystallinity without embrittlement, Oral *et al.* [771] proposed a remelting process under high pressure (200°C under 380 MPa for 5 h) to be performed after substantial cross-linking irradiation. According to this process, high oxidation resistance is also expected because the material is molten after crystallization at high temperature, therefore allowing the recombination of the residual free radicals from irradiation. The strategy followed in the most advanced UHMWPE liners nowadays manufactured aims at the same final result as in the study by Oral *et al.* [771], namely obtaining a relatively high degree of crystallization and of an *in vivo* stable microstructure with the concurrent annihilation of free radicals. However, this aim is not pursued by means of a high-pressure remelting process but by sequentially operating on the UHMWPE microstructure several partial steps of irradiation and annealing.

Two differently prepared raw components have been so far mainly used in the production of the UHMWPE liners of joint replacement prostheses: compression-molded sheets and extruded rods. The crystallographic textures developed in rods and sheets of UHMWPE are different and are sufficiently marked that they might eventually induce anisotropy in the macroscopic properties of polymers, such as modulus and yield stress. Both rods and sheets of UHMWPE reveal a discernible degree of preferred orientation of polyethylene chains within crystallites. However, according to Bellare and Cohen [772], a spatial variation in crystallographic orientation can be only observed in extruded rods. In particular, the direction of molecular chain alignment within crystallites located near the outer surface of rods is found to be orthogonal to the radial direction, whereas the chain direction is orthogonal to the axial or extrusion direction in crystallites located near the centerline of extruded rods. Crystallographic texture is instead conspicuously uniform (in three dimensions) in compression-molded sheets, with the chain direction within crystallites aligned orthogonal to the molding direction. Figure 6.1 shows a schematic of the microstructure of biomedical polyethylene and of the structural arrangement in the case of extruded rods and molded sheets. In both cases of manufacturing process, Bellare and Cohen [772] were capable to explain the induced crystallographic texture in terms of crystallization from an oriented melt. Their study, although conducted by X-ray diffraction techniques and, thus, with low spatial resolution, is important because it is the first study that foresees (and proves) a correlation between wear properties and the morphology of UHMWPE on the molecular scale. Indeed, molecular alignment strongly affects the wear resistance and the mechanical properties under biomechanical loading condition, especially in the presence of the multi-directional stress field that generates in the articulation of human hip joints [325]. High degree of molecular alignment has been reported to detrimentally affect the wear resistance of UHMWPE due to the occurrence of a phenomenon called strain softening (or weakening). It was proposed by Wang *et al.* [325] that stress components in a transverse direction to the oriented molecules can lead to shear rupture of long molecular chains and, ultimately, to the formation of fibrillar or filmy wear debris. Moreover, mechanical loading can be conductive below the articulating surface, and ultimately form a damaged layer as a consequence of irrecoverable plastic deformation [325, 772, 773]. All these notions point to the conclusion that it is mandatory to quantify the initial degree of molecular alignment near the sliding surface of the liner before implantation in order to consider the risk of strain softening assisted wear and to correctly predict the mechanical response and clinical performance of UHMWPE joint prostheses.

In this chapter, we shall examine three types of acetabular liners (all 28 mm inner diameter) that were prepared according to different raw components and manufacturing procedures. Of the three types of investigated UHMWPE liners, one was heated above the melting temperature (i.e., remelted) for stabilization of free radicals after exposure to electron beam radiation (henceforth also referred to as Liner A), while the remaining two (Liners B and C) were both heated below the melting temperature (i.e., annealed) after γ-ray irradiation according to a single step or to a sequential number of steps. A brief description of the processing procedure for the preparation of each investigated liner is given in Table 6.1. Liner A is the long-known brand Longevity^{TM} manufactured by Zimmer, Inc. (Warsaw, Indiana, USA), which represents a first-generation remelted liner, clinically introduced in the Trilogy acetabular cup design since 1999. Molded sheets, consolidated from GUR 1050 resin (5.5 to 6 million g/mol), are radiation cross-linked by electron beam with a total dose of 100 kGy and then remelted (>135°C) to quench residual free radicals.

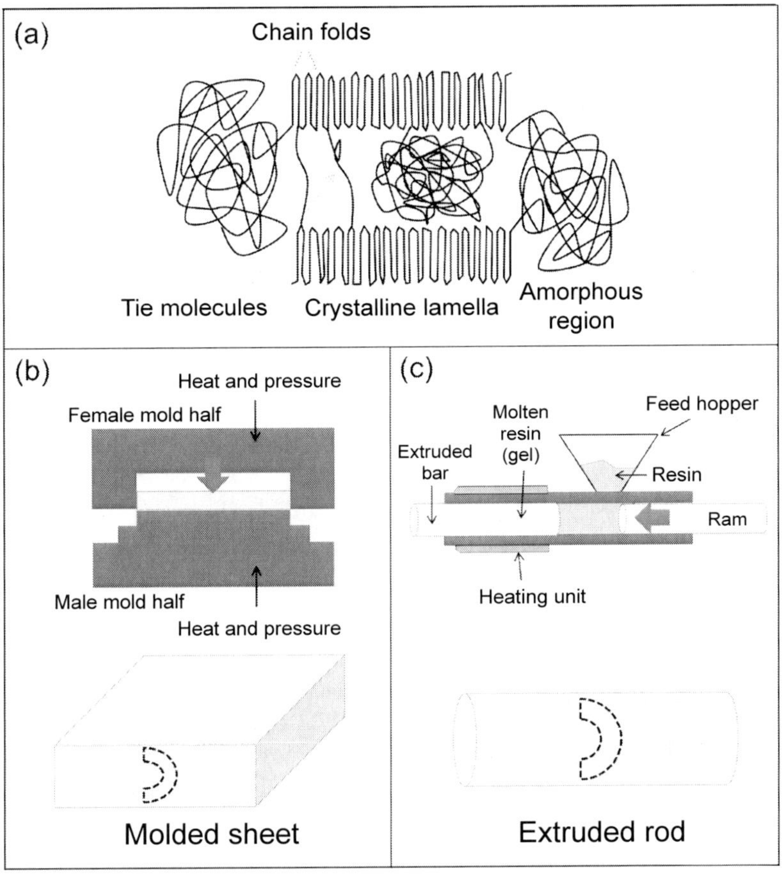

Figure 6.1 Comparison among processing steps in the manufacturing process of UHMWPE acetabular liners from different makers.

Liner B is the brand Crossfire^{TM} manufactured by Stryker Orthopedics, Inc. (Mahwah, New Jersey, USA), which also belongs to the first-generation of annealed liners. This liner was clinically introduced in 1998. The manufacturing procedure of Crossfire^{TM} also starts from GUR 1050 resin but the resin has the morphology of extruded rods. The rods are γ-irradiated with a nominal dose of 75 kGy and subsequently annealed at 130°C. After being machined into liner shape and then barrier packaged, Crossfire^{TM} is exposed again to γ-irradiation for sterilization purpose with the nominal dose of 30 kGy in nitrogen atmosphere.

Table 6.1 Salient details of the manufacturing procedures of Crossfire™ and X3™ liners

	Processing	Longevity™	Crossfire™	X3™
Step 1	Make from resin	GUR 1050 Molded sheets	GUR 1050 Extruded rods	GUR 1020 Molded sheets
Step 2	Irradiation	100 kGy Electron beam	75 kGy γ-irradiation	30 kGy γ-irradiation in 3 Steps (=90 kGy)
Step 3	Heat treatment	Remelting (>135°C)	Annealing (130°C)	Annealing after each γ-sterilization step (130°C)
Step 4	Maching sheets/rods on a lathe			
Step 5	Package			
Step 6	Steriliztion	Gas plasma	30 kGy γ-sterilization (N_2/Vac)	Gas plasma

Liner C is X3™ manufactured by Stryker Orthopedics, Inc. (Mahwah, New Jersey, USA), which belongs to a second-generation annealed liner and was clinically introduced in the Trident and Tritanium acetabular cup design in 2005. GUR 1020 (3.5 million g/mol) compression molded sheets are used after being γ-irradiated at the nominal dose of 30 kGy and then annealed at 130°C. The same procedure is sequentially repeated three times (i.e., the cumulative radiation dose being 90 kGy). For the same cumulative radiation dose, a more pronounced crystallization and cross-linking formation is expected through sequential irradiation and successive annealing steps, with a free radical concentration conspicuously lower than the standard single irradiation and annealing procedures. In the context of the complex background stated above, it should be noted that the X3™ liner undergoes a newly proposed process of sequential irradiation and annealing in order to improve the efficiency of free-radical elimination with concurrently maintaining all the possible positive aspects of the annealing process (i.e., as opposed to remelting) in terms of microstructural development. A recent hip simulator study [774] has preliminary shown that in addition to excellent mechanical properties, acetabular liners made from this new material also possess superior wear properties in comparison with conventional UHMWPE and to clinically successful first-generation highly cross-linked polyethylene materials. Owing to its recent introduction, there is only available a preliminary publication describing the clinical performance of the X3™ liner [775]. This recent study assessed the early clinical wear of a retrieved X3™ liner and compared its clinical performance with published results of both hip simulator tests and (retrieved) first-generation highly cross-linked polyethylene annealed liners. The wear rate was found to be less than the detection threshold for the employed software-assisted radio-stereometric technique. Such low level of wear is quite encouraging for the future clinical performance of this material. However, again the question here is what kind of microstructural characteristics and structural arrangement on the molecular scale have been achieved in the X3™ liner by means of the sequential irradiation/annealing process and how such microstructure might impact on the wear and creep performances of the material.

The purpose of this chapter is first to quantitatively unfold the three-dimensional crystalline morphology and the degree of molecular alignment of commercially available UHMWPE acetabular liners manufactured by remelting, by annealing, or by sequential annealing processes. The investigation starts from the consideration that the latest improvements in manufacturing process, as proposed by Stryker Orthopaedics, Inc., can actually produce a conspicuous increase in crystallinity and in the amount of preferential orientation of polyethylene molecules in the three-dimensional assembly of the X3™ acetabular liners, as compared with other liners. Different processing treatments should produce distinctive patterns in the final microstructures, in turn related to functional uniqueness and individuality during *in vivo* use. A second challenge pursued here is to precisely quantify the effect of crystallinity and of the extent of molecular alignment on the plastic creep response of different types of polyethylene hip liners. A non-destructive spectroscopic approach based on confocal/polarized

Raman spectroscopy is adopted throughout the evaluations. A schematic of the spectroscopic measurement protocol is given in Fig. 6.2. Five different areas were selected on the concave surface of each liner, locations (I), (II), (III), (II'), and (I') as shown in Fig. 6.2(a). The liners were placed on a rotation jig and polarized Raman spectra were collected at 19 different azimuthal angles selected within the interval $0° \leq \chi \leq 180°$, with sequential in-

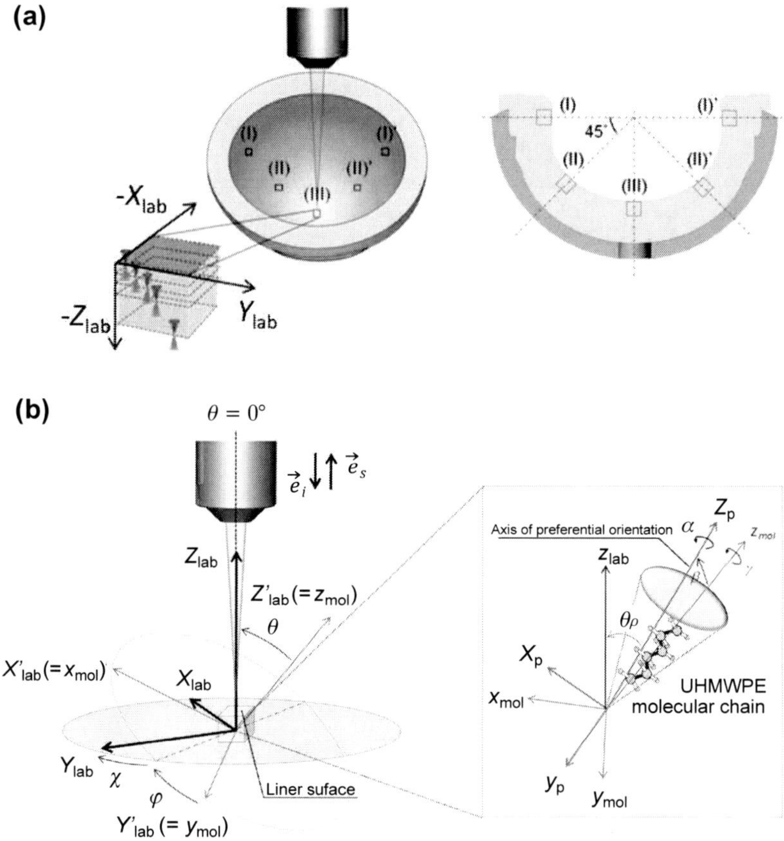

Figure 6.2 (a) Schematics of the selected measurement locations on the concave surface of the liner, and in-depth Raman mapping protocol using a confocal probe configuration in the selected five different areas. (b) Schematics of our choice of Cartesian reference systems and of the Euler angles governing their rotations in space, as explained in the text. The vertical arrows close to the electric vectors $\vec{e}_i$ and $\vec{e}_s$ represent the propagation directions of the incident laser and the scattered light, respectively.

plane rotational steps of 10° (Fig. 6.2(b)). The focal plane was eventually shifted toward the liner subsurface in order to non-destructively screen buried regions of material and to obtain a fully three-dimensional view of the microstructural and molecular arrangement in the investigated liners. Twenty locations were randomly selected for each of the five areas, each location consisting of a 100 × 100 μm^2 grid for each polarization choice, in order to secure an acceptable degree of statistical reliability in representing molecular arrangement. The total number of Raman spectra cumulatively collected on the three liners, including both in-depth and polarization analyses was in the order of 5 × 10^6. No statistically relevant differences were found between locations (I) and (I'), and (II) and (II') in any of the types of liner studied. Therefore, for each liner analyzed, data from locations (I) and (I'), and data from locations (II) and (II') will be presented as single sets of data (and referred to as locations (I) and (II), respectively).

6.2 Crystallinity, Molecular Arrangement and Their Spatial Variations

Figures 6.3(a)~(c) represent the in-depth profiles of average crystalline and amorphous phase fractions (α_c and $\alpha_{a,}$ respectively) as detected in Longevity™, Crossfire™, and X3™ acetabular cups, respectively. As seen, the content of crystalline phase on the surface of the liner (z_{lab} = 0) lies between 40% and 53% for all the three types of liner, being the lowest and the highest in Longevity™ and X3™, respectively. The surface crystallinity of Crossfire™ liner was the same as that of the X3™ liner. Moreover, both Crossfire™ and X3™ experienced a steep gradient of crystallinity along the first 20 μm in the sample subsurface, in contrast to the mild rising of crystallinity fraction recorded for Longevity™, which obeys a slaggy profile down to 100 μm in depth. The highest crystallinity value measured in this latter liner was only ≈50%. The saturated crystallinity value in the bulk of the liner was the highest (62%) in X3™ among all the investigated samples, while Crossfire™ saturated at around 55% in the bulk. The retrieved crystallinity profiles can be interpreted as the direct consequence of the selected processing (namely, reduced crystallinity by remelting (Longevity™) vs. substantial preservation of the as-irradiated structure upon annealing (Crossfire™ and X3™). Moreover, the collected data prove the high efficiency in the crystallization induced by an annealing process based on sequential steps compared with annealing performed

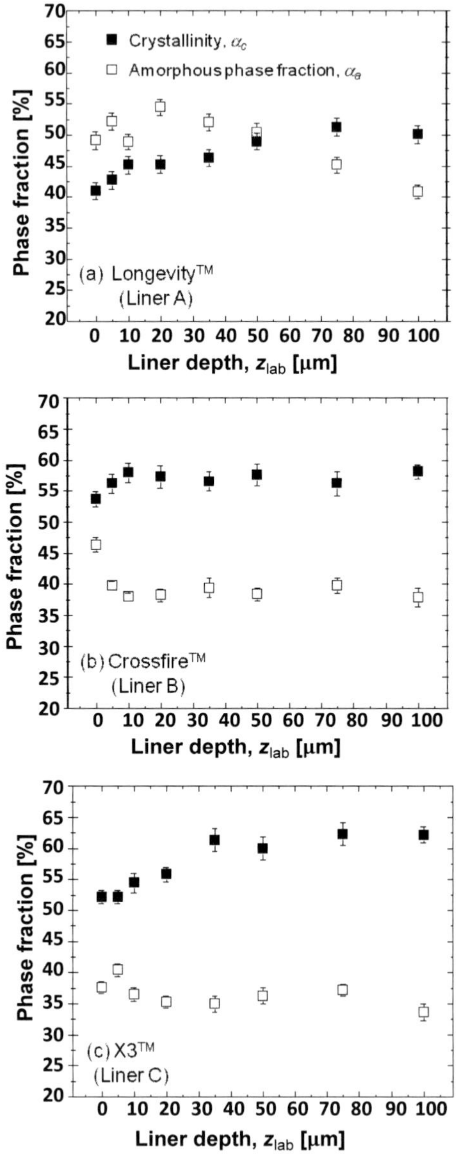

Figure 6.3 In-depth profiles of phase (volume) fractions as collected in the as-received liners (open and close symbols refer to amorphous phase fraction, α_a, and crystallinity, α_c, respectively).

in a single cycle. As a matter of fact, for a comparable dose of γ-irradiation, Crossfire™ and X3™ differ by about 7% in their bulk crystallinity. In other words, the manufacturing process of X3™ appears successful in obtaining an improved crystallinity upon cumulatively applying about the same irradiation dose. It should be also noted that in none of the examined liners traces of oxidation could be found at any location examined. A series of two-dimensional maps collected along the depth of different types of liner are shown in Figs. 6.4~6.6 for Longevity™, Crossfire™, and X3™ liners, respectively. The maps contained in each of the above three figures represent the volume fraction of the crystalline, α_c, (mainly orthorhombic) (a)~(h), of the amorphous, α_a (i)~(p), and of the third (or intermediate), α_t (q)~(x), phases at different depths from z_{lab} = 0 (liner surface) to z_{lab} = 100 μm. The maps in Figs. 6.4~6.6 give the statistical details of the stereological distribution of the constituent phases in the polymeric structure of UHMWPE in three dimensions. Figures 6.7(a)~(c), (d)~(f), and (g)~(i) display histograms of crystallinity fraction, α_c, at different depths for Longevity™, Crossfire™, and X3™ liners, respectively. The histograms are representative of the full set of statistical data collected on all the investigated liners of each type. The salient features revealed by a comparison among maps and histograms in Figs 6.4~6.7 can be listed as follows:

(i) The statistical trend for the degree of crystallinity at the surface of the Crossfire™ liner is represented by a relatively broad distribution compared with the Longevity™ and X3™ liners, although its mean value is comparable to that of the X3™ liner (and conspicuously higher than that of Longevity™). Unlike the Crossfire™ liner, both Longevity™ and X3™ liners preserved homogeneous histogram morphology throughout the sample depth.

(ii) The textures of the crystalline and amorphous phases in the Crossfire™ and X3™ liners appear to have the morphology of interpenetrated networks, while the stereological distribution of the constituent phases in the Longevity™ liner rather appears as that of isolated crystalline spots embedded into an amorphous matrix.

(iii) The amount of third phase (i.e., an intermediate phase between crystalline and amorphous) was clearly detectable in all samples at any location. However, it was particularly pronounced only in the bulk of the Longevity™ liner.

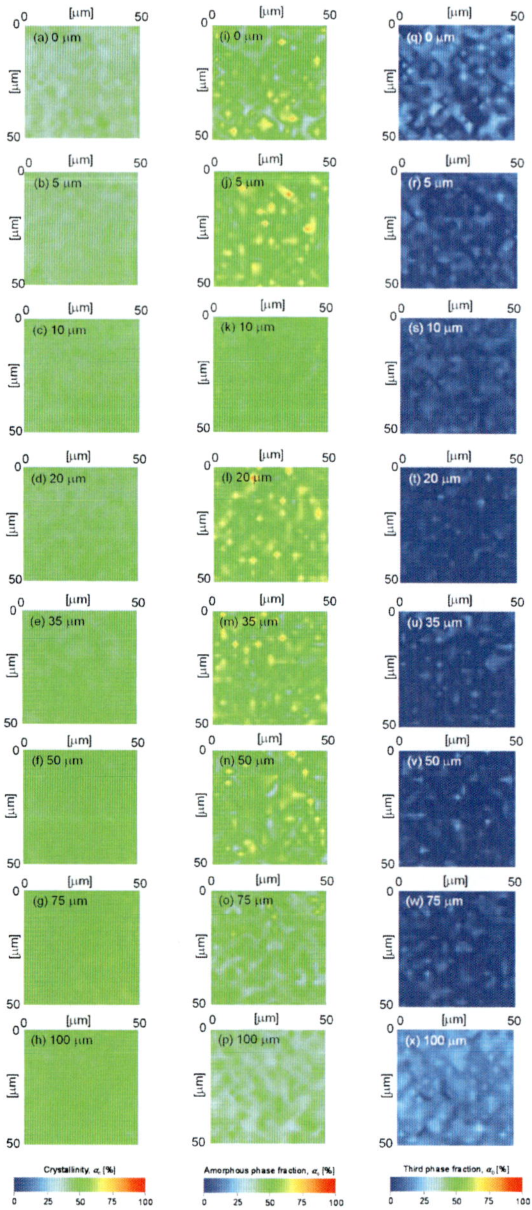

Figure 6.4 Maps of phase volume fractions collected at increasing depth of focal plane of Longevity^{TM} (liner A) ((a)~(h) for the crystalline phase fraction, α_c, (i)~(p) for the amorphous phase fraction, α_a, and (q)~(x) for the intermediate (third) phase fraction, α_t).

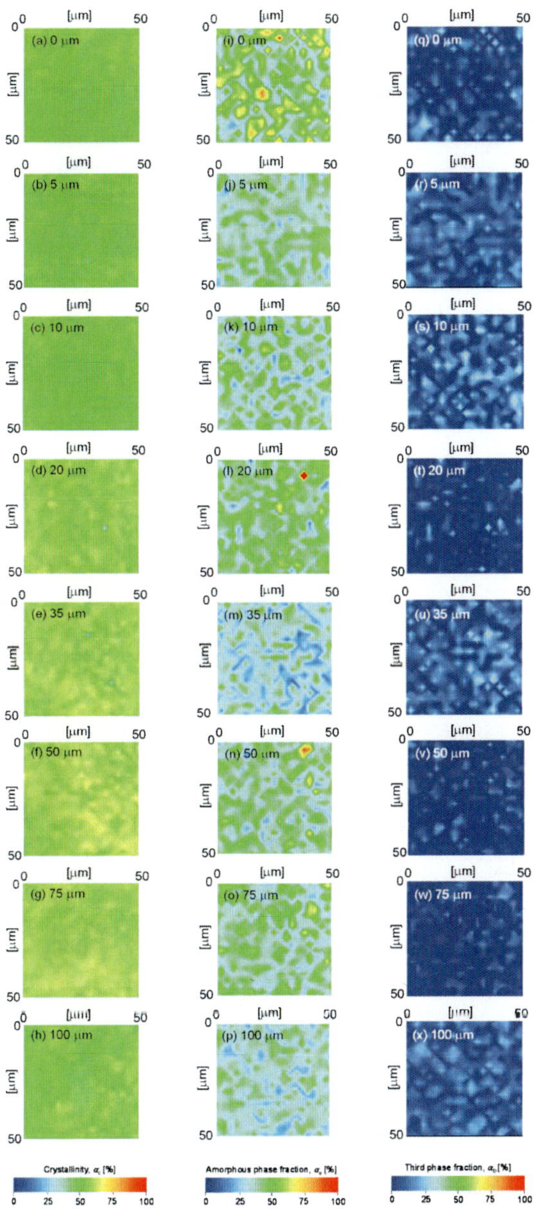

Figure 6.5 Maps of phase volume fractions collected at increasing depth of focal plane of Crossfire^{TM} (liner B) ((a)~(h) for the crystalline phase fraction, α_c, (i)~(p) for the amorphous phase fraction, α_a, and (q)~(x) for the intermediate (third) phase fraction, α_t).

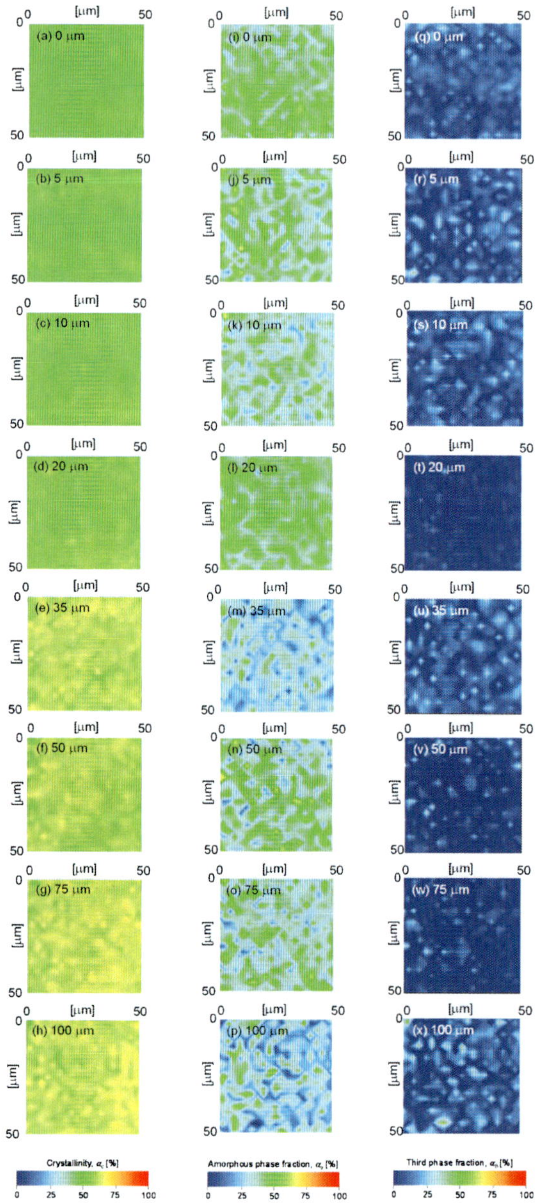

Figure 6.6 Maps of phase volume fractions collected at increasing depth of focal plane of X3^{TM} (liner C) ((a)~(h) for the crystalline phase fraction, α_c, (i)~(p) for the amorphous phase fraction, α_a, and (q)~(x) for the intermediate (third) phase fraction, α_t).

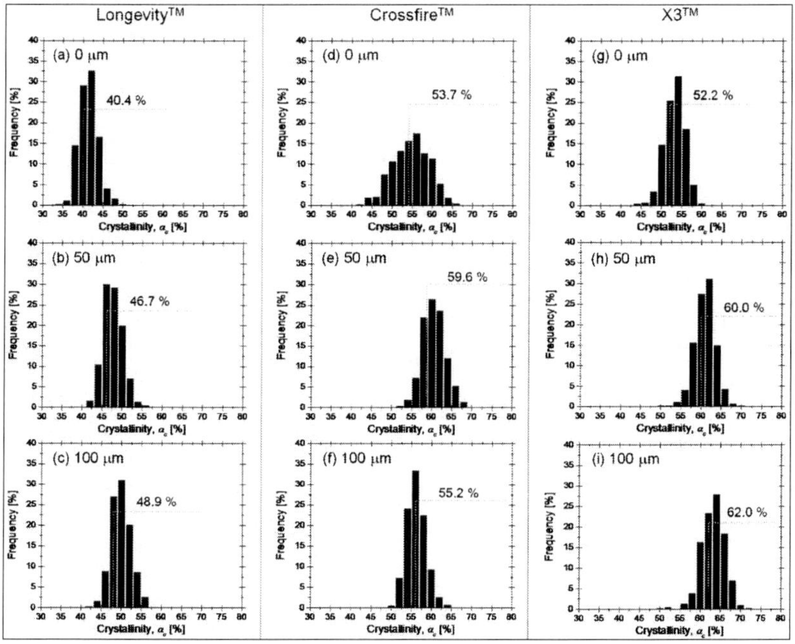

Figure 6.7 Histograms of crystalline phase fraction, α_c, (average values shown in inset), collected at different depths of the as-received liners.

At the nanometer length scale, UHMWPE is meanly a two-phase solid, consisting of crystalline domains embedded within an amorphous matrix. With increasing the amount of crystalline phase, the structure assumes the morphology of a two-phase interpenetrated composite. The crystalline phase of UHMWPE consists of folded rows of carbon atoms packed into lamellae, typically 10–50 nm in thickness and on the order of 10–50 μm in length (cf. Fig. 6.1). The crystalline morphology of UHMWPE encompasses a distribution of lamellar sizes within the polymer, although the typical interlamellar spacing is 50 nm, according to small-angle X-ray scattering measurements [776]. The amorphous phase consists of randomly oriented and entangled polymer chains traversed by tie molecules, which interconnect the lamellae. This latter phase is expected undergoing the main amount of internal deformation displacement under compression. Therefore, the high fraction of crystalline phase in the X3™ liner is expected to lead to high creep resistance. Furthermore, as mentioned in the introductive part of this report, cross-linking has been shown to dramatically improve the wear behavior of UHMWPE. This benefit to wear resistance, however, might be accompanied by a decrease in mechanical properties such as ultimate tensile strength, ductility, toughness and fatigue resistance. Degradation of such mechanical properties may have serious implications for the liner, owing to the high stress concentrations and large cyclic contact stresses produced by *in vivo* loading. A balanced microstructure combining the roles of an increased crystallinity and cross-linking should also be beneficial for the resistance to fatigue crack propagation, and a structure with these characteristics is also expected to possess high wear and creep resistances. X3™ seems to satisfy, from a microstructural view point, all these prerequisites, which confirms the reported wear data in hip simulator [774] and the preliminary report published on its *in vivo* performance [775].

As a first step in the assessment of molecular arrangement in the studied liners, the different crystallographic textures in liners obtained from ram-extruded rod stock and compression-molded sheets of UHMWPE were clarified. As already mentioned, the processing steps themselves induce a distinct crystallographic texture in the polymer structure, although the extent of such a texture might be less pronounced than that occurring after implantation due to loading/frictional effects in the joint [124]. The variation in the relative intensity of the 1170 and 1296 cm^{-1} Raman bands (i.e., those belonging to the orthorhombic structure of UHMWPE), which can be found upon collecting Raman spectra with varying the in-plane rotation angle, χ (also referred to as "azimuthal angle", henceforth), can be used to study the orientation of molecular chains in UHMWPE [123, 124]. The experimentally recorded dependence of the relative Raman intensities reveals periodic functions that can be fitted to a high degree of precision to a theoretical trial function for a selected configuration of the polarization filter. Figures 6.8(a)~(e), (f)~(j), and (k)~(o) show the angular dependences of normalized Raman intensities as retrieved along the in-depth direction at different locations (cf. draft in Fig. 6.2(a)) of the Longevity™, Crossfire™, and X3™ liners, respectively. Pronounced differences among different liners and among different locations within individual liners can be noticed in both periodicity and intensity variation of the angular profiles.

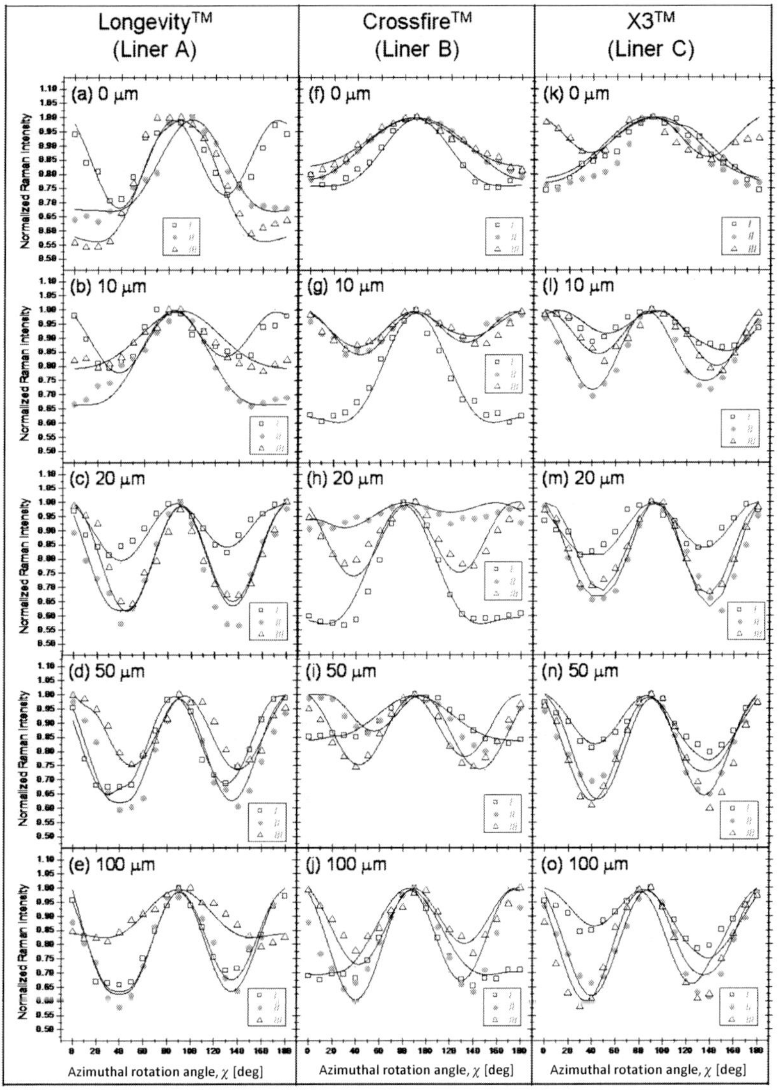

Figure 6.8 Experimental plots of the angular dependence of polarized Raman scattering intensities recorded upon in-plane rotation at different depths of the as-received liners ((a)~(e) for Longevity™ (liner A), (f)~(j) for Crossfire™ (liner B), and (k)~(o) for X3™ (liner C)). Different symbols are used to represent the measurement locations, (I)–(III) (cf. symbols in the legend). Full lines represent the results of best fitting to theoretical curves.

In this context, the salient feature is the change of periodicity from 180° to 90° observed in the plots at different locations along the sample subsurface. Such a change in periodicity is directly related to the out-of-plane variation of the mean orientation zenithal angle, θ, of the molecular chains. The set of data in Fig. 6.8 represents the basis for a three-dimensional analysis of the molecular structure in the three different types of liner.

Figure 6.9 shows the in-depth dependences at different locations of the liners of the zenithal angle, θ, (cf. Fig. 6.2(b)) describing the molecular orientation in the laboratory coordinate system, as retrieved from the best fitting of the data set in Fig. 6.8. The angular dependences were obtained by a least-square routine fitting. The salient notions that can be extracted from the plots in Fig. 6.9 can be summarized as follows:

(i) In all types of liner, independent of location on their concave surface, the molecular chains at the surface are mainly aligned along a direction parallel to the sample surface, but they tend to reach the direction perpendicular to the surface with proceeding along the subsurface. The trend of orientation parallel to the surface, commonly found on the surfaces of the investigated liners, is interpreted as being a direct consequence of the machining process.

(ii) In the X3™ liner, the in-depth variation of molecular orientation from parallel to perpendicular to the liner surface quickly occurs within the first 20 μm along the subsurface, independent of the probed location being the geometrical center of the liner or its lateral location. The steep and highly homogeneous trend found for the X3™ liner should also be related to the choice of compression-molded sheets as raw components, although conspicuously less homogeneous trend is found for the Longevity™ liner. On the other hand, the Crossfire™ liners, manufactured from extruded rods, showed molecular patterns aligned perpendicular to the sample surface only at their central location.

(iii) Despite being manufactured from highly homogeneous compression-molded sheets, the remelted Longevity™ liners showed large differences, both at the surface and in the subsurface trends, in molecular alignment among the investigated liners. This is considered being a consequence of the applied surface-machining procedure, with poor machining accuracy in areas close to the edge of the cup on which also less pressure is presumably applied.

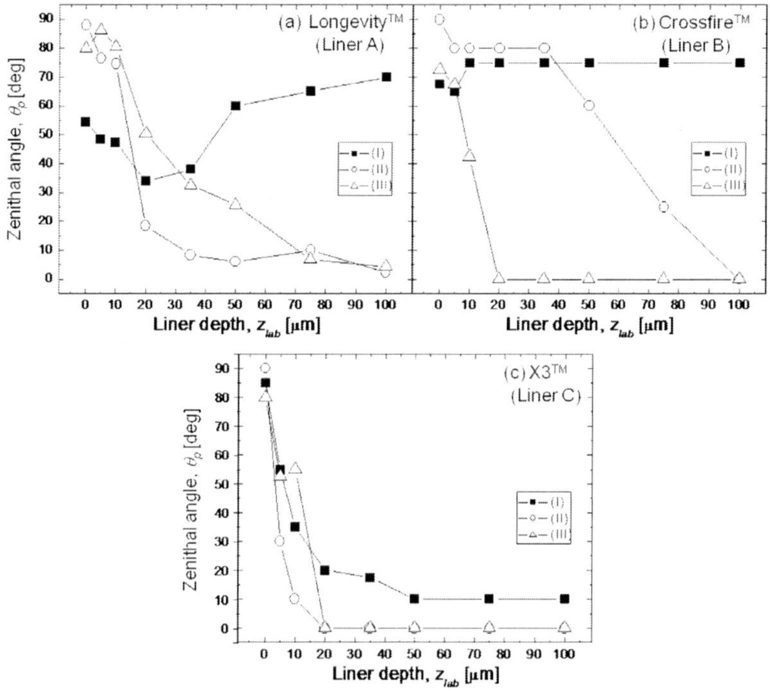

Figure 6.9 Plots of the mean zenithal angle, θ_p, calculated from the best fitting curves as shown in Fig. 6.8.

The orientation of the polyethylene molecule probed by Raman spectroscopy can be expressed in terms of Wigner functions that are reduced to Legendre polynomials after symmetry considerations [777,778]. This formalism leads to the determination of orientation distribution functions (ODF), $f(\beta)$, which express the probability that a molecular chain is aligned at a given angle, β, with respect to a preferential axis (cf. Fig. 6.2(b)), in turn expressed by the parameter, $\langle P_2(\cos\beta)\rangle$. The preferential axis is taken here as the mean zenithal angle, θ, plotted in Fig. 6.9. The order parameter $\langle P_2(\cos\beta)\rangle$ is also known as the Hermans orientation parameter. It assumes the value 0 when the orientation of the orthorhombic lamellae is fully random, while values 1 and −0.5 mean a perfect orientation along and perpendicular to a given axis (i.e., the axis of preferential orientation), respectively. The Hermans orientation parameter can be considered as the primary parameter to judge the alignment of UHMWPE orthorhombic lamellae. Additional order parameters display in the Legendre polynomial, which also contribute to describe the degree of orientation of the polymeric structure. However, the contribution of such additional parameters is less meaningful and straightforward than that of $\langle P_2(\cos\beta)\rangle$ [779]. Therefore, for the purpose intended here, it will suffice to discuss the degree of orientation of the investigated UHMWPE structures by only considering the Hermans parameter as an indicator of the degree of orientation of the structure.

The ODFs obtained for locations along the in-depth direction at different locations of the liner (cf. draft in Fig. 6.2(a)) are shown in Fig. 6.10 for the Longevity™ (Figs. 6.10(a)~(c)), Crossfire™ (Figs. 6.10(d)~(f)), and X3™ (Figs. 6.10(g)~(i)) acetabular cups,

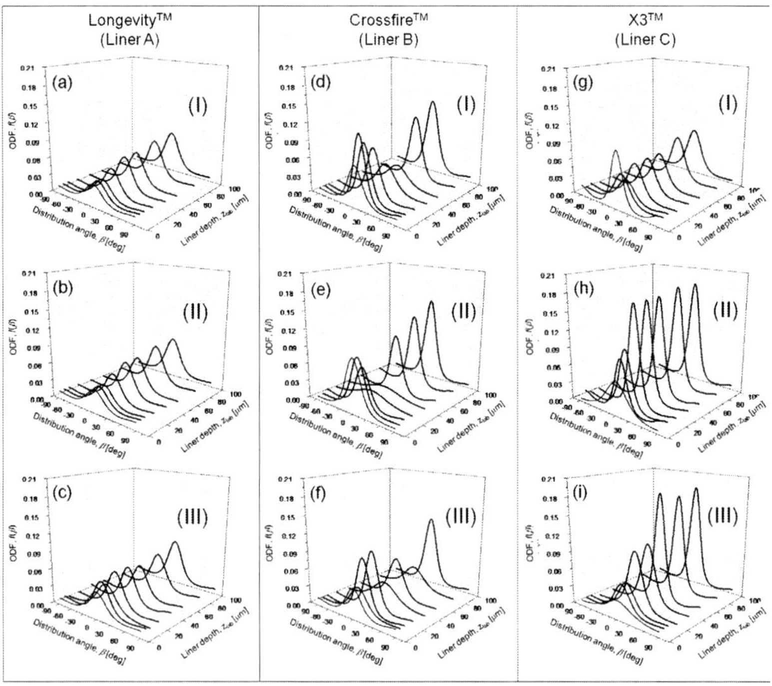

Figure 6.10 ODFs calculated at the different depth of the as-received liners ((a)~(c) for Longevity™ (liner A), (d)~(f) for Crossfire™ (liner B), and (g)~(i) for X3™ (liner C)).

respectively. Again, pronounced differences among different liners and different locations within individual liners can be noticed in the structure of $f(\beta)$. From a general viewpoint, the interpretation of the data in Fig. 6.10 can be facilitated by noting that for the same (mean) orientation angle, θ, the broader the ODF the less statistically aligned the structure. It immediately appears evident that the X3™ sample, compared with both Longevity™ and Crossfire™ samples, experiences by far the most statistically aligned structure for at least two of the three locations examined (i.e., locations II and III in Fig. 6.2(a)). From the set of data in Fig. 6.10 the Hermans parameter, $\langle P_2(\cos\beta)\rangle$, can be calculated, which describes the degree of alignment of the molecular structure in the three different types of liner. The results of this calculation are given in terms of plots $\langle P_2(\cos\beta)\rangle$ vs. z in Figs. 6.11(a), (b), and (c) for Longevity™, Crossfire™, and X3™ samples, respectively. The salient notions that can be extracted from the plots in Figs. 6.9~6.11 can be summarized as follows:

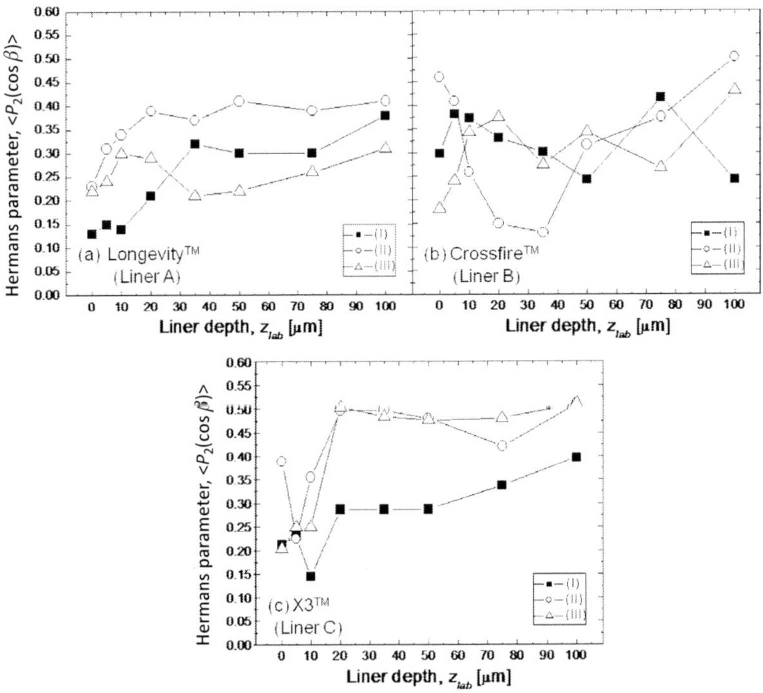

Figure 6.11 Plots of the Hermans parameter, $\langle P_2(\cos\beta)\rangle$, calculated from the best fitting curves as shown in Fig. 6.8.

(i) At the center/bottom surface location, all liners examined follow a similar statistical trend, with similarly high (mean) molecular orientation angles (i.e., comprised in the narrow interval $73° < \theta < 80°$, and thus conspicuously parallel to the sliding surface). Moreover, their molecular structure experiences a trend that is quite close to randomness ($0.18 < \langle P_2(\cos\beta)\rangle < 0.22$). Upon proceeding toward the depth at the same location, a relatively steep (i.e., within an interval $\Delta z_{lab} \approx 20$ μm) increase in the statistical degree of alignment of the X3™ liner (up to $\langle P_2(\cos\beta)\rangle = 0.5$) was recorded, while almost no change in the degree of randomness with increasing z_{lab} could be found in the Longevity™ liner. The trend recorded in the Crossfire™ samples was somewhat intermediate between the two above types of liner.

(ii) Screening the in-depth molecular orientation profile at different locations on the concave surface of the X3™ liner led to very close trends for locations II and III (steep change from $\theta = 0°$ to $\theta = 90°$ from the surface toward a depth of ≈20 μm, accompanied by an equally steep increase of the degree of orientation up to $\langle P_2(\cos\beta)\rangle \approx 0.5$ over the same interval, Δz_{lab}, of sample depth). The molecular trend at location (I) (i.e., in the peripheral zone close to the edge of the liner) displayed a similar average orientation angle, but also a conspicuously lower degree of molecular orientation. Such a reduced orientation pattern near the edge of the liner can be related to the machining procedure.

(iii) The Longevity™ liner generally showed a trend of low degree of orientation at any location of the liners with a relatively low increase as a function of the in-depth abscissa, Δz_{lab}. The maximum degree of alignment was found at the intermediate location (II) with $\langle P_2(\cos\beta)\rangle \approx 0.35$. The molecular orientation found for the Crossfire™ samples again appears to be an intermediate one between the Longevity™ and X3™ liners. However, a peculiarity of all the Crossfire™ samples was a high degree of randomness $\langle P_2(\cos\beta)\rangle \approx 0.12$) in the immediate subsurface ($20 < z < 35$ μm) of the intermediate location (II).

Schematic drafts that attempt to summarize the stereological assembly of the molecular structure (i.e., including both notions of average zenithal angle, θ, and Hermans parameter, $\langle P_2(\cos\beta\rangle$)

found in the different types of liner are given in Fig. 6.12. We shall hereafter refer to these simplified drafts for the purpose of a general discussion.

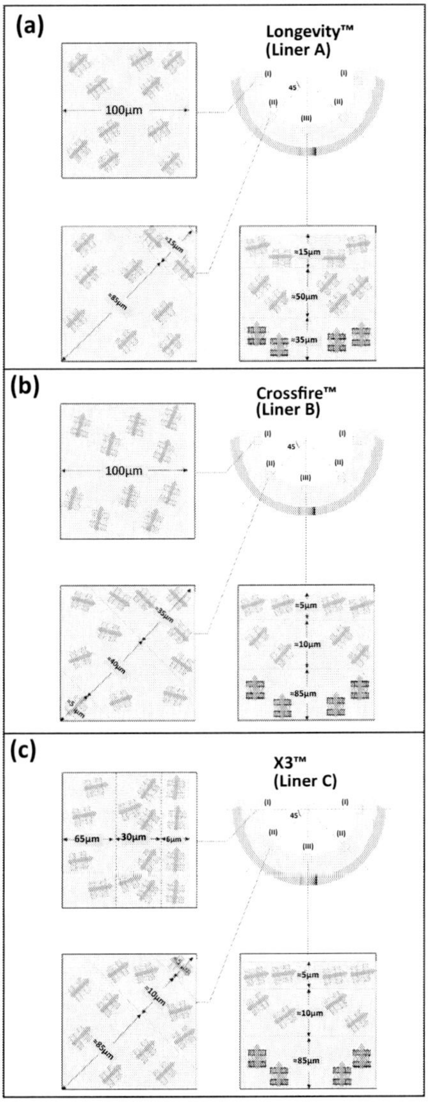

Figure 6.12 Structural model for the three as-received liners that experienced different processing steps in their manufacturing procedures. Arrows represent the preferential orientation of UHMWPE molecular chains.

As far as the expected wear resistance of the liners is concerned, early studies by Wang *et al.* [325,780] have documented in great details the interactions between contact stresses and the molecular structure of worn polyethylene surfaces. A strain softening-assisted adhesive wear model was proposed by which those researchers successfully clarified how crystalline anisotropy in the UHMWPE structure (i.e., as induced by different modes of sliding) could be responsible for a molecular reorganization process at the wear surface during sliding. This process is driven by plastic strain accumulation at the worn surface and arises from repeated cyclic asperity contacts. Unlike simply linear sliding contacts, in which UHMWPE molecules are stretched along the direction of sliding and undergo significant strain hardening, in multi-directional sliding contact such as that experienced in the natural human joints, molecular orientation actually leads to strain softening and weakening of the sliding surface. According to the Wang's model, the mechanism of wear debris generation in UHMWPE (in the absence of third-body particles) can be described as the sequential combination of rupture of transversely softened (oriented) molecular chains and shear rupture with formation of fibrillar wear debris. The most straightforward deduction that one can obtain from the pioneering studies of Wang *et al.* [325,780] is the positive effects of cross-linking on wear resistance (widely confirmed by a number of successive papers [781,782]), since cross-linking reduces molecular mobility and, hence, should also reduce the extent of molecular orientation that decreases the strength of the material in the transverse direction (experimentally confirmed in [783]). Moreover, the achieved physical insight into the effect of molecular orientation on wear resistance also implies that upon controlling (and engineering) the crystalline amount, the subsurface gradient, and the orientation of the oriented molecular chains, one can maximize the wear resistance by minimizing strain softening and the related weakening effects that occur upon sliding of the polyethylene surface. From a practical point of view, the findings by Wang *et al.* point to the most suitable direction for developing the most wear resistant UHMWPE as a material highly resistant to multiaxial stress-induced strain softening. To achieve high resistance to strain softening the adopted processing should allow maintaining a moderately crystallized and rigorously isotropic molecular structure at the load-bearing surface during sliding. Data in Figs. 6.3, 6.9, and 6.10 indeed clearly demonstrate that the X3™ liner possesses a unique surface structure with a 50% crystallized structure completely in plane oriented ($\theta = 0°$) with a two-dimensionally random texture. The orientation pattern was homogeneously obtained over the entire surface of each individual liner and found to be highly reproducible for a number of different liners of the same type. Such optimized surface structure is thus reliably engineered for providing the highest resistance to the multiaxial stresses developed *in vivo* in the hip joint.

Advanced Raman spectroscopic techniques are shown capable to reveal fundamental microstructural details of commercially available acetabular cups. The newest proposed process of sequential irradiation and annealing, as adopted by Stryker Orthopedics, Inc. in manufacturing the X3™ liner, offers an efficient way to obtain both surface and bulk UHMWPE structures potentially suitable for concurrently attaining high wear resistance and low creep deformation. At the molecular scale, the structure of the X3™ liner appears a peculiar one in its structural and stereological characteristics, and significantly improved compared with previously commercialized products by other makers.

The structural analysis by Raman spectroscopy at the molecular scale has clarified the following main points:

(i) Two-dimensionally, random in-plane orientation of the axis of UHMWPE molecules together with a moderate crystallinity is the main structure homogeneously achieved on all the surface of the X3™ liner. Such a structure showed minimum scatter among the investigated liners and realizes the best molecular assemblies for achieving high wear resistance, according to previously established knowledge by Wang *et al.* [325].

(ii) A steep gradient within the first 20 μm below the sliding surface in the UHMWPE structure in the X3™ liner leads to a very high degree of crystallinity (i.e., ≥60%), which is homogeneously preserved down to the bulk. Such a high level of crystallization is not achieved at any depth in commercially available UHMWPE liners belonging to the previous generation.

(iii) Besides high crystallinity, the Raman probe also detected a rigorous orientation of the molecular patterns orthogonal to the sliding surface (and thus to the direction of the applied compressive load) in the bulk of the X3^{TM} liner structure. Such orientation is quite homogeneously kept from >20 μm in depth from the surface down to the bulk. Such molecular structure, together with the high degree of crystallinity represents, according to the state-of-art knowledge in polymer deformation mechanics, the best-suited structure for achieving a superior creep resistance.

The vulnerability of UHMWPE acetabular liners to wear and creep has been long suggested to strongly depend on their molecular assembly and subsurface gradients. The Raman spectroscopic experiments shown here make clear how one could structurally differentiate liners from different makers. In other words, a detailed information about the liner structure on the molecular scale is now available and can be systematically related to the wear and creep performance of the liners after *in vitro* or *in vivo* exposure.

6.3 *In vitro* and *in vivo* Creep Behavior of Advanced UHMWPE Liners

Numerous papers are available in the literature about the effect of crystallinity and molecular orientation on the compressive creep of UHMWPE [215,784–791]. Concerning the effect of the degree of crystallinity in polyethylene structures on the macroscopic deformation behavior of the material, there is general agreement that an increase in crystallinity linearly increases the deformation yield of the material and that such relationship is rather insensitive to the conditions of crystallization [784–787]. Therefore, one should expect the highly crystallized bulk structure of the X3^{TM} liner minimizing creep deformation. With regard to molecular orientation issues, particularly relevant to the analysis of the X3^{TM} liner presented above is a study by Lee and Pienkowski [791], in which the static compressive creep behavior of UHMWPE was studied with machining the samples from the center or from the periphery of extruded GUR 4150HP rod stock. The amount and rate of creep strain varied with the radial position in the rod stock: specimens obtained from the periphery had 8~19% larger creep strain rates than did specimens obtained from the center. Note that the results of Lee and Pienkowski [791] are in agreement with general notions about compressive creep of polyethylene, as given in the classic studies by Lin and Argon [788] and by Philip *et al.* [789]. It was observed in the previous section that according to Bellare and Cohen [772], in extruded rods of UHMWPE a discernible degree of preferred orientation of molecular chains exists within crystallites. The direction of the axis of molecular chain alignment near the outer surface of the extruded rods is found to be orthogonal to the radial direction, whereas the molecular chain direction is orthogonal to the axial (or extrusion) direction in crystallites located near the centerline of the extruded rods. Merging the notions contained in the works by Lee and Pienkowski [791] and by Bellare and Cohen [772], we can thus state the following:

(i) A UHMWPE structure whose molecular chain axis is orthogonal to the applied compressive load (i.e., as in the case of samples obtained from zones near the centerline of extruded rods) should be more creep resistant than a structure with chain alignment parallel to the compressive loading direction (i.e., as the samples obtained from the peripheral zone of the extruded rod in the study of Lee and Pienkowski [791]). From this point of view, the bulk molecular structure of the X3™ liner appears to represent an optimum for maximizing the creep resistance of the liner.

(ii) A highly homogeneous structure within the liner with molecular chains uniformly aligned with their axis perpendicular to the liner surface should greatly help minimizing the azimuthally non-uniform deformation usually observed in retrieved acetabular cups. The highly homogeneous molecular structure of the X3™ liner, produced from compression-molded sheets, should thus effectively minimize azimuthal inhomogeneities in the liner deformation during *in vivo* exposure.

To prove the above statements, investigations were made of the modifications introduced at the molecular scale when uniaxial plastic compressive strain piled up in the microstructure of Crossfire™ and X3™ acetabular components. As already discussed, the two materials belong to different manufacturing generations, and the latter material represents the most advanced and recently launched γ-ray-irradiated polyethylene material in the worldwide hip implant market. Confocal/polarized Raman spectroscopy was systematically applied to characterize the microstructural response of the two different polyethylene materials to plastic deformation. For doing so, both bandwidth variation of the 1130 cm^{-1} Raman band (which is related to the C–C stretching vibration (A_g + B_{1g} mode)) and preferential orientation of molecular chains have been correlated to plastic strain magnitudes through preliminary calibration procedures based on one-dimensional relaxation tests applied to unused acetabular cups. Analyses of the *in vivo* deformation behavior of two short-term retrieved hip cups were also performed. According to the structural characteristics shown in the previous section, one would expect similar trends of preferential orientation of molecular chains as a function of residual strain for both materials, but clearly different in their developed extents. The sequentially irradiated material is expected to be more resistant to plastic deformation and to achieve, for the same magnitude of residual plastic strain, higher molecular chain orientation than the single-step irradiated one. These statements find a common rationale in the higher crystallinity and degree of cross-linking of X3™ compared with Crossfire™.

In order to calibrate the deformation response of the UHMWPE materials, the structural modifications induced by plastic deformation should be preliminary studied using a uniaxial relaxation test (in a compressive geometry) applied to samples obtained from unused liners. In the calibration experiments explained hereafter, samples were cut from the acetabular cups as received from the maker (Fig. 6.13(a)) into rectangular prisms 4 mm × 4 mm × 6 mm in dimension, suitable for uniaxial relaxation tests in compression (Fig. 6.13(b)). Particular care was taken in order to smooth down by polishing the four corners of the concave surface of the sample, which enabled us to obtain flat surfaces at the loading faces of the sample. In one-dimensional relaxation tests, the material was subjected to a sudden compressive strain of a predetermined magnitude, which was kept constant for 24 h in order to allow the full occurrence of stress relaxation possible in the microstructure. The strain field was then released and the sample allowed recovering of its anelastic strain for additional 24 h, so that only plastic strain remained stored in the microstructure. Compression test calibrations were repeated for each type of investigated material. Compressive load was applied stepwise. The samples were left unloaded for 24 h after each step of external compression. The residual (plastic) strain was measured along the sample long axis by means of a micrometer caliper, and the deformed samples analyzed by Raman spectroscopy. Spectroscopic characterizations served to analyze the modifications induced by compressive strain on the original microstructure of the acetabular component, phenomenologically reproducing the conditions encountered during *in vivo* loading. As a first step, the microstructures of the two types of investigated UHMWPE have been monitored in their as-received state with respect to their response to a constant state of compressive strain. The residual strain in each as-received material was assumed as $\varepsilon = 0$ and a constant (uniaxial) strain magnitude (i.e., referred to as true strain before recovery, ε_i) was increasingly applied at subsequent steps up to a level $\varepsilon_i \approx 32\%$. Figure 6.14 shows plots of true strain after recovery, ε_f as a function of externally applied strain, ε_i, for both Crossfire^{TM} and X3^{TM} materials. The $\varepsilon_f = \varepsilon_f(\varepsilon_i)$ plots obtained for both materials were linear in nature and their comparison revealed a distinct difference in slope (in inset), which was higher for Crossfire^{TM} compared with X3^{TM} material. In other words, for the same applied constant strain, ε_i, the X3^{TM} material revealed a higher capacity of recovery, thus incorporating a lower amount of plastic strain, ε_f. This experimental finding can be interpreted as a clear proof for a higher resistance to permanent deformation of the X3^{TM} microstructure compared with that of Crossfire^{TM}.

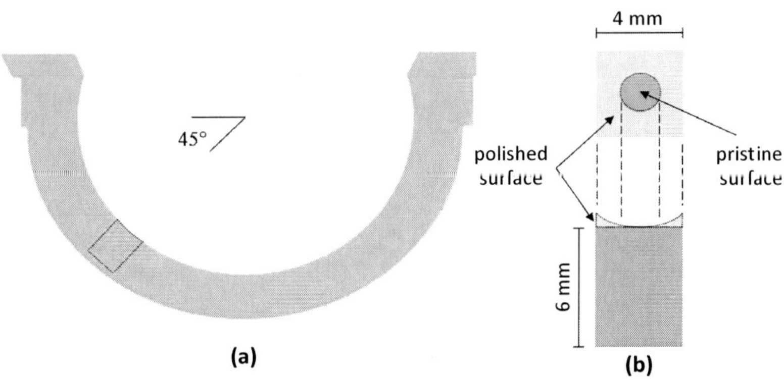

Figure 6.13 (a) Draft of the sample cutting procedure from acetabular cups as received from the maker; (b) rectangular prisms 4 × 4 × 6 mm in dimension used for uniaxial relaxation tests in compression.

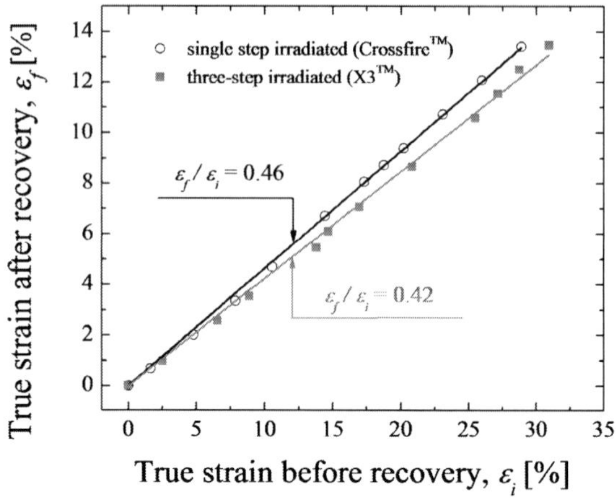

Figure 6.14 Plots of true strain after recovery, ε_f, as a function of externally applied (initial) strain, ε_i, are shown for Crossfire^{TM} and X3^{TM} materials. The slope of the linear plot was higher for the former material, as shown in inset.

In Fig. 6.15(a), experimental results are shown of band broadening ($\Delta\omega$ = FWHM) as retrieved from unpolarized Raman spectra at different values of residual compressive strain, ε_f, after strain recovery. The 1130 cm^{-1} band of the orthorhombic polyethylene structure was narrower in spectra collected from X3^{TM} compared with Crossfire^{TM}, due to the higher crystallinity of the former material (61.7% vs. 58%) [792, 793] and, as will be explicitly shown later, to its higher degree of molecular alignment. Both characteristics were a consequence of the three-step irradiation/annealing process followed in the liner manufacturing. The lower molecular weight of the starting resin of X3^{TM} (GUR 1020) compared with that of Crossfire^{TM} (GUR 1050) obviously had also a role in the formation of the recorded spectroscopic difference [794]. For better distinguishing the repercussions of external strain on microstructural rearrangement from the initial effects of the manufacturing procedures, the trends of band broadening observed in both types of material can be replaced with the bandwidth variation, $\Delta\omega - \Delta\omega_0 = \Delta FWHM$, with respect to the initial bandwidth value, $\Delta\omega_0$, in the as-received undeformed state. Accordingly, curves $\varepsilon_f = \varepsilon_f(\Delta FWHM)$ relating the plastic strain after recovery to spectroscopic features could be obtained, as shown in Fig. 6.15(b). Least-square fitting of the experimental data in Fig. 6.15(b) led to two phenomenological equations of a common cubic nature, as follows:

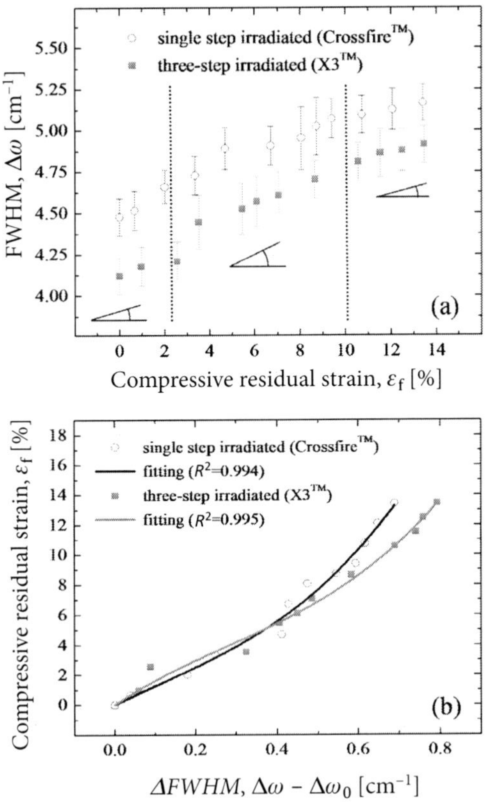

Figure 6.15 (a) Experimental plots of broadening, $\Delta\omega$ = FWHM, of the unpolarized 1130 cm^{-1} Raman band as a function of residual plastic strain, ε_f, after recovery are shown for Crossfire^{TM} and X3^{TM} materials. Both plots could be rationalized according to a division into three distinct deformation zones (separated by vertical dotted lines) with different slopes as shown in inset; (b) the experimental dependencies in (a) are re-plotted with taking the respective bandwidth variations with respect to initial bandwidth, $\Delta\omega - \Delta\omega_0 = \Delta FWHM$, in abscissa. This procedure enables to extract the effect of applied strain on the Raman band as distinguished from the initial difference arising from the different manufacturing procedures. Least-square fitting curves (correlation coefficients, R^2, in brackets in inset) are analytically represented by Eqs. (6.1) and (6.2) for X3^{TM} and Crossfire^{TM} liners, respectively.

$$\varepsilon_f = 18.05\Delta FWHM - 21.04\Delta FWHM^2 + 24.76\Delta FWHM^3 \quad (6.1)$$

$$\varepsilon_f = 13.11\Delta FWHM - 7.77\Delta FWHM^2 + 24.28\Delta FWHM^3 \quad (6.2)$$

in which $\Delta FWHM$ is expressed in units of cm^{-1}. Equations (6.1) and (6.2) refer to X3™ and Crossfire™ liners, respectively. The plots in Fig. 6.15(b) show that under the same level of applied strain, $\varepsilon_f > 5\%$, the Raman spectrum of the X3™ material undergoes a relatively higher broadening than that of Crossfire™. Figures 6.16(a) and (b) show examples of experimental angular dependencies of the $A_g + B_{1g}$ Raman mode on the azimuthal rotation angle, χ, obtained upon in-plane rotation at different stages of uniaxial deformation for the single-step and sequentially irradiated polyethylene structures, respectively. In both cases, with increasing the plastic strain stored in the material, a tendency to follow an angular periodicity of π rather than $\pi/2$ could be noticed, which was clearly a physical consequence of molecular alignment under strain. In particular, one could expect that under compressive load, the molecular arrangement tends to align in a plane perpendicular to the direction of the applied load. Values of preferential (out-of-plane) tilt angle, θ_p, and Hermans parameter, $\langle P_2(\cos\beta)\rangle$, can be obtained from the angular dependencies shown in Figs. 6.16(a) and (b) [123]. The dependencies of θ_p and $\langle P_2(\cos\beta)\rangle$ on deformation are plotted as a function of increasing plastic strain in Fig. 6.17(a) and Fig. 6.18, respectively, for both investigated materials. Upon subtracting the respective initial tilt angles, θ_{p0}, plots of $\varepsilon_f(\theta_p - \theta_{p0}) = \varepsilon_f(\Delta\theta_p)$ could be obtained for the two UHMWPE materials, as shown in Fig. 6.17(b). A comparison between the two plots in Fig. 6.17(b) clarifies that the X3™ material undergoes a higher tilting rotation at the molecular scale than Crossfire™ for the same magnitude of applied strain, $\varepsilon_f > 5\%$. Similar to the case of band broadening analysis, a least-square cubic polynomial fitting suitably applied to the observed experimental trends of molecular rearrangement, leading to the obtainment of two phenomenological curves, $\varepsilon_f = \varepsilon_f(\Delta\theta_p)$, as follows:

$$\varepsilon_f = 53.38\Delta\theta_p - 200.97\Delta\theta_p^2 + 488.32\Delta\theta_p^3 \quad (6.3)$$

$$\varepsilon_f = 42.45\Delta\theta_p - 83.05\Delta\theta_p^2 + 131.31\Delta\theta_p^3 \quad (6.4)$$

in which $\Delta\theta_p$ values are expressed in units of radiant. Equations (6.3) and (6.4) refer to X3™ and Crossfire™ liners, respectively. A clear difference could be found in the $\Delta\theta_p$ trends in the two investigated materials for $\varepsilon_f > 5\%$. At high plastic strains, the difference in the variation of out-of-plane tilt angle with respect to its value in original molecular orientation was more marked in the X3™ material, and the origin of such difference will be the object of the discussion presented hereafter.

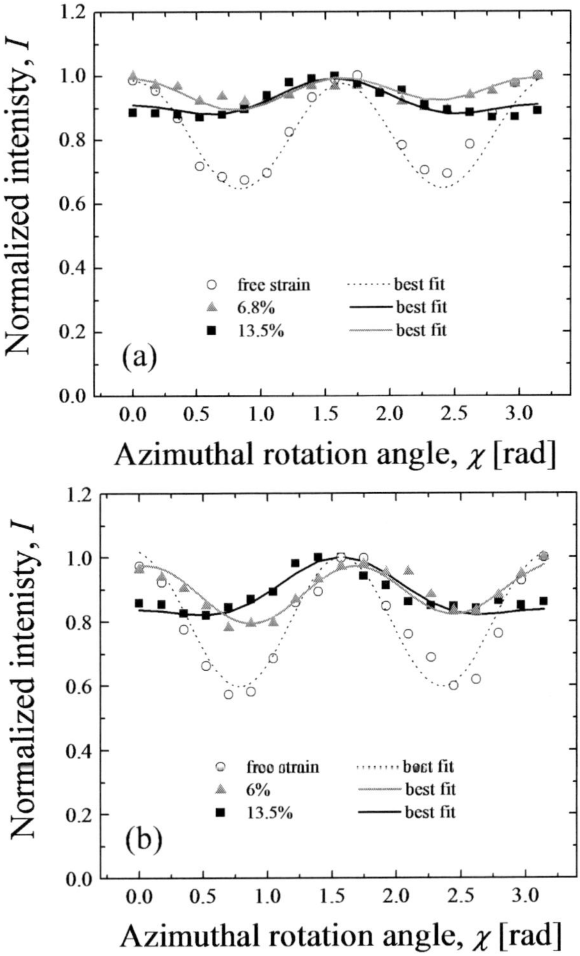

Figure 6.16 Experimental angular dependencies of the $A_g + B_{1g}$ mode Raman intensity on the azimuthal rotation angle, χ, obtained upon in-plane rotation at different stages of uniaxial deformation for Crossfire™ and X3™ materials (in (a) and (b), respectively).

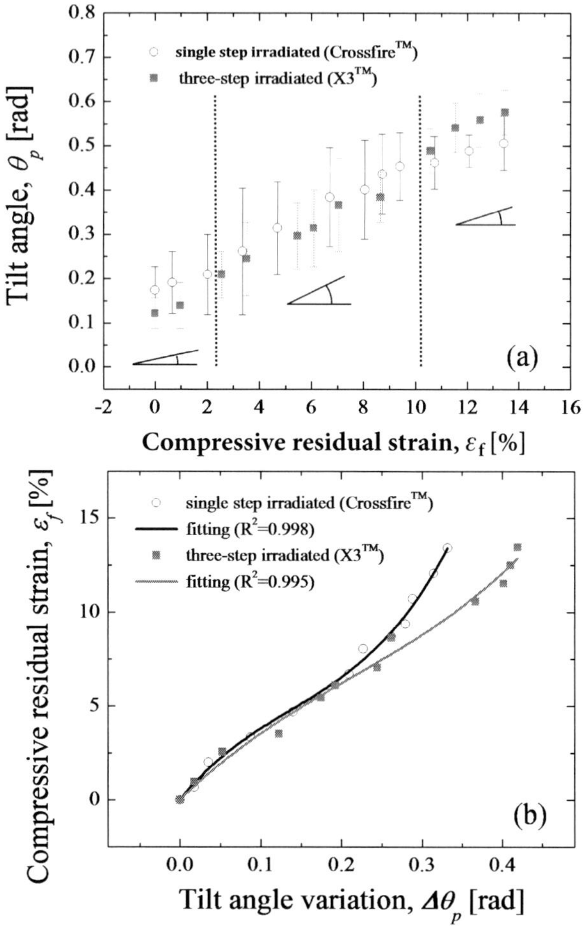

Figure 6.17 (a) Experimental plots of preferential tilt angle, θ_p, as a function of residual plastic strain, ε_f, after recovery are shown for Crossfire™ and X3™ materials. Similar to Fig. 6.15(a), both plots can be rationalized according to a division into three distinct deformation zones (separated by vertical dotted lines) with different slopes as shown in inset; (b) the experimental dependencies in (a) are replotted with taking the tilt angle variation, $\Delta\theta_p = \theta_p - \theta_{p0}$, in abscissa, thus separating the effect of applied strain on tilt angle from the effect of different manufacturing procedures. Least-square fitting curves (correlation coefficients, R^2, in brackets in inset) are analytically represented by Eqs. (6.3) and (6.4) for X3™ and Crossfire™ materials, respectively.

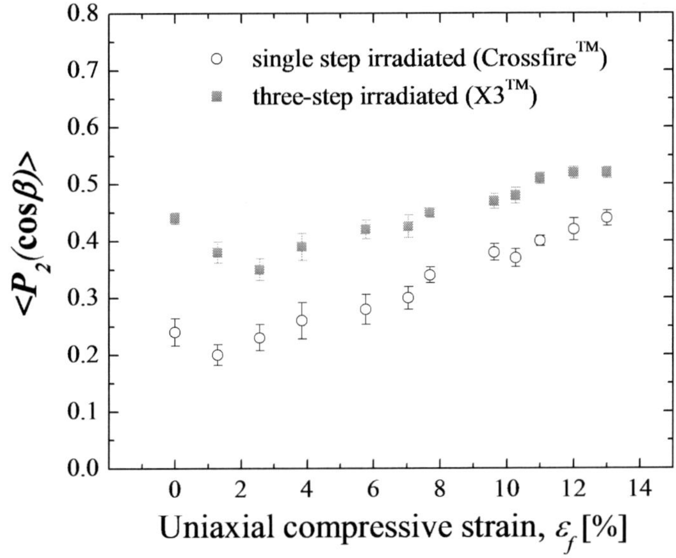

Figure 6.18 Plots of Hermans parameter, $\langle P_2(\cos\beta)\rangle$, as a function of residual plastic strain, ε_f, for both the investigated materials.

Based on the salient notions that can be extracted from the plots of Figs. 6.14~6.18, we can attempt to rationalize the origin of the microstructural modifications induced by uniaxial compression in bulk polyethylene and, ultimately, to discriminate the differences related to the particular processing that the polymer underwent to. Spectroscopic studies of deformation in highly crystalline and textured polymers (e.g., fibers) usually show the occurrence of both Raman band shift and bandwidth broadening, as a consequence of stretching of oriented molecules in both crystalline and amorphous regions [795–797]. Unlike those studies, in the experiment on bulk polyethylene shown here, the observed broadening of the 1130 cm^{-1} band was accompanied by a discernible statistical invariance of peak position (i.e., characterized by scattered values, but conspicuously constant in its average with increasing plastic strain). Spectral shifts of Raman bands under strain are expected to occur toward opposite directions for applied (uniaxial) strain magnitudes of tensile and compressive nature. The Raman band is also expected to only broaden (without shifting), when both types of deformation events (i.e., tensile and compressive) occur with the same statistical relevance at different locations within the probe volume. The tendency to band broadening without shifting under increasing plastic strain in biomedical polyethylene is reported in the literature [116]. A further step can be taken here in rationalizing the behavior under strain of UHMWPE by invoking a three-stage model, which could explain the sequence of microstructural modifications induced by uniaxial compressive load on the polymeric structure. The sigmoidal shape of the experimental curves in Figs. 6.15(a) and 6.17(a), which can be fitted to three distinct linear segments with different slopes, indeed suggests the existence of three stages in the overall deformation process. According to general notions in the field of deformation of bulk polymers [788,798], the inelastic response of semi-crystalline UHMWPE can be considered to begin with the main deformation process occurring within the amorphous regions of the polymeric structure, immediately followed by the activation of plastic deformation into the crystalline lamellae, predominantly via crystallographic slip mechanisms. Figure 6.19(a) show a schematic representing the microstructure of undeformed polyethylene, in which, according to measurements of tilt angle (cf. Fig. 6.17(a)), the preferential orientation of lamellar axes is broadly perpendicular to the bearing surface of the liners for both single-step and sequentially irradiated UHMWPE samples. This finding is in agreement with a previous study by Bellare and Cohen [772], who determined the nature of crystallographic texture in the bulk of ram-extruded rods and compression-molded sheets of UHMWPE. Both processing procedures indeed induced crystallographic texture in the polymer microstructures, although the compression-molded sheets employed for manufacturing X3™ displayed a higher degree of orientation, as revealed by the higher value of the Hermans parameter in Fig. 6.18 (i.e., at ε_f). The preferential orientation of molecular chains is a consequence of crystallization of the oriented polyethylene melt under a perpendicular compressive stress. In the amorphous phase surrounding the crystalline orthorhombic lamellae, due to the high molecular weight of polyethylene and to the high irradiation dose applied, the concentration of tie molecules, entanglements and cross-links is high and affects the response of the microstructure to the applied external load. During the first stage of deformation (i.e., up to ≈2% plastic strain, as shown in Figs. 6.15(a) and 6.17(a)), the molecular chains present in the amorphous phase are those mainly undergoing deformation. However, the important characteristic since the initial stage of deformation is that the strain locally stored in the structure is not necessarily compressive in nature, due to the high concentration of entanglements and cross-links throughout the disordered (amorphous) phase (cf. Fig. 6.19(b)). At this initial stage, rotation of crystalline lamellae is barely activated by the external compressive load, as demonstrated by only a slight increase of the tilt angle, θ_p (cf. Fig. 6.17(a)). The decrease of Hermans parameter during the initial deformation stage, consistently recorded for both the investigated materials (cf. Fig. 6.18), rather suggests the development of a higher state of disorder in the structure. The increasing presence of strain gradients within the probe volume, especially in the amorphous fraction of the materials, explains the incipient occurrence of band broadening (as shown in Fig. 6.15(a)). During the stage of secondary deformation (i.e., in the range $2\% \leq \varepsilon_f \leq 11\%$; cf. Figs. 6.15(a) and 6.17(a)), both materials showed the most remarkable variations in θ_p and $\Delta FWHM$. Significant band broadening, due to overstressed tie molecules, entanglements and cross-links between crystalline and amorphous regions, arose from steeper strain gradients of both tensile and compressive nature (Fig. 6.19(c)). Moreover, as shown by the pronounced rising of the $\langle P_2(\cos\beta)\rangle$ parameter (cf. Fig. 6.18), crystalline lamellae underwent significant rotation in this secondary stage of deformation, with a larger population of crystallites experiencing preferential orientation and aligning along a plane parallel to the sample surface. The rotation of lamellae should be massively activated by the previously mentioned exacerbation of tensile and compressive strain gradients in the amorphous phase (cf. Fig. 6.19(c)), while also a mechanism of structural rearrangement of intra-lamellar sliding concurrently takes place on the crystalline side of the structure [799]. By comparing the secondary stage of deformation as occurring in the two different liners, we have already noticed that the increase in tilt angle starts to be more pronounced in X3^{TM} than in Crossfire^{TM}. This finding suggests a higher concentration of cross-links in the amorphous phase of the former material, although the cumulative dose of irradiation was the same for both materials. In fact, as proved by Bartczak [790] and Boontongkong *et al.* [800], when subjected to the same strain magnitude in a range of relatively low deformations, highly entangled and/or highly cross-linked polyethylene structures achieve a higher degree of crystallographic orientation compared with less cross-linked and/or less entangled structures. In other words, if the concentration of cross-linking is high, the molecular chains in the amorphous region might quickly become fully stretched to their maximum limit, i.e., even at relatively low strain magnitudes. Such microstructural circumstance in turn triggers a faster reorientation of the crystalline lamellae according to the mechanism shown in Fig. 6.19. In the last (third) stage of compressive deformation (i.e., true strains in the interval, $11\% \leq \varepsilon_f \leq 13\%$), the observed variations of bandwidth and molecular orientation became milder than those in the second deformation stage (cf. lower slopes in Figs. 6.15(a) and 6.17(a), respectively). Such a mitigation of the process of molecular rearrangement concurs with the saturation of the rotation process, with a large population of molecular chains now experiencing preferential orientation at maximized tilt angle variations, $\Delta\theta_p$. Further plastic flow among crystalline lamellae is hampered by the onset of strain hardening correlated to the presence of cross-links. Above this stage, only chain slip within individual crystallites can be expected to become active as an intrinsic deformation mechanism. Crystalline slip occurs along the [001] direction of the orthorhombic structure (i.e., which corresponds to slip along the most closely packed crystallographic plane) [799]. In other words, strain hardening becomes the preponderant effect and should also be responsible for the milder band broadening shown by both materials in Fig. 6.15(a) at $\varepsilon_f \geq 11\%$. Such high levels of plastic strain, however, are not expected to occur under the mere effect of creep deformation in acetabular cups. On the other hand, the severe damage induced by abrasive/adhesive wear might locally produce extreme elongations in the lamellae, with the microstructure developing a texture similar to that of a single crystal (fibrillar structure) [799]. At these extreme levels of deformation, the effect of strain hardening induced by cross-linking should also be maximized. At the compressive strain levels experienced by the two investigated materials during the present characterization of plastic deformation, one could only detect, to a lower extent, the difference in strain hardening effect between X3™ and Crossfire™ materials. Nevertheless, it is clarified that sequentially irradiated UHMWPE, despite being produced from a lower molecular weight resin (i.e., with an expectedly lower initial concentration of molecular entanglements), shows a higher resistance to plastic deformation and a larger recovering capacity, and undergoes a faster molecular orientation at the initial deformation stage (i.e., up to 11% compressive plastic strain) compared with single-step irradiated polyethylene. Such properties, which should also involve an earlier strain hardening effect at higher strain levels, are representative of an improvement in deformation behavior as a consequence of the sequentially applied irradiation/annealing manufacturing procedure.

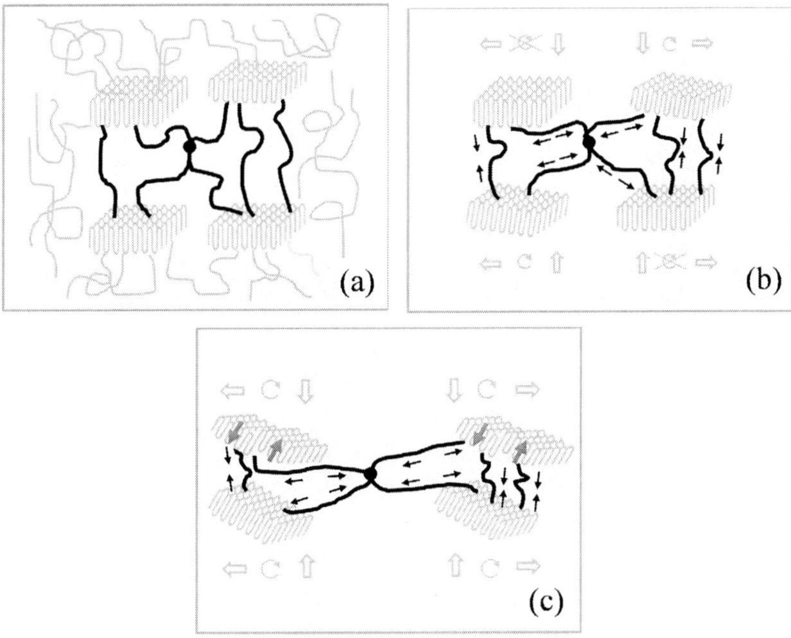

Figure 6.19 Schematics explaining the local development of both compressive and tensile strain gradients upon application of compressive external load on the composite (amorphous/crystalline) structure of UHMWPE ((a) unloaded, (b) and (c) at increasing levels of external strain). The local presence of both types of strain gradient leads to the observed (and calibrated) Raman band broadening (cf. Fig. 6.15).

Two short-term acetabular cup retrievals were investigated immediately after their respective revision surgeries in comparison with pristine unused samples of the same types. One cup (referred to as Retrieval #1, henceforth) was of the Crossfire™ type and was implanted in the patient's body for 7 months. Another cup (referred to as Retrieval #2, henceforth) was of the X3™ type and was implanted in the patient's body for only 3 months. In both cases, the total hip replacement was made with using a cementless stem. Figure 6.20 shows the results collected on Retrieval #1 (Crossfire™). In (a), a histogram of residual (plastic) strain is given as calculated from Raman bandwidth data according to Eq. (6.2), which was retrieved at a fixed location 50 μm below the surface of the main wear zone; and, in (c), the results of Raman intensity variation upon in-plane rotation at the same subsurface location with the determinations of the average tilt angle of the molecular chains, its average variation with respect to the molecular arrangement in the as-received cup, and the average Hermans parameter in the main wear zone (all parameters shown in inset in Fig. 6.20(c)). In Figs. 6.20(b) and (c), similar results are presented for Retrieval #2 (X3™). Comparing the histograms in Figs. 6.20(a) and (b), one could notice a 21% lower average plastic strain, $\overline{\varepsilon}_f$, and a less broad strain distribution in the X3™ liner compared with the Crossfire™ liner. The lower average strain could also be related to the shorter implantation time of Retrieval #2, while the sharper distribution is a clear consequence of a more homogeneous microstructure both in terms of crystallinity and molecular alignment. The value obtained for the average tilt angle in the X3™ liner was about half that found in the Crossfire™ one ($\overline{\theta}_p = 0.16$ vs. 0.31 rad; cf. inset values in Figs. 6.20(c) and (d), respectively), consistent with the initial difference in molecular alignment in the as-received cups (cf. Fig. 6.17(a)). Very low variations in tilt angle, $\overline{\Delta\theta_p}$, were detected in both retrievals, while the average value of Hermans parameter, $\overline{\langle P_2(\cos\beta)\rangle}$, was discernibly higher in the X3™ retrieval as found for the unused cups. These characteristics confirm that both the *in vivo* exposed UHMWPE structures were yet in their quite early stages of plastic deformation. Interestingly, the average tilt angles found in both retrievals were slightly higher than those obtained *in vitro* for the same amount of plastic strain. This is probably due to the influence of frictional sliding on molecular assembly, which, unavailable in static tests conducted *in vitro*, might promote some additional effect on the rotation of lamellae also in the material subsurface. According to the shown results, after few months of *in vivo* implantation, the two retrievals experienced comparably low levels of creep strain and quite low variations in rotation angles of molecular chains towards directions perpendicular to that of applied load.

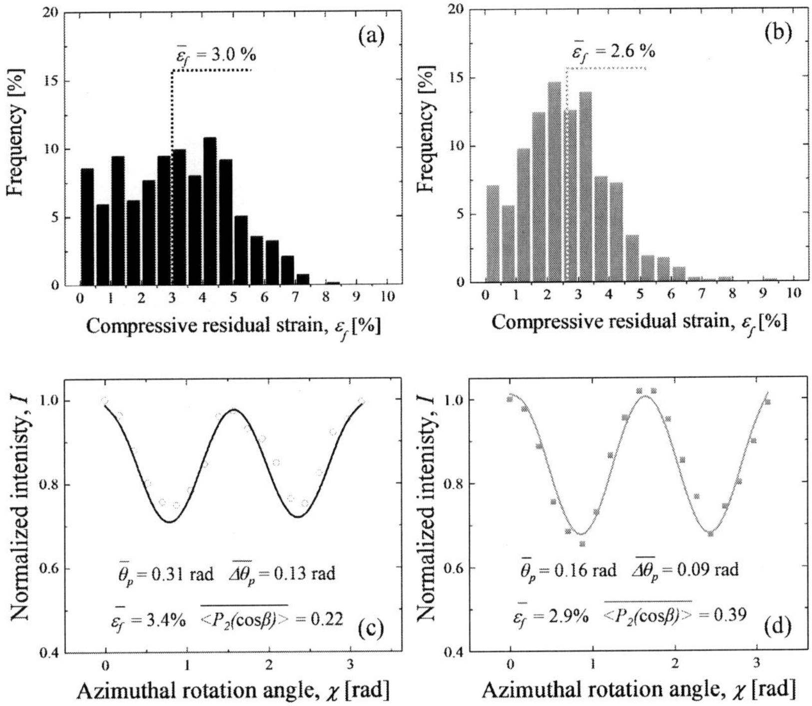

Figure 6.20 In (a) and (b), histograms of residual (plastic) strain, ε_f, as statistically retrieved from Raman bandwidth data, *ΔFWHM*, in the main wear zone of the Crossfire™ and X3™ short-term retrievals, respectively; in (c) and (d), results are shown of Raman intensity variations upon in-plane probe rotation in the main wear zone of the Crossfire™ and X3™ short-term retrievals, respectively. Azimuthal angle rotation results were used for the determinations of average tilt angles, $\overline{\theta}_p$, and average tilt angle variations, $\overline{\Delta\theta_p}$, of the molecular chains, and average Hermans parameter, $\overline{\langle P_2(\cos\beta)\rangle}$ (all parameters shown in inset together with the average plastic strain, $\overline{\varepsilon_f}$, obtained from the histograms in (a) and (b)).

In this section, phenomenological correlations enabling non-destructively assessments of residual compressive strain in polyethylene hip cups by Raman spectroscopy have explicitly been determined for two UHMWPE materials belonging to two successive design generations of γ-irradiated materials. Polarized Raman spectroscopy was also applied to retrieve variations in tilt angle occurring upon loading and representing the main microstructural rearrangement occurring during static deformation. The material manufactured by sequentially applied irradiation/annealing steps was more resistant to plastic deformation than the one irradiated with the same dose and annealed by a single-step procedure. Based on the calibration results collected *in vitro* on the as-received materials, quantitative analyses were also conducted of the plastic compressive strain generated in the main wear zone during short-term *in vivo* loading. A comparison between retrievals made of single-step and sequentially irradiated liners revealed comparably low levels of creep strain and quite low amounts of tilting rotation of molecular chains under body weight.

6.4 Differentiating the Roles of Creep, Wear and Oxidation on Long-Term *in vivo* Degradation

Wear of polyethylene acetabular cups in patients subjected to total hip arthroplasty is routinely deduced from the penetration of the femoral head into the acetabular liner as observed in the radiographs. However, the linear penetration thus measured represents the cumulative contribution of two components, one due to wear, and the other due to creep (or irreversible deformation) of the polyethylene structure. The (erroneous) attribution to wear of the entire penetration displacement of the head in the cup might lead to misinterpretation of the actual performance of acetabular cups. Raman spectroscopy procedures might enable to differentiate and to quantify the head displacement components due to wear and to creep, as they occur *in vivo* in acetabular cups, and relating them to the oxidation state of the material. Particular insightful is a comparison between the behaviors on the molecular scale of acetabular cups subjected to different sterilization procedures (e.g., γ-ray irradiation vs. ethylene oxide treatment). Creep and wear represent the two main degradation mechanisms found in various kinds of UHMWPE acetabular cups and responsible for their failure [801–803]. From a phenomenological viewpoint, creep refers to the permanent deformation that occurs under the effect of body weight and does not recover after load release, while wear involves both delamination and progressive peel-off of surface polyethylene flakes, resulting in the formation of minute and highly reactive debris. In the latter case of degradation phenomena, oxidation was found to play a main detrimental role in triggering wear, since oxidized molecules might delaminate faster due to the embrittlement of the polymeric network [804]. The two degradation mechanisms of creep and wear might negatively interact and converge toward a cup loosening effect, which mandatorily requires revision surgery. Unlike wear, creep is not accompanied by any irreversible mass loss from the material, but it involves packing and adjustment of polyethylene molecules in their reciprocal positions under pressure. Despite the different physical origin of these two main degradation mechanisms, from a phenomenological point of view, they both manifest themselves with a reduction in cup thickness, whose total extent is routinely measured both *in vivo* and on cup retrievals, and cumulatively recorded in clinical data.

Some of early generations of polyethylene acetabular cups have been sterilized by ethylene oxide gas (EtO), while the majority of the conventional acetabular cups were sterilized by γ-irradiation in air. Sterilization by γ-irradiation in air causes the highest potential risk of oxidative degradation, despite the occurrence of cross-linking, which improves the wear-resistant property of polyethylene [805,806]. Therefore, most of the manu-facturers in the late 1990s changed the procedure to γ-sterilization in inert gas or to gas plasma sterilization without radiation, after having realized that the shelf-time of polyethylene after γ-sterilization in air affects their oxidized state. However, there is still nowadays a concern regarding residual free radicals, which may oxidize polyethylene *in vivo*. Accordingly, the impact of polyethylene oxidization on clinical results is strongly dependent on the microstructural design of polyethylene bearings [769,807,808]. Hence, polymer scientists and technologists have long studied and continue to study methods to concurrently improve wear resistance, deformation/fracture resistance and oxidative stability of polyethylene materials through the application of different manufacturing procedures. In particular, treatments of UHMWPE have been the object of intensive research in order to maximize the creep resistance of the material without inducing tangible oxidation, embrittlement effects and wear enhancement [805,809–812]. However, yet a lack of clarity can be found in examining the vast available literature, since one may came across several aspects of the functional response of different polyethylene types that are somewhat contradictory and represent a main concern for the objects of the artificial joint research:

(a) Systematic measurements of the *in vitro* quasi-static tensile and compressive creep (bulk) properties of UHMWPE have reported that cross-linking by γ-irradiation might significantly devalue the creep properties [813]. This negative data on the "intrinsic" mechanical behavior is in contrast to some reports on hip simulator experiments [814] and, in general, to positive literature reporting that cross-linking reduces the head penetration rate *in vivo* (and enhances the wear resistance of the polymer [815]).

(b) A significant effect was noted in a change of the pressure dependence of the wear rate on the γ-irradiation dose under inert atmosphere [816]. Thus, whether or not a sterilizing (or resterilizing) dose measurably enhances wear rate shall strongly depend on contact stresses. In their hip simulator study, Dowson and Jobbins [817] have indicated that creep can account for an appreciable portion of the total penetration in 22 mm cups within the first few million cycles. However, a method for precisely assessing the actual fraction of displacement due to creep in acetabular cups exposed *in vivo* is still lacking.

The basic importance and the practical implications of the complex time- and load-dependent *in vivo* results, together with a need to clarify several discrepancies between the intrinsic and the extrinsic properties of various polyethylene grades employed in hip arthroplasty, call for a better understanding of the relations between molecular structure and mechanical properties, including a substantial improvement in the methods of characterization.

In this section, advanced techniques of confocal Raman spectroscopy are employed as a non-destructive tool for non-destructive oxidation analysis and for differentiating, from the overall thickness decrease observed in acetabular cups exposed *in vivo*, the contributions respectively arising from creep and from wear. Additionally, we validate here (i.e., by means of case-by-case calibrations) a reliable and non-destructive method for measuring the residual strain profile along the cross-section of acetabular cups using spatially resolved Raman characterizations. Concurrently, the oxidation state of the material is monitored through a comparative analysis of Raman spectral regions representing vibration twisting and wagging of the $-CH_2-$ bond of the polyethylene structure [98, 116]. A comparison is carried out between two types of polyethylene cups, which were originally subjected to different sterilization procedures, namely EtO gas treatment vs. γ-irradiation, and exposed *in vivo* up to 25 years. The large body of information obtained through Raman spectroscopy helps shedding some light on the discrepancies found in the literature on the performance of liners made of different grades of polyethylene. The Raman method gives direct access to the vibrational response of the molecular structure of polyethylene and might provide a rational guide, compared with other available evaluation methods, for surgeons and technologists in quantitatively evaluating the true structural performance of polyethylene cups fabricated by different manufacturers.

A total of 16 retrieved acetabular cups were obtained at the time of the respective hip arthroplasty revision surgeries (the majority of them in a quite recent and narrow interval of time; cf. Table 6.2): 14 cups were long-term (>7.5 years; <25.3 years) *in vivo* exposed and 2 cups short-term (>0.7 years; <1.8 years) exposed. Among the long-term–exposed liners, seven cups were made of the same grade of a conventional polyethylene material (GUR 412) and sterilized in EtO gas (Kyocera Co.), while the remaining seven cups were from different makers (cf. Table 6.2), but they were all cross-linked UHMWPE with surface irradiated by γ-rays. The available seven retrievals sterilized in EtO represented a quite homogeneous sampling, not only because they were made of the same material and belonged to the same type of implant, but also because they were all implanted by cemented THA against alumina-based materials, and were all retrieved for the same reason (aseptic loosening) after long-term exposure *in vivo* (i.e., in the interval between 16.8 and 25.3 years). Among the seven EtO-sterilized samples, six belonged to female patients in the age between 49 and 74 at the time of the revision surgery. All the γ-irradiated UHMWPE acetabular cups analyzed in this section were from cementless THA; five of them were employed against CoCr femoral heads, while the remaining four cups were employed against alumina ceramic heads. Regarding to the age and sex of the patients, sampling for the γ-irradiated cups was statistically similar to that of the EtO-sterilized ones except for one short-term implanted sample that belonged to a rather young (32 years old) female patient. The two short-term (<2 years) *in vivo* exposed cups were both γ-irradiated (the shortest term exposed cup (0.7 year) was retrieved due to fracture/dislocation). Acetabular components revised for aseptic loosening had prerevision radiographs, from which the head migration displacements were calculated. Such linear displacements were also measured in all the studied cups directly on the retrievals using a micrometer screw to obtain the cup thickness at the exact locations where spectroscopic assessments were made in the main-wear zone. Linear displacements (cf. variations in thickness, Δt, in Table 6.2) were then obtained by subtracting the (average) thickness measured in the main-wear zone from the nominal thickness of an unused sample. Linear displacements in the main-wear zone and other salient details related to the clinical history of the retrievals are specified in Table 6.2. It should be emphasized that from the viewpoint of the polyethylene performance, none of the 14 long-term exposed retrievals examined was defective, except for one of the γ-irradiated samples, which was retrieved for excessive liner wear (cf. sample No. 14 in Table 6.2). In other words, the majority of the employed materials performed according to standards and respected the expectations for *in vivo* trends in terms of wear rate.

Table 6.2 List of 16 retrieved acetabular cups including fourteen cups long-term (>7.5 year; <25.3 year) exposed and two cups short-term (>0.7 year; <1.8 year) exposed

Sterilization	Sample no.	Age	Gender	Follow-up [y]	Manufacturer	Cup material	Total radiation dose [kGy]	External diameter [mm]	Δt [μm]	Δt_c [μm]	Femoral head	Cause of revision
EtO	1	49	Female	25.3	Kyocera Co.	GUR 412	0	42	5410	130	28 mm Alumina (AY7)	Cup loosening
	2	60	Female	24.5	Kyocera Co.	GUR 412	0	44	2500	59	28 mm Alumina (AY7)	Cup loosening
	3	67	Female	22.2	Kyocera Co.	GUR 412	0	42	3650	163	28 mm Alumina (AY7)	Cup loosening
	4	51	Female	22	Kyocera Co.	GUR 412	0	42	3760	262	28 mm Alumina (AY7)	Cup loosening
	5	77	Male	21.1	Kyocera Co.	GUR 412	0	46	3430	292	28 mm Alumina (AY7)	Cup loosening
	6	52	Female	17.9	Kyocera Co.	GUR 412	0	50	1700	129	28 mm Alumina (AY7)	Cup loosening
	7	74	Female	16.8	Kyocera Co.	GUR 412	0	44	3330	210	28 mm Alumina (AY7)	Cup loosening
γ-ray	8	70	Female	20.8	Zimmer	GUR 415	25–40	48	1490	132	28 mm Alumina Biolox II	Cup loosening
	9	64	Female	20.2	Stryker	GUR 415	25–40	44	4250	111	22 mm CoCr	Cup loosening
	10	65	Female	19.9	Stryker	GUR 415	25–40	48	3700	167	26 mm CoCr	Cup loosening
	11	48	Female	15.7	Zimmer	GUR 415	25–40	52	870	141	28 mm Alumina Biolox II	Stem breakning
	12	73	Female	15.2	Zimmer	GUR 415	25–40	52	1600	228	28 mm Alumina Biolox II	Cup loosening
	13	55	Male	11.1	DePuy	GUR 415	25–40	44	4260	307	22 mm CoCr	Cup loosening
	14	60	Female	7.5	Zimmer	GUR 1050	90–110	46	2330	501	26 mm CoCr	Liner breakning
	15	32	Female	1.8	Stryker	GUR 1050 Cross-fire	105	50	130	129	32 mm Alumina Biolox®*forte*	Cup loosening
	16	68	Male	0.7	Stryker	GUR 1050 Cross-fire	105	58	310	307	32 mm CoCr	Fracture dislocation

Note: Among the long-term exposed liners, seven cups were made of a conventional polyethylene material (GUR 412) sterilized in EtO gas, while the remaining seven cups were all cross-linked UHMWPE with surface irradiation by γ-rays.

The dependence of selected Raman bands on applied strain was preliminary calibrated by using a uniaxial compression jig [116]. A controlled (uniaxial) state of strain was applied to a calibration sample of each polyethylene type (3 mm × 3 mm × 6 mm in dimension) obtained from a virgin cup, while monitoring the variation in width of a selected Raman band from the polyethylene spectrum. The obtained calibration plots of bandwidth vs. applied strain, typically linear in nature up to relatively high strain values, were then used to analyze the unknown strain fields that remained stored in the retrieved acetabular cups. Assessments of oxidation index, OI, from the relative intensity of selected bands of the Raman spectrum of polyethylene have been fully validated by means of "control" experiments using both Raman and infrared spectroscopy exactly on the same samples [98]. All the Raman measurements on retrievals were made in a fully non-destructive way, without any sample manipulation, by focusing the confocal probe on both main-wear and non-wear zones of the studied acetabular cups. Figures 6.21(a) and (b) show a draft of the locations in the retrieved acetabular cups object of the Raman assessments and the related protocol for *in-depth* (non-destructive) evaluations by means of a Raman microprobe, respectively. Exploiting the high transparency of polyethylene, non-destructive in-depth scans enabled to retrieve detailed subsurface profiles of both strain and oxidation index along the entire thickness of the retrieved cups. In the experimental practice, an automated sample stage with submicrometric step precision was employed, making it possible to record spectra at each depth with focusing below the sample surface, and to map spectra with lateral line scanning on the sample surface and subsurface. Maps 30 μm × 30 μm were typically recorded at each location and depth and their spectra (900 spectra for each map) averaged to give the molecular vibrational modes of the polyethylene structure at each selected *in-depth* location. Measurements of subsurface profile properties were eventually repeated at tens of locations in the main-wear zone, in order to obtain a statistical validation of the states of strain and oxidation for each of the retrievals investigated. The total number of collected Raman spectra on all the retrievals (including both main-wear and non-wear zones) was in the order of 1.5×10^6 for a total measurement time of ≈4200 h.

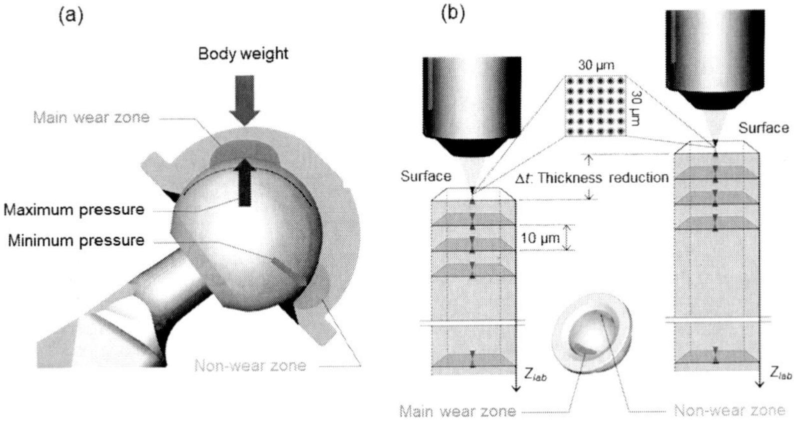

Figure 6.21 (a) Schematic showing the mechanics of acetabular cup deformation due to creep; (b) protocol for in-depth Raman mapping using a confocal probe configuration in both main-wear and non-wear zones.

In the molecular structure of polymers, an applied stress is directly translated into internal strain (in both bond angles and lengths) of the polymer backbone. Due to the anharmonicity of the atomic bonds, this circumstance brings about changes in the vibrational spectra, which can be probed by Raman spectroscopy. In general, a compressive strain causes a shift of Raman bands to higher wavenumbers, whereas the reverse effect is observed in tension [818]. Extensive literature has been reported about the dependence on strain of the Raman spectrum of polyethylene fibers and oriented films [795, 819]. However, unlike linearly elastic materials, polyethylene shows a complex and strongly non-linear dependence of the Raman spectrum on strain. This circumstance makes it difficult a quantitative assessment of strain from band shift in the wide interval of (plastic) strains experienced by *in vivo* exposed acetabular cups. Fortunately in the case of polyethylene an additional phenomenon is observed: both C–C asymmetric stretching mode B_{1g} (1060 cm^{-1}) and symmetric stretching mode A_g (1127 cm^{-1}) bands split under strain into two components, which originates a broadening of the Raman bands. This has been interpreted as being due to a bimodal stress distribution of the C–C bonds in the material [796, 818, 820, 821]. Both tensile

[822] and compressive [116] plastic strains have been measured in medical grades of UHMWPE by using a direct proportionality relationship between uniaxial strain and the increase in full width at half maximum (FWHM) of a selected Raman band located at 1127 cm^{-1} (A_g vibrational mode). The rationale for bandwidth being a sensor of strain in the polymeric network resides in it reflecting the degree of disorder of the network and the degree of molecular orientation, which both are affected by strain. The increase in structural disorder under compressive strain is reflected in a broadening of the Raman band due to inter- and intra-lamellar slip processes. Additional phenomena leading to Raman band broadening have also been indicated, as the beginning of crystallite fragmentation, fibril formation, and chain disentanglement [823]. Broadening of the symmetric-stretching A_g band as a strain sensor has been selected here as a sensor of strain because, unlike band spectral shift, experiences a conspicuously linear dependence on plastic strain up to quite large values (e.g., in the order of the tens of percent). However, despite such a straightforward relationship, a drawback of the Raman assessment of plastic strain by band-broadening method resides in its dependence on the individual polyethylene structure investigated. In other words, a lack of generality might be found in the proportionality factor relating bandwidth to strain, which necessarily requires preliminary case-by-case calibrations of the (compressive) strain dependence of the Raman spectrum for each polyethylene grade investigated. Strain calibration plots, as obtained for all the investigated polyethylene materials, are shown in Fig. 6.22. Broadening of the symmetric C–C stretching Raman band (located at 1127 cm^{-1}) under compressive strain followed a clearly detectable (linear) trend for all the investigated materials (e.g., cf. sequence of spectra in Fig. 6.22(a) for the EtO-sterilized polyethylene), although the slopes of the respective plots were different as a result of the aforementioned structural dependence of the obtained plots. Calibration lines are explicitly given for all the investigated polyethylene structures in Fig. 6.22(b). A full description of the origin of the different slopes recorded in differently manufactured materials is beyond the scope of this book. However, we can attribute to both a higher degree of molecular alignment and to a lower structural disorder the lower (unstrained) C–C stretching bandwidth generally recorded in γ-irradiated

compared with EtO-sterilized materials. On the other hand, a higher slope found in the plots of FWHM vs. strain is believed to capture the essence of a better shear-activated stress transfer

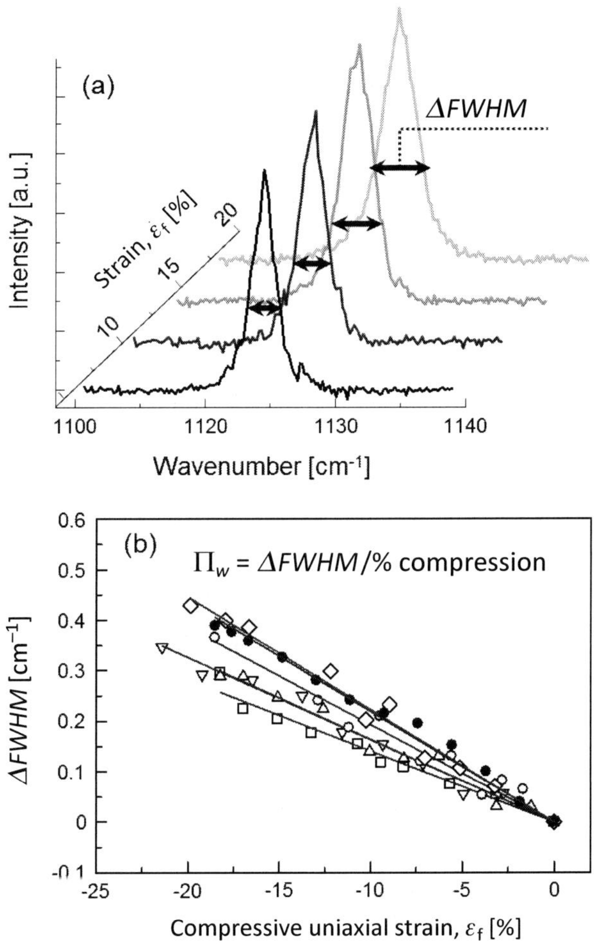

Figure 6.22 (a) Spectral band broadening as detected upon increasing the externally applied compressive strain for the EtO-sterilized polyethylene; (b) comparison among FWHM/strain calibration plots performed on all types of investigated polyethylene materials. The slope of the linear plots correspond to: (●) –0.0219 (Kyocera Co. GUR412); (◇) –0.0223 (Stryker GUR 415); (○) –0.0193 (Stryker GUR 1050 Crossfire); (Δ) –0.0164 (Zimmer GUR 415); (∇) –0.0163 (Zimmer GUR 1050); (□) –0.0141 (Depuy GUR 415).

mechanism, as already suggested by Tarantili *et al.* [818]. Note that the strain assessments by Raman require a choice of a standard (minimum) width for the symmetric C–C stretching band of polyethylene. The width of a band retrieved from the core of unused (and unloaded) acetabular cups of each type was selected here. The plots of FWHM vs. strain given in Fig. 6.22(b) represent the basis for investigating the profiles of permanent strain stored after long-term *in vivo* exposure in acetabular cups obtained from different manufacturers, which are presented hereafter.

In Figs. 6.23(a)~(g) and (h)~(n), strain profiles are shown, which were non-destructively collected at increasing probe depths in both main-wear and non-wear zones (a)~(g) and (h)~(n) for EtO-sterilized and γ-irradiated long-term exposed retrievals, respectively). In this figure, the number assigned to each sample corresponds to the sample number given in Table 6.2; it is thus increasing with decreasing exposure time *in vivo*. Each data point in the plots represents an average value retrieved over an area of ≈900 μm^2 at each subsurface depth. We plotted the strain profiles with placing a common origin for the plots on the internal surface of the acetabular cup at the time of measurement. For this reason, plots representing main-wear and non-wear zones correspond to the same probing depths but refer to different thicknesses of the liners. The thickness reductions, Δt, that cumulatively arose from both creep deformation and wear abrasion (i.e., as they piled up during the *in vivo* lifetime) are listed in Table 6.2. The Δt values could be retrieved because precise assessments of cup thickness in the main-wear zone were available from post-surgical measurements. It immediately appears that a rational trend in terms of the measured (overall) reduction of cup thickness indeed exists for the main wear zone as a function of service time *in vivo*, the longer the service time the higher Δt. However, there are exceptions to this trend, especially in the γ-irradiated samples. This latter observation, which will be expanded in a later discussion, clearly reflects a long idiosyncratic difficulty in quantitatively assessing and rationalizing the actual *in vivo* performance of acetabular cups from different makers in terms of structural stability and rate of reduction of their initial thicknesses.

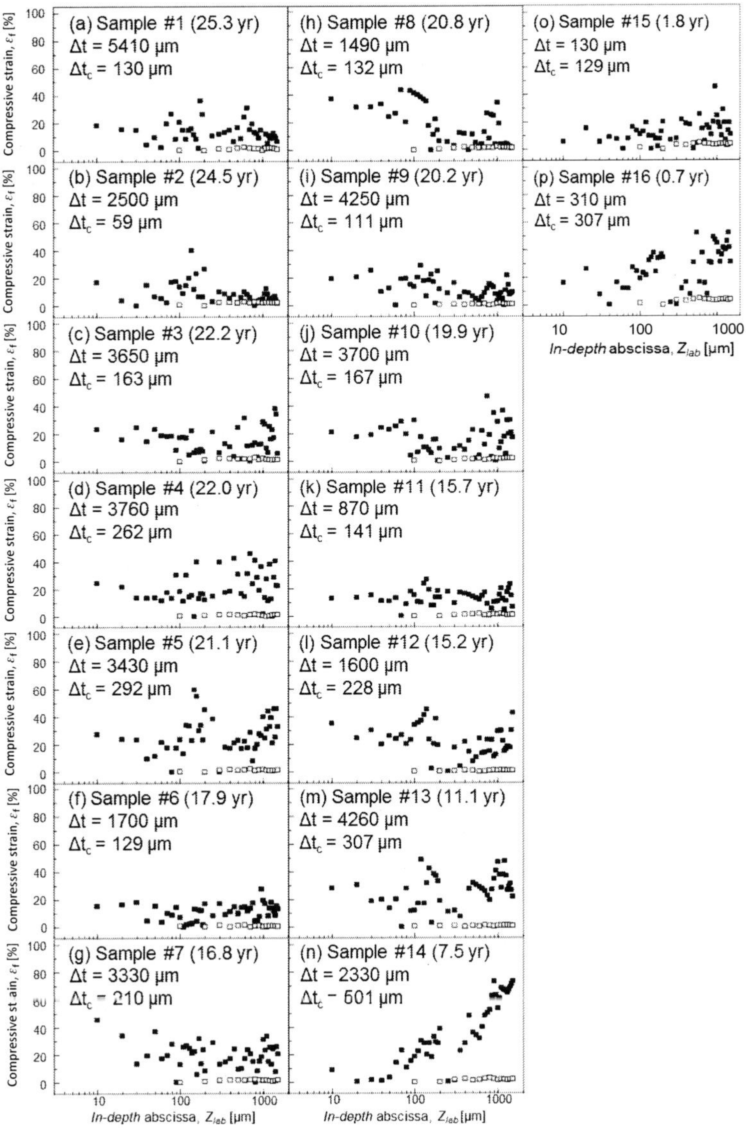

Figure 6.23 In-depth strain profiles collected on retrievals as listed in the respective insets and in Table 6.2 (open and close circles refer to non-wear and main wear zones, respectively). In (o) and (p), in-depth strain profiles are shown as collected in short-term retrievals sterilized by γ-rays (open and close symbols refer to non-wear and main wear zones, respectively).

In the remainder of this section, we shall take the creep profiles detected in the non-wear zone as representative of the residual state of strain in the main-wear zone before implantation, namely in the implants as-received from the maker. As a general trend, all the investigated cups were typically (residual) strain-free at the time of implantation. However, in comparing main-wear and non-wear zones in all samples, Raman experiments always revealed a significant increase in the amount of residual strain stored in polyethylene structures belonging to main-wear zones. The average uniaxial strain was typically in the order of 20% (in compression) for the EtO treated implants (with only cup No. 5 in Table 6.2 showing a higher value (cf. Fig. 6.23(e)). The average residual strain stored in the γ-irradiated samples after joint explantation was similar in magnitude but more scattered than that observed in the EtO treated implants. This data scatter should depend on the type of cross-linked polyethylene analyzed and on the homogeneity/accuracy of the adopted cross-linking process. Interestingly, strain maxima were not found in correspondence of the very surface of the material but at depths of both several tens and several hundreds of μm. These results help visualize the creep contribution to the *in vivo* penetration of femoral component into the polyethylene liners and enable one to quantify the thickness reduction due to creep. In order to estimate the head-penetration component, Δt_c, due to creep at the time of the explantation of the liner, a numerical integration of the strain profile in the main-wear zone was performed over the entire thickness of the liner [116]. The results of this calculation are shown in Table 6.2. A general conclusion can be drawn from an examination of Δt_c data in comparison with the overall displacements, Δt: at the time of explantation, the creep contribution to the overall femoral head (linear) displacement onto the liner was always by far (i.e., from one to two orders of magnitude) lower than that due to wear (i.e., $\Delta t_W = \Delta t - \Delta t_c$). Figures 6.23(o) and (p) show the residual strain profiles stored into two γ-irradiated samples that were implanted for only for 1.8 and 0.7 years, respectively (samples No. 15 and 16 in Table 6.2). The head-penetration component, Δt_c, due to creep at the time of the explantation of those short-term exposed liners was found to be comparable to that of the long-term implanted liners and with the total migration displacement of the head, Δt. These findings clearly show that the head displacement onto the liner is creep-dominated in the initial period of implantation and limited to a relatively small fraction of the overall linear migration after long-term *in vivo* exposure.

The oxidation state of the polyethylene structure can be non-destructively evaluated from a comparative analysis of the Raman spectrum of the material in the two spectral regions of $-CH_2-$ twisting vibration (at around 1300 cm^{-1}) and of $-CH_2-$ bond wagging (between 1350 and 1500 cm^{-1}). In particular, the Raman intensities of the bands located at 1414 cm^{-1} (characteristic of the orthorhombic crystal polymorph) and at 1293 cm^{-1} (representing the overall degree of crystallinity of the polyethylene structure) are used for this evaluation. The Raman method for oxidation assessments in polyethylene has been validated in comparison with infrared spectroscopy data [98], and only the outputs of oxidation assessments in the studied samples are shown in this book without further validation of the assessment method. Figures 6.24 (a)~(g) and (h)~(n) show OI profiles non-destructively collected at increasing depths in both main-wear and non-wear zones for EtO-sterilized and γ-irradiated retrievals, respectively. Average OI values in the main- and non-wear zones ($\overline{OI}_m$ and $\overline{OI}_n$, respectively) are also explicitly shown in each plot. As in the case of creep strain profiles, the order of the plot is dictated by the decrease of their elapsing time of exposure *in vivo*, according to Table 6.2. It should be noted that nearly all the long-term implants examined here matched the lifetime expectations given by the respective makers. Nevertheless, from a comparison among the 14 profiles shown in Fig. 6.24, three striking features could be noticed: (i) the OI values measured in the non-wear zones were in general much more pronounced in γ-irradiated samples than in the EtO-sterilized ones; (ii) for both types of implants, the overall amount of oxidation did not significantly increase after even very long *in vivo* exposures; and, (iii) the OI values in the main-wear zones were slightly lower for EtO-sterilized retrievals compared with the γ-irradiated ones.

Maxima of OI could be found not only in the far depth of the thickness, as widely reported and explained in terms of delamination in artificial joints [824–827], but also in the immediate subsurface profiles of the retrieved cups, at locations roughly coincident with the depths at which maxima were observed in the profiles of compressive strain. A comparison can again be made

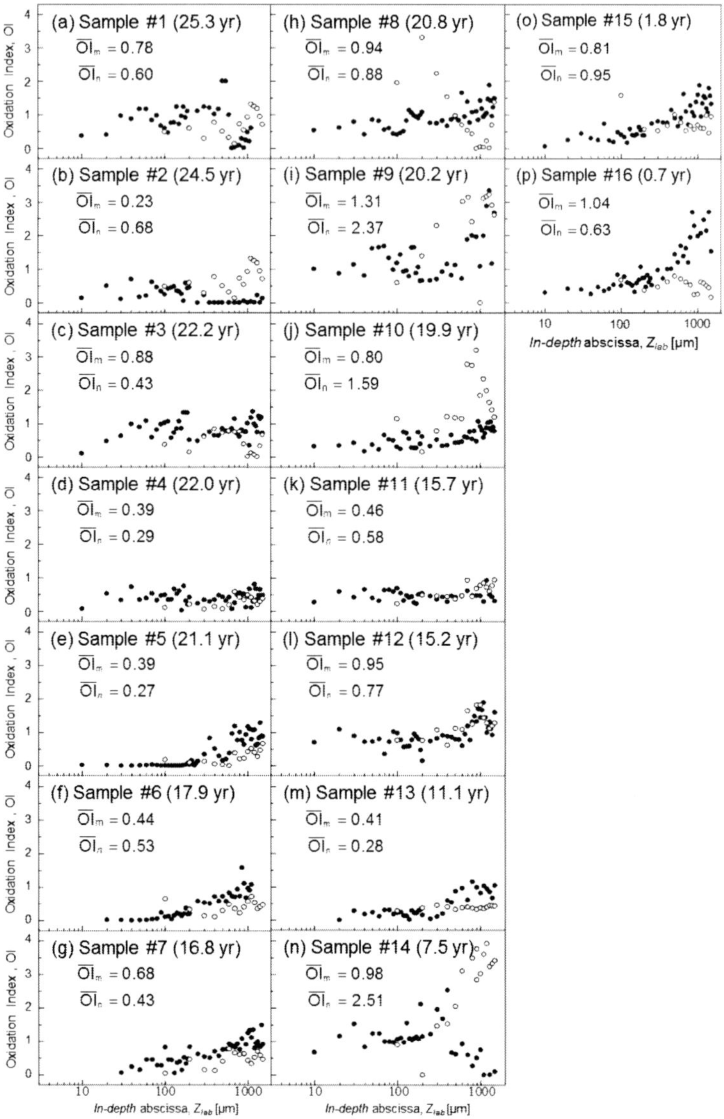

Figure 6.24 In-depth oxidation profiles collected on retrievals as listed in the respective insets and in Table 6.2 (open and close circles refer to non-wear and main wear zones, respectively). In (o) and (p), in-depth oxidation profiles are shown as collected in short-term retrievals sterilized by γ-rays (open and close symbols refer to non-wear and main wear zones, respectively).

with the oxidation profiles observed in the short-term exposed acetabular cups (samples No. 15 and 16 in Table 6.2). The oxidation profiles measured by Raman in the main-wear and non-wear zones for these latter two samples are shown in Fig. 6.24(o) and (p), respectively. Profiles of OI were similar in main-wear and non-wear zones for both samples and the maximum OI value was similar to those detected in the main-wear zones of long-term exposed γ-irradiated cups, although the profile morphology as a function of in-depth abscissa was different (i.e., monotonically increasing and not showing intermediate maxima).

According to the new information provided here by means of highly spatially resolved Raman spectroscopy, the occurrence of severe oxidation paths just below the exposed surface of *in vivo* exposed polyethylene components calls for a reconsideration of the kinetics of the oxidation processes compared with previous literature, and in particular on the peculiar role of compressive strain on the oxidation process.

In a recent randomized clinical study, Glyn-Jones *et al.* [828] have analyzed the creep and wear behavior of highly cross-linked and standard polyethylene liners over a short-term implantation time (i.e., 3 years) using radio-stereometric analysis. These researchers showed that penetration of the femoral head onto the liner was creep-dominated in the first six months of implantation; while, after 1 year, the creep component of the overall migration displacement saturated and virtually all the additional penetration was due to wear. The conclusion of that study was that highly cross-linked polyethylene experienced a 60% lower rate of wear than standard polyethylene, from which it was extrapolated that cross-linked polyethylene will probably perform better in the long term. The outputs of our Raman studies on retrieved polyethylene liners can be used to validate those conclusions. We have indeed found that the creep Δt_c component was the dominant contribution to the overall migration displacement of the femoral head in short-term *in vivo* exposed retrievals, but it represented a minor part of the overall displacement Δt measured at the time of explantation. On the other hand, the wear Δt_w component represented by far the dominant fraction of the overall head displacement Δt in long-term exposed liners at the time of explantation. The unavailability of short-term retrievals for

EtO-sterilized liners does not allow us a direct comparison with assess the contribution of the initial creep displacement on the overall linear migration of the femoral heads measured at the time of revision surgery. However, the amount of residual strain stored in the EtO-sterilized liners showed no statistical difference in comparison with γ-sterilized liners at the time of revision surgery (the exceptional strains recorded in sample No. 5 can be attributed to a larger clearance in this implant, as suggested by finite element simulation studies by Bewill *et al.* [829]). As anticipated earlier in this section, increased radiation doses to achieve a high level of cross-linking might reduce some of the intrinsic mechanical properties of γ-irradiated materials [813], including elastic modulus and yield strength, thus increasing creep displacements. However, our study did not reveal any substantial difference between creep displacements measured in EtO- and γ-sterilized liners. In other words, the present spectroscopic data validate the numerical and experimental analyses of contact stress recently published by Plank *et al.* [830], showing that the use of relatively large femoral heads can confine contact stresses below a threshold value for structural yielding even in highly irradiated (i.e., with intrinsically lower deformation resistance) polyethylene liners.

In vivo oxidation of polyethylene occurs in the presence of unstabilized radicals within the polymer and molecular oxygen uptake from body fluids and tissues [831]. The results of detailed investigations have suggested that an OI > 3 is associated with a "critical" step in the loss in mechanical properties and a propensity for fatigue damage *in vivo* [832]. Accordingly, OI ≤ 1 can be interpreted as insignificant levels of oxidation and would not affect the ultimate mechanical performance of polyethylene. Furthermore, a lack of correlation found in the literature between oxidation state and clinical performance also suggests that level of oxidations OI > 3 should be reached to compromise the mechanical performance of polyethylene. From this latter point of view, none of the OI profiles reached, at the time of explantation and for both types of liner investigated, a level of oxidation for which a substantial degradation of mechanical properties could be suspected. On the other hand, it is remarkable that four of the eight investigated γ-irradiated samples were heavily oxidized (OI > 3) in their non-wear zones, thus suggesting that they might have been already highly oxidized at the time of primary surgery. In these cases of faulted components, the initial wear rates could have been significantly accelerated by an embrittlement of the oxidized polyethylene structure. Another possibility is that a chemically activated oxidation process preferentially takes place in the non-wear zone.

Since it remains the suspect that the short-term exposed samples could be faulted samples at the time of implantation, a comparison of creep and oxidation profiles in main-wear and non-wear zones of short-term and long-term γ-irradiated samples unfortunately cannot be used here to substantiate that creep occurs before oxidation in normally performing liners. However, additional information is obtained here on the role of excessive initial oxidation on the wear performance. Near-surface oxidation is known to contribute accelerating wear mechanisms in polyethy lene acetabular cups during service [804]. Buchanan *et al.* [833] reported that accelerated aging of ultra-high molecular weight polyethylene in pressurized oxygen results in peaks of polymer density and degree of oxidation up to 500 μm below the polymer surface. Shelf and *in vivo* aging was also found leading to density increases (i.e., mainly arising from changes in crystallinity) below the sample surface. Formation of microscopic cracks may occur *in vivo* in regions of maximum crystallinity, assisted by the presence of high subsurface (contact) strain gradients. In highly oxidized zones, the microscopic elongation needed to locally break the polyethylene structure decreases [834], thus wear results accelerated. We found here that at least four out of the eight investigated retrievals of γ-irradiated liners presumably experienced an OI ≥ 3 either at the time of implantation in the patient or they developed oxidation in a very early stage of implantation. These liners, all retrieved because of aseptic loosening, showed abnormal head migration displacements onto the liner, namely which degraded the structural performance of these liners below the standard performance of liners made of a less advanced EtO-sterilized polyethylene. Finally, a striking finding was the observation of an oxidation process in EtO-sterilized acetabular cups. If γ-irradiation is responsible for free-radicals formation and, thus for successive oxidation *in vivo*, why could EtO-sterili-zed cups, deficient in free radicals, oxidize? Enhanced oxidation of polyethylene components due to chemical species such as cholesterol, fatty esters of cholesterol and squalene, originating from synovial liquid could be the answer. Such species, which were found in the bulk of retrieved acetabular samples, experienced concentrations depending on the individual patient [835]. Most recent experiments proved the strong oxidative effect of squalene [836].

In this section, quantitative methods of Raman spectroscopy have been applied to describe and to compare the magnitude of residual creep strain and the oxidation index in acetabular liners made of different polyethylene grades. Exploiting the main advantage of a non-contact and spatially resolved (confocal) probe enabled us to assess the correct in-depth morphology of strain and oxidation profiles stored in both main-wear and non-wear zones of liners sterilized with EtO gas or γ-irradiated. The main outcomes of the investigation can be summarized as follows:

(i) Creep contributes the dominant portion to the overall migration displacement of the femoral head in short-term *in vivo* exposed retrievals, but it represents only a minor part of the overall displacement measured at the time of explantation.

(ii) Independent of sterilization procedure, the wear component represent by far the dominant fraction of the overall head displacement in long-term exposed liners at the time of explantation.

(iii) The use of relatively large femoral heads confines the magnitude of contact stresses below a threshold value for structural yielding in highly irradiated polyethylene liners, thus making their creep performance comparable to that of EtO-sterilized liners.

(iv) A large fraction (50%) of the investigated γ-irradiated samples were heavily oxidized (OI > 3) in their non-wear zones (presumably since the time of primary surgery or very early after implantation). Such faulted components experienced wear rates comparable or even below those of standard EtO-sterilized liners.

(v) EtO-sterilized acetabular cups were also oxidized *in vivo*, despite they conspicuously lacked of free radicals. The oxidative process can be attributed to the detrimental effect of squalene and/or other lipids present in the synovial fluid.

6.5 Use of Vitamin E Infusion to Counteract Oxidation in UHMWPE Liners

In the last 15 years, cross-linked polyethylene has been introduced in the orthopedic market to counteract the formation *in vivo* of polyethylene wear debris, responsible for a cascade of biological reactions ultimately leading to osteolysis and to the need of revision surgery [764,837]. According to available statistics, this detrimental effect yet represents the most critical issue in hip arthroplasty and it was found to be the most limiting factor in the longevity of artificial hip implants (cf. also Fig. 1.4 and discussions in Chapter 1) [756]. Cross-linking polyethylene molecular chains, which can be promoted upon exposure to high-energy irradiation (e.g., by γ-rays), can greatly increase wear resistance, thus reducing debris formation and, with it, the probability for osteolysis to occur. The main shortcoming of this procedure is that cross-linking also unavoidably involves the formation of free radicals, which remain trapped in a chemically unstable equilibrium with in the material microstructure after irradiation [838]. If left unstabilized, free radicals could be highly reactive to oxygen, which eventually starts a chain reaction ultimately causing oxidative degradation over time. Following the above notions, modern UHMWPE hip components can be classified according to the specific method used by manufacturers to counteract oxidation degradation processes in presence of residual free radicals. Some manufacturers proposed to reduce the free-radical concentration by reheating above the melting temperature (i.e., remelting) the material after cross-linking. Remelting would allow substantial recombination of the free radicals and thus reduces free-radical concentration below detectable levels, which in turn increases oxidation resistance. However, remelting can be detrimental to the structural properties of polyethylene, which manifests with a drop down in tensile strength and fatigue resistance [18,839,840]. As an alternative processing procedure, annealing of the polyethylene structure below its melting temperature (i.e., after cross-linking) was also found to produce annihilation of free radicals while also allowing for the detainment of strength and fatigue resistance properties. However, with simply annealing the polyethylene liner, there is no guarantee that all the free radicals trapped at the microstructural scale could recombine and, therefore, a residual fraction of free radicals eventually remains in the liner, which oxidizes *in vivo* (cf. also discussions in Section 6.4) [112,841,842]. In Section 6.2, we have discussed about the structural improvements achieved through an optimized multiple-step (sequential) annealing process without terminal γ-sterilization, which has been recently proposed and shown to greatly increase oxidative stability above the previous generation of conventionally annealed polyethylenes [792,793]. As an alternative procedure to sequential annealing, polyethylene liners have been processed below the melting temperature in order to maintain unchanged the structural characteristics of irradiated samples but, concurrently, vitamin E has also been infused in their microstructure [843,844]. Vitamin E is a collective term for the group of tocopherols, of which α-tocopherol shows the best properties as an antioxidant, namely a substance that stabilizes free radicals and prevents oxidative degradation [843–846]. According to the above reasoning, sequential annealing and E-vitamin infusion are nowadays the two most advanced processing options that can be offered by manufacturers for elongating the lifetime of irradiated UHMWPE liners. In other words, these two options represent the cutting edge technological developments in microstructural design of biomedical polyethylene.

In this section, we build upon the reported notion of anti-oxidative effects by vitamin E-infused polyethylene liners and further inquire about the structure of this newly developed material at the molecular scale. Infusing vitamin E into irradiated polyethylene is claimed to annihilate free radicals in the polyethylene by donating a hydrogen atom from the OH^- group of its ring structure and thus transferring the free radicals from the polyethylene chain to the vitamin E molecule [843–849]. However, while the "chemical" rationale supporting the anti-oxidative capacity of vitamin E-infused (or blended) liners is clearly stated in the published literature, the material remains almost completely unexplored with respect to its actual three-dimensional structure on the molecular scale. Moreover, its microstructural response to externally applied (compressive) load, which quantitatively reflects the degree of mobility of its molecular assembly, is yet conspicuously unknown. We attempt here to provide those missing notions and show spectroscopic characterizations of the newly launched vitamin E-infused liners in comparison with a model (i.e., commercially unavailable) polyethylene liner made from the same resin (undoped and unirradiated/un-cross-linked) and conventional UHMWPE liners subjected to the same γ-sterilization procedure (i.e., with a dose of 33 kGy) as the vitamin E-infused liners. These undoped liners represent the previous generation UHMWPE acetabular components commercialized by the same maker. The spectroscopic comparison will clarify the effect of the vitamin E dopant on the developed material microstructure and on its deformation response to external load. The present structural characterizations are similar to those shown in Section 6.3 for the newly launched liners sequentially annealed (without terminal γ-sterilization).

Three types of liners have been analyzed, which differed for the respective manufacturing procedures. All liners had a diameter of 32 mm and were provided by Biomet Inc., Warsaw, IN, USA. One type of liner was the newly launched liner E1®, available on the international market since 2007. Another type of component belonged to a former generation of polyethylene, the brand ArCom®, which was clinically introduced in 1995 and it is currently commercially available. For comparison, we also examined a model liner, which underwent no irradiation, no anti-oxidative stabilization, and no sterilization. The model liner, the brands ArCom® and E1® will be henceforth referred to as Liner A, B, and C, respectively. Manufacturing of all three types of liner commonly started from isostatically compression molded GUR 1050 resins. In the case of Liner B, no γ irradiation and no anti oxidative stabilization were made, but terminal γ-ray sterilization with 33 kGy was made in argon gas. Liner C was preliminary subjected to γ-irradiation with 100 kGy, then it was subjected to vitamin E infusion by annealing at 130°C, and was finally sterilized with a dose of 33 kGy in argon gas, similar to Liner B. Table 6.3 summarizes the processing procedures followed for manufacturing the three types of investigated UHMWPE liner. Spectroscopic analyses of the components were made on five different samples for each type of liner.

Table 6.3 Comparison of the processing steps followed in manufacturing the three different UHMWPE acetabular liners investigated

	Processing	Liner A	Liner B	Liner C
Step 1	Make form resin	GUR 1050 Isostatically compression molded	GUR 1050 Isostatically compression molded	GUR 1050 Isostatically compression molded
Step 2	Irradiation (Crosslinking)	None	None	100 kGy γ-irradiation
Step 3	Stabilization process	None	None	Vitamin E infusion followed by annealing (130°C)
Step 4	Fabricate bearing			
Step 5	Package			
Step 6	Sterilization	None	33 kGy γ-sterilization (Argon)	33 kGy γ-sterilization (Argon)

The structural modifications associated with plastic deformation were studied using uniaxial relaxation tests in a compressive geometry, which were applied to samples obtained from the liners as-received from the maker. The procedure followed for examining the compressive deformation behavior of the materials was the same as that described in Section 6.3. Compression tests were systematically performed on five samples for each type of investigated material and the compressive load, applied stepwise, was set to achieve predetermined levels of plastic strains. The residual (plastic) strain was measured along the sample long axis by means of a micrometer caliper, and the deformed samples analyzed by Raman spectroscopy. Spectroscopic characterizations revealed the modifications induced by compressive strain on the original microstructure of the acetabular components, phenomenologically reproducing the conditions encountered during *in vivo* loading. Deformed UHMWPE samples were investigated by a confocal Raman probe at successive levels of deformation. The focal plane of the confocal probe was gradually shifted down to several hundreds of micron below the sample surface to non-destructively obtain spectral profiles toward the central region of the sample [98]. For each type of studied polyethylene, the results of confocal Raman assessments were averaged on five different samples compressively loaded in order to achieve the same deformation displacements.

Volume fractional assessments of amorphous (α_a) and crystalline (α_c) phases were made using the relative intensity of vibrational bands located at 1080, 1293 and 1305 cm^{-1}, as obtained from unpolarized Raman spectra. The band located at 1080 cm^{-1} arises from C–C stretching vibrational mode, while the two bands at around 1293 and 1305 cm^{-1} are related to –CH– twisting vibrational modes. The intensity of the peak located at 1293 cm^{-1} was used to approximate the overall degree of crystallinity of the UWMWPE structure [821,850,851]. Note, however, that specific vibrational modes are not directly related to long-range 3-D order, but they are related to conformational state populations, which may lead to 3-D crystallinity. Therefore, the crystallinity fraction mentioned here refers to cumulative conformational populations that might be present in both crystalline and non-crystalline regions of the material. On the other hand, the intensity of the band located at around 1080 cm^{-1} reflects the fraction of amorphous phase contained in the microstructure. Computations of phase fractions were made according to the method given by Strobl *et al.* [850], Maxfield *et al.* [851], and Rull *et al.* [821]. The sum ($\alpha_a + \alpha_c$) might locally be slightly <1, because of the possible presence of a minor fraction of matter in an anisotropic intermediate disordered state (i.e., usually referred to as the "third phase" [852]). Locations at which ($\alpha_a + \alpha_c$) results slightly >1 instead reflect the experimental error involved with fractional measurements by Raman spectros copy (in the order of $<0.5\%$). Microstructural modifications induced by uniaxial plastic strain could be monitored as a function of depth below the concave surface of each sample. Assessments of preferential molecular orientation were performed by analyzing the spectroscopic behavior of the Raman band located at

1130 cm^{-1}, which is related to the C–C stretching vibration ($A_g + B_{1g}$ mode). The statistical distribution around the preferential orientation axis of the molecular structure was evaluated by determining the structure of the ODF, $f(\beta)$, as obtained from Raman spectra collected in confocal/polarized configuration at different azimuthal angles, χ, using a rotating jig placed under the micro-probe (cf. Fig. 6.2(b)). The procedures and the definitions of the measured angles and parameters were the same as those described in Section 6.3. Similar to what previously discussed with examining step-wisely annealed samples, in the conventions adopted in this book, the angle, θ_p, represents the out-of plane tilt angle with respect to the uniaxially loaded surface of the polyethylene bearing. This angle, thus, gives a direct indication of the main microstructural modification expected to occur in the polymeric structure subjected to a compressive strain field applied along a direction perpendicular to the bearing surface.

As a first step, the evolution of amorphous and crystalline phase fractions contained within the microstructures of the three types of investigated UHMWPE liners has been monitored with respect to their response to compressive strain fields of increasing magnitude. The as-received materials were assumed to be in a residual strain-free state, while a static (uniaxial) strain magnitude was increasingly applied in order to reach, after unloading and successive strain recovery, two sequential levels of plastic deformation at around 5 and 10% strain (i.e., henceforth simply referred to as true strain after recovery, ε_f). Displacements in the order of ≈300~600 μm were achieved upon plastic deformation (i.e., ≈5~10% residual strains of the 6 mm liner thickness), which can be considered to be comparable to those expected to occur *in vivo* under the effect of body weight. Figure 6.25 shows plots of amorphous phase fraction, α_a, (data for Liners A, B, and C in (a), (b), and (c), respectively) and crystalline phase fraction, α_c, (data for Liners A, B, and C in (d), (e), and (f), respectively) at three successive levels of true strain, ε = 0, ≈5%, and ≈10% after recovery. Data are plotted as a function of the in-depth abscissa, z_{lab}, taken along the sample subsurface with origin on the concave surface of the liner. The obtained $\alpha_a(z_{lab})$ and $\alpha_c(z_{lab})$ plots were markedly non-linear in all the investigated materials and experienced distinct variations of property gradients among each other. Their comparison clearly revealed the somewhat competitive effect of γ-irradiation and vitamin E infusion on the final material microstructure. The main items that can be evinced from examining the plots in Fig. 6.25 can be summarized as follows:

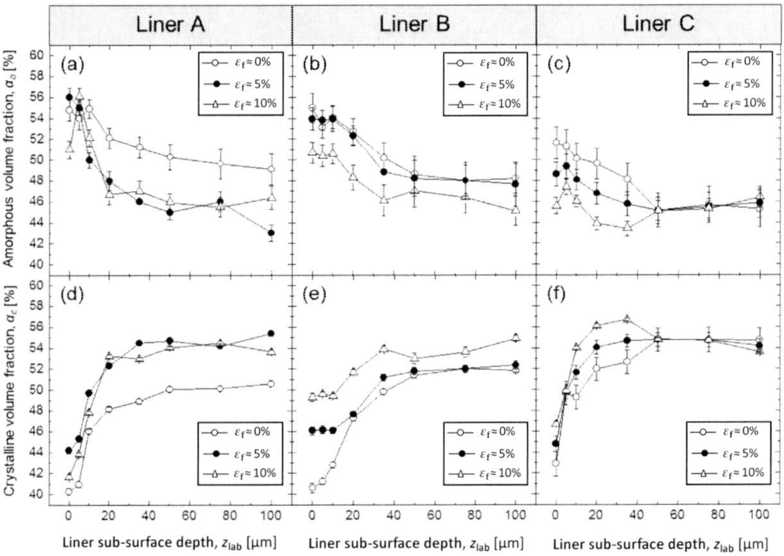

Figure 6.25 Depth profiles of phase volume fraction for Liners A, B, and C, as recorded upon different values of applied compressive strain ((a)~(c) amorphous fraction, α_a, and (d)~(f) for crystalline fraction, α_c).

(i) All as-received liners experienced the lowest degree of crystallinity (≈40~43%) on their concave surfaces. This common effect is interpreted as a consequence of surface machining, which was the same for all the investigated liners.

(ii) The crystalline phase fraction in the sample bulk rose up to about 50% (beyond a subsurface depth of about 35 μm) and then saturated in Liner A, which reflects the characteristic structure of the resin GUR 1050 commonly selected as a starting material. On the other hand, the as-received Liners B and C, although prepared from the same starting resin as Liner A, reached higher crystallinity values (in the order of 52 and 55%, respectively) in their bulk ($z_{lab} \geq 50$ μm). When comparing the processing procedures among the three investigated liners, as listed in Table 6.3, their crystallinity differences can be attributed to the effect of the different γ-irradiation doses received by the different liners. Liner C exhibited the highest degree of crystallinity, owing to the fact that it received the highest irradiation dose (totally 133 kGy) among the three investigated liners. However, the terminal (sterilizing) irradiation of 33 kGy for Liner C might not significantly contribute to crystallization and formation of cross-linking because of an obstructive effect of infused vitamin E with respect to radiation cross-linking efficiency. Barron and Birkinshaw [794] showed 53.7% as crystallinity value of 100 kGy-irradiated GUR 1050 by using Raman spectroscopy, which is a level of crystallinity comparable to the present data measured on Liner C. This fact seems to suggest that there is no loss of crystallinity in Liner C after vitamin E infusion and the subsequent homogenization heating treatment below its melting point (at 130°C).

(iii) Liner A, which received no irradiation dose, showed large increases in crystallinity (especially in its bulk) with increasing the magnitude of plastic strain. A small phase-structure variation was seen within the first 10 μm below the surface upon increasing the level of externally applied plastic strain. On the other hand, large fluctuations were observed in its bulk, beyond a subsurface depth of about 20 μm. However, the impact of plastic strain on the crystallinity of Liner A was insignificant within the studied strain interval $\varepsilon \approx 5{\sim}10\%$.

(iv) Liner B, which only received 33 kGy irradiation dose as a sterilization process, showed the largest fluctuations (within the first 35 μm below the surface) among the three liners, and a significant increase in crystallinity upon increasing plastic strain. This is an expected trend, which is a consequence of the breakage of long polymeric chains with subsequent increase in their mobility and, thus, a better capacity of molecular rearrangement to form crystalline structures [229,793]. Below 50 μm in depth, only small crystallinity variations were observed, meaning that strain did not significantly affect the bulk structure of the liner.

(v) The small crystallinity fluctuations ($(\Delta\alpha_c)_{max} \approx 4\%$) that were observed in Liner C were confined to a depth <35 μm, while the bulk behavior was almost constant upon increasing strain magnitude. This observation suggests that phenomenologically, the impact of plastic strain on the microstructure of Liner C was mitigated by the presence of cross-linking.

(vi) Plots of amorphous (Figs. 6.25(a), (b), and (c)) and crystalline (Figs. 6.25(d), (e), and (f)) phase fractions, as detected either before or after plastic deformation, represented independent spectroscopic measurements and showed good consistency, the former plots decreasing while the latter increasing with increasing sampling depth. In all cases, the fractional amount of the third (semi-crystalline) phase was found to be of a negligible entity.

The conclusive statement from the outputs of this section is that vitamin E-infused UHMWPE liners experience a crystallographic phase structure in their as-received state and an evolution in microstructural trend under plastic deformation mainly dictated by the initial processing step involving 100 kGy cross-linking irradiation.

Figures 6.26(a)~(d), (e)~(h), and (i)~(l) show the experimental angular dependencies at different subsurface depths of the 1130 cm^{-1} band ($A_g + B_{1g}$ Raman mode) on the azimuthal rotation angle, χ, obtained upon in-plane rotation at different stages of uniaxial deformation for the polyethylene structures of Liners A, B, and C, respectively. The key to interpret the azimuthal angular plots in Fig. 6.26 resides in considering the tendency to follow angular periodicities of $\pi/2$ and π for out-of-plane molecular alignments parallel ($\theta_p = 0°$) and perpendicular ($\theta_p = 90°$) to the liner surface, respectively. On the other hand, an increasing tendency toward a constant angular dependence of the Raman intensity on rotation angle indicates an increased degree of randomness in the molecular arrangement. With these notions in mind, the following discussion can be made from the plots in Fig. 6.26:

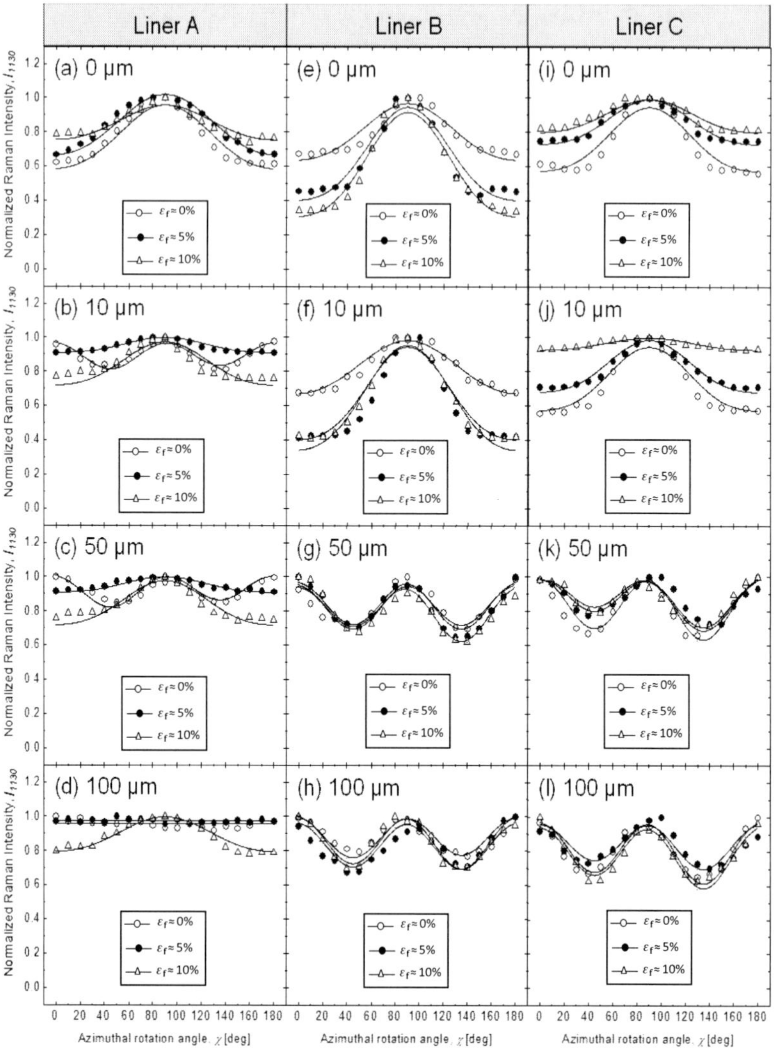

Figure 6.26 Experimental plots of angular dependence of the polarized Raman scattering intensities recorded upon in-plane rotation (angle, χ) at different depth of Liners A, B, and C ((a)~(d) for Liner A, (e)~(h) for Liner B, and (i)~(l) for Liner C). Full lines represent the results of best fitting to the experimental data.

(i) Liner A (Figs. 6.26(a)~(d) presents a sharp (i.e., within the first 10 μm below the surface) transition from a molecular alignment parallel to the sample surface to a random distribution, which is in fact the molecular pattern expected for a isostatically compression molded resin. The π periodicity is rather weak (i.e., with low amplitude) also on the very surface of the sample and, similar to what we already observed for the crystallinity fraction in Fig. 6.25(d), the effect of uniaxial compressive strain does not appear very effective in altering the plot toward a higher amplitude, namely toward a molecular pattern possessing a higher degree of orientation parallel to the sample surface.

(ii) Liners B and C (Figs. 6.26(e)~(h) and Figs. 6.16(i)~(l), respectively) showed very similar trends, with exactly the same $\pi/2$ periodicity and amplitude below a subsurface depth of 50 μm. Above such depths, a compressive strain field in the range applied in this study appears to have almost no effect on the molecular alignment of both materials. However, the strain behaviors in the first 10 μm of subsurface depth were inherently different between the two materials. While in Liner B strain consistently enhanced the amplitude of the π-periodic dependence on azimuthal angle (thus pushing, as expected, a larger fraction of molecular chains to align their long-axis in a configuration parallel to the sample surface), in Liner C the applied compressive strain first pushed the surface molecular arrangement from π periodicity toward a random configuration (straight line), as an intermediate step to further achieve, beyond 10 μm, a $\pi/2$ periodicity.

A numerical procedure of least-square fitting to the collected experimental trends of (polarized) Raman intensities (cf. full lines in Fig. 6.26), as described in Ref. [123], enabled us to retrieve plots of preferential (average) tilt angle, θ_p (Fig. 6.27), and Hermans parameter, $\langle P_2(\cos\beta)\rangle$ (Fig. 6.28), as a function of sample depth and for increasing level of plastic strain in the sample microstructures. Figures 6.27(a), (b) and (c) show tilt-angular plots for Liners A, B, and C, respectively. A comparison between the three investigated materials better visualizes the strong similarity between the behaviors of Liners B and C, both materials undergoing sudden tilting rotation at the molecular scale along the subsurface in order to develop textures perpendicular to the surface. When translated in terms of tilting angles, the differences in periodicity induced by strain between Liners B and C (cf. Fig. 6.26) appear to fall into negligible differences in angular intervals. In the context of tilting angle variations, Liner A appears to possess by far the most pronounced dependence on strain among the investigated liners, with showing a progressive textural alignment parallel to the sample surface with increasing the magnitude of compressive plastic strain stored in the material microstructure. It should be noted, however, that average angles are indeed representative of

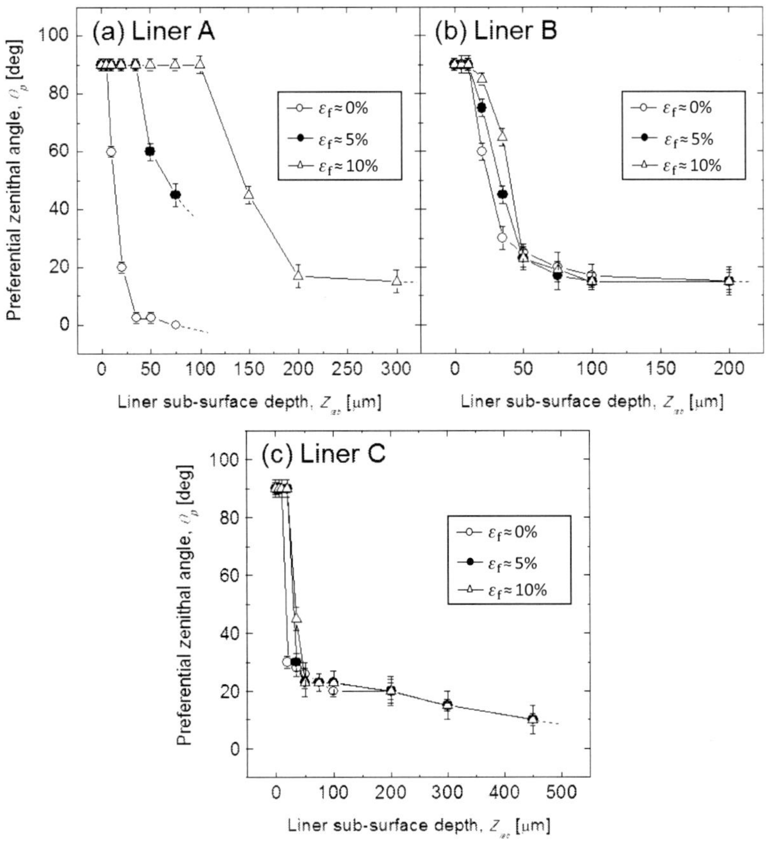

Figure 6.27 Depth profiles of average zenithal angle, θ_p, as calculated from the best fitting curves shown in Fig. 6.26 (data for Liners A, B, and C in (a), (b), and (c), respectively). Plots were interrupted at shallower depths when a full randomness was achieved in the molecular structure.

the texture but give no statistical information about the actual molecular population that experiences the observed textured pattern in the polymer microstructure. The missing information can be obtained from plots of Hermans parameter (in Figs. 6.28(a), (b), and (c) for Liners A, B, C, respectively), as well as from drawing the full ODF distribution (Fig. 6.29) as the function representative of the statistics of molecular tilt angles in the solid angle around the respective average values plotted in Fig. 6.27. The model Liner A (Fig. 6.28(a)), which lacked of cross-linked molecular chains, strikingly responded to strain on the molecular scale with a significant increase of the textured population parallel to the sample surface down to a depth of 100 μm. However, the overall ODF patterns for Liner A (cf. Figs. 6.29(a)~(c)), with or without in corporating plastic strain, always resulted much broader, and thus with textures much less relevant, than the other two liners under any strain condition. $\langle P_2(\cos\beta)\rangle$ plots in Figs. 6.28(b) and (c) revealed similar orientation homogeneity on the surface and in the immediate subsurface between the as-received Liner B and Liner C, although beyond 50 μm in depth Liner C appeared to retain a slightly higher degree of alignment. New physical insight, however, could be obtained in comparing the statistical evolutions of the molecular orientation patterns found in Liners B and C, when they incorporated increasing amounts of plastic strain. While in the microstructure of Liner B the compressively strained molecular chains tended to gradually and consistently align parallel to the sample surface with increasing strain magnitude (cf. plots in Fig. 6.28(b) and the sharpening of the near-surface ODF distributions in Figs. 6.29(e) and (f) compared with (d)), the opposite trend was observed for Liner C (Figs. 6.28(c)), in which plastic strain seemed instead to have the effect of pushing the pre-existing texture toward more random patterns (i.e., $\langle P_2(\cos\beta)\rangle$ tending to zero). This effect was significant only within the first 50 μm below the sample surface, as could be easily visualized in the gradual smearing out over broader angular populations of the ODF distributions in Figs. 6.29(h) and (i) compared with (g). The presented structural data represent the underlying foundation of the discussion given hereafter, which aims at interpreting the impact of different microstructural characteristics on the functionality of the liners.

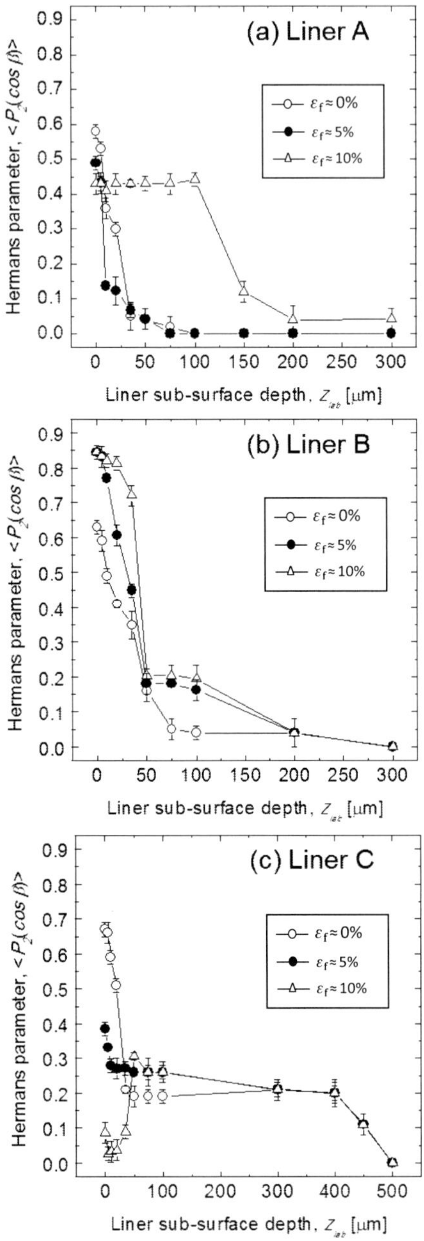

Figure 6.28 Depth profiles of Hermans parameter, $\langle P_2(\cos\beta)\rangle$, as calculated from the best fitting curves shown in Fig. 6.27 (data for Liners A, B, and C, in (a), (b), and (c), respectively).

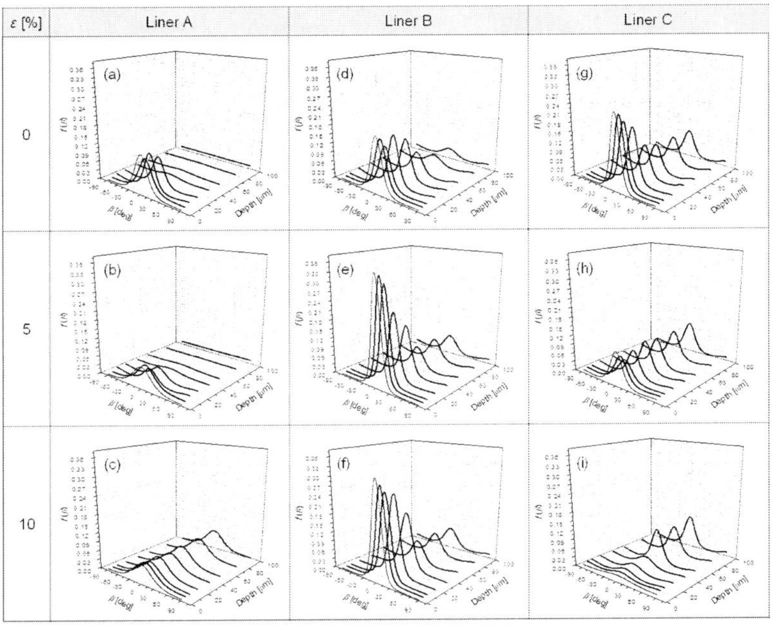

Figure 6.29 ODF at different depths in Liners A, B, and C, as retrieved after introducing different magnitudes of compressive strain in the microstructures ((a)~(c) for Liner A, (e)~(f) for Liner B, and (g)~(i) for Liner C).

According to the salient notions that could be extracted from the plots in Figs. 6.25, 6.27, and 6.29, we have so far phenomenologically clarified the salient structural differences induced by different processing steps involved with the respective manufacturing procedures of the studied liners. Moreover, clear differences came into view regarding the response of different microstructures to uniaxial compressive strain. However, in the two previous sections, a fundamental question was left unanswered, which deals with the structural reason behind the different impact of plastic strain on both crystallinity and molecular chain orientation observed in different liners.

Liner C, even after infusion of vitamin E, seems to preserve an acceptable level of crystallinity, achieved upon the 100 kGy irradiation dose injected in the liner before vitamin E infusion. Any obstructive effect on crystallization by vitamin E could only have taken place during application of the final sterilization γ-ray dose of 33 kGy. Oral *et al.* [853] discussed in detail about the phenomenon of diffusion of vitamin E into irradiated UHMWPE. The crystalline phase of the polymer was considered to be conspicuously impermeable to large molecules like α-tocopherol, and the diffusion of vitamin E was assumed to primarily occur through the amorphous phase. Moreover, the presence of crystalline regions hindered (although with an effect conspicuously independent of irradiation dose) the diffusion of molecules by restricting diffusion pathways, which in turn produced a further decrease in magnitude of diffusion coefficient through the amorphous network of the semicrystalline polymer compared with a bulk amorphous material. Given these physical circumstances, it follows that promoting appreciable diffusion of vitamin E through the bulk of a semicrystalline UHMWPE liner would require enhancing temperature with eventually applying external pressure. The most obvious procedure to overcome the difficulty encountered in diffusing the antioxidant phase through the UHMWPE bulk was proposed by Wolf *et al.* [854]. Those researchers introduced a homogenization step in inert atmosphere and super-critical carbon dioxide at temperatures above the melting point of cross-linked UHMWPE (>135°C). However, such procedure is not viable in advanced liners because it would just lead to remelting the material, thus conspicuously invalidating any positive effect of the irradiation dose superimposed prior to homogenization. Oral *et al.* [853] further inquired about the possibility of developing a homogenization method to penetrate vitamin E in highly cross-linked UHMWPE joint components without remelting the material. Homogenization at 120°C in inert gas, thus well below the melting point of the polymer, was found capable to diffuse vitamin E down to several millimeters below the surface of highly irradiated liners. The maker of the vitamin E-infused Liners C studied here indicated an annealing temperature of 130°C (cf. Table 6.3), but did not disclose the full details of the homogenization process. Therefore, we have no way to know to which extent the followed process was different from that described by Oral *et al.* [853]. However, what we have experimentally observed in analyzing Liner C is that its crystallinity preserved a value comparable to the crystallinity level of 100 kGy-irradiated GUR1050 UHMWPE [794], namely without any remelting effect of UHMWPE during homogenization heat treatment (cf. Fig. 6.25(f)). This fact can be considered as being evidence that no significant changes of microstructure (and perhaps mechanical properties) occurred during the homogenization procedure.

Regarding the effect of plastic strain on the material microstructure, as stated in the above point (ii), the differences found in comparing Liners B and C were substantial. Data in Fig. 6.29 show that the profile trends reached in Liner C at increasing levels of plastic strain were rather similar to those displayed by Liner A than reflecting those recorded for Liner B. Liner C showed an increasing degree of randomness with increasing compressive strain (cf. Figs. 6.29(g), (h), and (i)). This characteristic greatly contrasts with the significant sharpening of zenithal angle observed in Liner B under compressive strain (cf. Figs. 6.29(d), (e), and (f)).

According to general notions from the field of deformation of bulk polymers [788, 798], the response of semi-crystalline UHMWPE to strain should be considered to begin with a main deformation process occurring within amorphous regions, immediately followed by the activation of plastic slips inside the crystalline lamellae. In the initial stage of deformation, no significant rotation of crystalline lamellae should be found, with all the strain absorbed by microscopic displacements within the amorphous regions. After saturation of such displacements, crystalline lamellae start zenithal rotations toward a configuration perpendicular to the applied compressive load. The ability of responding to compressive strain with a geometrical rotation is a measure of the overall chain mobility. Bartczak [790] and Boontongkong *et al.* [855] have shown that in UHMWPE materials strained to a relatively low range of deformation, the microstructural texture experiences a higher degree of crystallographic orientation when it possesses a higher degree of cross-linking. This is because, in presence of a high degree of cross-linking, the molecular chains in the amorphous region might quickly become fully stretched to their maximum limit. With amorphous regions incapable to incorporate additional displacements on the microscopic scale, strain is thus transmitted to crystalline lamellae that under its effect, reorient perpendicular to the applied load. Data presented for Liner A and B indeed agrees with the microstructural model proposed in Refs. [790] and [800, 855], showing the most insensitive response to strain in the unirradiated (and therefore lacking of cross-linking) Liner A, and with Liner B, which possesses a higher degree of cross-linking, showing higher microstructural mobility compared with Liner A (cf. angular distribution trends in Fig. 6.29). However, Liner C, which presumably possesses the highest degree of cross-linking, did not follow the above mentioned model, and in fact, the microstructural response to strain (i.e., the increasing randomness observed upon strain application) of Liner C was closer to that of an unirradiated material than to that of an irradiated one. This behavior may indicate that the chain mobility of polyethylene became significantly lower by infusing α-tocopherol. The above notions are summarized in Figs. 6.30(a) and (b), which show drafts describing the deformation behavior under compressive load of Liners B and C, respectively.

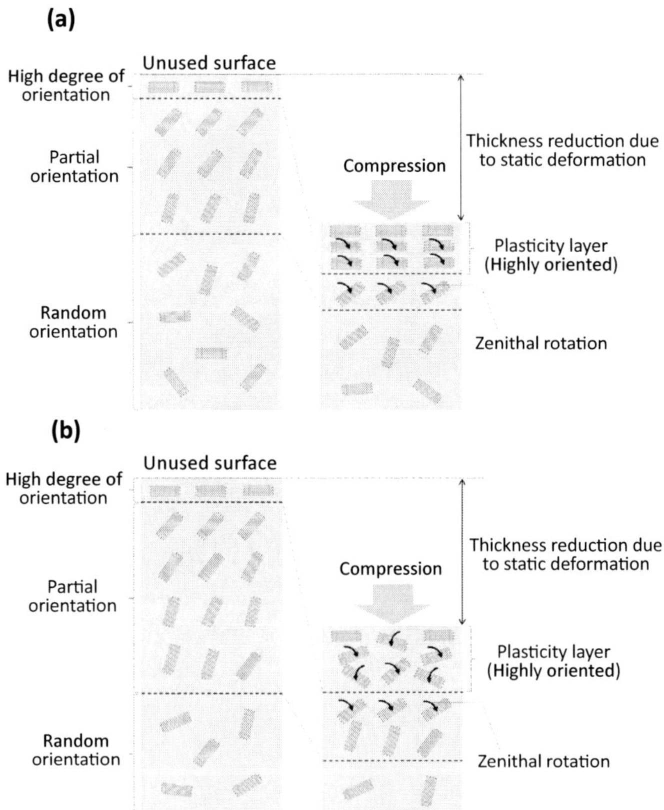

Figure 6.30 Schematics of molecular orientation pattern in Liners obtained from isostatically compression molded UHMWPE resin. The deformation models in (a) and (b) refer to Liner B and C, respectively.

In their seminal contribution on the effect of molecular orientation on the wear behavior of UHMWPE, Wang *et al.* [856] showed that in the multi-directional stress field experienced in hip joints, the UHMWPE bearing surface might undergo a strain-softening (weakening) effect related to structural anisotropy, which results in shear rupture and in the formation of fibrillar or filmy wear particles of UHMWPE. In order to minimize the detrimental effect that this phenomenon induce on wear behavior, a homogeneous and isotropic structure should be created at the surface of the liner and maintained during its functional activity. From this point of view, the low degree of molecular orientation of Liner C in its as-manufactured state and the further increase in material isotropy detected under the effect of compressive strain, might render the surface of this liner ideal to resist wear degradation (i.e., as suggested by the nearly tenfold reduction in volumetric wear-rate published by the maker in comparison with the previous product, Liner B [857]).

So far, very few studies have been published on the possible effects of vitamin E addition on wear of UHMWPE without confounding factors related to irradiation and cross-linking. *In vitro* knee simulator study performed by Teramura *et al.* [858] have proved that wear performance can be consistently improved by just adding vitamin E into un-cross-linked polyethylene. However, the reason for such improvement remained unclear in that paper. Interestingly, our microstructural assessments under static strain application between Liner B and C could help in the interpretation of the wear behavior reported in Ref. [858], showing an increase in orientational randomness as induced by the presence of vitamin E after plastic deformation. This phenomenon can reduce the risk of wear associated with strain softening. Recent clinical study reported by Glyn-Jones *et al.* [828] have elucidated the creep and wear behavior of conventional and highly cross-linked polyethylene liners over a short-term implantation time (i.e., 3 years) using radio-stereometric analysis. These researchers showed that penetration of the femoral head onto the liner was creep-dominated in the first six months of implantation; while, after 1 year, the creep component of the overall migration displacement saturated and virtually all the additional penetration was due to wear. This indicates that superior wear performance of Liner C can be expected also in *in vivo* use in comparison with Liner B, owing to a lowered risk of strain softening. However, *in vivo* studies for Liner C are still unavailable, and a concern arises from the isotropically random molecular orientation of its bulk structure. A marked reduction in creep resistance in isotropic polyethylene compared with oriented polyethylene represents a long known notion [859], as well as the marked improvement in creep behavior achieved in oriented polyethylene structures compared with isotropic ones is also well established [789]. From this point of view, the poor texture in Liner C induced by isostatically compression molding does not appear to have been properly designed to maximize creep resistance. The "molecular randomization" effect caused by plastic deformation in Liner C could be a positive effect in minimizing microscopic wear phenomena as mentioned above, but large deformations, which also lead to dimensional change in liner curvature and joint clearance, can also trigger macroscopic wear enhancements due to the formation of a shape mismatch between femoral head and acetabular liner. Therefore, as long as we can judge from the present data, superior *in vivo* performance could be expected in Liner C only compared with the conventional product Liner B produced from the same isostatic polyethylene bar with poor texture. A final conclusion on whether the new material of Liner C could be more advanced compared with other highly-cross-linked UHMWPE currently available on the market remains thus to be validated when the respective retrievals will become available to researchers.

The presented spectroscopic investigation builds upon the nowadays established chemical notion that vitamin E molecules potentially stabilizes free radicals throughout the structure of UHMWPE liners, allowing for vigorous γ-irradiation without increasing the risk of oxidative degradation. We further inquired here about the consequences involved, on the microstructural and molecular scale, with the manufacturing choice of infusing an antioxidant substance in the UHMWPE structure. In particular, the two topics assessed in this section deal with structural items related to the effect of vitamin E diffusion on crystallinity and molecular assembly. The studied UHMWPE structure was subjected to a 100 kGy irradiation prior to vitamin E infusion and to a standard (33 kGy) sterilization/irradiation process after it. The obtained results can be summarized as follows:

(i) With respect to the crystallinity ratio found on the sample surface and their profile along the subsurface, vitamin E-infused liners showed no loss of crystallinity due to homogenizing the antioxidant substance.

(ii) In terms of microstructural texture, reflections of the orientation patterns induced by γ-irradiation actually remained in the average tilt-angle profile along the subsurface of the vitamin E-infused liner. However, the statistical distributions around such preferential orientation angles were completely annihilated by the effect of compressive loading, which is beneficial to avoid strain-softening assisted wear phenomenon. This findings, revealed by means of advanced Raman spectroscopic assessments, call for a prompt and detailed confirmation of the static and dynamic deformation behavior of this newly launched UHMWPE component.

(iii) The poor molecular texture observed in all the liners investigated in this study, which is a direct consequence of the choice of isostatically compression molded raw-material bars, could be detrimental to creep resistance *in vivo*, which might lead to macroscopic wear enhancements due to a morphologic mismatch between the curvature of the femoral head and acetabular liner.

In highly cross-linked UHMWPE liners, energy inputs from mechanical stressing are generally assumed to produce only minor changes in mechanical and physical properties. Accordingly, in hip-joint applications, the changes in material properties arising from in-service dynamic loading are generally assumed to be negligible when compared with changes arising from chemically initiated aging processes (i.e., oxidation). Besides the experimentally proved truthfulness of this notion, the molecular texture of the studied vitamin E-infused UHMWPE (Liner C) does not appear to possess structural characteristics belonging to the class of highly creep resistant polyethylene structures. This finding thus calls for a prompt and detailed confirmation of the static and dynamic deformation behavior of this newly launched E1® UHMWPE component.

6.6 In-Plane Molecular Rearrangements in Hip Joints Exposed *in vivo*

The most applied type of prosthesis in total hip arthroplasty (THA) consists of a system with a femoral head made of a metal alloy (e.g., CoCr) impinging against an ultra-high molecular weight polyethylene (UHMWPE) acetabular cup. We have already discussed that in hip joint systems, the UHMWPE acetabular cup undertakes the multiple roles of body-weight bearing, low-friction sliding surface, and impact absorber. Accordingly, it is liable to experience extensive creep and wear damages with the concurrent formation of polyethylene debris, which eventually leads to joint loosening and osteolysis (i.e., to the need for a revision surgery) [860, 861]. In other words, UHMWPE components unavoidable degrade both chemically and mechanically during *in vivo* implantation. In an attempt to both clarify the origin of implant degradation and propose methods for elongating their lifetime, a number of Raman studies have been carried out focusing on phenomena of chemical and structural degradation (e.g., oxidation and degree of crystallinity) in the polyethylene structure [115, 804, 862–864]. On the other hand, Raman measurements of residual strain in UHMWPE acetabular cups have provided, as discussed in the previous section, an effective tool for the quantitative assessment of mechanical degradation in terms of residual strain [116, 822]. In particular, this latter Raman spectroscopic method provided one with an experimental path to separate creep and wear contributions from the dimensional change experimentally observed in *in vivo* exposed acetabular cups. Inasmuch as Raman studies of chemical, structural, and mechanical alterations greatly contributed to advance our knowledge of degradation processes in biomedical UHMWPE grades, yet a long way seems to be left until the development of a rigorous spectroscopic protocol for *in vivo* lifetime prediction of biomedical components will eventually become available. The reason for such a lack of information might partly reside in often neglecting an additional structural factor (i.e., besides crystallinity) as important as the chemical and the mechanical ones: the occurrence of local crystallographic alignment of the polyethylene lamellae. Polarized Raman spectroscopy possesses the potential to quantitatively unfold the missing crystallographic information by screening with a laser microprobe the molecular orientation patterns developed on the surface of acetabular components [851,865–869]. However, such an evaluation represents a formidable experimental and computational task. Crystalline (e.g., mainly orthorhombic) phases in UHMWPE might be randomly oriented within the amorphous matrix or be preferentially oriented as a consequence of the manufacturing process. However, the orientation of crystalline lamellae is sensitive to mechanical and frictional loading [870–872]. Therefore, the lamellae will unavoidably tend to preferentially orient themselves on the surface of UHMWPE acetabular cup during *in vivo* loading. This molecular rearrangement reflects both primary and secondary motions generated at the contact surface in artificial hip joints, thus representing an important mechanism, precursor to the formation of wear debris throughout the loading history.

In this section, we focus on a spectroscopic method aimed at quantifying the degree of molecular orientation and the angular distributions of orthorhombic lamellae on the surface of UHMWPE. The method is based on theoretical developments and experimental validations of the Raman selection rules and of the Raman tensor elements intrinsic to the orthorhombic structure of polyethylene, respectively. Orientation distribution functions [873–875] are also incorporated, similar to what described in Sections 6.2 and 6.3, into the mathematical algorithm of Raman crystallographic orientation analysis in order to quantify the local degree of alignment of the structure concurrently to the orientation in space of the *c*-axis of the orthorhombic cell. According to the knowledge of both intrinsic vibrational parameters and orientation distribution functions, one could quantitatively discuss the orientation of orthorhombic lamellae from relative changes in intensity of selected Raman bands in selected polarization geometries. Accordingly, areas from main wear and non-wear zones can be characterized in comparison with unused acetabular cups, and the effect of wear on molecular orientation clarified.

Four different acetabular cups are investigated in this section, which were all retrieved from left-side hip joints in the respective patient bodies at Tokyo Medical University. These acetabular cups will be also referred to as short-term (2.4 and 2.8 years) and long-term (10.3 and 12.2 years) retrievals, respectively. The short-term retrieved acetabular components were both made of highly cross-linked polyethylene, manufactured from 1900H bar stock by isostatic compression molding (with no addition of calcium stearate) (ArCom®, Biomet Japan Inc., Tokyo, Japan) and sterilized by γ-ray irradiation with a dose of 33 kGy. One cup belonged to a 61-year-old male patient for which the cause of revision was infection with a follow-up period of 2.4 years, while the other cup belonged to a 53-year-old female patient for which the cause of revision was infection dislocation with a follow-up period of 2.8 years. On the other hand, two long-term retrievals were made from GUR4150 bar stock by Ram extraction molding (calcium stearate was added in these case) and sterilized with a dose of γ-ray radiations ranging between 25 to 37 kGy. One cup (manufactured by Zimmer Inc., Tokyo, Japan) belonged to 47-year-old male patient, while the other cup (ArCom®, Biomet Japan Inc., Tokyo, Japan) belonged to a 60-year-old female patient. Both cups were retrieved due to aseptic loosening and the follow-up period was 10.4 and 12.2 years, respectively. For comparison, an unused acetabular cup was investigated, which was also from the Biomet manufacturer and possessed the same manufacturing characteristics of the short-term retrieval described above. Locating the main wear zone on both short-term and long-term retrievals could be pursued in a relatively easy way by the naked eye, owing to a slight difference in surface roughness (and, thus, in sample translucency) compared with the non-wear zone. On the other hand, an exception was the short-term retrievals exposed *in vivo* for 2.8 years, for which such an observation was difficult. In this latter case, we assumed the main wear zone to be located within the angular interval 30°~40° from the location of cup dome, in analogy with the other retrievals studied.

The relationship between the observed Raman bands and the vibrational modes of the orthorhombic polyethylene structure is amply documented in the pre-existing literature [116,851]. Briefly here, we summarize the main features found in the Raman spectrum of UHMWPE in the 1000~1500 cm^{-1} spectral region, which are also explicitly listed in Table 6.4. The Raman spectrum can be subdivided into three main regions: region (I) in the interval 1000~1200 cm^{-1}, which is dominated by C–C stretching vibrations; region (II) at around 1300 cm^{-1}, which is dominated by $-CH_2-$ twisting vibrations; and, region (III) in the interval

1400 and 1500 cm^{-1}, which is dominated by $-CH_2-$ wagging vibrations. In dealing with a highly crystallized structure, as in the case of the fiber sample, the vibrations with tensor axis coincident with the axes of the crystalline orthorhombic units are expected to contribute the most relevant part of the detected Raman intensity. In other words, the modes with A_g, B_{2g}, and B_{3g} symmetry (cf. Table 6.4), which satisfy this requirement, should have a dominating effect on the polarized Raman spectra of the UHMWPE structure studied here as compared with the B_{1g} mode (i.e., mainly related to the amorphous structure). Two broad bands located at 1080 and 1310 cm^{-1} are also assigned to the amorphous (matrix) phase. In the case of all the UHMWPE samples investigated here, the intensities of these bands were conspicuously weak (and vanishingly low in the fiber sample) as a consequence of a high degree of crystallinity and highly aligned molecular structure. Nevertheless, we have assessed the degree of crystallinity using the relative intensity of the band located at 1296 cm^{-1} (representing the crystalline part of the structure) vs. the band located at 1310 cm^{-1} (representing the amorphous structure), according to the equation given by Mutter *et al.* [876].

Table 6.4 Raman bands and respective vibrational modes in UHMWPE

Wavenumber, cm^{-1}	Phase	Mode	Symmetry
1060	*C*(*A*)	ν_{as}(C–C)	$B_{2g} + B_{3g}$
1080	*A*	ν(C–C)	—
1130	*C*(*A*)	ν_s(C–C)	$A_g + B_{1g}$
1170	*C*(*A*)	$\rho(CH_2)$	$A_g + B_{1g}$
1296	*C*	$\tau(CH_2)$	$B_{2g} + B_{3g}$
1310	*A*	$\tau(CH_2)$	—
1370	*C*(*A*)	$\omega(CH_2)$	$B_{2g} + B_{3g}$
1418	*C*	$\sigma(CH_2)$	A_g
1440	*A*	$\sigma(CH_2)$	$A_g + B_{1g}$
1460	*A*	$\sigma(CH_2)$	$A_g + B_{1g}$

C, crystalline; *A*, amorphous; ν, stretching (s, symmetric; as, asymmetric); ρ, rocking; σ, bending; τ, twisting; ω, wagging.

Note: Spectral locations are explicitly indicated together with the related phases, vibrational modes and symmetries (in round brackets are the specific molecular species involved with individual vibrational modes).

The band located at 1170 cm^{-1} possesses $A_g + B_{1g}$ symmetry and results from the CH_2 rocking mode. The 1130 cm^{-1} band, also with $A_g + B_{1g}$ symmetry, mostly arises from the crystalline part of the polymer, but the trans C–C bond in the amorphous phase are also expected to contribute to the scattering intensity at this frequency. Maxfield *et al.* [851] have used this band to calculate the orientation of the crystalline part of low-density polyethylene. This band is clearly visible in the Raman spectra of standard polyethylene samples, but in the acetabular cups, its intensity was very low and this hampered a precise characterization of intensity variations as a function of polarization angle. The origin of bands related to CH_2 bending modes at around 1450 cm^{-1} is the most ambiguous in polyethylene because of the possibility of Fermi resonance between the Raman active CH_2 bending modes and its first overtones and the possible combinations of the infrared active CH_2 rocking modes [865]. In addition, combinations with infrared active CH_2 rocking modes cannot be ruled out. All this body of reasons, suggest not selecting bands belonging to CH_2 bending modes for our Raman polarization analyses.

According to the Raman polarization technique, visualization of the crystallinity and the near-surface molecular orientation is possible in UHMWPE acetabular cups retrieved after different periods of *in vivo* exposure, according to spectral mapping procedure applied to both main wear and non-wear zones. For comparison, maps can also be collected at similar locations in unused UHMWPE acetabular cups. On the other hand, the mean molecular orientation of the orthorhombic cell in the Raman probe at each location of the maps and its distribution function can be retrieved from polarization experiments. For this latter purpose, angular in-plane rotations need to be performed at each location to retrieve molecular orientation Euler angles and orientation distribution functions. Figures 6.31(a)~(e) and 6.32(a)~(e) show typical maps (100 μm × 100 μm, in dimension) of crystallinity and molecular orientation patterns, respectively, as collected at the same locations for both wear and non-wear zones. In the above figures, maps in (a), (b), (c), (d), and (e) refer to the unused cup, and to cups retrieved after 2.4, 2.8, 10.3, and 12.2 years, respectively. In the maps of Figs. 6.32(a)~(e), an orientation of the *c*-axis of the orthorhombic structure corresponding to a reference angle of molecular alignment, $\chi = 0$, is taken in correspondence of a straight line separating the anterior–superior (A–S) zone of the cup from its posterior–inferior (P–I) zone (i.e., the axis shown in Fig. 6.32). Positive angles are then counted anti-clockwise. Figures 6.33(a)~(e) display histograms of crystallinity, α_c, and of molecular orientation angle, χ, which are representative of the full set of statistical data collected on five 100 μm × 100 μm maps per each zone of each cup. The salient features revealed by a comparison among maps and histograms in Figs. 6.31~6.33 can be listed as follows:

(i) The statistical trend for the degree of crystallinity in the unused cup was uniformly represented (i.e., over the entire surface of the cup) by a relatively broad distribution, whose mean value was determined as about 54%. However, as a general trend, all crystallinity histograms of the *in vivo* exposed cups appeared to be smeared over a much wider interval of α_c values. As a result, the mean values were only slightly shifted towards higher fractions. Irrespective of exposure time *in vivo* and of whether they belonged to main wear or non-wear zones, the α_c histograms collected on the bearing surface of the UHMWPE cups appeared significantly altered by *in vivo* implantation with the formation of "hot spots" of crystallinity reaching values as high as 80~85%.

(ii) The unused cup showed a weak pattern of molecular alignment on its surface, with a quite low value of Hermans parameter, $\langle P_2(\cos\beta)\rangle = 0.40$ (cf. histogram in Fig. 6.33(a) and Table 6.5). The partial alignment was most likely a consequence of the manufacturing process.

(iii) Unlike the unused cup, the distribution of the in-plane molecular orientation angle, χ, on the surfaces of the retrievals was always bimodal. In other words, the exposure *in vivo* appeared to introduce a new population of oriented orthorhombic lamellae sharply clustered at orientation angles around 30°. This new angular population grew at the expenses of the originally homogeneous angular population oriented at around 68° as observed in the unused cup. The strongly bimodal character of the angular distribution was a common feature to all maps collected on retrievals as can be easily perceived by the conspicuous absence of gray zones (i.e., the predominance of black and white regions) in the related maps.

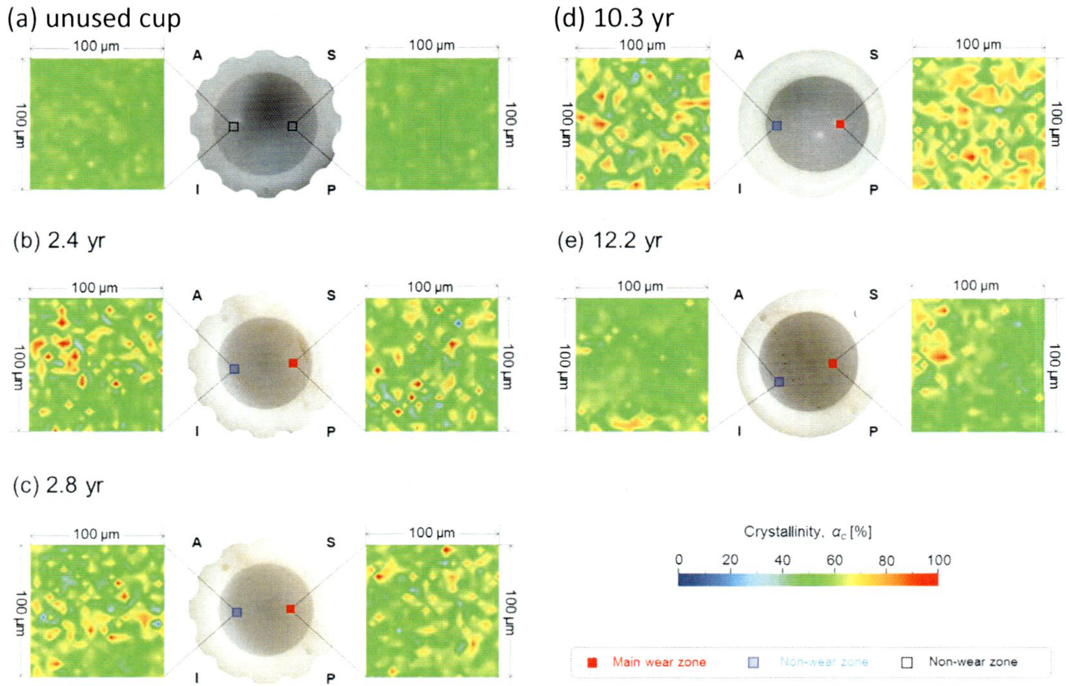

Figure 6.31 Typical maps of degree of crystallization, α_c, as revealed by Raman scattering intensities on selected areas of the four investigated retrievals in comparison with the unused acetabular cup. Left and right sides of each retrieved cup are from non-wear and main wear zones, respectively. In analogy, maps were collected at two similar locations also in the unused cup.

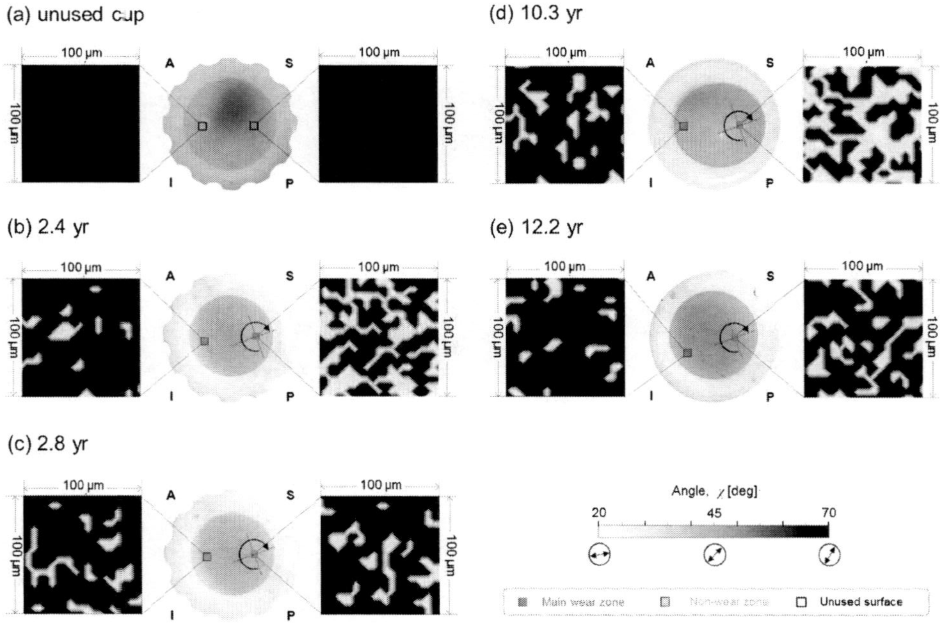

Figure 6.32 Typical maps of molecular orientation patterns as revealed by polarized Raman scattering intensities on selected areas of the four investigated retrievals in comparison with the unused acetabular cup. Left and right sides of the maps in the retrieved cups are from non-wear and main wear zones, respectively. In analogy, maps were collected at two similar locations also in the unused cup. Full and broken lines drawn on each retrieved cup represent the approximate direction of gait motion and the mean molecular orientation direction detected in the white areas of the maps, respectively. The arrowed rotation indicates a secondary displacement by torsion that might be at the origin of the observed molecular alignment.

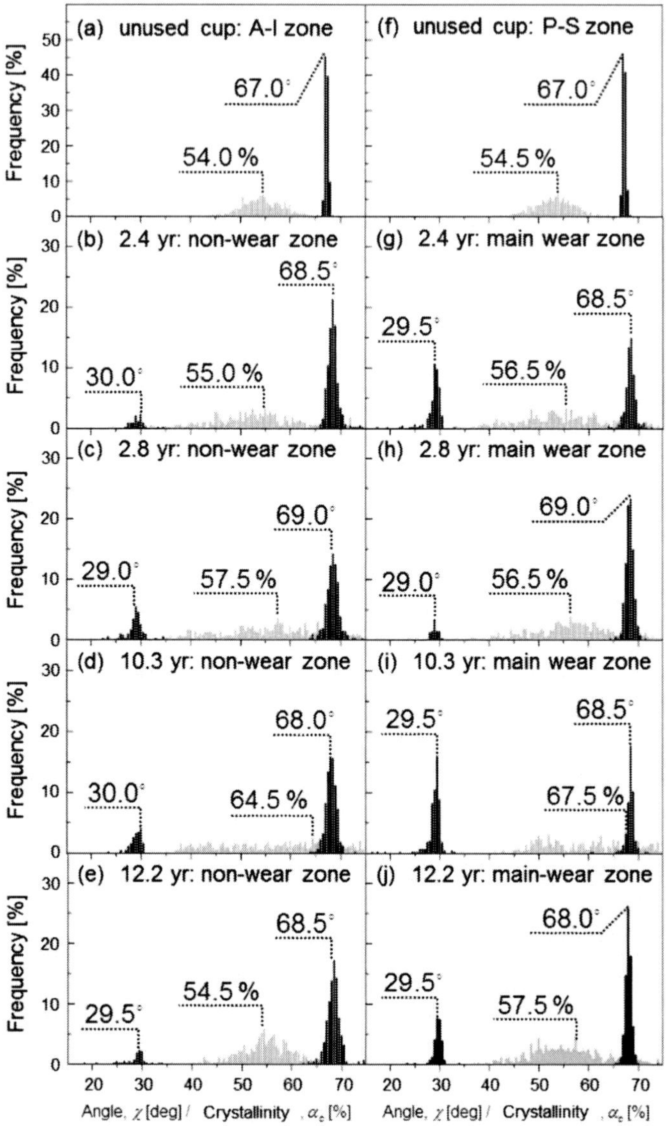

Figure 6.33 Histograms of the degree of crystallinity, α_c, and of c-axis orientation angle, χ, for both main and non-wear zones of short-term and long-term retrievals as compared with the as manufactured material. Note the homogeneous structure of this latter sample in both anteroinferior and posterosuperior zones (in (a) and (f), respectively). Each histogram is representative of a surface area of 5×10^4 μm^2.

Table 6.5 Numerical parameters characterizing the orientation distribution functions plotted in Fig. 6.34

Sample	$\langle P_2(\cos\beta)\rangle$	$\langle P_4(\cos\beta)\rangle$	A	λ_2	λ_4
Fiber	0.97	0.92	3.29×10^{-9}	−10.00	−10.00
Main wear zone <long-term >	0.88	0.78	7.51×10^{-4}	−1.70	−5.00
Main wear zone <short-term>	0.73	0.60	3.18×10^{-3}	−1.65	−3.00
Non-wear zone	0.58	0.44	5.94×10^{-3}	−1.50	−2.00
Unused cup	0.40	0.19	9.10×10^{-3}	−1.50	−0.65

Note: The parameters listed in the above table refer to an ODF structure given as: $f(\beta) = A[-(\lambda_2 P_2(\cos\beta) + \lambda_4 P_4(\cos\beta))]$, with the parameters $\langle P_2(\cos\beta)\rangle$ and $\langle P_4(\cos\beta)\rangle$ being the average coefficients of a series expansion in Legendre polynomials as explained in details in Ref. [124]. In this formalism, the parameter $\langle P_2(\cos\beta)\rangle$ (i.e., the Hermans parameter) is by far the most representative in statistically describing the preferential orientation of the molecular array, and we have discussed, for simplicity's sake, only this parameter throughout the text. The parameters of the ODF function representing a highly aligned polyethylene fiber structure are also shown for comparison.

(iv) Black regions in the maps of angle, χ, represent the original orientation of the orthorhombic cell on the cup surface after manufacturing. While the distribution of white regions appeared to be random on the analyzed surfaces, the molecular alignment within those zones conspicuously differed from the direction of sliding displacements (gait motion) at the contact surface between femoral head and acetabular cup (cf. displacement and *c*-axis orientation directions in Fig. 6.31) during walking. This is an important feature, which suggests that also secondary motions (e.g., torsions) play an important role on surface molecular alignment. Analyses of local orientation distribution in non-wear zones showed that the black regions maintained quite low values of the Hermans parameter (i.e., in the narrow range $0.4 \leq \langle P_2(\cos\beta)\rangle \leq 0.47$, cf. Table 6.5) as in the case of the unexposed material. The low degree of alignment in non-wear zones can be also confirmed by comparing the angular dependences of Raman intensity in these zones with those in the unused cup. Interestingly, as far as main wear zones were concerned, white regions in the χ maps often (but not necessarily) corresponded to highly crystallized regions, while no such relationship could be observed in the non-wear zones, despite they also showed some increase in degree of crystallinity compared with the unused cup. In the main wear zones, the degree of in-plane angular orientation was by far more pronounced, and the white areas in the χ maps could locally reach $\langle P_2(\cos\beta)\rangle$ values as high as 0.90.

(v) No clear trends for an increase in both crystallinity and Hermans parameter as a function of *in vivo* exposure time could be obtained in this study. In particular, the long-term retrieval in Figs. 6.31(e) and 6.32(e) showed significantly lower degrees of crystallinity and molecular alignment as compared with the other long-term retrieval in Figs. 6.31(d) and 6.32(d). The values were comparable to those of the short-term exposed cups. While a lack of statistics hampers any final conclusion regarding the relationship between the degree of crystallinity/alignment and *in vivo* exposure time, we can only speculate here that the presumed lower activity of a 60-year-old female patient vs. that of a 49-year-old male patient could be, for the otherwise exactly same type and size of implant, the reason for the observed structural differences.

Despite such a lack in statistics, the experimental data clearly suggest that the observed variation of structural patterns in the main wear zone, namely both the fractional increase of orthorhombic lamellae population and their clustering around an orientation different from the direction of gait motion in the hip joint, visualizes the occurrence of wear damage on the UHMWPE bearing surface. In other words, the highly crystallized/aligned zones (i.e., the "hot spots" observed in the α_c maps) formed as a result of prolonged and repetitive sliding motion of the femoral head along the direction of gait motion and are likely to detach from the surface, thus becoming wear debris (in agreement with the phenomenological description given in previous literature [812]). Data obtained by shifting the focal plane of the confocal probe along the subsurface of the acetabular cups (i.e., with steps of 1 μm) revealed detectable spectral variations (i.e., toward the original structure of the unexposed material) starting from a depth z_0 = 5~8 μm, while the full restoration of the original structure occurred from depths at around 20 μm.

Average orientation distribution functions, as obtained for the non-wear and main wear zones of the long-term retrieval in Figs. 6.31(d) and 6.32(d) and the short-term retrieval in Figs. 6.31(c) and 6.32(c), are plotted in Fig. 6.34. For comparison, the functions retrieved for highly crystallized and molecularly oriented polyethylene fiber sample and for the unused cup are also shown as an upper and lower boundary for the degree of orientation of a UHMWPE structure, respectively. All the parameters characterizing the orientation distribution functions are explicitly listed in Table 6.5. The plots in Fig. 6.34 represent the probability of finding a molecule oriented at an angle, β, with respect to the average in plane angle, χ, the broader the function the closer the distribution to a random one. Data are representative of about 2200 spectra over a total area of $\approx 10^5$ μm^2 per each zone of the investigated cup. The degree of alignment can be clearly visualized by the narrow peak centered at $\beta = 0$, the higher the peak the higher the degree of alignment. Results confirm that the probability of

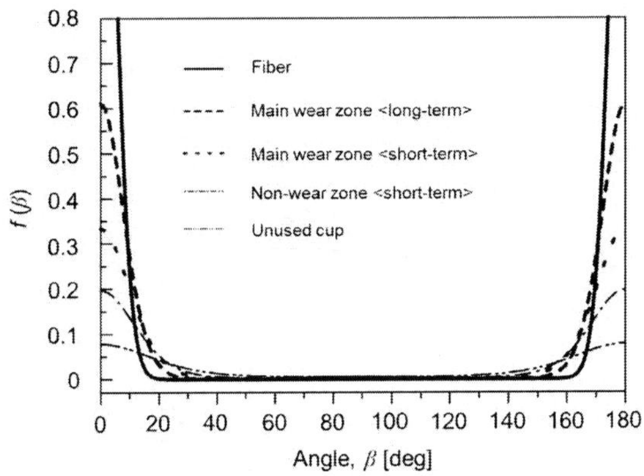

Figure 6.34 Orientation distribution functions as calculated from experimental data for the main wear zones of the 10.3 year long-term retrieval and of the 2.8 year short-term retrieval are plotted in comparison with the functions retrieved for the fiber sample and for the unused cup as an upper and lower boundary for the degree of orientation of a UHMWPE structure, respectively. The functions for the non-wear zone between the 10.3 and 2.8 year retrievals in their respective non-wear zone were almost coincident and are represented by the same plot. The ODF function representing a highly aligned polyethylene fiber structure is also plotted for reference in the figure. Each function is representative of Raman spectra averaged over an area of 5 × 10^4 μm^2.

finding UHMWPE lamellae oriented along the direction of gait motion in the hip joint was the highest in the main wear zone of the cup sample exposed for long time *in vivo*, although such a degree of orientation was far from reaching the extremely high value found for the UHMWPE fiber along its long axis. On the other hand, some increase in the degree of alignment was visible upon exposure *in vivo* even in the conspicuous lack of mechanical load (i.e., in the non-wear zone), as compared with the unused cup (i.e., $\langle P_2(\cos\beta)\rangle = 0.58$ vs. 0.40).

From a general perspective, the present structural analysis by Raman spectroscopy confirms and quantifies how the degree of alignment of the orthorhombic structure on the surface of *in vivo* exposed UHMWPE acetabular cups depends on loading history and, thus, suggests that the Hermans parameter can be seen as a measure of both cumulative wear history and effective lifetime in acetabular cups exposed *in vivo*. The developed Raman methodology coupled with the ODF formalism provides direct access to the appropriate length scale for quantitative structural assessment in UHMWPE and, thus, gives scientists and technologists a chance to experimentally verify the performance and to rationalize the *in vivo* lifetime of UHMWPE components for biomedical applications.

6.7 Out-of-Plane Molecular Rearrangements in Knee Joints Exposed *in vivo*

The response to applied strain of EtO-sterilized and γ-irradiated polyethylene materials belonging to tibial inserts can be studied by polarized Raman spectroscopy in a way similar to that shown for hip acetabular cups in the previous section. Initial calibrations on samples as received from the makers can be employed to preliminary clarify the rearrangement of molecular chains under strain, as expressed in terms of Euler angular displacements in space and ODF. This body of information can be then applied to quantitative analyses of tibial inserts retrieved after *in vivo* exposures. Similar to the case of acetabular cups, the main object of the research efforts resides in avoiding *in vivo* generation of polyethylene debris, which are unquestionably the most commonly encountered issues affecting the durability of knee joint

[802, 877]. The cyclic sliding motion between femoral condyle and polyethylene tibial insert components induces wear and fatigue damage that can lead to separation of micrometric particles of polyethylene from the surface or even, in the most unfortunate cases, to fracture of the bearing parts [801–803, 877, 878]. The sub-products of wear degradation then produce a body reaction leading to osteolysis and, ultimately, to revision surgery [9, 17, 92, 879]. Even if the knee joint forces are comparable to those developed at the hip cup, due to a nonconformity between the surfaces of tibial and femoral components, the external cyclic load applied to the tibial plate is distributed over a more limited area than the hip, generating a level of stress that could easily exceed the polymer yield strength [880, 881]. Therefore, building a clear picture of the structural changes occurring during *in vivo* loading in the "soft" components of artificial knees represents a mandatory step to understand and to improve total knee arthroplasty procedures.

The texture of a structurally complex material like biomedical polyethylene, namely the orientation distribution of crystalline lamellae and molecular chains, has been deeply studied [772, 882, 883]. Such microstructural features play a crucial role in both wear resistance and strength properties. Several studies can be found in the available literature, reporting about structural modification induced by processing on polyethylene components. We have already discussed in Section 6.2 how samples produced by extrusion and by compression molding possess different textures as a consequence of different processes of plastic deformation. Song *et al.* [884] investigated samples of high-density polyethylene produced either by rolling or by channel-die compression. The orientation of orthorhombic crystallographic planes was evaluated by means of wide- and small-angle X-ray scattering, and a preferential distribution of c-axis along the plastic flow direction was noticed. Moreover, also a tendency of the orthorhombic α-axis to orient toward the loading direction was reported. The microstructural modifications induced by uniaxial compression in high-density polyethylene have also been studied by Bartczak *et al.* [885] at different stages of deformation. In this latter study, the change of morphology in the polymer structure was monitored to values of true strain up to 2. As revealed by microscopy assessments, the initial spherulitic superstructure was completely random and, during deformation, the lamellae rotated away from the loading direction. Moreover, from the very beginning of plastic deformation process, it was confirmed a tendency of the *a*-axis to align along the loading direction. In this section, we build upon the assessments of molecular orientation shown in the previous section for acetabular cups of hip joints and use polarized Raman micro-spectroscopy to quantitatively assess the microstructural modifications induced by plastic deformation in polyethylene bearing components used in knee replacements. Tibial inserts are hereafter analyzed, which underwent plastic deformation (i.e., in addition to that initially stored in the samples upon processing) *in vivo*, in comparison with the respective unused samples as received from the makers. The plastic strain stored in the material can be correlated to the out-of-plane variation of tilt angle in the polyethylene chains and to the variation of statistical ODF parameters.

A total of seven UHMWPE tibial plates were characterized, three as received from the makers and four retrieved after total knee arthroplasty revision surgery. Regarding the four retrieved UHMWPE tibial plates, two were manufactured by Japan Medical Materials (JMM, Osaka Japan) and sterilized by ethylene oxide (EtO) gas (henceforth referred to as sample A and B), while the remaining two, referred to as sample C and D, were commercially distributed by Stryker K. K. (Tokyo, Japan) and Smith & Nephew Orthopedics (Tokyo, Japan), respectively. The tibial plate C was Vacuum/N_2-flush-packaging followed by irradiation by γ-ray (33 kGy) was applied for the tibial plate sample C, while EtO-sterilization was applied to the plate D. Sample A belonged to a 73-year-old female patient for which the cause of revision was aseptic loosening with a follow-up period of 5 years 8 months. Sample B belonged to a 77-year-old female patient. Also for this latter patient, the cause of revision was aseptic loosening after a follow-up period of 4 years 7 months. Samples C and D were both retrieved from female patients whose ages were 83 and 81 years, respectively. In the former case, the cause of revision was aseptic loosening after an implantation period of 4 years, while for the latter the cause was malpositioning after a follow-up of only 7 months. All patients were old and not so active but all were ambulating. Table 6.6 gives a summary of the investigated cases, including manufacturing characteristics and clinical data. The three unused tibial plates were of the same type as the retrieved ones, one from each manufacturer. All three types of tibial plate were machined from compression-molded sheets. For the as-received samples, the same letters are used as those locating the retrieved plates, and indicate manufacturing by the same maker. Samples were probed on their surfaces by visually selecting the locations under the optical microscope. Twenty locations for Raman assessments were randomly selected in both main wear and non-wear zones of each *in vivo* exposed tibial plate. Unlike EtO sterilization, γ-irradiation is known to generate cross-linking and, concurrently, also to produce some amount of free radicals [16,90,98]. Such major alterations of the polymeric structure are known to strongly affect the macroscopic strain behavior. For this reason, calibrations under compressive load were repeated for each type of tibial insert.

Table 6.6 Manufacturing characteristics and clinical data of the four investigated knee retrievals

Case	Name of implant (Maker)	Resin	Processing	Sterili-zation	Size	Patient	Follow-up	BMI
A	KU3(JMM)	GUR 1050	Compression molding	EtO	Small 9 mm	73 yr female	5 yr 8 mo	22.0
B	KU3(JMM)	GUR 1050	Compression molding	EtO	X-small 9 mm	77 yr female	4 yr 7 mo	23.6
C	Scorpio NRG (Stryker)	GUR 1020	Compression molding	γ-ray (33 kGy)	8 mm with stabilizer	83 yr female	4 yr	23.1
D	Smith & Nephew (Genesis II)	GUR 1020	Compression molding	EtO	9 mm H/F	81 yr female	7 mo	25.8

Figure 6.35(a) shows the dimensions of the samples and the location in the unused tibial components from which samples for uniaxial strain-calibration testing were obtained. The choice of the cut configuration was made for representing as much as possible the conditions of *in vivo* loading. Particular care was taken in order to cut the tibial insert in a position in which the bearing surface is almost parallel (misalignment always $< 4°$) to the lower surface of the insert itself. The effect of the curvature upon loading the 3×3 mm square face obtained after cutting was in this case negligible. The surface of the sample was then investigated by confocal Raman

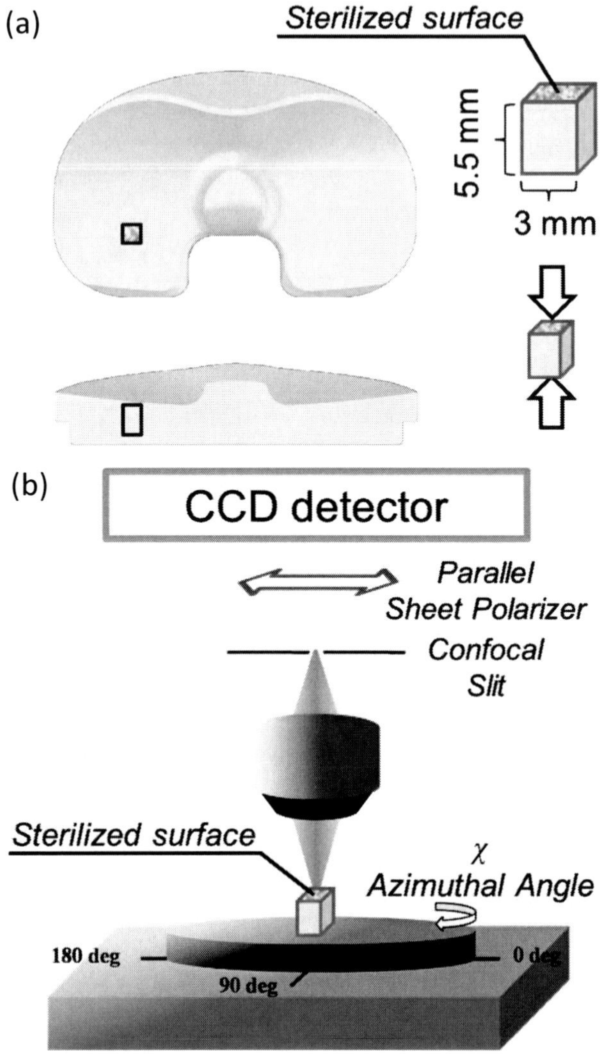

Figure 6.35 (a) Geometry of the tested samples and the location in the unused tibial components from which they were extracted for performing uniaxial strain testing. Compressive load was applied parallel to the long axis of the sample. In (b), a schematic draft of the experimental set-up adopted for in-plane rotation assessments. Raman spectra were collected using sheet polarizers in parallel configuration with respect to the incident laser polarization vector and filtered by means of a confocal pinhole placed across the backscattered emission.

spectroscopy (Fig. 6.35(b)). For each type of tibial insert, two rectangular bars were loaded at different steps. Compressive load was applied parallel in a way similar to the case of *in vivo* loading, by means of a uniaxial compressive jig. In order to assess only the plastic component of strain, after each step of compression, we left the sample unloaded for 24 hours until a complete recovery of the anelastic strain component in the polymer structure was reached. The compressed surface was analyzed with placing the sample in a rotation jig and collecting polarized Raman spectra at different azimuthal angles, χ. In Fig. 6.35(b), a schematic draft is shown that explains the experimental set-up adopted for in-plane rotation assessments. Raman spectra were collected using sheet polarizers in parallel configuration with respect to the incident laser polarization vector. Particular care was taken in order to align the axis of the microscope with the axis of the rotation jig. For each point under investigation, Raman polarized spectra were collected at 19 different azimuthal angles within the interval $0° \leq \chi \leq 180°$, with sequential steps of 10°. The same procedure was adopted to analyze both wear zones and non-wear zones in the retrieved tibial plates. In spectroscopic strain calibrations, we monitored the polyethylene microstructures from its as-received state (i.e., at residual strain assumed as $\varepsilon_f = 0$) up to $\varepsilon_f = 12\%$ of uniaxial compressive true strain. Since there was no appreciable difference between the behaviors of the two EtO-sterilized materials produced from different makers, we shall show and discuss the strain calibration results by simply comparing EtO-sterilized and γ-irradiated samples. Examples of experimental angular dependencies obtained upon in-plane rotation at different stages of uniaxial deformation for EtO-sterilized samples are shown in Fig. 6.36(a), while the results of best fitting and the calculated ODFs are reported in Figs. 6.36(b) and (c), respectively. Similarly, experimental results of polarized Raman intensity as a function of in-plane rotation, the related best fitting curves, and ODFs are reported for the γ-irradiated sample in Figs. 6.36(d), (e) and (f), respectively. The periodical trend found for the Raman intensity of the $A_g + B_{1g}$ mode upon in-plane rotation is independent of uniaxial strain applied along a direction perpendicular to the sample surface. Independent of the adopted sterilization procedure, the in-plane Euler angle locating the preferential orientation on the surface of the sample was measured as $\chi_p \approx \pi/5$ and it was invariant with increasing the magnitude of applied (static) strain. On the other hand, as a general rule, an increase of applied strain led to a larger population of molecular chains experiencing preferential orientation, as shown by the increasingly pronounced maximum in the calculated ODF (cf. Figs. 6.36(c) and (f) for EtO-sterilized and γ-irradiated materials, respectively). However, such a trend appeared more pronounced in the EtO-sterilized material as compared with the γ-irradiated one. Important to the present context is that the experimental plots in Fig. 6.36, also contain information about the out-of-plane molecular orientation angle, θ_p. Figure 6.37 shows values of θ_p (a) and Hermans parameter, $\langle P_2(\cos\beta)\rangle$, (b) as retrieved from best fitting of the full set of strain dependence curves (of which a selection is shown in Figs. 6.36(b) and (e) for EtO-sterilized and γ-irradiated samples, respectively). The salient notions that can be extracted from the plots in Fig. 6.37 are summarized as follows: (i) the molecular chains were initially aligned along a direction nearly perpendicular ($\theta_p \approx \pi/12$) to the sample surface in a similar way for both types of sample, with a commonly low statistical frequency ($\langle P_2(\cos\beta)\rangle \approx 0.25$); (ii) the tilt angle, θ_p, locating the direction of the long axis of the molecular chains gradually increased up to $\theta_p \approx \pi/5$ (with a slope similar for both types of material) under application of strain; and, (iii) unlike the γ-irradiated sample, which showed a comparatively low statistical degree of alignment ($0.25 \leq \langle P_2(\cos\beta)\rangle \leq 0.4$) over the entire interval of investigated strain, the EtO-sterilized sample showed an abrupt increase in the Hermans parameter (i.e., up to $\langle P_2(\cos\beta)\rangle \approx 0.7$) starting from a threshold value of strain at around 7.5%. As far as the above point (i) is concerned, the finding is in agreement with the study of Bellare and Cohen [772] on compression-molded sheets, a similar angular population for EtO-sterilized and γ-irradiated samples in their as-received state conceivably arising from the samples being manufactured from rods obtained by the same procedure. It should also be reasonable that uniaxial strain tends to align the molecular chains onto a direction parallel to the surface, i.e. perpendicular to the direction of the applied compressive load. Galeski *et al.* [799] have given a comprehensive interpretation of morphological alteration of the polyethylene structure during plane strain compression. At the initial stage of deformation, the main mechanism of structural rearrangement was described as mainly consisting of interlamellar sliding, while chain slip within individual crystallites become active in a subsequent stage, when the lamellae start "feeling" shear strain and molecular chains become prone to slip along the [001] direction of the orthorhombic structure

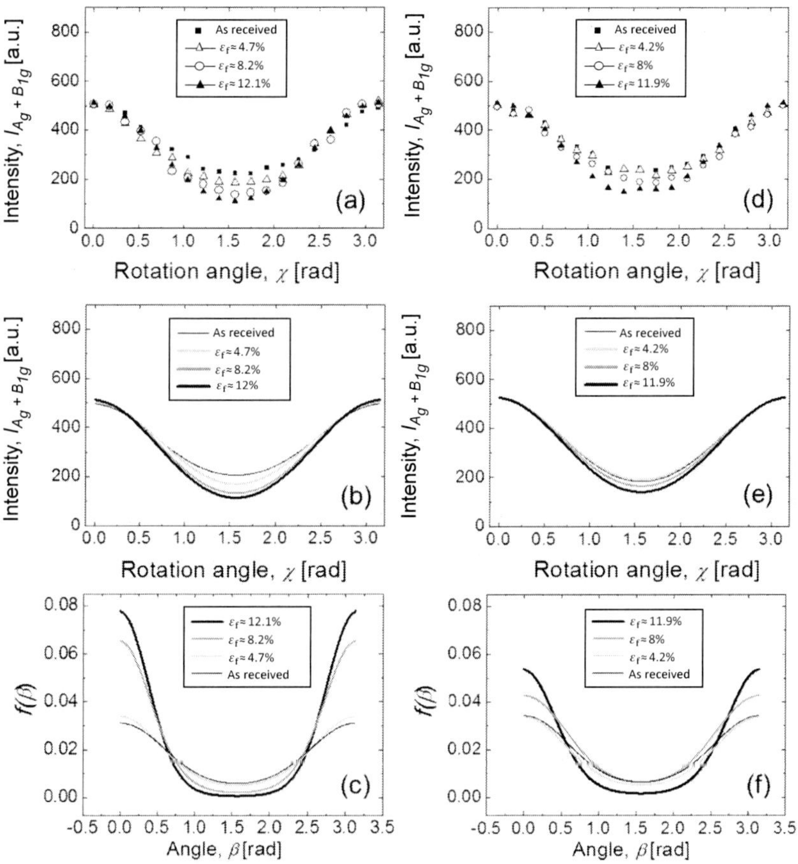

Figure 6.36 Experimental azimuthal angular dependencies obtained upon in-plane rotation at different stages of uniaxial deformation for EtO-sterilized samples (a). The results of best fitting to the experimental data and the calculated ODFs are reported in (b) and (c), respectively. Analogous plots are also shown for the case of γ-irradiated sample in (d), (e) and (f), respectively.

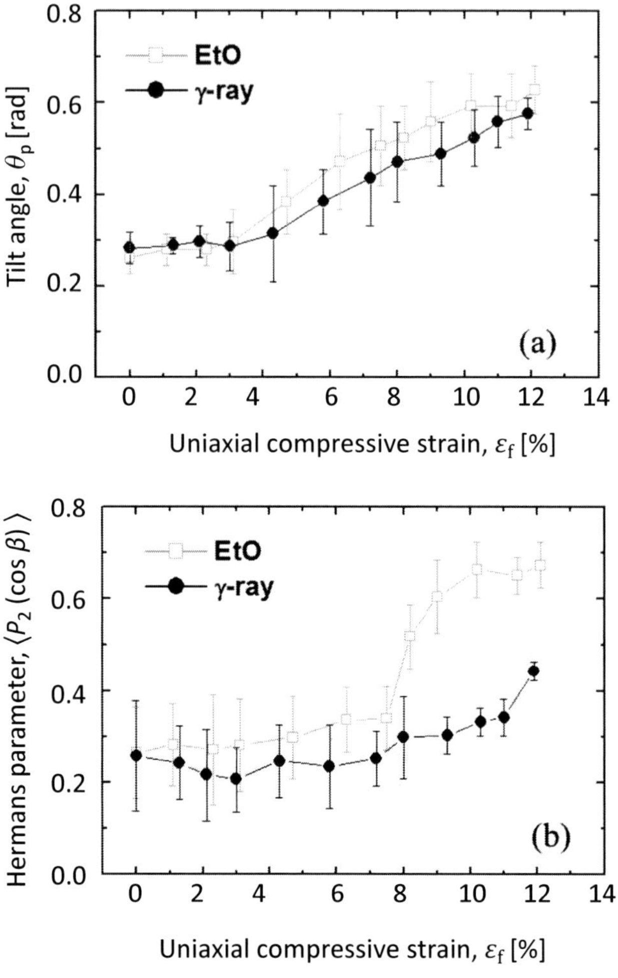

Figure 6.37 Values of θ_p (a) and Hermans parameter, $\langle P_2(\cos\beta)\rangle$, (b) as retrieved from the best fitting curves as those shown in Figs. 6.36(b) and (e) for EtO-sterilized and γ-irradiated samples, respectively. Error bars represent the standard deviation of the measurements.

(i.e., which correspond to a slip along the most closely packed crystallographic plane). At higher deformation levels, the lamellae are more and more elongated and a thickness decrease is also observed. This latter structural modification is due to the movement of chains, which are, to this extent, forced to align along the direction of plastic flow. It has been postulated that at rather elevated level of strain, the microstructure of polyethylene can develop a texture that is similar to that of a single crystal [798]. According to our results (cf. trends of θ_p angles in Fig. 6.37(a)), the onset strain for obtaining a modified texture appears at values 3~4% for EtO-sterilized UHMWPE, while in γ-irradiated polyethylene such a strain threshold seems to be somewhat delayed (or, for the same strain threshold, the θ_p gradient appreciably lower). This observation, together with the different trends of ODF (cf. Figs. 6.36(c) and (f)) between γ-irradiated polyethylene and the EtO-sterilized one, might confirm the findings of Bartczak [790] and Boontongkong *et al.* [800], which can be summarized as follows. Highly entangled and highly cross-linked polyethylene achieves higher crystallographic orientation when subjected to the same strain as less cross-linked and/or less entangled polyethylene. This is because the initial deformation accommodated by the amorphous regions below the yield stress results in macromolecules getting extended and "locked" prior to activation of slip systems in the lamellar regions. If the polyethylene is cross-linked then its gets fully stretched to its maximum limit at lower strains and begins to reorient the lamellae. Thus macromolecular orientation is faster (at lower strains) in cross-linked polyethylene. The observations of this study that irradiated polyethylene has lower orientation is not a result of lower molecular mobility but probably because highly cross-linked and/or more entangled polyethylene materials, upon unloading, have higher strain recovery than polyethylene that is less entangled and has lower or no cross-linking. Presumably, during the initial stage of plastic strain, only the amorphous phase undergoes plastic deformation, while the crystalline orthorhombic phase becomes involved with the structural rearrangement process only at higher values of strain. During the secondary deformation stage, i.e., in the range of ε between 4 and 12%, we observed the most remarkable variation of out-of-plane tilt angle, θ_p, which suggests the observed strain threshold being related to a homogeneous tendency of orthorhombic molecules to align along a plane parallel to the sample surface. The observed trends of molecular rearrangement in both types of sample can be expressed according to phenomenological curves, $\varepsilon_f = \varepsilon_f(\Delta\theta_p)$, as shown in Figs. 6.38(a) and (b) for EtO-sterilized and γ-irradiated samples, respectively. The $\Delta\theta_p$ trends represent the variation of out-of-plane tilt angle with respect to the original orientation direction before loading. The plots in Fig. 6.38 are different for EtO and γ-irradiated materials; however, a procedure of least-square fitting led to two equations of a common cubic nature, as follows:

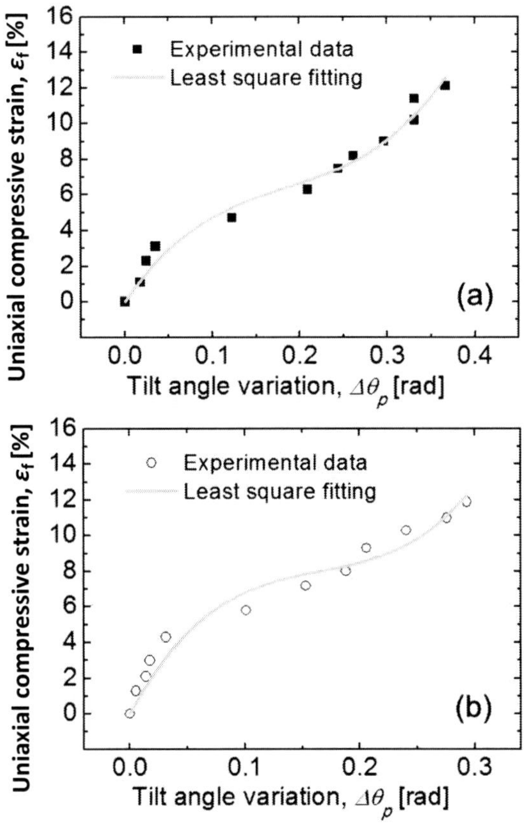

Figure 6.38 Relationships between compressive strain and variation of out-of-plane tilt angle, $\Delta\theta_p$, are reported for EtO (a) and γ-ray (b) sterilized UHMWPE, respectively. Compressive residual strain has been expressed as a function of $\Delta\theta_p$ by means of cubic interpolation functions. The least-square fitting results are represented by the Eqs. (6.5) and (6.6) for (a) and (b), respectively.

$$\varepsilon_f = 71.96\Delta\theta_p - 302.72\Delta\theta_p^2 + 546\Delta\theta_p^3 \quad (6.5)$$

$$\varepsilon_f = 119.47\Delta\theta_p - 643.82\Delta\theta_p^2 + 1293.28\Delta\theta_p^3 \quad (6.6)$$

(with angular variations expressed in radians) for EtO and γ-irradiated materials, respectively. The correlation factor R^2 obtained for the fitting of the experimental curves to cubic polynomials was 0.993 and 0.987 for Eqs. (6.5) and (6.6), respectively. Such equations are important because they link the residual strain stored in the sample to a measurable microstructural parameter (i.e., $\Delta\theta_p$) and thus can be used to quantitatively discuss the amount of residual strain stored in tibial inserts during *in vivo* exposure.

Investigating molecular orientation in retrievals represents a quite challenging computational problem because, unlike unused samples that were only statically loaded, retrievals have been concurrently subjected to forces of compressive and frictional nature. It follows that local variations of χ_p cannot be neglected and, thus, the computational analysis of Raman intensities upon in-plane sample rotation should be applied with considering the concurrent variations of two Euler angles, θ_p and χ_p. However, in analyzing retrievals, we can take advantage of the two phenomenological Eqs. (6.5) and (6.6) in order to quantify the amount of compressive residual strain stored in the retrieved tibial plates. The results of polarized Raman analysis of four retrievals (i.e., as listed in Table 6.6) are summarized in Figs. 6.39 and 6.40 in terms of in-plane and out-of-plane Euler angles (i.e., χ_p and θ_p, describing the preferentially oriented long axis of the molecular chains) and residual strain, ε_f, respectively. Looking first at the data in Fig. 6.39, one might note that θ_p values collected in the non-wear zones were all very close to the χ_p and θ_p values observed in the unused plates (i.e., $\chi_p = \pi/5$ and $\theta_p \approx \pi/12$), independent of sterilization process and as dictated by the common manufacturing process of the compression molded sheets. In other words, the microstructures in the non-wear zone looked very much the same as those of the as-received samples, independent of exposure time *in vivo* and sterilization process. On the other hand, in the main wear zone of the retrieved tibial plates, locations at which the highest compressive and frictional load was applied *in vivo*, the angles of molecular orientation, χ_p and θ_p, showed appreciable changes with respect to the as-received state. In the three EtO sterilized samples, the tilt angle, θ_p, was found to commonly lie in a narrow interval at around $\pi/8$, despite the quite different exposure time *in vivo* (i.e., significantly shorter for sample D compared with samples A and B). The tilt angular rearrangement, $\Delta\theta_p \approx \pi/22$, for these three samples corresponds to surface strains comprised in the narrow range, ε_f = 5.0~5.5% (cf. Fig. 6.40). This finding seems to confirm that the most significant amount of plastic deformation in polyethylene components occurs during the first year of implantation, as previously reported by other authors [828, 886]. It should be noted that load displacement curves obtained by Edidin *et al.* [887] have shown higher strain hardening of GUR 1050 compared with GUR 1020. This means the relatively lower amount of residual

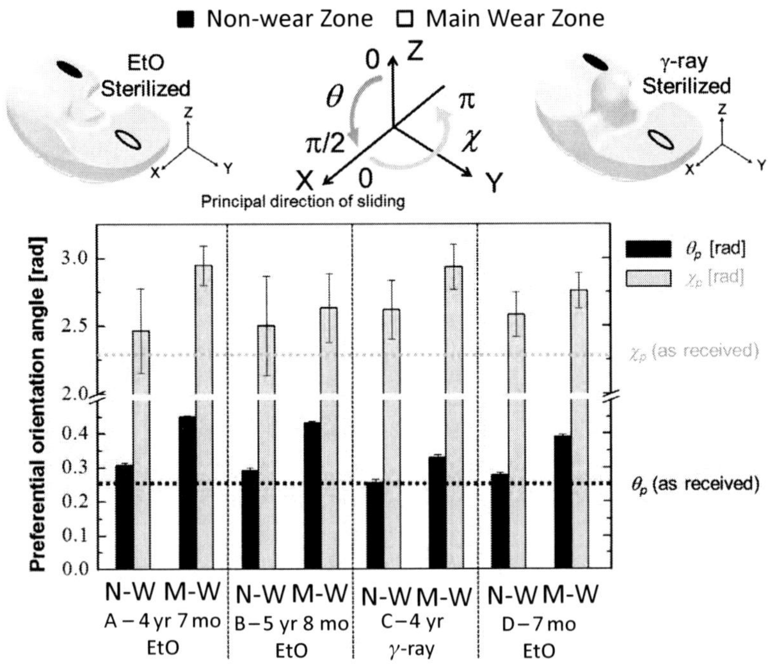

Figure 6.39 Average preferential out-of-plane tilt angle, θ_p, and azimuthal in-plane angle, χ_p, as calculated from the main wear zone and non-wear zone of each of the four analyzed retrievals. The two dotted lines represent the average values of θ_p and χ_p as obtained from virgin samples. Error bars represent the standard deviation of the measurements.

plastic strain in sample D compared with samples A and B might be partly due to a difference in type of resin. Some residual strain seems to accumulate also in the non-wear zone, despite the conspicuously load-free conditions of such a part of the knee joint upon normal walking activity. Note that the conspicuous absence of wear in the non-wear zone during *in vivo* service does not necessarily mean also absence of load, which is the main cause of creep and thus molecular realignment. However, the calculated amount of residual strain is very low and within the experimental scatter. On the other hand, the γ-irradiated sample C, despite its comparatively long-term exposure *in vivo*, experienced quite low tilt angle variation for a similar amount of plastic strain (i.e., $\Delta\theta_p \approx \pi/40$ and ε_f = 6%; cf. Figs. 6.39 and 6.40). This confirms a higher strain hardening of the γ-irradiated sample compared with EtO-sterilized samples, which was also observed during static loading experiments.

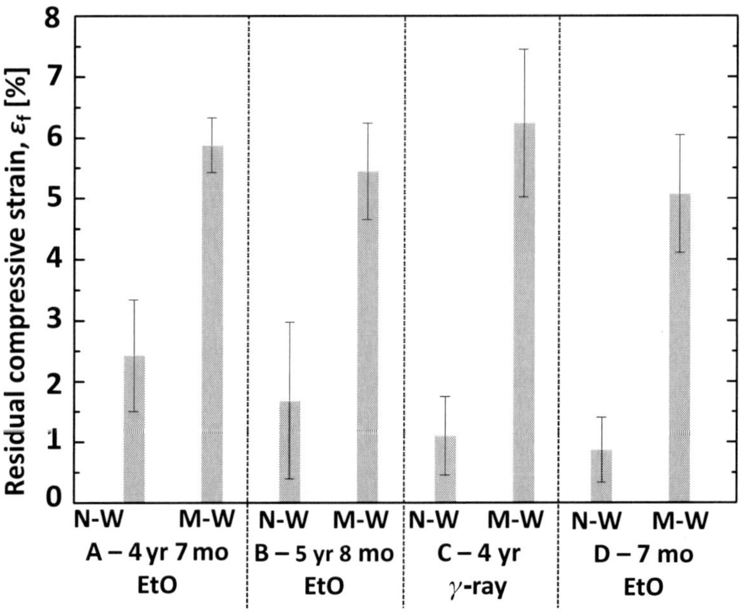

Figure 6.40 Residual strain, ε_f, as calculated from the main wear and non-wear zones of the four investigated retrievals. Assessments were made using phenomenological Eqs. (6.5) and (6.6). Error bars represent the standard deviation of the measurements.

Unlike the relatively straightforward outputs of the Raman analysis regarding the effect of compressive load on the surface of tibial insert retrievals, the analysis of in-plane molecular displacements appears to be more complex and difficult to rationalize. Sample A, for example, although being implanted for a period of time 13 months longer than sample B, showed less in-plane alignment along the direction of primary motion or principal direction of sliding (as shown in Fig. 6.39) (i.e., $\chi = \pi$) (cf. Fig. 6.39). It is indeed conceivable that in elapsing longer periods of exposure time *in vivo*, the long axis of the polyethylene molecules tends to align on the surface with the direction of primary motion. Note that such a molecular alignment process has been reported to produce a partial reduction in wear resistance on the sample surface [888, 889]. However, such a mobility process should strongly depend on both activity and body weight of the patient. Unlike χ_p angular displacements, clear differences could be found between ODFs calculated in the main wear zone and in the non wear zone of each sample (Figs. 6.41(a), (b), (c), and (d) for samples A, B, C, and D, respectively). Plots in Fig. 6.41 were obtained by considering average ODF parameters for each investigated area, while the Hermans parameters associated to each $f(\beta)$ distribution curve are explicitly shown in inset to each plot. It can be noted that although a preferential orientation of polyethylene chains has also been observed in non-wear zones, the distribution of molecular directions in these zones was always quite broad. On the other hand, by comparing ODFs in the main wear zone of EtO-sterilized samples (i.e., samples A, B, and D) with that of the γ-sterilized one (i.e., sample C), a significant difference could be found, thus confirming that γ-ray sterilized UHMWPE possesses a more "rigid" microstructure and, thus, it is less prone to increase its degree of texture as a consequence of the occurrence of plastic deformation *in vivo*.

In conclusion, polarized Raman spectroscopy can be quantitatively applied to detect the molecular rearrangements and the residual strain correlated to the plastic flow that occurs *in vivo* in tibial inserts of artificial knee joints. The Raman procedure again coupled with the ODF formalism appears capable to describe the molecular population obeying a given set of Euler angles in space. Raman assessments based on this algorithm reveal clear changes in molecular orientation patterns both in main wear and non-wear zones of tibial insert retrievals. Variations of out-of-plane and in-plane Euler angles, characteristic of the preferential orientation of the long axis of polyethylene chains, were found to mainly obey compressive and frictional forces, respectively. Visualization of structural parameters like molecular chain rearrangement and texture, so far only qualitatively discussed in the majority of the literature regarding biomedical grades of polyethylene, led to the following conclusions: (i) γ-irradiated samples, compared with EtO-sterilized samples, experienced lower texturing on the molecular scale likely due to a higher strain recovery capability; and, (ii) independent of sterilization method, the amount of plastic strain was mainly developed in early *in vivo* implantation times, within which out-of-plane molecules rotated under load onto planes parallel to the sample surface until reaching a saturation of their angular displacements.

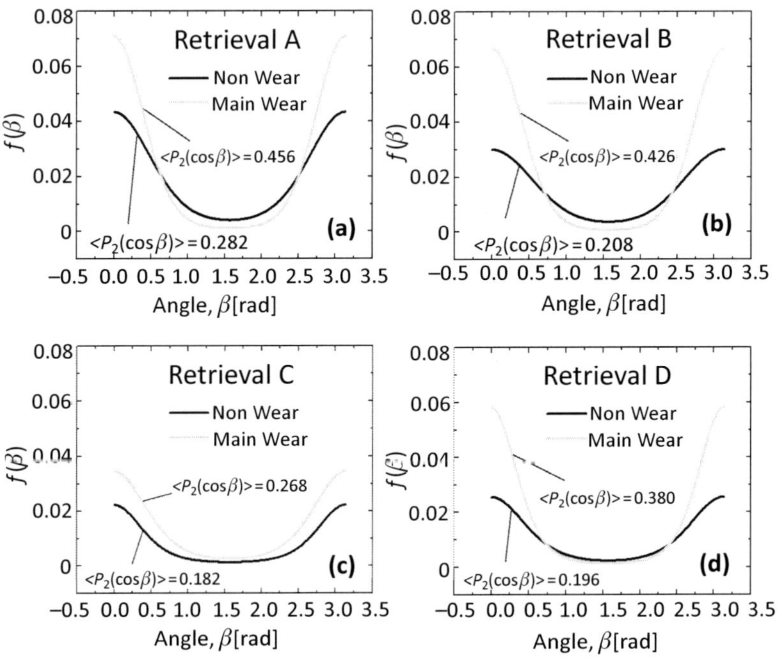

Figure 6.41 ODFs calculated in the main wear zone and in the non-wear zone of each sample (i.e., (a), (b), (c), and (d) for samples A, B, C, and D, respectively). Each plot was obtained considering ODF parameters averaged over the investigated area. Hermans parameters associated to each $f(\beta)$ distribution are explicitly shown in inset to each plot.

6.8 Failure of Ceramic-on-Ceramic Hip Implants Due to Polyethylene

Through the relatively long history of ceramic-on-ceramic hip implants, the cases of fracture reported with relatively high rates can systematically be associated to design failures [7]. French statistics from the early 1970s [20,890,891] reported a 2% fracture rate for alumina-on-alumina implants due to an unreliable fixation method adopted on the cup side. In Germany, an early design with a skirted head mated with a bulky monoblock screw cup (i.e., also referred to as the Mittelmeier design) led to fracture incidences up to 0.8% [892–894] and was abandoned by the maker in 1991. More recently, in Japan, a high fracture incidence rate in alumina ceramic-on-ceramic implants has been found for a particular "sandwich" design (Fig. 6.42), which included the insertion of an adaptive layer of UHMWPE between the ceramic liner and the metal shell [895]. In the period between 1998 and 2001 (after which the maker interrupted the supply), about 5500 hips were replaced by using this system. Since then, several authors reported about catastrophic fractures at the alumina-bearing surface (ABS) of the sandwich-type implants from the cup side [60,62,896–899]. Owing to the phenomenological aspects of the described cases, the failures of sandwich-type implants have commonly been referred to in the published literature as "ceramic failures" [60,62,896,899]. Suzuki *et al.* [896] described problems of fracture and dislocation with the ceramic liner and Amino [897] reported on 5500 cases of ABS cup (January 1998 to July 2000) with 16 fractures by January 2002. Kitajima and Hotokebuchi [898] also reported more than 60 fractures by January 2003. Similarly, fractures of modular ceramic acetabular components with a sandwich polyethylene insertion were recently also reported by German surgeons [434]. While fracture of the ceramic liner component certainly represents the most evident and catastrophic phenomenon observed in a retrieved sandwich-type implant, there are two important details suggesting that the origin of implant failure does not necessarily resides in a poor structural behavior of the ceramic cup component. On the one hand, the quality of the latest generation of alumina components (e.g., those manufactured by Kyocera Co.) could be considered to be excellent. As a matter of fact, although it is obviously impossible to completely eliminate the risk of fracture in brittle ceramic components as hip heads and liners, thorough data reviews (excluding sandwich-type implants) indeed show that the fracture rate of third-generation alumina-bearing couples is usually reported at extremely low levels [7, 434]. On the other hand, ceramic cups usually possess by far more load-bearing capacity than the mating ceramic heads, not only because cups are mainly loaded in compression but also because, unlike balls that necessarily contain taper edges, the cup morphology can be accurately designed in order to conspicuously avoid stress intensification. Accordingly, among the sporadic events of fracture reported in the literature [724, 898, 900–903], a large majority rather concerns fractured ceramic heads than ceramic liners. So, if the poor strength (or brittleness) of alumina ceramic would actually be located as the cause of failure in sandwich-type implants, it could be difficult to explain why fracture systematically occurred on the less-stressed liner side instead of hitting at the corners of the head taper.

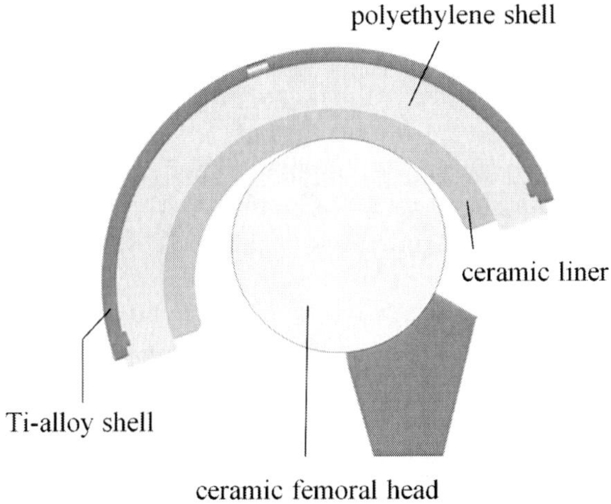

Figure 6.42 Alumina ceramic-on-ceramic implants has been found for a particular "sandwich" design, which includes the insertion of an adaptive layer of UHMWPE between the ceramic liner and the metal shell [894].

The so-called sandwich cup configuration, with its ceramic liner locked into an adaptive layer of polyethylene, was originally conceived in order to reduce the rigidity of the ceramic-on-ceramic coupling and to prevent impingement between the rim of the ceramic liner and the metal neck of the femoral stem. Various surgeons, who reported about sandwich implant failures, observed that the liner had rotated during gait by about 90° inside the metal shell and the ball head has been displaced in superolateral direction [60, 432]. The ball head eventually entered into contact with the metal shell in the superolateral area and in a number of cases the ceramic liner fractured. In one case, fracture and fragmentation of the ceramic cup was reported [60], while in another report the liner was found yet unfractured despite the implant having undergone liner rotation [432]. In reviewing the published literature, one might intuitively feel consensus toward authors hinting that the fault of sandwich implant failure arises from brittleness of the ceramic components [62, 899]. The squatting attitude of Asian patients was also reported to be an exacerbating factor in the fracture process [62]. However, a clear and final explanation of the implant failure mechanism(s) is still missing in the literature. In this section, several cases of sandwich-type implant failure are revisited with focusing on the specific role played by the polyethylene shell component in the overall process of implant failure. The opinion of the writer is that the published descriptions of ceramic liner fracture in sandwich-type implants are indeed phenomenologically correct. However, experimental proofs exist that it was not the structural inadequacy of the alumina components the factor actually originating failure in sandwich-type implants, but rather a structural defeat by creep deformation on the polyethylene side of the implants, as a consequence of the flawed joint design.

Six cases of sandwich-type implant failure were examined, whose clinical details are summarized in Table 6.7. All retrieved implants were of the sandwich type ABS HA Shell (CH 46)/ABS Liner (28–46)/Ball Head (28N: –4)/Perfix Stem #12-M, produced by Kyocera Co., had cementless fixation, and belonged to female patients. The *in vivo* implantation lifetime of the devices ranged between 2 years 11 months and 9 years 8 months, for an average follow up of 6 years 9 months. No traumatic event as possible cause of failure was encountered in all patients. The time delay between symptoms of failure and revision typically ranged between few days and few weeks. Except for the shortest follow up (Case IV in Table 6.7), all the studied retrievals showed dislodgment of the liner at the time of revision surgery. However, in two of the six studied retrievals (Cases 2 and 3) the ceramic liner did not fracture. Among the four cases in which the ceramic liner fractured, Case IV was completely different from the other cases because it showed fragmentation of the ceramic liner into many small pieces. Anteversion and inclination angles are also listed in Table 6.7, as obtained from radiographic analyses immediately after primary surgery. As far as inclination angles are concerned, a range comprised between 30° and 50° is considered to be a safe zone for avoiding dislocation, while for anteversion the angular range is between 5° and 25° [449, 904]. Therefore, only Case IV, for which radiographic analyses showed an inclination angle of 59° (cf. Table 6.7), should be considered affected by the effects of an excessive inclination. Values of anteversion angle, which could not be considered in the safe zone, included Cases I, VI and VI. In particular, the anteversion angle ≈ −5° of Case I clearly represented an implantation error.

Table 6.7 Clinical details of the six cases of sandwich-type implant failure examined in this study

Case	Gender	Follow-up	Cause	Pristine PE thickness [μm]	Side	Inclination [deg]	Anteversion [deg]
I	Female	4 y 8 mo	Dislodgement	3000	Left	42	-5
II	Female	9 y 3 mo	Dislodgement	5000	Right	43	16
III	Female	9 y 8 mo	Dislodgement	5000	Right	50	24
IV	Female	2 y 11 mo	No-dislodgement Destruction	2000	Left	59	41
V	Female	4 y 11 mo	Dislodgement Fracture	2000	Right	45	25
VI	Female	9 y	Dislodgement Fracture	3000	Left	51	51

Similar to the experiments shown in the previous sections of this Chapter, retrieved UHMWPE shells were investigated by employing a confocal Raman probe focused at different radial locations. Variations of FWHM with respect to a virgin sample reflected the microstructural modifications induced by body weight, namely by the uniaxial plastic strain piled up in the polymeric structure. The width of the Raman band located at 1130 cm^{-1} ($A_g + B_{1g}$ mode or symmetric stretching of C–C bonds [796, 820]) was selected as a sensor for plastic strain in the polymeric network because it reflects the degree of disorder of the polymeric network and its degree of molecular orientation, which are both directly affected by strain. The increase of structural disorder under compressive strain in turn reflects in a broadening of the Raman band due to inter- and intra-lamellar slip processes. Additional phenomena leading to broadening of the Raman bands have also been indicated, including crystallite fragmentation, fibril formation, and chain disentanglement [823]. However, all these microstructural modifications can only appear at strain level much higher than those of interest here and will thus be neglected in this investigation. As a matter of fact, broadening of the 1130 cm^{-1} band obeyed a conspicuously linear dependence up to quite large strain values (e.g., in the order of the tens of percent). Band-width/strain calibrations have explicitly been shown in previous papers [116,217,822]. Exploiting the high transparency of polyethylene, non-destructive in-depth scans allowed us to retrieve detailed subsurface profiles of spectral properties along the entire thickness of the polyethylene shells. In the experimental practice, an automated sample stage with submicrometric step precision was employed, making it possible to record spectra at each depth with focusing below the sample surface, and to map spectral features with lateral line scanning on the sample surface and along the subsurface. Maps 30 μm × 30 μm were typically recorded at 50 different depths for each polar angle of the shell, and the collected spectra (900 spectra for each map) averaged to give the representative molecular vibrational modes of the polyethylene structure at each selected in-depth location. Measurements of subsurface profile properties were eventually repeated at nine polar angles across the main-wear zone in addition to the geometrical center of the shell, in order to obtain statistically validated polar plots of the state of strain for each of the investigated retrievals.

The photographs in Figs. 6.43(a)~(f) represent the ceramic-cup/polyethylene-shell components of the investigated failed implants after being retrieved from the patients' body. The results of radiographic examinations immediately before revision surgery are shown for each of the studied Cases in Figs. 6.44. Case I in Table 6.7 (Figs. 6.43(a) and 6.44(a)) was revised after dislodgment (namely a clearly visible shift of the joined ceramic/polyethylene parts out of the metal shell). The cause of failure was simply classified as "dislodgment", although the retrieval also showed a clear-cut circumferential fracture trajectory dividing the ceramic liner into two distinct parts of about the same size (cf. Fig. 6.43(a)). The two Cases labeled II and III in Table 6.7 were revised due to liner dislodgment (cf. Figs. 6.43(b) and (c), respectively, with radiographic analyses in Figs. 6.44(b) and (c)), and showed no fracture of the ceramic liner. Among the remaining three cases, Case IV showed no visible dislodgment (Figs. 6.43(d) and 6.44(d) for Case IV), but its ceramic liner fractured with extensive fragmentation (cf. photograph of the broken pieces of the ceramic liner in inset to Fig. 6.43(d)). The many broken ceramic pieces needed to be retrieved separately from the implant in the body of the patient. Cases V and VI both underwent dislodgment (Figs. 6.43(e) and (f), respectively; radiographs shown in Figs. 6.44(e) and (f), respectively) and fracture of the respective ceramic liners. However, important differences could be noted in comparing the fracture patterns of these latter two ceramic liners compared with the other fractured liners. Cases V showed three broken (chipped) pieces at the rim of its ceramic liner, but unlike Case I no circumferential fracture path. On the other hand, the fracture pattern in Case IV was somewhat merging the patterns found in Cases I and V, with displaying both edge chipping (into two pieces) and a main circumferential fracture path. The different fracture pattern represents an important difference, which differentiated the mechanisms leading to the catastrophic failure events occurred *in vivo* in different implants, and which will be discussed in a later paragraph of this section. In all cases of dislodgment, there was never observed any (even local) detachment between the UHMWPE shell and the ceramic liner. Both components thus shifted with remaining integer to each other. Except for Cases I and IV, the polyethylene shells showed significant damages, including severe abrasive wear especially localized at the rim area, in which significant plastic deformation also locally occurred, possibly due to creep. In a purely mechanistic view, the damages appeared similar to those reported earlier by Messieh *et al.* [905] in describing wear debris originated from the contact of a bipolar cup with the femoral neck. Some circumferential cracks were also visible near the edge of the polyethylene shell belonging to Cases V and VI. Cases II, III, and VI showed severe delamination and flaking of the polymeric structure mainly at the contact area between shell and stem, but also in other zones around the circumference of the shell. Kaku *et al.* [906] described phenomenologically similar micro-fracture events and damages for the polyethylene liner of a bipolar femoral head. Moreover, our data seem to confirm a thesis put forward by Yamaguchi *et al.* [907]. In reviewing a large number of acetabular components, these researchers found that cups with impingement were systematically more anteverted than those without impingement. As a matter of fact, we also found significant UHMWPE damage due to impingement in Cases IV and VI, which were the implants with the highest anteversion angle in the studied series of retrievals. Besides promoting subluxation and dislocation of the femoral head, prosthetic impingement was reported to significantly contribute to implant loosening by imparting eccentric loads to the cup and by the direct production

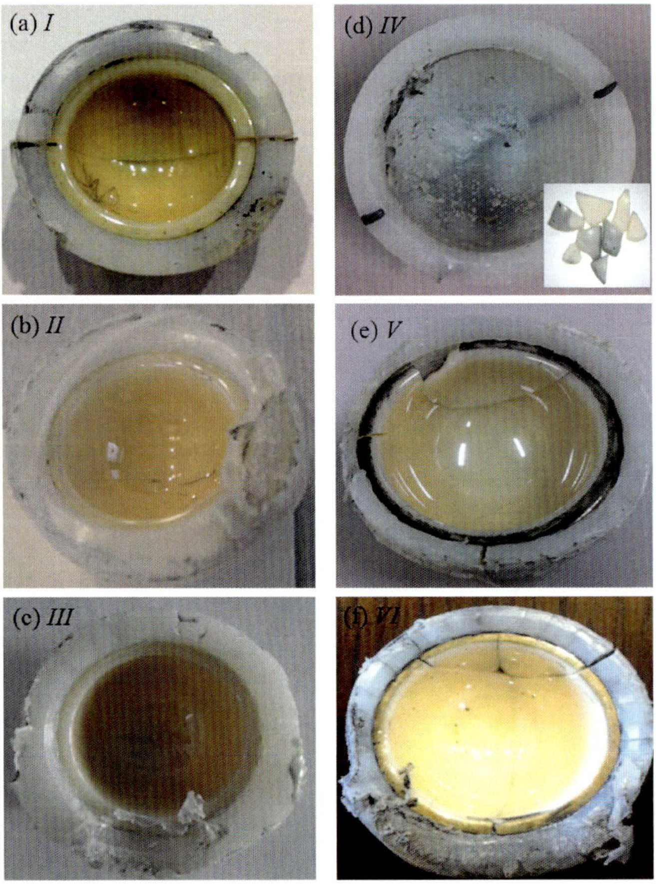

Figure 6.43 Photographs of the ceramic-cup/polyethylene-shell components of the investigated sandwich-type implants after being retrieved from the patients' body. In Case IV, destruction of the ceramic liner occurred *in vivo* (cf. photograph of the ceramic broken pieces in inset to (d)).

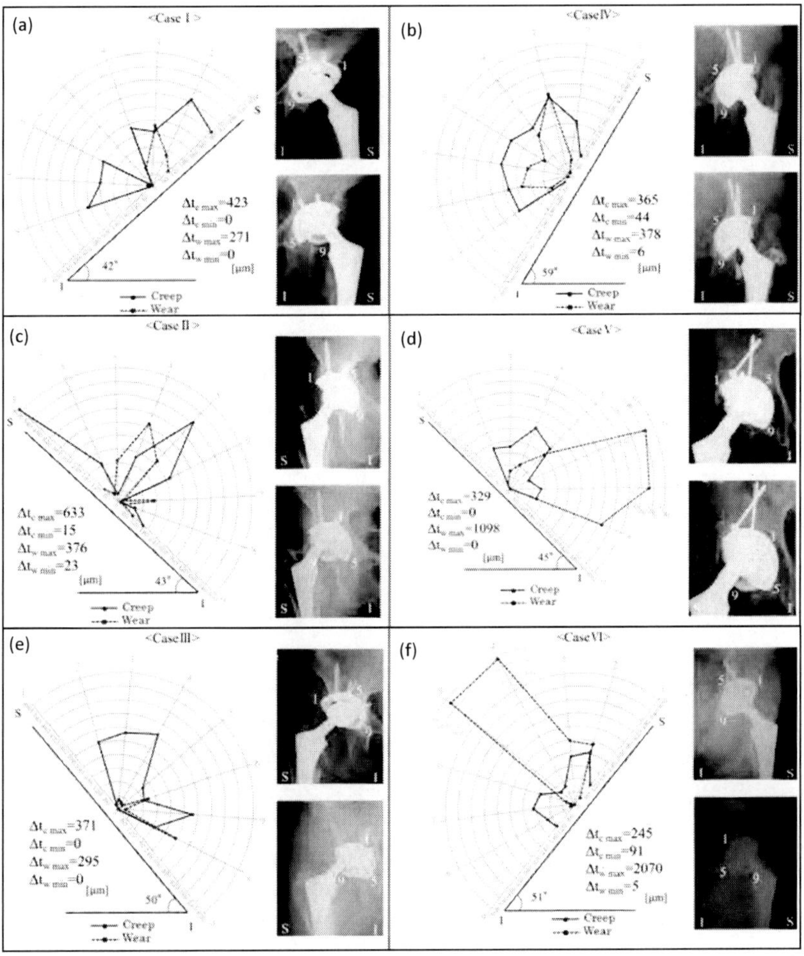

Figure 6.44 Polar plots of the total creep and wear displacements recorded along a circumferential path of the UHMWPE shell of the investigated implants. Inclination angles are also shown for better clarity. Radiographic analyses are shown as collected immediately before revision surgery. The numbers shown in inset to the radiographs correspond to the numbers locating the radial directions in each polar plot.

of polyethylene wear debris [908–910]. It is shown later that impingement might have played a role also in sandwich-type implants by promoting sliding of the UHMWPE and ceramic shells and, thus, the observed dislodgment. As far as the inclination angle was concerned, it is conceivable to expect a higher creep deformation in the zone near the edge of the UHMWPE liner in the implants with high inclination angle.

Following the Raman confocal procedures described above, spatially resolved profiles of the strain field that permanently remained stored in the UHMWPE shells of the retrieved sandwich-type implants could be measured and displayed in polar plots as a function of sample depth along the entire thickness of the shells. Note (from Table 6.7) that the pristine thickness of the UHMWPE shell was different for different implants, despite all implants being from the same maker. An intermediate thickness of 3 mm (Cases I and VI), a minimum thickness of 2 mm (Cases IV and V) and a maximum thickness of 5 mm (Cases II and III) were the three patterns available in the examined retrievals. In Fig. 6.44, polar plots are shown, for each of the examined retrieval, of the total creep displacements recorded along a typical circumferential path of the UHMWPE shell. The examined circumferential path crossed the main wear zone of the bearing surfaces. Creep displacements could be obtained by numerically integrating over the entire thickness of the shell the respective in-depth strain profiles, according to the same procedure followed in Section 6.4 [116, 217]. In-depth strain profiles were in turn non-destructively retrieved from FWHM data analyses of the Raman band of UHMWPE representing symmetric stretching of the C–C bonding. In the polar plots, the inclination angle of the acetabular cup of each implant is also represented for better clarity, as given in Table 6.7. It was already mentioned that the numerical integration, performed for calculating local creep displacements, encompassed profiles of fifty points for each polar angle, while data points at each depth represented an average value retrieved over 900 spectra. The thickness reductions that arose from creep deformation, Δt_c, and wear abrasion, Δt_w, as they piled up during the *in vivo* lifetime are represented in Fig. 6.44 by full and broken lines, respectively. Numerical displacement values are also explicitly listed for better clarity in Table 6.8. The Δt_W values were obtained by subtracting the measured, Δt_c, from the pristine cup thickness at each location of the polar plot. It was previously described that no detachment between the UHMWPE shell and the ceramic liner was observed in the investigated retrievals. Therefore, different from the usual definition of abrasive wear between ceramic and polyethylene bearings, the wear damages reported in this paper unequivocally refer to the occurrence of backside wear due to friction between the Ti-metal shell and the UHMWPE shell. It is anticipated at the outset that a comprehensive interpretation of the data shown in Fig. 6.44 might result quite complex due to the fact that we could only access to final thickness variations, without knowledge of the temporal sequence at which such variations occurred (i.e., in particular at which stage of dislodgment they occurred). Moreover, different implants showed quite different patterns of creep and wear damages in terms of the respective thickness reductions. Nevertheless, some important evidences could be collected, which can be summarized as follows:

Table 6.8 Numerical displacement values of UHMWPE shells at different polar locations, as due to creep and backside wear, which were measured in the six failed sandwich-type implants examined

Wear [μm]

		Measurement point								
		1	2	3	4	5	6	7	8	9
Case	I	108	161	271	95	0	16	17	17	0
	II	93	46	186	376	257	23	170	24	92
	III	0	29	57	33	25	147	40	295	0
	IV	6	79	378	234	137	189	226	103	15
	V	0	30	95	121	240	1098	1052	503	0
	VI	37	285	296	1614	2070	45	19	25	5

Creep [μm]

		Measurement point								
		1	2	3	4	5	6	7	8	9
Case	I	363	423	257	275	0	250	240	316	0
	II	633	185	42	223	485	250	15	80	156
	III	0	304	345	371	160	122	345	181	0
	IV	112	250	365	276	305	307	283	275	44
	V	0	220	215	329	290	117	163	157	0
	VI	119	245	214	99	91	177	188	149	121

(i) In comparing different retrievals, it immediately appears evident that the thickness reductions due to backside wear in Cases V and VI were exceptionally high compared with the other retrievals examined. However, while in Case VI the maximum wear damage measured ($\Delta t_{\mathrm{w\ max}}$ = 2.070 mm) occurred in correspondence of a location where one would approximately expect the occurrence of the main wear zone, in Case V the maximum wear damage ($\Delta t_{\mathrm{w\ max}}$ = 1.098 mm) occurred at a location corresponding to what one would expect to be the non-wear zone of the cup at the time of implantation. Both implants indeed showed substantial dislodgment, but the difference in the observed locations of wear patterns suggest that unlike Case VI, abrasive backside wear in the UHMWPE shells of Case V occurred after slip of the UHMWPE shell out of the Ti-alloy shell. This speculation is partly confirmed by the fact that in Case VI significant damage of the UHMWPE shell appeared in the rim area as a consequence of stem impingement during gait (after rotation of the ceramic/UHMWPE components inside the metal shell), while the shell in Case V showed no damage at its rim but it was severely abraded in its backside zone due to impingement on the edge of the metal cup after dislodgement.

(ii) Both Cases II and III, which by design incorporated the thickest UHMWPE component in their pristine state, showed significant abrasive damage at the rim of the UHMWPE shell (i.e., by impingement of the stem). The *in vivo* times of these two implants were nearly the same and also the longest in the studied series. Both implants showed pronounced dislodgment at the time of revision surgery, but no fracture of the ceramic cup. The occurrence of backside wear was quite limited and localized in both implants, suggesting that dislodgement occurred suddenly. However, peculiar to Case II, was a quite high creep displacement at the upper edge of the UHMWPE shell, due to severe impingement by the femoral head at the onset angle for subluxation.

(iii) Case IV, which showed no dislocation and destruction of the ceramic liner, was the only implant in which creep deformation was quite homogeneous in the polar rotation interval encompassing gait motion (all other implants showed inhomogeneous distributions of creep displacements with maximum values at variable inclination angles). We shall associate the lack of localized deformation in the UHMWPE shell of Case IV to the absence of dislodgement. Despite being the implant with the shortest exposure *in vivo*, the implant of Case IV showed creep displacements comparable to those measured in the long-term retrievals analyzed. This observation confirms the notion that creep deformation in polyethylene hip components mainly occurs during the initial time (<2 years) from primary surgery [828,829].

The results shown in Fig. 6.44 help visualizing a significant creep contribution to the *in vivo* penetration of ceramic liner component into the Ti-metal shell as a consequence of local flattening of the polyethylene shell. The general conclusion drawn from the examination of Δt_c data in comparison with the overall displacements, Δt, is that at the time of explantation, the creep flattening contribution in the UHMWPE shell could be locally as large as one third of the entire UHMWPE shell thickness. Such large creep displacements were responsible not only for the linear penetration of the ceramic liner into the metal shell, but also for the successive patient weight redistribution with application of an asymmetric (incorrect) loading to the ceramic liner.

In a recent paper, Dalla Pria *et al.* [911] have reviewed the topic of breakage of ceramic-on-ceramic hip couples. Although none of the reviewed implants belonged to the sandwich-type studied here, extensive discussions and classifications were given of fracture patterns in ceramic liners, which present interesting aspects and represent guidance in the context of this paper. Two main types of fracture mode were reviewed: (i) the so-called "undetected fracture" of the liner, in which circumferential fracture occurred into two parts above the conical coupling, with no fragments [912]; and, (ii) the rim fragmentation (or chipping) fracture which arises from neck impingement against the rim of the ceramic liner upon subluxation [62,913]. The above-referred type (i) of fracture is quite unusual and was not observed in our investigation. In type (ii), even assuming the ceramic liner being correctly positioned in the metal shell, a combination of shocks and edge loading by the ceramic head was designated as responsible for rim breakage, which is indeed what we have observed in Cases V and VI (cf. Figs. 6.43(e) and (f)). Chipping of the liner has been reported to occur when the inclination angle is too steep or when the anteversion angle is out of the safe zone [449, 913, 914]. This was obviously the case in retrieval Case VI, which showed both inclination and anteversion angles at the limit of the safe zone. On the other hand, in Case V, the cup was initially positioned in a correct way (cf. angles in Table 6.7). However, from the backside abrasive damage pattern on the UHMWPE shell, we could deduce that the ceramic liner worked for a non-negligible period of time after having been rotated by about 45° into the metal shell (cf. thickness reductions by wear in Fig. 6.45(e)), thus dramatically increasing the risk of subluxation and head impingement. It should be indeed after liner rotation had already occurred that rim chipping presumably happened.

In Cases I and VI, we additionally observed a completely different pattern of fracture that can be considered to be peculiar to the sandwich-type liner. This is a circumferential crack path spanning over the entire cup, which in turn resulted in splitting of the ceramic liner into two broken hemispheres (cf. Figs. 6.43(a) and (f)). In Case VI, this fracture pattern was additive to rim chipping. The origin of such different crack path has not yet been discussed in the published literature. We newly suggest here that it arose from localized loading (in bending) of the convex surface of the ceramic cup after its rotation into the metal shell. The effects on fracture paths of this kind of localized loading applied on the pole of a curved brittle system with unsupported margins has been studied in detail by Rudas *et al.* [915] by means of a boundary element analysis. This analysis indeed predicted (and experimentally validated) the formation of cracks, which nucleated at the pole of the cup and extended toward the dome base. Figure 6.45 shows a series of drafts that attempts to comprehensively describe the sequence of degradative events that led to the observed fracture patterns. Figure 6.45(a) shows a hip joint correctly implanted, in which the body weight selectively induces creep deformation in a limited interval of radial angles in the UHMWPE shell (Fig. 6.45(b)). Under the effect of an increased tangential force due to the local deformation of the polyethylene shell, dislodgment eventually occurred (Fig. 6.45(c)), and such an incorrect implant configuration exacerbated impingements of both femoral head on the upper rim of the ceramic liner (i.e., in a state of subluxation) and stem neck on the lower rim of the UHMWPE shell (cf. Figs. 6.45(d) and (e)). In addition, Fig. 6.45(f) schematically shows the state of localized loading on the (rotated) pole of the ceramic cup (integer to the UHMWPE shell). The loading configuration indeed foresees polar loading (at location A in Fig. 6.45(f)) with bending of the curved cup component upon loading reactions at the supporting points B and C in Fig. 6.45(f), which corresponded to the rim impingement locations of the femoral head and of the stem neck, respectively. Such loading configuration ultimately led to a single circumferential crack starting from the pole of the ceramic liner and propagating toward the cup base.

The complex sequence of mechanisms shown in Fig. 6.45 can rationally explain the phenomenological observation made on all the analyzed retrievals, with the exception of Case IV. As a matter of fact, the occurrence of multiple crack paths, the observation of no dislodgment in the radiographic preoperative exam, and the lack of any abrasive damage in the UHMWPE shell clearly reveal the occurrence of a different failure mechanism. The ceramic liner was indeed backed by the thinnest among the UHMWPE shells employed by the maker and the fracture pattern suggests a compressive fracture event [916, 917], presumably amplified by shocks of the femoral head against the ceramic cup. Recently, Uribe *et al.* [918] have presented a focused modeling study of shock-induced damages in ceramic hip prostheses. In this study, the shock-induced stress was determined numerically using finite element analysis and demonstrated that even a minor microseparation effect in an all-ceramic hip implant could cause a severe shock on the bearing surface when heel touch the ground. Such shock can be as high as nine times the body weight. Under such conditions and owing to the presence of crack initiation sites on the bearing surface as a consequence of wear scars, it is conceivable to conclude that the thickness of the ceramic liner could have been designed too thin to guarantee structural integrity under gait conditions in presence of microseparation.

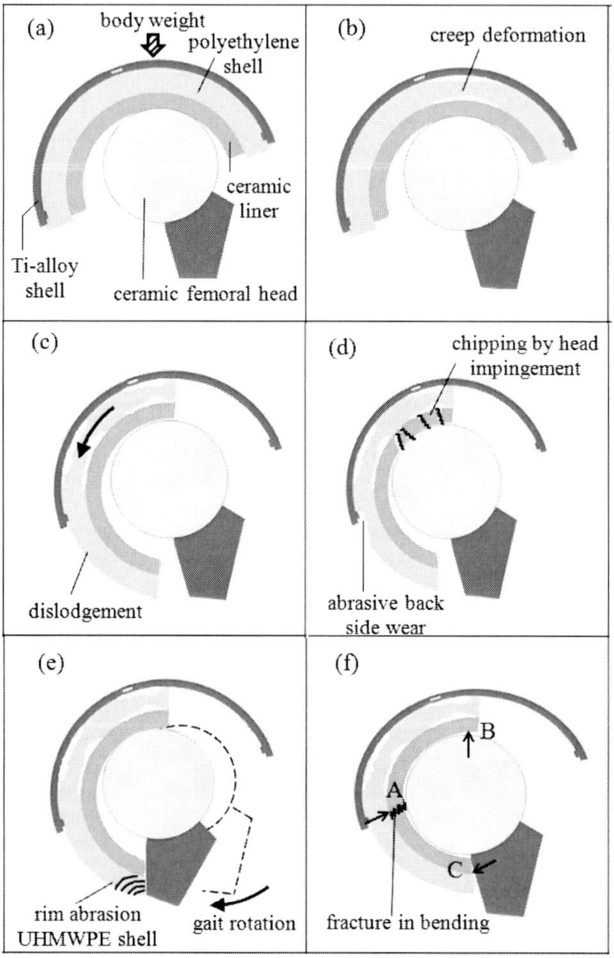

Figure 6.45 Drafts describing the sequence of degradative events that led to the observed liner fracture patterns: (a) sandwich-type hip joint correctly implanted; (b) creep deformation in a limited interval of radial angles of the UHMWPE shell due to body weight; (c) occurrence of dislodgment upon rotation of UHMWPE shell/ceramic liner inside the metal shell; (d) impingement of femoral head on the upper rim of the ceramic liner (i.e., in a state of subluxation) producing chipping of the ceramic liner; (e) impingement of the stem neck on the lower rim of the (rotated) UHMWPE shell, which in turn produced severe abrasions to the shell rim; and, (f) polar loading (at location A) producing bending of the curved cup component constrained by the supporting points B and C.

In conclusion, a series of six (failed) sandwich implants with *in vivo* lifetimes ranging between 2 and 9 years (average follow up of 6 years 9 months) was studied in order to rigorously classify their mechanisms of failure and the related causes. Among the investigated implants, four implants showed fracture of the ceramic liner. Three different patterns of liner fracture could be located: (i) chipping into several pieces of the rim of the ceramic liner due to subluxation accompanied by impingement and shock of the femoral head against the liner (two cases); (ii) fracture of the liner into two hemispheres by a single circumferential crack path spanning over the entire cup (two cases, of which one also included the pattern in (i)); (iii) fragmentation fracture of the ceramic liner into a large number of small pieces (one case). In the case of pattern (iii) (i.e., in only one case), dislodgement of the UHMWPE shell/ceramic liner was not observed in preoperative radiographic analyses. An analysis of the failure events showed that with the exception of the fracture pattern (iii), all the other ceramic fracture cases were a consequence of dislodgment or of implantation errors. In particular, creep of the polyethylene shell was found to be the triggering phenomenon for dislodgment and, thus, the origin of the overall sequence of failure events. The results of accurate spectroscopic investigations suggest that a failure classification of the sandwich-type implant as a "ceramic fracture failure" could be misleading and definitely represent a confounding factor in judging about the reliability of modern ceramic implants. We propose instead that failure cases of sandwich-type implants should be classified as design failures rather than ceramic-on-ceramic fractures since no material could stand in its bearing functions when loaded in the incorrect geometry that arose from such a malfunctioning implant mechanics

Chapter 7

Future Trends in Joint Arthroplasty

7.1 Innovative Metal/Ceramic Hybrid Joint Components

A novel approach has recently been proposed for obtaining artificial hip and knee joint components that could combine the superior structural reliability of metallic components (including their highly reliable strength behavior and high toughness) with the advantages of oxide ceramics as articulating surfaces, including their greater lubricity and superior resistance to abrasive wear. This new approach exploits the simple idea of using a joint bearing component, metallic in its bulk but covered with a strong ceramic layer, which would conceivably consent to retain the benefits of ceramic surfaces wedded to the mechanical resiliency of a bulk metallic component. In the (so far only one) successful example of hybrid metal/ceramic joint implants discussed in this section, the ceramic surface layer is actually not a coating but an intrinsically formed oxidation layer on the bulk metal surface. The idea of creating a metallic bulk component with a ceramic surface is

Advanced Materials for Joint Implants
Giuseppe Pezzotti

ISBN 978-981-4316-88-0 (Hardcover), 978-981-4364-39-3 (eBook)
www.panstanford.com

indeed a quite straightforward one but, as in the case of many other apparently self-evident scientific concepts, it involves a number to technological issues of not so obvious manufacturing realization. As the design of mechanically strong interfaces between metals and ceramics yet remains a long debated issue and lacks a general solution in the field of materials science [918], no previous successful case of bioceramic coating on metal surfaces has been reported in the literature. So, it is quite intriguing for scientists to clarify for which physical and chemical reasons an intrinsically formed oxidation layer works structurally better than a coating on a load-bearing metal surface.

A massive production of scientific literature has been published on various applications for both oxide [919–922] and non-oxide [923–927] coatings deposited on metallic surfaces. Many of the published investigations clearly demonstrated the practical difficulties that technologists have long encountered in optimizing the many physical and chemical parameters taking part in the development of a strong metal/ceramic interface [928]. One main issue resides in the residual stress field of thermal nature, which develops at the metal/ceramic interface due to a mismatch in thermal expansion between the ceramic layer and the metallic bulk. A thermal expansion coefficient of the metallic bulk phase higher than that of the ceramic layer represents a quite common technological case and might lead to the development of residual stresses of a compressive nature in the ceramic layer, the higher the thermal expansion mismatch the higher the residual stress magnitude. Compressive residual stresses stored at the material surface could be considered beneficial in enhancing both wear resistance in ceramics and ceramic coatings [929,930]. However, a quite steep residual stress gradient might develop along the subsurface of the ceramic layer, which might experience a conspicuous intensification of its magnitude at the ceramic/meal interface. Beyond a threshold value of in-plane compressive residual stress, the ceramic/metal interface could undergo spontaneous failure by buckling and delamination [931,932] and, even below such a threshold, the ceramic layer could break under the compressive load exerted during service by a hard counterpart. In other words, the price to be paid in order to achieve beneficial effects in terms of wear resistance at the material surface might involve a substantial risk for delamination to occur at the ceramic/metal interface. Another issue, equally important although relatively less investigated, resides in the influence induced by the metallic material on the stoichiometry of the ceramic layer, including both diffusion of ions from the metal bulk toward the ceramic side through the ceramic grain boundaries [933] and the concurrent formation of vacancy sites and complexes in the oxygen sublattice of the ceramic phase [934]. Hence, local off-stoichiometry might also be expected to tangibly contribute to either a release or an enhancement of the residual stress field at the interface, in addition to produce a stoichiometry-assisted gradient in thermal expansion coefficient within the ceramic phase itself. Design experts conceivably fear that uncontrolled residual stress fields and stoichiometry gradients, combined with the extreme thermomechanical conditions under which bearing surfaces work in human joints, might trigger high risks of structural failure in the actual application of ceramic coatings to metallic joint components. Accordingly, alternative technological solutions have been searched for obtaining synergistic coupling between metals and ceramics with safer characteristics of structural reliability. As mentioned above, the most successful solution realized so far has been that of processing metallic bulk components so that the metallic surface is transformed by means of a suitable oxidation process into a strong and abrasion-resistant ceramic oxide layer [935,936]. In this case, as previously stated, the oxide layer is not an externally applied coating, but rather represents the result of an inherent transformation of the original metal surface into a ceramic oxide. Therefore, different from a coating, the obtained ceramic layer is somewhat "native" to the metal phase, which can greatly help minimizing (through the occurrence of diffusive phenomena) the unwanted excess in compressive residual stresses and local chemical mismatches localized at the metal/ceramic interface. According to a suitable oxidation process, an oxidized layer formed on the surface of a selected zirconium alloy could be obtained with the characteristics of a monoclinic zirconia ceramic phase, which was found beneficial in substantially reducing wear when articulating against UHMWPE [937]. Such oxidized zirconia layer has also been shown to be very durable and extremely adherent to the underlying metal substrate [938–942]. Joint components consisting of oxidized zirconium alloy has been manufactured by the reconstructive orthopedic surgery division of the medical device company Smith & Nephew under the name of OXINIUM™ and, so far, commercialized both as knee femoral condyle components (GENESIS™ II Total Knee System) and hip femoral head components (VERILAST Technology, OXINIUM Hip Implants). Based on laboratory investigations and early clinical results [938–943], it appears that the combination of properties displayed by OXINIUM™ might actually contribute to an effective reduction of wear-related complications in arthroplasty. According to the National Joint Registry of England and Wales (JREW) published in the year 2011 [944], on a total of 67590 condylar knee brands for primary total knee procedures performed during 2010, a fraction of 8% (5235) were GENESIS™ II Total Knee System. Among a total number of 20580 patients who received through the years the GENESIS™ II Total Knee System, only fractions of 0.26, 1.05, and 1.65% underwent revision (excluding revisions due to infection) after 1, 3, and 5 years implantation, respectively [945]. These statistical data support the thesis of an improved performance of such innovative knee implants. Regarding artificial hip joints, which include OXINIUM™ femoral heads sliding versus highly cross-linked polyethylene, the latest Annual Report from the Australian Orthopaedic Association National Joint Replacement Registry (i.e., containing statistical data from September 1999 to December 2010) lists quite excellent results, which include the highest survivorship of all hip-bearing categories at 7 years (97.8%) [946]. Indeed OXINIUM™ exhibits 4900 times less volumetric wear and 640 times less deep scratches in laboratory wear testing compared with traditional cobalt-chromium alloys [947]. Moreover, the oxidized surface hardly chips off or wears away, even when a strip of oxide is intentionally removed perpendicularly across the wear track before testing [948], thus demonstrating that the grown oxide layer can easily tolerate localized damage or material losses without any risk of catastrophic failure by spalling or delamination. However, despite the superior abrasive wear resistance of the zirconia layer, the bulk zirconium alloy is relatively soft (Vickers hardness of 285 Kg/mm^2) when compared with standard cobalt-chrome alloy femoral heads (Vickers hardness of ~420 Kg/mm^2). Accordingly, a retrieval study, published in 2007, suggested that OXINIUM™

femoral heads might deform under abnormal conditions of impinging contact against acetabular shell materials (Vickers hardness of ~350 Kg/mm^2), e.g., in the case of hip dislocation [949]. In the same study, surface damage was found to occur not only upon dislocation but also when performing closed joint reduction operations. A more recent paper [950] reported about a case of early retrieval of a damaged OXINIUM™ femoral head, with occurrence of extensive damage also to the polyethylene liner after only 48 h after the primary hip replacement. Both the above reports indeed describe implant failures that seem rather related to abnormal conditions, like as unfortunate (and rare) dislocation cases and surgery failures, than to a defective performance of the OXINIUM™ femoral head itself as a biomaterial component. However, as elaborated in the final part of this section, the origin of these negative circumstances can be located in a strong mismatch in elastic properties between the stiff ceramic oxide layer and the soft bulk substrate. As far as the clinical performance of OXINIUM™ is concerned, data collected since its market release and spanning more than 8 years confirm that the oxidation scale of OXINIUM™ components remains adherent to its metal bulk in service and maintains full integrity under service load. In the reminder of this section, building upon already published reports, deeper investigations are reported, which were undertaken to further characterize the physical and chemical characteristics of the oxide scale formed on the surface of OXINIUM™ femoral head components, as well as the intrinsic and the extrinsic toughness of the monoclinic zirconium oxide layer itself. Raman and cathodoluminescence spectroscopic techniques were employed here, which enabled to clarify important stoichiometric details so far missing in specifying the physical origin of the superior structural behavior of OXINIUM™ components. The shown spectroscopic outcomes are helpful in discussing and rationalizing the actual physical and chemical reasons behind the proved integrity of the ceramic/metal interface, which is responsible for both the good adherence and the surface durability reported in prosthetic applications of OXINIUM™ components. In particular, combined spectroscopic methods enable to answer the basic question of why an oxidation layer of inherently brittle monoclinic zirconia ceramic works better than a common coating. Hints can also be obtained about the possibility of further improving the structural performance of "native" ceramic layers adhering to the surface of metallic phases.

Spectroscopic analyses, based on both Raman and cathodo-luminescence approaches, and indentation testing were conducted on 28 mm femoral heads made of OXINIUM™ (Smith & Nephew, Memphis, TN). The OXINIUM™ heads were studied in their as-received state from the maker and after increasingly longer autoclave cycles in water vapor, in order to assess the structural stability of the material in hydrothermal environment. Autoclave cycles were run at 132°C under 2 bar pressure, up to exposures of 100 h. A typical unpolarized Raman spectrum, collected with focusing a confocal laser beam (wavelength 488 nm) on the surface of an OXINIUM™ head, is compared in Fig. 7.1(a) with a Raman spectrum collected under exactly the same experimental conditions on a high-purity monoclinic zirconia (baddeleyite) single-crystal. The comparison shows that all the vibrational peaks observed in the single crystal, as labeled with respect to their vibrational origin in Fig. 7.1(a), were also found in the oxidized zirconia layer, thus confirming that the oxidation products consisted almost exclusively of a monoclinic zirconia polymorph. Regarding the possible presence of a minor fraction of tetragonal polymorph in the oxidized zirconia layer, data found in the literature are spread and controversial. Godlewski *et al.* [951] performed Raman investigations on zirconium alloy oxide films formed in autoclave at 400°C. They found that the oxide layer mainly consisted of a monoclinic phase, but a minor phase fraction was found to be tetragonal. Three zones were found in the oxidation layer: the zone closest to the ceramic/metal interface, namely a very thin layer (about 100 nm in thickness), possessed a high concentration of the tetragonal phase (about 40%); then, an intermediate plateau area was recorded that contained about 15% of tetragonal phase; and, finally, near the oxide free surface, only a very low fractional level of tetragonal phase could be recorded. On the other hand, Cox [952] studied some oxide layers formed on different zirconium alloys in water with, in some cases, addition of lithium. Oxidized layers about 5 μm in thickness, which formed in hot steam, contained tetragonal zirconia at their surface, contrarily to what was observed in

Ref. [951]. This discrepancy is not surprising, since it is well known that even tiny compositional differences could lead to quite different stoichiometry and microstructural features in the grown oxide layer [951, 953]. The origin of the differences found in the studies by Godlewski *et al.* [951] and Cox [952] could obviously reside in the different phase composition of the bulk alloy and in the thermodynamical conditions under which the oxide layer formed, which we could not judge how different they were from those of OXINIUM^{TM}. OXINIUM^{TM} prosthetic components are produced from a wrought zirconium alloy (Zr-2.5%Nb) that is oxidized by thermal diffusion in heated air at 600°C [938, 954], in order to create a zirconium oxide surface of about 5 μm in its average thickness. The main reason why a small amount of niobium has been selected for alloying the zirconium metal (i.e., besides exploiting the high biocompatibility of Nb ions) is clearly not only that of controlling the microstructure of the alloy, but also the properties of the oxidized layer for its optimized response in orthopedic prostheses. However, from both basic physics and chemistry viewpoints, the rationale behind the obtainment of such an exceptionally strong ceramic/metal interface (e.g., clearly stronger than in a conventional coating) and the high wear resistance of the OXINIUM^{TM} surface remains yet unclear. Qualitatively speaking, it is known that the presence of Nb element can infer significant stoichiometric alterations to the oxygen sublattice of zirconium oxide with locally introducing strong gradients of oxygen interstitials and vacancies in its structure [106, 955–957] Such gradients in turn affect local oxygen overcrowding around the Zr^{4+} ions, on which polymorphic transformation strongly depends [246]. In Chapter 4, we have discussed how tetragonal zirconia might become unstable as the tetragonality of its lattice cell increases toward 1.020, which corresponds to the value experienced by a monoclinic cell at room temperature. On the other hand, stability increases as the tetragonality decreases toward unity, which corresponds to the establishment of a cubic cell. This relationship allows for the classification of oxide dopants into either stabilizers (i.e., decreasing the cell tetragonality) or destabilizers (i.e., increasing the cell tetragonality) for the tetragonal phase [106, 955–957]. As it will be discussed more in detail later in this section, pentavalent ions (e.g., Nb^{5+}) substituting for Zr^{4+} in the zirconia lattice are positively charged, and thus tend to annihilate oxygen vacancies and promote oxygen overcrowding [958]. The main consequence of such electrical-neutrality-induced effect is a destabilization of the tetragonal phase in favor of monoclinic phase formation and, thus, it represents the main reason for its conspicuous suppression from the final oxide layer microstructure. The above reasoning represents the basis for explaining the outcomes of the present Raman data on OXINIUM™ femoral heads. In this study, any presence of the tetragonal polymorphic structure could not obviously be revealed in the oxidized layer by unpolarized (confocal) Raman spectroscopy (i.e., all the bands labeled in Fig. 7.1(a) belongs to the monoclinic polymorph). The collection of cross-polarized spectra at different in-plane rotation angles (Fig. 7.1(b)) helped improving signal-to-noise ratio and revealed quite weak traces of the most intense Raman band of the tetragonal structure located at ~260 cm^{-1} (cf. arrowed frequency in Fig. 7.1(b)). This weak tetragonal band was sporadically found in spectra collected from the top surface, and it eventually disappeared at a large number of locations of spectral acquisition randomly selected on the femoral head surface. Moreover, given the conspicuous band weakness, no clear phase-composition gradient could be revealed by performing confocal scans by the Raman probe along the cross-section of the oxide layer as a function of distance from the ceramic/metal interface. As only traces of the 260 cm^{-1} band could be detected, the commonly used Raman algorithms for phase fraction characterization, which utilize the relative intensity of the 145 cm^{-1} tetragonal band (ubiquitously undetectable in OXINIUM™) to the monoclinic doublet located at 179 and 190 cm^{-1} ([227], also cf. Eq. (5.13)), could not be applied. Accordingly, no tetragonal phase fraction in OXINIUM™ femoral heads could be quantitatively determined. In other words, such fraction, if any, lied below the resolution limit of our Raman spectroscopic assessments (i.e., <3 vol.%). This result is in agreement with X-ray diffractometric results by Hobbs *et al.* reporting fractions of tetragonal phase <5 vol.% for the OXINIUM™ knee [936]. We interpret the conspicuous absence of tetragonal-to-monoclinic partly transformed regions in the oxide layer as a positive output, since such mixed structures might come locally accompanied with strong stress gradients (i.e., strongly tensile in the untransformed tetragonal phase; cf. Chapter 4), which could eventually weaken the overall oxide layer.

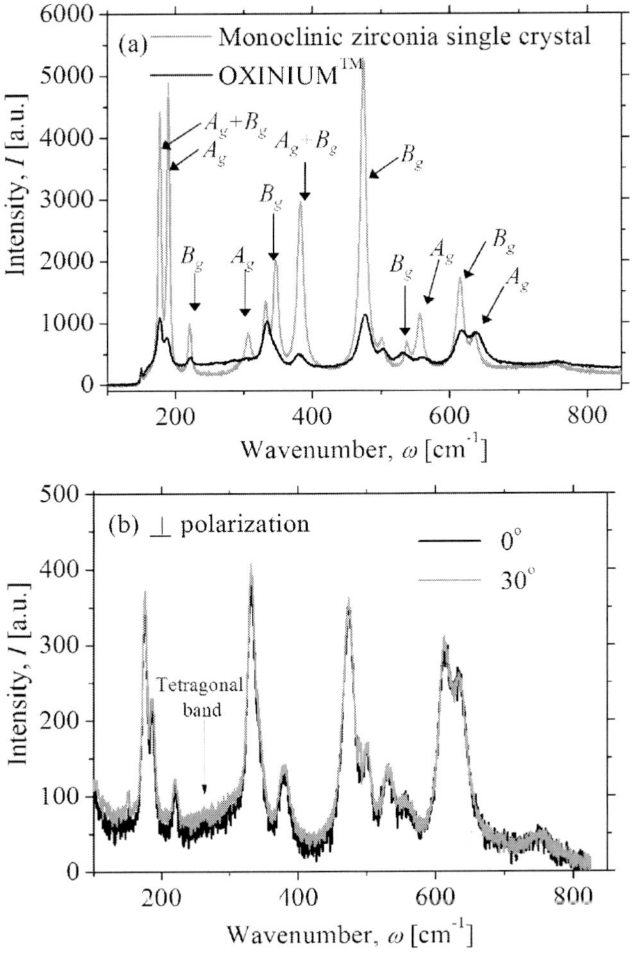

Figure 7.1 (a) Unpolarized Raman spectra of OXINIUM^{TM} femoral head and of high-purity monoclinic zirconia single crystal. All the vibrational peaks are labeled with respect to their vibrational origin; (b) cross-polarized spectra sporadically revealed a quite weak band at ~260 cm^{-1}, which represent the most intense Raman band of the ZrO_2 tetragonal structure (cf. arrow). The angles shown in inset represent the angular in-plane rotation between an arbitrary direction in the fixed laboratory frame and the rotating sample.

Additional information that could be obtained from collecting polarized spectra at different in-plane rotation angles (as shown in Fig. 7.1(b)) showed that the oxidized layer was conspicuously free of crystallographic texture, no spectral changes in relative peak intensity being found upon angular rotation of the sample with respect to the laser polarization axis. Hobbs *et al.* [936] reported about the microstructures of oxidized layers obtained from different types of bulk Zr-based metallic alloys, which underwent different processing conditions, and found significant differences in the textures developed in different oxidized layers. As a general feature for oxidized Zr-alloys, the oxide layer was found to form by inward oxygen diffusion, which is a consequence of zirconia being an excellent oxygen conductor. From a microstructural viewpoint, the main consequence of this phenomenon is the complete absence of porosity in the structure of the oxide layer. Electron diffraction patterns and X-ray diffractometry consistently revealed preferred crystallographic orientations of fine (i.e., diameter typically in the order of the tens of nanometer) columnar lath-like oxide grains for the OXINIUM^{TM} structure. However, two different fiber textures were found to occur with similar probability, whose preferred lath axes approximately lied along the [111] and [001] crystallographic directions of the monoclinic cell. Such dual orientation pattern might be the reason why we hardly detected any distinct angular dependence in polarized Raman rotation experiments. More quantitative details about morphological characteristics of individual bands in the collected Raman spectra will be given in a forthcoming paragraph of this section, dealing with the stoichiometry characteristics of the oxide layer.

The presence of Nb ions diffused from the bulk metal toward the oxidized layer of OXINIUM^{TM} could be clearly substantiated by energy dispersive X-ray elemental analyses performed in the scanning electron microscope. Figure 7.2(a) shows a micrograph of the cross section of the OXINIUM^{TM} femoral head in an oxidized area about 7 μm in thickness, in which elemental analyses relative to O, Zr, and Nb were performed (in Figs. 7.2(b), (c), and (d), respectively). The elemental map reporting the Nb concentration in Fig. 7.2(d) unequivocally shows the presence of this element for fractions in the order of <2 wt.% in the oxidized layer (i.e., together with Zr and O), although the resolution of the energy dispersive

X-ray analysis at such low elemental concentrations did not allow us for any direct quantification of possible stoichiometric gradients along the layer thickness. Due to the intrinsically low sensitivity of energy dispersive X-ray analyses with respect to light elements like oxygen, no information about oxygen stoichiometry gradients could be directly obtained by direct elemental analyses. Galetz *et al.* [954] have reported about elemental depth profiling experiments performed with both glow discharge optical emission spectroscopy and energy dispersive X-ray spectrometry in a portion of OXINIUM™ oxidized layer with a thickness similar to that analyzed in Fig. 7.2. Also these researchers detected the Nb element with a constant profile (of an unspecified low amount) across the layer thickness. Moreover, the oxide layer in the vicinity of the free surface was found to be a ZrO_2 phase in an almost stoichiometric state (with some niobium incorporated). But, a clear gradient in the oxygen content with a concentration minimum in the immediate depth of the free oxide surface was found with scanning across the oxidized layer. From a stoichiometric

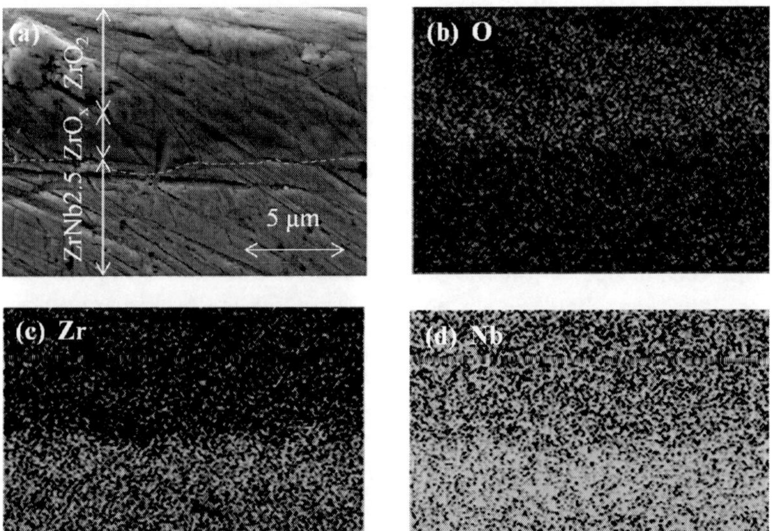

Figure 7.2 (a) Micrograph of the cross section of the OXINIUM™ femoral head in an oxidized area about 7 μm in thickness; (b), (c), and (d) give the results from the area in (a) of elemental analyses relative to O, Zr, and Nb, respectively.

viewpoint, Nb ions might dissolve into ZrO_2 and are expected to have diametrically different effects on stoichiometry (and oxygen diffusivity) depending on their incorporated valence. The lowest valence Nb^{2+} dissolves into the zirconia lattice with an accompanying defect reaction that enhances oxygen vacancy concentration and accelerates oxygen diffusivity (in Kröger–Vink notations [575]):

$$NbO \xrightarrow{ZrO_2} Nb''_{Zr} + O^{\times}_{O} + V^{\bullet\bullet}_{O} \tag{7.1}$$

On the other hand, Nb ions incorporated as Nb^{5+} consume oxygen vacancies and reduce oxygen diffusivity according to the following defect reaction:

$$Nb_2O_5 + V^{\bullet\bullet}_{O} \xrightarrow{ZrO_2} 2Nb^{\bullet}_{Zr} + 5O^{\times}_{O} \tag{7.2}$$

The equilibrium oxygen partial pressure (pO_2) at the Zr-alloy/ZrO_2 interface (10^{-56} atm at 600°C [954]) is lower than that required for oxidizing Nb. Therefore, excess oxygen vacancies arising from niobium dissolution as Nb^{2+} are expected to form in that portion of the layer. Oxygen vacancies will tend to diffuse toward regions closer to the free surface of the oxide layer, where oxygen is abundant; Nb^{4+} and Nb^{5+} are thus stable, and $V^{\bullet\bullet}_{O}$ depressed. This phenomenon of inward oxygen transport, which is the main factor responsible for the growth of the oxide layer, also creates, at equilibrium, an oxygen distribution gradient with a concentration minimum reached in the subsurface. Of interest here is that the zirconium oxide layer near the free surface is quite stable and nearly stoichiometric (thus, one could expect a better wear performance), while the oxide possesses a functional vacancy gradient with progressing toward the ceramic/metal interface, which will be shown later to play a role in partly releasing the thermal residual stress field developed near the interface (therefore, reducing the risk of surface delamination and spalling of the oxide layer). In this study, new evidence for the oxygen vacancy gradient stored in the oxide layer of OXINIUM™ femoral components could be obtained by spatially and spectrally resolved cathodoluminescence spectroscopy. As we have already extensively discussed in Chapters 4 and 5, the cathodoluminescence emission from zirconia ceramics is a direct consequence of the several types of oxygen deficient centers present in the lattice. Figure 7.3 shows a comparison among the average cathodoluminescence spectra of the OXINIUM™ oxidized layer (taken on the material surface), of a monoclinic ZrO_2 single-crystal (i.e., a baddeleyite crystal), and that of a 3 mol.% Y_2O_3-doped polycrystalline (tetragonal) zirconia (3Y-TZP, henceforth) also used in femoral head biomedical implants. In Fig. 7.3, the absolute intensities of the three spectra are compared as collected under exactly the same experimental conditions (i.e., 5 kV, 200 pA). One peculiarity of the cathodoluminescence emission of zirconia resides in the fact that its intensity increases with decreasing concentration of oxygen vacancies [666, 737]. Vacancy annihilation leads to an increase in CL intensity since producing an increase in Zr–O bond stretching (i.e., as a consequence of oxygen overcrowding), which in turn enables a more efficient emission compared with oxygen vacancy sites themselves. In other words, the intensity of the cathodoluminescence emission is directly proportional to the local oxygen (rather than vacancy) content, and thus it represents a *lack* of vacancy sites in the lattice. According to this notion, we can now comparatively interpret the cathodoluminescence spectra shown in Fig. 7.3, which represent the stoichiometric state of both sample surface and immediate subsurface (i.e., as a consequence of both electron scattering and zirconia transparency to visible light). The spectrum collected from the monoclinic single-crystal sample (i.e., by far the most intense, with one order of magnitude higher intensity than the other two samples) proved that a quite low amount of oxygen vacancies was present in this sample. A quite low intensity could be expected for the spectrum collected from the 3Y-TZP sample, due to its relatively high vacancy concentration, a direct consequence of the high concentration of the subvalent Y^{3+} ions substituting for Zr^{4+}. The cathodoluminescence emission collected on the OXINIUM™ oxidized layer was the lowest among the investigated samples, meaning that this sample indeed contained a quite high oxygen vacancy concentration in its immediate subsurface, compared with a nearly stoichiometric single-crystal sample. Keeping in mind the above qualitative discussion of emission intensity features, establishing a link between intrinsic and extrinsic sources of cathodoluminescence and the morphology of the observed emission spectrum is crucial to the effective application of this method to biomaterials analysis. For doing so, we need to inquire more deeply into the physics of the cathodoluminescence emission with further discussing about the morphological details of the emitted spectra. In Fig. 7.4, the cathodoluminescence (average) spectra shown in Fig. 7.3 are normalized to their respective maxima for a better morphological comparison. Figures 7.4(a), (b), and (c) refer to the monoclinic ZrO_2 single-crystal, to the 3Y-TZP biomedical grade (tetragonal) zirconia, and to the OXINIUM™ oxidized layer, respectively. Three main spectral features appear from the comparison:

(i) The spectrum collected from the OXINIUM™ oxidized layer resulted significantly broadened on both its low- and high-energy sides with respect to both spectra from monoclinic single-crystal and 3Y-TZP polycrystalline samples.

(ii) Spectra from the single crystal and the 3Y-doped polycrystal, despite belonging to different polymorphic structures, experienced their respective maxima at exactly the same wavelength and very similar morphologies, except for two distinct features at around 320 and 700 nm, only present in the latter spectrum.

(iii) The low-energy profile of the monoclinic single-crystal spectrum displayed a small but distinct shift toward higher energies compared with that of the 3Y-TZP polycrystal.

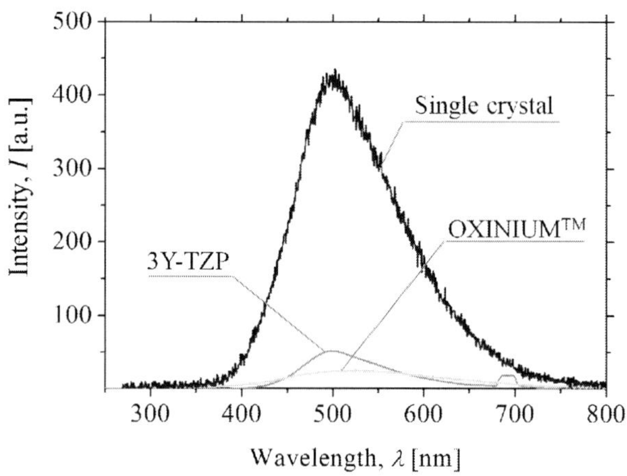

Figure 7.3 Comparison among the average cathodoluminescence spectra of the OXINIUM™ oxidized layer, of the monoclinic ZrO_2 single-crystal, and of a biomedical grade 3Y-TZP. Absolute spectral intensities are compared as collected under electron-beam conditions of 5 kV and 200 pA. In all cases, the spectra were collected from the top surface of the samples.

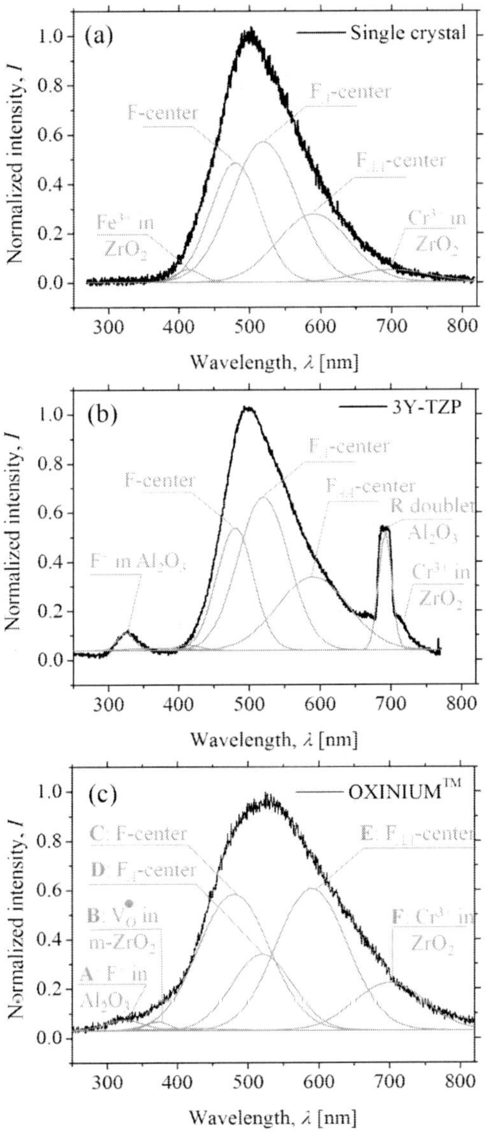

Figure 7.4 The average cathodoluminescence spectra in Fig. 7.3 are normalized to their respective maxima for better morphological comparison. Monoclinic ZrO_2 single-crystal, 3Y-TZP, and OXINIUM™ oxidized layer in (a), (b), and (c), respectively. Deconvolution into sub-band components of Gaussian nature are given of the respective cathodoluminescence spectra, according to the criterion described in the text.

Figures 7.4(a), (b), and (c) also show deconvolutions into sub-band components of Gaussian nature of the respective cathodoluminescence spectra. General observations of luminescence emission from zirconia materials, as found in the literature [664–666], consistently report a broad emission band (peaking at around 500 nm) independent of lattice polymorphism, which well agrees with what is found in the present investigation. Embedded in such a broad emission spectrum and partly overlapping to each other, three distinct sub-bands of Gaussian nature are reported to be located at around 460 nm (2.69 eV), 520 nm (2.25 eV), and 600 nm (2.07 eV) [665]. The sub-band located at 460 nm represents a component of intrinsic nature and it is usually referred to as a "neutral" vacancy center; namely, a singly occupied anion vacancy site with four Zr^{4+} ions nearest neighbors to an oxygen vacancy ($V_O^{\times}$) (F-center) [664]. As also extrinsic oxygen vacancies might generally form in the presence of subvalent substitutional cations (i.e., in order to maintain charge neutrality), associated defects (complexes) can be created. In this latter type of defects, both the number of subvalent cations at the associated defect site and the degree of aggregation of these types of defect increase with increasing substitutional concentration. The simplest complex site, which has been widely studied, is referred to as the F_A-center and contains one three-valent ion (e.g., Y^{3+}) nearest neighbor to an oxygen vacancy with three Zr^{4+} ions at nearest-neighbor positions to the oxygen vacancy. Such complex should be close in energy to that of the intrinsic site, $V_O^{\times}$, since both are neutral, but a slightly lower energy could be expected since the extrinsic site contains only one electron (whence, the sub-band location at around 520 nm) [959]. An additional type of complex, the F_{AA}-center, is then associated to the presence of two three-valent ions and two Zr^{4+} as nearest neighbors to one oxygen vacancy. This lattice configuration forms a complex with two electrons, and thus is characterized by a lower energy compared with the F_A-center (i.e., the sub-band located at around 600 nm) [664, 666]. The deconvoluted spectrum of the 3Y-TZP polycrystal (Fig. 7.4(b)) can indeed be well explained according to the presence of F, F_A, and F_{AA} centers, in addition to emissions related to the presence of a fraction of Al_2O_3 dopant (i.e., an additive phase intentionally introduced into 3Y-TZP polycrystalline biomaterials in order to better stabilize its tetragonal polymorph [960]) and its natural impurity Cr^{3+}. As discussed in details in Chapters 3 and 5, the cathodoluminescence spectrum emitted from Al_2O_3 mainly also consists of emission from oxygen vacancy centers, in addition to that from substitutional Cr^{3+} cation sites. Two spectrally close lines (i.e., the ruby lines) result from non-phonon radiative transitions from the first excited state ($2\bar{A}$ and $\bar{E}$ doublet) to the ground state of substitutional Cr^{3+} ions ($^4A2$), present as a natural impurity in the alumina lattice [738]. The R-doublet is typically located at 692 and 694 nm (1.79 and 1.78 eV, respectively), and it is present in the luminescence spectrum of Al_2O_3 as an extrinsic feature, even if no addition of Cr-ions is intentionally made. Red emission could distinctly be observed in the spectrum of Fig. 7.4(b), although the doublet could not be clearly resolved in the spectrum due to an insufficient grating in spectral analysis. On the other hand, the presence of oxygen vacancies in the Al_2O_3 lattice involves extra luminescence emission, which can be observed in the ultra-violet region upon high-energy excitation [471]. Such emission, which is related to the optical activity of F^+-center, is identified with a band located at around 325 nm (3.8 eV). Both R-lines and F^+-center emission from the alumina lattice are not directly related to the present purpose of discussing the oxygen sublattice characteristics of ZrO_2, and, thus, will be left aside in the remainder of this section. An additional feature in the red interval of the spectrum, which also covers marginal importance in the present discussion, is a broad transition located at around 700~750 nm, which is originally a broad singlet related to the luminescence activity of Cr^{3+} in the ZrO_2 lattice, as located according to a study by Alonso *et al.* [961]. If one takes aside the emission features arising from the Al_2O_3 phase and the luminescence activity of Cr^{3+} in the ZrO_2 lattice, the cathodoluminescence spectrum of the monoclinic zirconia single-crystal (Fig. 7.4(a)) is found to possess morphology very similar to that of the 3Y-TZP polycrystal. The main impurity ions contained in the natural baddeleyite single-crystal investigated here were: Nb_2O_5 (0.4 wt.%), TiO_2 (1.1 wt.%), HfO_2 (1.5 wt.%), FeO (0.8 wt.%), Y_2O_3 (0.3 wt.%), and other oxide impurities including SiO_2, MnO, MgO, and CaO (respective contents $\leq$0.1 wt.%). We shall exclude, in first approximation, luminescence contributions related to isovalent substitutional ions in the cathodoluminescence spectrum of the single-crystal sample, as well as those from ions with too low concentrations. Possible candidates for producing additional emission bands could be substitutional Fe^{3+} and Mn^{2+} centers, which were reported to emit in the zirconia lattice at 3.0 and 3.1 eV, respectively [962]. Berry *et al.* [963] proved the presence of interstitial Fe^{3+} ions coupled with oxygen vacancies in iron-zirconium oxide compounds by a combination of spectroscopic techniques including electron diffraction and iron-57 Mössbauer spectroscopy. However, we could only detect a weak emission from Fe^{3+} centers in the single crystal examined in the present study, probably because it was mainly incorporated in the zirconia lattice as FeO, and thus with a valence lower than the reported Fe^{3+}. The main discussion in comparing the spectra of baddeleyite single crystal and 3Y-TZP (in Figs. 7.4(a) and (b), respectively) should then be focused on interpreting the intensity balance among intrinsic and extrinsic band components arising from different oxygen-vacancy centers in the ZrO_2 lattice. Interestingly, both samples contained Y^{3+} ions, although in quite different fractions, and one should thus expect a common presence of F_A and F_{AA} centers in both spectra. However, the concentration balance of various types of oxygen-vacancy defect was slightly altered, showing a somewhat higher amount of F_A centers in the 3Y-TZP sample compared with single crystal. Such difference can be attributed to the lower amount of Y_2O_3, as well as to a possible vacancy-annihilation effect associated with the concurrent presence of Nb^{5+} impurity in the ZrO_2 single-crystal lattice (absent in 3Y-TZP). In a basic study on photo-stimulated emission from extrinsic vacancy centers in Fe-doped yttria-stabilized zirconia, Nakajima *et al.* [964] found that the presence of iron alloyed in the ZrO_2 lattice does not alter intrinsic and extrinsic defect structures, but only partly quenches the intensity of their emissions. Therefore, we should also rule out the effect of iron on the relative intensity of different sub-bands related to oxygen-vacancy sites. Moreover, the relative balance between intrinsic F-center and F_{AA}-center concentration was conspicuously the same in both single-crystal and 3Y-TZP samples.

Based on the interpretation given for the reference spectra shown in Figs. 7.4(a) and (b), we can now attempt a deeper discussion on the stoichiometry structure of the oxidized zirconia layer at the surface of OXINIUM™ components. We have already mentioned about the dual nature of the Nb ions diffused in the oxidized zirconia layer with reference to their electrical charge, and the possible interplay of their different valences (i.e., either of sub- or supervalent nature) at sites substitutive for Zr^{4+} in the monoclinic structure of the zirconia lattice. Accordingly, specific contributions to the spectral morphology of the cathodoluminescence emission should be expected to arise from both subvalent Nb^{2+} substitutional sites, which can create extrinsic oxygen-vacant sites, and super-valent Nb^{5+} sites, which instead annihilate oxygen vacancies. The cathodoluminescence spectrum of OXINIUM^{TM} (Fig. 7.4(c)) obtained from the top surface of the as-received hip component could be deconvoluted into six sub-band components. Starting their description from the high-energy side of the spectrum, a weak band was seen at around 320 nm (also referred to as sub-band **A**, henceforth), which, as in the case of the 3Y-TZP polycrystal, could be assigned to F^+-center emission from Al_2O_3. Isolated Al_2O_3 grains could indeed be observed in the OXINIUM^{TM} microstructure, as shown in Fig. 7.5 (cf. (a), (b), (c), and (d) for a scanning electron image and O, Al, and Zr elemental analyses, respectively). Another weak band could additionally be separated at around 370 nm (referred to as band **B**), which, together with the contribution of sub-band **A**, led to the overall broadening of the low-wavelength side of the OXINIUM^{TM} spectrum compared with that of the monoclinic ZrO_2 single crystal. Sub-band **B** is believed to arise from defect-transitions peculiar to the monoclinic ZrO_2 phase. Foster *et al.* [965] performed a detailed theoretical study of point defects in monoclinic zirconia. The results demonstrated that interstitial oxygen atoms ($O_i^{\bullet}$ and O_i'' in different charge states) and positively charged oxygen vacancies ($V_O^{\bullet}$ and $V_O^{\bullet\bullet}$ for singly and doubly charged sites, respectively) could trap electrons from the bottom of the zirconia conduction band. Energetically favorable defect associations might then occur according to the following stoichiometry reactions:

$$O_i^{\times} + V_O^{\times} \rightarrow O_i' + V_O^{\bullet} \tag{7.3}$$

$$O_i' + V_O^{\bullet} \rightarrow O_i'' + V_O^{\bullet\bullet} \tag{7.4}$$

$$O_i^{\times} + V_O^{\times} \rightarrow O_i'' + V_O^{\bullet\bullet} \tag{7.5}$$

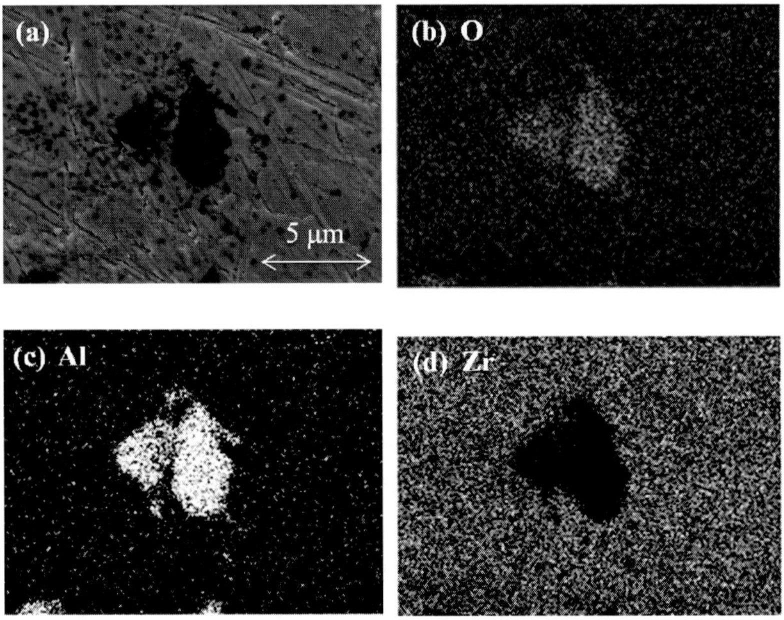

Figure 7.5 Isolated Al_2O_3 grain observed in the OXINIUM™ microstructure; (a), (b), (c), and (d) represent a scanning electron micrograph and O, Al, and Zr elemental analyses, respectively.

Cathodoluminescence emission for such transitions is expected in a relatively narrow interval just below the band gap of ZrO_2 (i.e., emitted with low efficiency at ~5.0 eV [966] and undetectable in this study), according to a series of weak sub-bands located at around 268 nm (O_i'), 332 nm ($O_i^{\times}$), 350 nm ($V_O^{\bullet\bullet}$), and 372 nm ($V_O^{\bullet}$). The occurrence of the defective reaction expressed by Eq. (7.2), according to which Nb^{5+} enters the ZrO_2 lattice, was also substantiated in a study by Petrik *et al.* [967], based on water radiolysis experiments in comparison with pure ZrO_2. The presence of Nb^{5+} in the ZrO_2 lattice might impose the formation of oxygen interstitials for charge neutrality condition to be satisfied. Migration of intrinsic anionic defects could then involve extensive defect association with $V_O^{\bullet}$ emission at 372 nm, according to Eq. (7.3). We could indeed observe the weak sub-band **B** around this wavelength in the cathodoluminescence spectrum of OXINIUM™ but not in that of the monoclinic single crystal (cf. Figs. 7.4(c) and (a), respectively), which also contained a (minor) fraction of

Nb-ion impurity. A theoretical study by Foster *et al.* [968] on pure monoclinic hafnia suggests that O_i' is energetically not favored at any Fermi level in a monoclinic lattice, which appears to be the case here for the spectrum in Fig. 7.4(a). Therefore, the present results on the OXINIUM^{TM} sample suggest that the presence of interstitial oxygen sites in the monoclinic ZrO_2 lattice might depend on the balance of different defect sites, which was different between OXINIUM^{TM} and single-crystal samples as discussed hereafter.

The sub-bands labeled **C**, **D**, and **E** in Fig. 7.4(c) are representative of the stoichiometry of the oxygen sublattice, as discussed above for other representative spectra from the ZrO_2 lattice. In the deconvoluted spectrum of OXINIUM^{TM}, one could find an amount of neutral vacancy F-centers (sub-band **C**) comparable with that in the monoclinic ZrO_2 single crystal, while the emission from F_A-centers (sub-band **D**) resulted strongly attenuated compared with reference spectra in Figs. 7.4(a) and (b), both collected from samples containing Y^{3+} dopant. On the other hand, the relative contribution from F_{AA}-centers (sub-band **E**) to the overall emission spectrum of the OXINIUM^{TM} sample was significantly higher than in the case of both single-crystal and 3Y-TZP samples. In the monoclinic ZrO_2 lattice, Zr atoms have coordination number 7, which relates to two types of oxygen sites: the O^I sites, which are triangularly coordinated to Zr and lie approximately parallel to the (100) plane of the monoclinic cell, and the O^{II} sites, which are coordinated nearly tetrahedrally in a distorted square also parallel to the (100) plane. At room temperature, the Zr atom is located between two oxygen atomic layers, respectively formed by the triangular O^I and the tetrahedral O^{II} series of atoms (with distances from the Zr atom of 0.205~0.216 nm and 0.215~0.229 nm, respectively) [969]. For such crystallographic structure, experimental and theoretical evidence has been provided [583, 970, 971] suggesting that substitutional subvalent cations with an ionic diameter larger than that of Zr^{4+} might favor formation of oxygen vacancies at next-nearest-neighbor sites, while cations with an ionic diameter smaller than that of Zr^{4+} preferentially create oxygen vacancies at nearest-neighbor sites. The ionic radius of the Nb^{2+} ion (0.085 nm) (i.e., unlike that of Y^{3+}, which is larger (0.134 nm)) is nearly the same as that of the host Zr^{4+} (0.084 nm). Therefore, while it is clear that each Nb^{2+} ion should require the formation of one oxygen vacancy in the monoclinic

ZrO_2 lattice for maintaining charge neutrality (cf. Eq. (7.1)), it is difficult to infer *a priori* whether such oxygen vacancy should be located at next-nearest-neighbor (like in the case of Y^{3+}) or at nearest-neighbor locations at triangularly or tetrahedrally coordinated sites. Accordingly, one cannot obviously predict any preponderance in the emission contributions from different defect-complex centers in the spectrum emitted from the surface of the OXINIUM™ sample. Moreover, the crystallographic assembly created by doping with divalent substitutional cations (Me^{2+}) in the $Zr_{1-x}Me_xO_{2-x}$ lattice could be quite different from that of Y^{3+}. According to a theoretical study by Stefanovich *et al.* [972], at $x \geq 0.1$, the impurity-vacancy dipoles are located very close to each other and the anion vacancies are quite mobile. Therefore, it is not possible to distinguish between different modes of charge compensation. For instance, vacancies could occupy both the nearest neighbor and the next-nearest-neighbor sites with respect to a divalent impurity ion. Accordingly, substitutional (divalent) cation impurities and oxygen vacancies have been considered as nearly randomly distributed among the available lattice sites. Our choice of spectral deconvolution for the cathodoluminescence spectrum acquired from the free-surface neighborhood of OXINIUM™ (Fig. 7.4(c)), which is comprehensively based on the physical background available from previously published experimental and theoretical studies on luminescence emission from the ZrO_2 lattice, proves a strong preponderance of F_{AA} sites in an overall strongly non-stoichiometric oxygen sublattice. The broad additional sub-band, which is located in the red emission zone of the spectrum beyond 700 nm (i.e., labeled **F** in Fig. 7.4(c)) and enables to fully fit the low-energy side of the spectrum, can be attributed, in analogy to the case of the 3Y-TZP sample (cf. Fig. 7.4(b)), to the presence of Cr^{3+} diffused from the bulk Zr-alloy metal [953] through the ZrO_2 lattice [961].

The spectroscopic features dealing with oxygen off-stoichiometry in the cathodoluminescence spectrum of OXINIUM™ could be further discussed by examining the cathodoluminescence spectral morphology recorded at different locations on a cross-sectional profile of the oxidized layer. Spatially resolved cathodoluminescence line scans across a selected cross-section profile of the oxidation scale (i.e., along the in-depth abscissa, *z*, with origin at the sample surface) showed a great variation in the stoichiometric balance achieved within the oxidation layer. A scanning electron micrograph of the analyzed location and a typical cathodoluminescence intensity profile, as detected in the studied OXINIUM^{TM} femoral components, are reported in Figs. 7.6(a) and (b), respectively. Since the cathodoluminescence intensity is inversely proportional to oxygen vacancy concentration [666, 737] and, thus, directly proportional to local oxygen content, the overall intensity profile along the oxide scale suggests that the surface of OXINIUM^{TM} is closer to oxygen stoichiometry than its subsurface. At the very surface of the sample, the intensity emission greatly increases toward that of a highly stoichiometric single-crystal sample (cf. Fig. 7.3). On the other hand, a vacancy-rich zone was restored in the immediate sample subsurface down to about 2 μm in depth, followed by a gradual stoichiometry recovery down to a depth of about 6 μm. Finally, an abrupt increase in the concentration of oxygen-vacancy sites (i.e., a decrease in cathodoluminescence intensity) could also be recorded in the transition layer of ~1 μm in thickness at the interface between the oxide scale and the bulk metal-alloy structure. For comparison, the oxygen profile detected by Galetz *et al.* [954], according to glow discharge optical emission spectroscopy, on an OXINIUM^{TM} sample is also plotted in Fig. 7.6(b). Indeed, the two spectral profiles, obtained according to completely different physical principles, showed excellent agreement in their overall morphology. It should also be noted that the resolution of both spectroscopic analyses was comparably high (i.e., in the nanometer scale), which enabled a direct comparison between the two respective stoichiometric profiles, but the profiles being recorded at different locations and the inherently different response functions of the two probes give rise to some morphological differences in the recorded profiles, especially in the zone near the free surface and in the immediate neighborhood of the oxide/alloy interface. Nevertheless, the qualitative agreement with data by Galetz *et al.* [954] supports the outputs of our cathodoluminescence analysis.

Elemental analyses in Fig. 7.2(d) could detect no gradients in the amount of Nb-ions present in the oxidized layer. But, thermodynamic considerations about the oxygen stoichiometric equilibrium developed during oxidation reaction and leading to oxide layer formation strongly suggested the development of steep gradients in the valence associated to the diffused Nb ions [954]. Super-valent substitution of Nb^{5+}, expected to occur more frequently near the surface of the oxidized OXINIUM™ layer, induced conspicuous annihilation of oxygen-vacancy sites, while subvalent Nb^{2+}, abundant in the neighborhood of the metal alloy/oxide interface, favored the formation of oxygen vacancies in the monoclinic ZrO_2 lattice. The morphological features of cathodoluminescence spectra from selected locations on the scanning profile in Fig. 7.6, which are compared in Fig. 7.7, further prove the structural model proposed at the beginning of this section. As a general trend, the spectra in the profile, independent of vacancy concentration, experienced similar morphologies with a general preponderance of the band related to F_{AA}-type centers on other bands from different types of defect (cf. Figs. 7.7(a), (b), and (c), corresponding to locations on the cross-section scan at $z = 0$, 2.0, and 4.2 μm, respectively; data corresponding to the shown spectra are encircled for better visualization in the plot of Fig. 7.6(b)). However, in correspondence of the interface between the oxide scale and the intermediate layer (e.g., at $z = 6.17$ μm), F_A-center sites became preponderant (cf. Fig. 7.7(d)). It should be noted that substitution of each Nb^{2+} for one Zr^{4+} involves the formation of one oxygen vacancy for charge compensation, while substitution of each Nb^{5+} for Zr^{4+} requires only ½ zirconium vacancy (i.e., provided that a defect complex $2Nb^{5+}_{Zr}$-V_{Zr} might exist). Therefore, since the probability of finding two Nb^{5+} ions binding together close to an oxygen vacancy is much higher than that involved with a single Nb^{2+} ion, the F_{AA} band can be considered mainly contributed by a singly occupied oxygen vacancy with two Nb^{5+} and two Zr^{4+} ions neighbors to the oxygen atom. On the contrary, the F band can be considered to arise from two kinds of origin: (i) an occupied oxygen vacancy surrounded by one Nb^{2+} and three Zr^{4+} ions; and, (ii) an occupied oxygen vacancy with one Nb^{5+} and three Zr^{4+} ions neighbors to the oxygen atom. As a further feature, the broad band with quite low intensity, emitted at around 410 nm, became more clearly visible at depths $z \geq 2$ μm (cf. spectral deconvolution in Figs. 7.7(b)~(d). This band could be assigned to substitutional Fe^{3+} centers [962]. Iron is indeed present by ~0.22 wt.% in the bulk Zr-alloy from which OXINIUM™ is manufactured [953]. Similar to Nb ions, Fe ions are also expected to diffuse from the bulk metallic alloy during the oxidation process [737]. However, the rather weak emission from iron centers, observed by collecting spectra near the sample free surface, suggests that during manufacturing iron could hardly diffuse through the full thickness of the oxide layer.

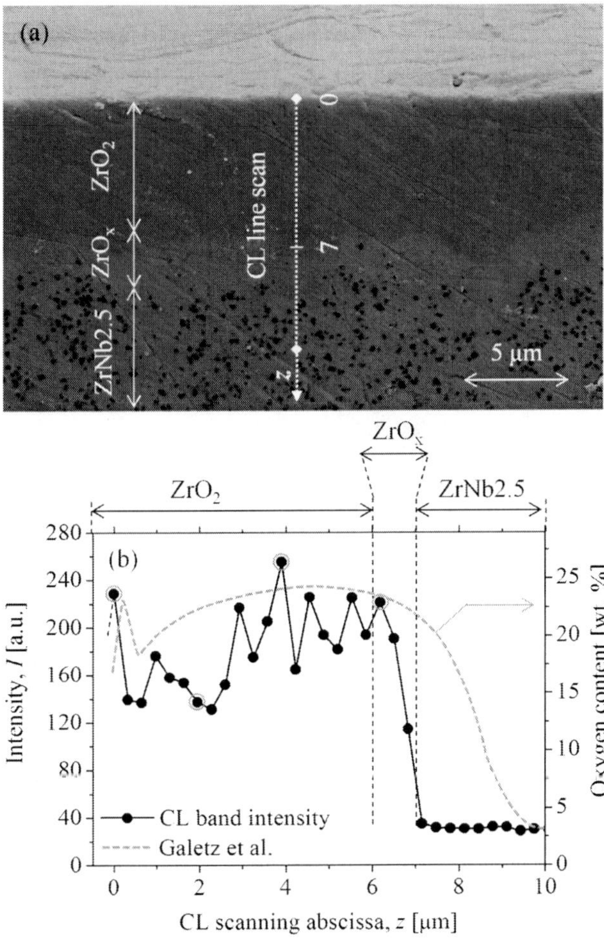

Figure 7.6 A scanning electron micrograph of the cross-section of the OXINIUM™ femoral component (a), and a typical cathodoluminescence intensity profile (b). The oxygen profile detected by Galetz *et al.* [954] on OXINIUM™, according to glow discharge optical emission spectroscopy, is also plotted for comparison.

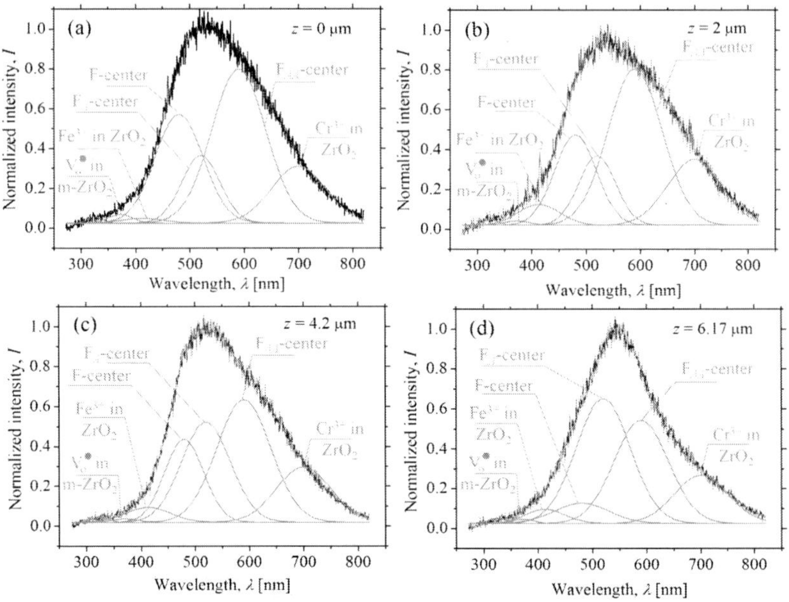

Figure 7.7 Morphological features of the cathodoluminescence spectra collected at selected locations on the scanning profile on sample cross section (i.e., encircled locations in Fig. 7.6(b) and depths, z, in inset to each plot in Fig. 7.7). The intensity of different sub-bands represent the population of different families of lattice defects, as discussed in the text.

The biological environment, in which the bearing surface of a joint prosthesis is embedded, is quite demanding: saline (~2 mol/l NaCl), marginally basic in healthy joints (pH ≈ 7.35~7.45), but quite acidic in osteoarthritic patients [973], and definitely oxidative ($pO_2 \sim 5 \times 10^{-2}$ atm). Preliminary evaluations of the chemical stability of OXINIUM™ hip components could be obtained by accelerating the eventual occurrence of degradation effects in a controlled and severe hydrothermal environment. Figure 7.8 shows the relative variation of the overall intensity of cathodoluminescence emission and, with it, the variation in oxygen sublattice stoichiometry, before and after long-term exposure to water vapor autoclave environment (i.e., 100 h at 132°C). Remarkably, almost no change was found in the OXINIUM™ sample, meaning that the concentration of oxygen vacancies near the material surface remained conspicuously unchanged. This behavior was very different from that of the

3Y-TZP sample (also shown in Fig. 7.8), which instead showed a five-fold intensity increase and, thus, significant annihilation of oxygen vacancy sites near the surface of the as-received sample. The peculiar stoichiometric structure of the oxidized ZrO_2 layer of OXINIUM™, which stands in a stable monoclinic state and conspicuously lacks vacancy sites at its very surface, can be interpreted as a strong protective barrier against environmentally assisted wear. The origin of environmental stability and wear properties of OXINIUM™, therefore, partly resides in the stoichiometric characteristics of its surface ZrO_2 lattice. In other words, the presence of super-valent Nb^{5+} ions at the material surface enables to conspicuously suppress vacancy formation not only during manufacturing, but also during interactions with aggressive environment. Moreover, it is confirmed that doping with an even small amount of Nb^{5+} ions has the remarkable effect of suppressing water adsorption on the surface of monoclinic ZrO_2 [967]. As we have already discussed in Chapter 5, water adsorption is the primary cause of surface degradation in biomedical ZrO_2. In thermally activated processes in moist environment, oxygen vacancies at the surface of partially stabilized tetragonal ZrO_2 annihilate at lattice locations where water radicals are strongly adsorbed (cf. 3Y-TZP sample in Fig. 7.8). Annihilation of vacancies occurs with oxygen from the environmental water atmosphere filling vacancy sites, while hydrogen is placed at adjacent interstitial sites. Such process destabilizes the tetragonal lattice and triggers polymorphic transformation to the monoclinic phase. Nb^{5+} ions incorporated into the ZrO_2 structure annihilate all the oxygen vacancies at the OXINIUM™ surface and, with this action, completely suppress the presence of tetragonal phase in the sample after manufacturing and, with it, any water adsorption during successive exposures to hydrothermal environment. For this reason, we could observe a complete stoichiometric inertness of the oxygen sublattice at the OXINIUM™ surface upon long-term exposure in autoclave. Finally, it should also be noted that in the context of environmentally driven off-stoichiometry effects, the OXINIUM™ surface should be considered even more bioinert than polycrystalline Al_2O_3 biomaterials. As we have previously discussed in Chapter 3, polycrystalline Al_2O_3 shows a marked tendency to accumulate oxygen vacancies in its surface layer when exposed for increasing periods to a hydrothermally activated environment, with a direct impact on its wear resistance.

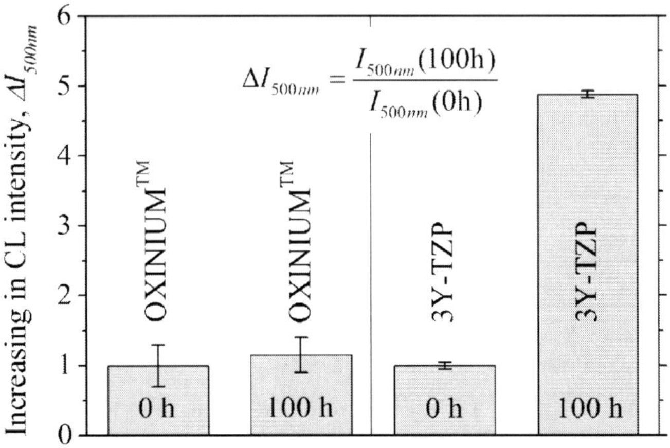

Figure 7.8 Relative variation of the overall intensity of cathodoluminescence emission (i.e., variation in oxygen sub-lattice stoichiometry) before and after long-term exposure to water vapor autoclave environment (i.e., 100 h at 132°C) for OXINIUM™ and 3Y-TZP samples.

Additional quantitative information about the oxygen vacancy distribution developed upon manufacturing within the surface oxidation layer of OXINIUM™ can, in principle, be obtained by means of Raman spectroscopy. For doing so in a quantitative manner, however, a deeper interpretation of the physical origin of the vibrational behavior of monoclinic ZrO_2 is needed, together with a quantitative estimation of the morphological effects that its Raman spectrum experiences when the monoclinic lattice becomes affected by an increasing concentration of oxygen vacancy. Li *et al.* [974] have recently published a detailed study based on lattice dynamics calculations about phonon anharmonicity of the ZrO_2 lattice in its monoclinic polymorphic structure. The calculations were used to identify the individual motions of metal and oxygen atoms in the different Raman modes and confirmed that vibrational modes involving changes in oxygen-oxygen bond length were the most anharmonic. This finding indeed proved that selected Raman bands, showing measurable peak broadening and shift, could be used as sensors for oxygen stoichiometry. Essential to our analytical implementations, detailed information about density of states (*DOS*) as a function of Raman frequency, ω, was also provided for the monoclinic ZrO_2 polymorph. From the $DOS(\omega)$ function calculated by Li *et al.* [974], we could extract the normalized O-projected morphology for a pure and vacancy-free crystal as a best fitting function, $g_0(\omega)$, in the frequency interval between 0 and 400 cm^{-1}, as follows:

$$g_0(\omega) = \sum_{m=1}^{6} D_{A,m} \times \exp\left[\frac{-2(\omega - \omega_{f,m})^2}{D_{B,m}^2}\right] \tag{7.6}$$

where the constants, $D_{A,m}$, and, $D_{B,m}$, and the frequencies, $\omega_{f,m}$, of the individual vibrational bands in the studied frequency interval are listed in Table 7.1. According to the physical information available from Eq. (7.6), we can attempt to simulate the morphological variations occurring to the Raman doublet located at 179 and 190 cm^{-1}, which belongs to the $A_g + B_g$ and A_g vibrational modes, respectively, and involve displacements of oxygen atoms in the monoclinic ZrO_2 lattice [658]. These two vibrational bands were selected not only because they involve quite stoichiometry-sensitive oxygen vibrational displacements, but also because they show no overlaps with Raman bands emitted from the tetragonal ZrO_2 polymorph. A valuable guidance in the procedure for simulating the morphological variations of Raman bands from the function $g_0(\omega)$ in Eq. (7.6) is provided in an early study by McBride *et al.* [975], who succeeded in simulating the effect of oxygen vacancy on the Raman spectrum of cerium oxide. According to general notions, the Raman lines are expected to lose intensity, to broaden, to shift, and to become asymmetric as the concentration of oxygen vacancies increases, e.g., concurrent with the introduction into the lattice of an increasing amount of subvalent cations, substitutional for Zr^{4+}. This effect can be substantiated by a calculation of the effects of oxygen vacancies on the Raman spectrum, which, although somewhat simplified with respect to a full computational procedure [975], uses a Green's function technique with the vacancies treated as point defects with zero mass. Note that the identification of a Raman signature for oxygen vacancies involves fundamental implications in characterizing ZrO_2-containing biomaterials, since cathodoluminescence is yet hardly quantitative and X-ray diffraction is generally insensitive to oxygen vacancy concentration. Following McBride *et al.* [975], we could first set the average Green's function for ZrO_{2-y}, according to a self-energy ansatz and then, with it, describe the Raman intensity of a selected band, $I_R(\omega)$, from an area with constant oxygen vacancy concentration, as follows:

$$I_R(\omega) = \sum_{l=1}^{2} -\mathrm{Im} \frac{C_l(y)}{\omega^2\left[1-\sigma(\omega)\right]-\omega_{R,l}^2} \tag{7.7}$$

$$\sigma(\omega) = \frac{y/2}{1-\omega^2\left[\int_0^{+\infty} \frac{g_0(\eta)}{\eta^2-\omega^2} d\eta - i\pi \frac{g_0(\omega)}{2\omega}\right]} \tag{7.8}$$

Table 7.1 Constants describing the best fitting function, $g_0(\omega)$, in the frequency interval between 0 and 400 cm^{-1}, as represented by Eq. (7.6)

m	$D_{A,m}$	$D_{B,m}$ (cm^{-1})	$\omega_{f,m}$ (cm^{-1})
1	1.923×10^{-3}	120	175
2	1.923×10^{-3}	8	155
3	1.923×10^{-3}	150	185
4	1.154×10^{-3}	13	190
5	5.769×10^{-3}	200	350
6	7.692×10^{-4}	60	300

where $C_l(y)$ represents a function of concentration that differs for the individual Raman bands present in the studied interval of frequency (i.e., here, we shall set $l = 2$ since the studied interval was confined to the frequency interval 160~220 cm^{-1}); η is an integration variable, and Im and i are used in their usual meaning of imaginary part of a complex number and imaginary unit, respectively. The Raman frequency, $\omega_{R,l}$, associated to each Raman band, is a function of vacancy concentration, y, and can be given as follows:

$$\omega_{R,l}(y) = \omega_{0,l}\left[1-\frac{3K}{\omega}\times\left(\frac{\partial\omega}{\partial p}\right)_l \times L_v y\right] \tag{7.9}$$

where K = 155 GPa is the bulk modulus reported for monoclinic ZrO_2 at room temperature [976,977]; the lattice variation, $\Delta a = L_v y$, is assumed to be linear through a coefficient, L_v, to vacancy concentration, y; and, the coefficient $(\partial\omega/\partial p)_l$ describes the dependence of Raman frequency on pressure, p, for the l-th Raman band, which in turn is linear with pressure up to pressures of several GPa [978–980]. The hydrostatic coefficients, $(\partial\omega/\partial p)_l$, taken as three times the linear stress/shift coefficients measured for a uniaxial stress state [117], were −2.7 and −2.4 cm^{-1}/GPa for the 179 and 190 cm^{-1} bands of monoclinic ZrO_2, respectively. Equations (7.7)~(7.9) represent the basis for morphological computations on the doublet located at 179 and 190 cm^{-1} in the monoclinic ZrO_2 spectrum emitted from a homogeneous sample with constant vacancy concentration. Along a cross-sectional profile of the oxidized surface of OXINIUM^{TM}, however, the vacancy distribution is a function of the in-depth abscissa, z, while the Raman probe experiences a response function of Gaussian nature [202]. Therefore, the Raman intensity, $\bar{I}_R(\omega, z_0)$, observed with a probe centered at a location, z_0, along the cross-section profile in an area containing a gradient in vacancy concentration is expressed as:

$$\bar{I}_R(\omega, z_0) = \int_0^T I_R(\omega, z)\left\{\exp\left[\frac{-2(z - z_0)^2}{B^2}\right]\right\}dz \tag{7.10}$$

with $\bar{I}_R(\omega, z)$ being the local contribution to Raman emission from each location z, T the thickness of the oxidation scale, and the exponential function in brackets giving the Gaussian distribution of Raman intensities within the probe. The constant B can be measured according to preliminary calibrations [208] (i.e., in this case, B = 2.6 μm). Substituting in Eq. (7.10) for $I_R(\omega, z)$ from Eq. (7.7), and considering that in Eq. (7.7), the presence of a gradient in vacancy concentration can be represented by the function of in-depth abscissa, $y = y(z)$, one can simulate the intensity variation of the Raman doublet located at 179 and 190 cm^{-1} along the cross-section profile, as it is expected to arise from the presence of an off-stoichiometry gradient. A full assessment of the morphology of the Raman doublet (i.e., assumed as Lorentzian functions) requires summing the contributions of the two partially overlapping bands, according to the two following equations:

$$\bar{I}_R(\omega, z_0) = \sum_{l=1}^{2} \frac{I_{0,l}}{\left[\omega - \left(\omega_l + \Delta\omega_{l,\text{tot}}\right)\right]^2 + \left(\Gamma_l/2\right)^2} \quad (7.11)$$

$$\Delta\omega_{l,\text{tot}} = \omega_{l,\text{tot}} - \omega_{0,l} = \Delta\omega_{l,s} + \Delta\omega_{l,c} \quad (7.12)$$

where $I_{0,l}$ and $\omega_{0,l}$ are the intensities and the spectral locations at maximum, respectively, of individual Raman bands when emitted from a perfectly stoichiometric and stress-free sample; $\omega_{l,\text{tot}}$ is the phonon frequency of the l-th band maximum as altered by the concurrent presence of both stress and oxygen vacancies; Γ_l is the full width at half maximum (FWHM) of each individual Raman band in the studied frequency interval. The total observed shift in Raman frequency with respect to a perfectly stoichiometric and stress-free sample, $\Delta\omega_{l,\text{tot}}$, in turn consists of two separate components, $\Delta\omega_{l,s}$, and $\Delta\omega_{l,c}$, which represent the frequency shifts associated with the presence of residual stress (or "mechanical" shift) and oxygen vacancies (or "chemical" shift) in the lattice, respectively. A best-fitting computational routine was run in search for a match to 100 experimental spectra collected along a cross-section profile of the oxide scale of the OXINIUM^{TM} sample. Iterative computations allowed retrieving the two functions $C_l(y)$ for the bands located at 179 and 190 cm^{-1} and the vacancy concentration profile, $y = y(z)$, for which all the 100 experimental Raman spectra could be best fitted. The character of a trial function in search for the vacancy concentration profile in the oxide scale of OXINIUM^{TM} was selected according to the experimental CL data in Fig. 7.6(b). Figure 7.9(a) shows a series of 4 selected experimental Raman spectra in the region 160~210 cm^{-1}, as collected at different locations, z_0, along a cross-section profile in the OXINIUM^{TM} sample. The results of the best fitting were computed according to Eqs. (7.6)~(7.12), as shown in Fig. 7.9(a) (in terms of Raman spectra), and in Figs. 7.9(b) and (c) in terms of band-intensity and FWHM profiles, respectively. The full lines represent best fitting curves to the experimental data after convolution within the finite size of the Raman probe according to Eqs. (7.10) and (7.11) for Figs. 7.9(b) and (c), respectively. As can be seen, best-fitting spectra describe with acceptable accuracy the morphological changes of the Raman spectrum along the profile, except for their band-shift characteristics. This observation confirms the presence of an additional and

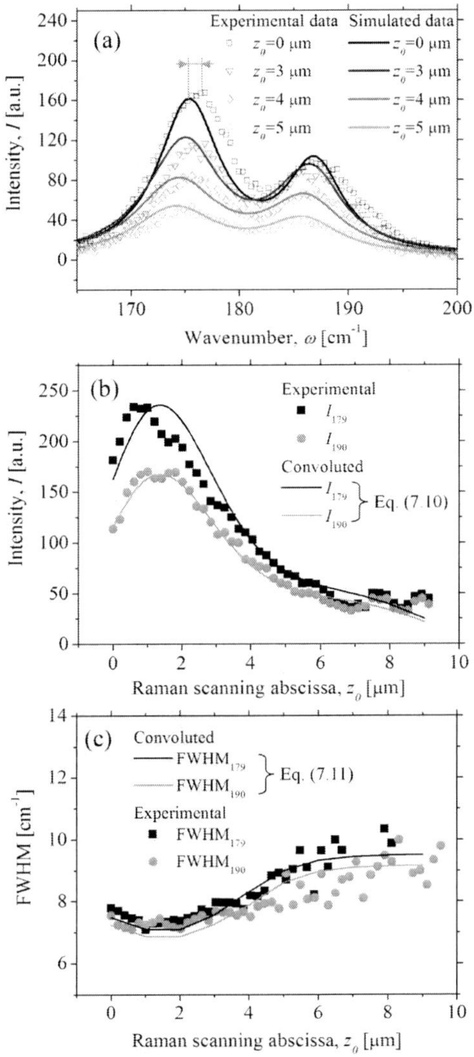

Figure 7.9 (a) A series of four selected experimental Raman spectra in the region 160~210 cm^{-1}, collected at different locations, z_0, along a cross-section profile of the OXINIUM^{TM} sample. The results of the best fitting (full lines) were computed according to Eqs. (7.6)~(7.12). In (b) and (c), plots are given of band-intensity and FWHM profiles, respectively. In these latter plots full lines represent best fitting curves to the experimental data after probe convolution according to Eqs. (7.10) and (7.11), respectively.

non-negligible band-shift contribution arising from a residual stress field stored in the oxide layer. Data for Raman band intensity, $I_l(z)$, and full width at half maximum, $\Gamma_l(z)$, are plotted in Figs. 7.10(a) and (b), respectively, after deconvolution of local spectra from the Gaussian filter of the probe. From these latter plots, it is possible to retrieve the relationships that relate Raman band intensity and FWHM to oxygen vacancy concentration, y, as shown in Figs. 7.10(c) and (d), respectively. The mathematical expressions retrieved from the best-fitting procedure for the oxygen vacancy profile, $y = y(z)$, (plotted in Fig. 7.11(a)) and for the functions, $C_l = C_l(y)$, in Eq. (7.7) are given in the following:

$$y(z) = 0.1794 - \frac{3.694 \times 10^{-5}}{(z-0.15)^2 + 2.5 \times 10^{-3}} + 5.175 \times 10^{-2} \times \exp(-0.9z)$$
$$-3.401 \times 10^{-2} \times \mathrm{acrtan}\,(4.808 - 1.923z) \quad (7.13)$$

$$C_{179}(y) = 8.4 \times 10^5 \times \{\exp[-(0.693 + 1.54 \tan z)]\}^{0.85} \quad (7.14)$$

$$C_{190}(y) = 4.5 \times 10^5 \times \{\exp[-(0.687 + 1.58 \tan z)]\}^{0.80} \quad (7.15)$$

where the subscripts on the left side of Eqs. (7.14) and (7.15) represents the unperturbed frequencies, $\omega_{0,l}$, of the studied monoclinic Raman doublet. Note that the computations involving Raman band intensity and width have been carried out under the assumptions that band intensity is only affected by the off-stoichiometry of the crystal and that the effect of oxygen vacancies on band broadening is largely preponderant compared with the effect of gradients in the residual stress field stored in the oxide scale. Such an assumption can be justified by considering that even the steeper stress gradient developed at the tip of a crack in the oxide layer material lead to a broadening in the order of 10^{-1} cm^{-1} (as discussed later in this section), thus much smaller than the "chemical" broadening we could observe in the present experiments (cf. Fig. 7.9(c)). On the other hand, Eq. (7.12) states that band shifts of chemical and mechanical origin are both important and should concurrently be considered in band-shift analysis. The convoluted Lorentzian contributions that represent the local Raman signal at each location along the line-scan profile (i.e., plotted as fitting spectra in Fig. 7.9(a)) experience distinct shifts with respect to the reference spectrum of a stoichiometric sample located at $\omega_{0,l}$. However, the obtainment of the true band-shift profile that develops along the thickness of the oxide layer, $\Delta\omega_{l,c}(z) = \omega_{l,c}(z) - \omega_{0,l}$, also requires a Gaussian deconvolution with respect to the spatial abscissa, z, as follows:

$$\overline{\Delta\omega_{l,c}}(z_0) = \overline{\omega_{l,c}}(z_0) - \omega_{0,l} = \frac{\int_0^T \left[\omega_{l,c}(z) - \omega_{0,l}\right] I_l(z) \times \exp\left[\frac{-2(z-z_0)^2}{B^2}\right] dz}{\int_0^T I_l(z) \times \exp\left[\frac{-2(z-z_0)^2}{B^2}\right] dz} \quad (7.16)$$

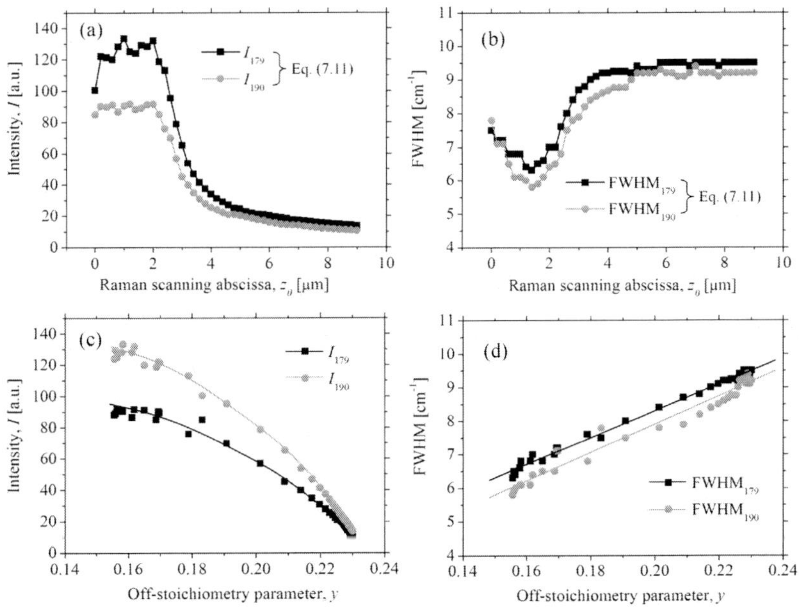

Figure 7.10 In (a) and (b), plots as a function of in-depth abscissa, z, for local Raman band intensity and FWHM, respectively, after deconvolution from the Gaussian filter of the Raman probe. Relationships between Raman band intensity and FWHM to oxygen vacancy concentration, y, are shown in (c) and (d), respectively. The full-line curves represent best fits to the experimental trends.

The convoluted spectral shifts, $\overline{\Delta\omega_{l,c}}(z_0)$, represent the chemical contribution to the experimentally observed frequency shifts (i.e., as arising from the oxygen vacancy profile depicted in Fig. 7.11(a)) of each individual Raman band. Chemical shifts, $\Delta\omega_{l,c}$, are plotted after Gaussian deconvolution in Figs. 7.12(a) and (b) as a function of in-depth abscissa, z, and vacancy concentration, y, respectively. The spectral shift profile expected by the effect of a gradient in the residual stress field stored along the oxide scale thickness, $\overline{\Delta\omega_{l,s}}(z)$, can then be computed by subtracting the convoluted chemical shift profile due to oxygen off-stoichiometry, $\overline{\Delta\omega_{l,c}}(z = z_0)$, from the overall experimentally observed shift profile, $\Delta\omega_{l,tot}$ (cf. also Eq. (7.12)). Under the usual assumption made for isotropic thin films that the residual stress field stored in the oxide layer is of an equi-biaxial nature [981–983], we can now compute the convoluted residual stress profile, $\overline{\sigma_R}(z)$, according to the usual proportionality relationship to Raman frequency shift [117]:

$$\overline{\sigma_R}(z) = \overline{\sigma}_{xx}(z) + \overline{\sigma}_{yy}(z) = \frac{1}{3}\left(\frac{\partial\omega}{\partial p}\right)_l^{-1} \overline{\Delta\omega_{l,s}}(z) \tag{7.17}$$

where $\overline{\sigma}_{xx}(z)$ and $\overline{\sigma}_{yy}(z)$ represent the two in-plane components of the residual (equi-biaxial) stress field stored in the oxide film. According to a Gaussian deconvolution procedure similar to that described by Eq. (7.16), the true (i.e., deconvoluted) profile of residual stress, $\sigma_R(z)$, stored in the oxide layer of OXINIUM™ can finally be plotted as shown in Fig. 7.11(b). The mathematical expression, which describes the residual stress profile, $\sigma_R = \sigma_R(z)$, stored after manufacturing in the strongly non-stoichiometric ZrO_{2-y} oxide layer (i.e., as plotted in Fig. 7.11(b)), is given by:

$$\begin{aligned}\sigma_R(z) = &-3.2\times10^3\times\exp(0.15z - T) + 38.0\times\exp(0.65z - T)\\ &+0.9\times\exp(-0.9z) - 0.5\arctan(1.5 - z) - 0.57\end{aligned} \tag{7.18}$$

The stress magnitude determined by Raman spectroscopy in this work is in excellent agreement with the average residual stress measured by Hobbs *et al.* [936] at room temperature according to X-ray diffractometry (i.e., compressive stress equal –670 MPa). A closer examination of stoichiometry and stress results, as plotted in Figs. 7.11(a) and (b), respectively, suggests that the zirconium oxide surface layer formed in OXINIUM^{TM} joint components indeed possesses quite peculiar characteristics in both oxygen off-stoichiometry and residual stress. Moreover, the morphological similarity between the vacancy concentration and the residual stress profiles in Fig. 7.11 suggests a role of the former in the development of the latter distribution. In other words, peculiar mechanochemical characteristics could develop during the manufacturing process owing to two distinct but deeply intertwined elementary processes: (i) a differential shrinkage between bulk and surface due to a strong thermal expansion mismatch; and, (ii) the formation of a gradient in oxygen vacancy concentration, assisted by a valence switching effect in the thermally diffused Nb-ions. In this context, it should be noted that the lower thermal expansion coefficient of the oxide layer compared with the metal bulk introduces a residual stress component of compressive nature in the oxide film whose magnitude is directly proportional to the thermal expansion mismatch. On the other hand, diffusional effects concurrently take place to partly release such stress by means of the formation of a strong chemical gradient in the oxygen stoichiometry profile. Note that not only the formation of vacancies itself can partly relieve the compressive residual stress field, but also the increase in thermal expansion coefficient associated with an increase in oxygen vacancy concentration in the ZrO_{2-y} lattice [984,985] might lead, as a second-order effect, to reducing the thermal expansion mismatch between the oxide layer and the bulk metallic alloy. A fully quantitative rationalization of the contribution of different phenomena to the experimentally determined residual stress profile represents a quite formidable task and it would require a comparison among samples prepared by altering the processing parameters. What can be clearly stated here is that the mechanical stress state of the "native" ZrO_{2-y} oxide layer is quite peculiar and inherently different from that expected for a coating made of the same surface and bulk phases, but in the conspicuous absence of diffusional processes. When the residual stress is mainly dictated by a thermal expansion mismatch between film and substrate, no significant stress relaxation can be expected at the interface, as instead observed in OXINIUM^{TM}. Rather, stress intensification could be expected at the interface [918,986,987]. In other words, the obtainment of a strong compressive stress at the ceramic sample surface, which we have discussed above as being a quite desirable characteristic for achieving high wear resistance, will necessarily involve similarly strong shear stresses at the interface, thus increasing the possibility of local delamination and successive spalling of the coating during service. In conclusion, the spectroscopic results shown in this section not only demonstrate the uniqueness of OXINIUM™ as a structurally engineered and greatly innovative material for joint components, but also, as a general design concept, confirm the possibility of optimizing lattice stoichiometry gradients and residual stress fields at the bearing surface in order to concurrently achieve ceramic bearings with superior characteristics of wear resistance and environmental stability. This concept, which was already introduced in Chapter 5 in discussing bulk ceramic hip components, represents the key for future improvements of ceramic bearings in joint arthroplasty.

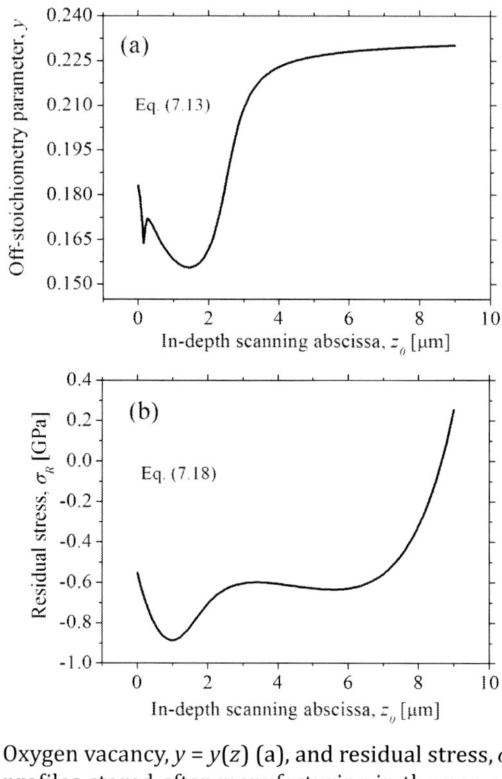

Figure 7.11 Oxygen vacancy, $y = y(z)$ (a), and residual stress, $\sigma_R = \sigma_R(z)$ (b), profiles stored after manufacturing in the non-stoichiometric ZrO_{2-y} oxide layer.

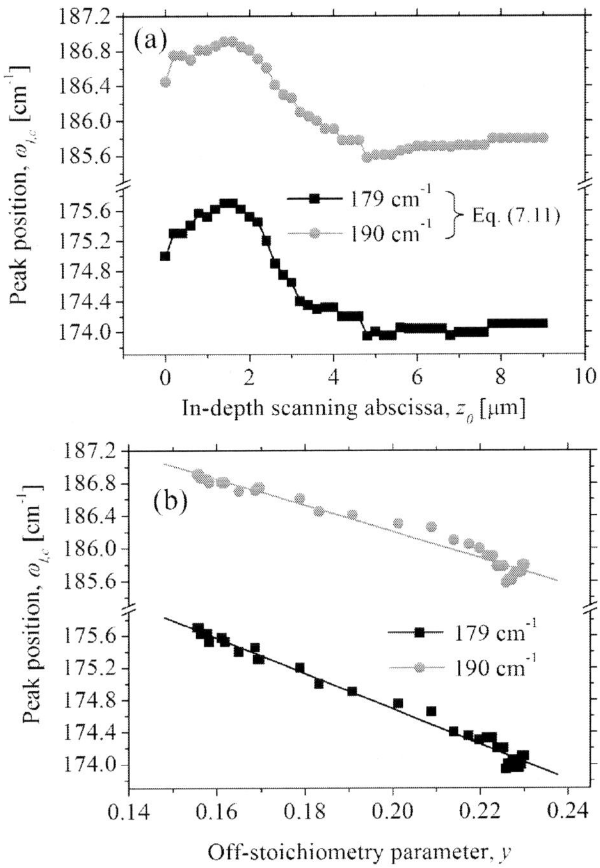

Figure 7.12 Chemistry-related variations in Raman band frequency, $\omega_{l,c}$, after Gaussian probe deconvolution in (a) and (b) as a function of in-depth abscissa, *z*, and vacancy concentration, *y*, respectively. The full lines in (b) represent best fits to the experimental trends.

In the introductive part of this section, we have mentioned about some potentially negative effects related to the excessive ductility of the Zr-2.5%Nb metal alloy that constitutes the bulk region of OXINIUM^{TM} hip components. Deformation and fracture modes of hard thin films bonded to soft substrates were studied by Hutchinson and Suo [988] and by Drory and Hutchinson [989] in their full theoretical and applicative details, respectively. Splitting and spalling/delamination of the film were located as the main failure mechanisms, whose occurrence is largely affected by the nature and by the magnitude of the residual stress field piled up during manufacturing. Compared with other possible combinations in which film and substrate possess similar characteristics of elastic deformation, the above failure mechanisms might result severely exacerbated during service loading for a soft substrate supporting a stiff film. This is, for example, the case of the strong mechanical contacts developed in the case of hard-on-hard bearing couples. One material parameter playing a fundamental role in maintaining the structural integrity of the ceramic oxide surface layer is its intrinsic fracture resistance (or toughness), whose quantitative characterization represents the first step in the assessments given hereafter.

The fracture toughness of a brittle and thin oxide layer cannot be evaluated by the standard fracture mechanics tests usually applied to bulk materials (cf. description in Section 2.6). On the other hand, micromechanical assessments need to be employed that locally analyze microcracks of controlled morphology, propagated within a tiny portion of surface material. One possibility is to use the local surface stress field developed by a pyramidal (i.e., Vickers) indentation. Upon indenting a brittle and homogeneous material, microscopic crack propagation usually occurs from the corners of the indentation print, and is locally driven by the elastoplastic strain components developed in the material beneath and immediately around the pyramidal indenter [295]. The elastic strain field acting upon an indented semi-infinite body greatly diminishes after unloading the indenter, but a residual driving force persists on the propagated crack even after load is removed. Such driving force arises from the local plastic deformation generated during contact between the indenter and the sample. If one considers that the generated microcrack is exactly arrested at the critical stress intensity factor, K_{IC}, which should be exceeded for obtaining its further opening and propagation [298], it follows that a quantitative evaluation of the local crack-tip K_{IC} parameter can directly lead to the assessment of material toughness. Two fully quantitative methods have been proposed for such fracture mechanics evaluation: (i) measurements of crack-opening displacements (COD) in a region close to the crack tip in the scanning electron microscope [296–298]; and, (ii) measurements of Raman wavenumber shifts by operating a line scan ahead of the indentation crack with operating a translation of the center of the laser probe along a selected direction with displacements of submicrometric precision [282,990–992]. Fracture toughness assessments by the two methods listed above should be considered as complementary to each other, since the COD profile developed behind the crack tip and the stress profile developed ahead of it actually represent two different aspects of the same quasi-equilibrium phenomenon of a surface crack on the verge of its extension. However, while in a bulk material the K_{IC} value measured at equilibrium unequivocally represents the intrinsic toughness of the material, for a crack embedded in a thin layer of material bonded to a soft substrate, the measured K_{IC} value might be affected by extrinsic effects related to the properties of the substrate material and their mismatch with those of the film. This assertion will be further substantiated later in this section. Here, we shall first apply the two methods (i) and (ii) mentioned above to measure the *extrinsic* toughness properties of the zirconium oxide scale on the surface of the OXINIUM^{TM} hip components. The term *extrinsic* is then used for emphasizing that the toughness value retrieved by those methods does not represent the intrinsic fracture resistance of the oxide material, but is affected by the presence of a relatively soft substrate in the particular geometry of the oxide film. Figure 7.13(a) shows a portion of Vickers indentation printed on the surface of the OXINIUM^{TM} component with a load of 50 N, while the enlarged scanning electron micrograph in Fig. 7.13(b) represents a magnified part of the near-tip profile of the small crack in Fig. 7.13(a), propagated from the corner of the indentation. From the micrographs, one could notice that despite the non-negligible magnitude of the indentation load applied to the brittle oxide layer, crack propagation resulted in a quite short length (e.g., the same indentation load applied to a baddeleyite single-crystal sample would result in several times longer crack-length propagation). The amount of crack extension developed on the surface of the OXINIUM^{TM} hip component still results in almost one order of magnitude longer propagation than the thickness of the oxide layer, but the limited crack propagation length observed in the inherently brittle oxide layer represents indeed the consequence of an extrinsic effect that should be attributed to the presence of the compliant metallic substrate. A proof for such assertion can be obtained by examining cracks propagated under different indentation loads. While Vickers indentations printed with loads $P < 50$ N led, as expected, to the development of shorter cracks, further increases in indentation load beyond 50 N produced cracks whose length tended to saturate at around 40 μm (cf. Fig. 7.13(c)). Moreover, when the equilibrium stress intensity factor was measured by the COD method (i.e., the above method (i)) on shorter cracks, it displayed apparently lower toughness values. Obviously, the crack morphology obtained by indenting a brittle and thin oxide layer bonded to a tough and compliant metallic substrate is quite different from the fully developed half-penny-shaped crack that could be obtained upon indenting a bulk ceramic sample. The shallow crack developed by indenting the oxide film is expected to span with similar length the entire film depth, but then to arrest at the ceramic/metal interface due to the high resilience of the bulk metallic alloy. Figure 7.14(a) shows a direct comparison between two COD profiles collected in the scanning electron microscope from cracks propagated under 10 and 50 N indentation loads. Anomalous crack geometry is expected for the indentation cracks propagated in the oxide film compared with the customary median-crack morphology of fully developed indentation cracks. Nevertheless, according to Fett [993], crack-tip K_{IC} computations are still possible for the very near-tip COD profile by following an approximate fracture mechanics procedure. Such computational procedure is based on using only a discrete number of initial terms for expressing the exact fracture mechanics solution in terms of a power series expansion of the crack length variable, r (i.e., with origin at the crack tip). The COD profiles, $2U(r)$, in Fig. 7.14(a), can then be rationalized by means of Fett's formalism, as follows:

$$2U(r) = K_{IC}(c)\frac{2\sqrt{c}}{\sqrt{\pi E'}}\ln\frac{c+\sqrt{c^2-(c-r)^2}}{(c-r)} = K_{IC}\Psi(r) \qquad (7.19)$$

where c is the length of the crack departed from the indentation corner and for the in-plane Young's modulus, $E' = E/(1 - \nu)$, (with ν being the Poisson ratio) a value should be selected that takes into account the composite nature of the sample. Regarding this latter parameter, it could be computed according to the following equation (cf. Appendix A in Ref. [994]):

$$E = E_s + \frac{2h}{\pi c}(E_f - E_s) \qquad (7.20)$$

where h is the average film thickness (i.e., 5 μm), and E_S and E_f are the Young's moduli of the metal alloy substrate and of the oxide film, respectively (i.e., 88 and 200 GPa, respectively).

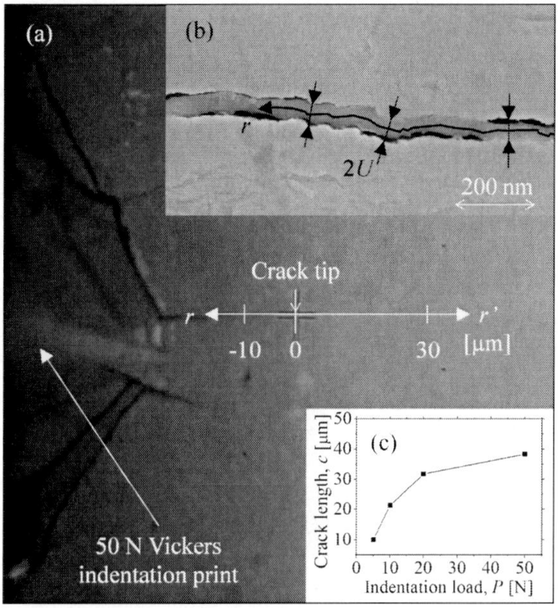

Figure 7.13 (a) Portion of Vickers indentation printed on the surface of the OXINIUM™ component with a load of 50 N; (b) COD displacements on enlarged scanning electron micrograph of the near-tip profile of the crack in (a) propagated from the corner of the indentation; and, (c) crack length as a function of indentation load.

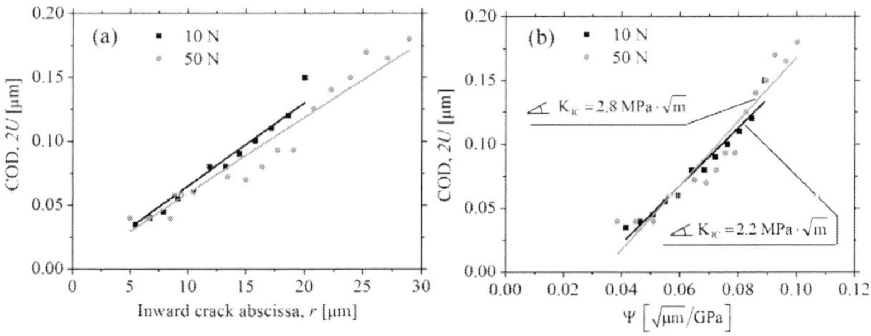

Figure 7.14 (a) Direct comparison between two COD profiles collected in the scanning electron microscope from cracks propagated under 10 and 50 N indentation loads. In (b), the data in (a) are replotted according to the formalism put forward in Eq. (7.19), in order to directly obtain apparent toughness values from the slopes of the plots. Full lines represent the results of a least square fitting routine applied to the respective sets of experimental data.

According to Eqs. (7.19) and (7.20), the plots shown in Fig. 7.14(a) could be converted into plots of $2U$ vs. Ψ, as shown in Fig. 7.14(b). From the respective slopes of these latter plots, we could retrieve constant values of K_{IC} = 2.2 and 2.8 MPa × $m^{1/2}$ for cracks propagated under indentation loads of 10 and 50 N (i.e., with crack extensions from the indentation corner of 21 and 38 μm), respectively. In other words, the toughness data showed a clear dependence on crack length, the longer the crack the higher the toughness. Figures 7.15(a) and (b) show the results of Raman scans for bands located at 179 and 190 cm^{-1}, as obtained along a straight line ahead of the tip of the crack in Fig. 7.13(a) (i.e., propagated from a 50 N-indentation corner). Unlike band broadening results, which showed negligible variations for both Raman bands, distinct band shifts could be recorded as a consequence of the residual stress gradient developed at the crack tip. Applying the usual proportionality relationship between stress and Raman frequency shift [117] in Eq. (7.17), stress-induced frequency shifts could be promptly converted into equi-biaxial stress magnitudes. The equi-biaxial stress field, $\sigma_{eq}(r')$, developed straight ahead of the crack (i.e., where an abscissa is now taken as, $r' = -r$) can be expressed according to the following equation [548, 995–997]:

$$\sigma_{eq}(r') = \frac{K_{IC}}{\sqrt{2\pi r'}} + \tilde{\Omega}(r') \tag{7.21}$$

where $\tilde{\Omega}(r')$ represents higher order terms that are negligible in the immediate neighborhood of the crack tip [996]. Given the steep stress gradient involved with Raman shift characterizations ahead of the crack tip, a Raman probe convolution procedure is needed for fitting the experimental results collected in Fig. 7.15. The spectral convolutive algorithm can be set, as follows [202, 203, 233, 990]:

$$\overline{\Delta\omega_l}(r_0', z_0) = \frac{\int_0^{+\infty}\int_0^{T} \wp(r_0', z_0, r', z) I_{l,c}(z) \left\{ \left[\frac{1}{3}\left(\frac{\partial\omega}{\partial p}\right)_l \frac{2K_{IC}}{\sqrt{2\pi r'}} \right] + \left[\omega_{l,c}(z) - \omega_{0,l} \right] \right\} dr'dz}{\int_{-\infty}^{+\infty}\int_0^{T} \wp(r_0', z_0, r', z)\, I_{l,c}(z) dr'dz} \tag{7.22}$$

where $\Delta\overline{\omega_l}\,(r_0', z_0) = \overline{\omega_l}\,(r_0', z_0) - \overline{\omega}_{0,l}$ is the frequency shift observed for the l-th Raman band at each location of the geometrical center of the Raman probe with respect to the frequency recorded at an unperturbed location far away from the indentation crack, $\overline{\omega_{0,l}}$; $I_{l,c}(z)$ and $\omega_{l,\mathrm{tot}}(z)$ are the deconvoluted profiles of Raman intensity and frequency shift along the thickness of the oxide scale for the *l*-th Raman band; and, the three-dimensional response function for the Raman probe is given as:

$$\wp(r_0',z_0,r',z)=\left\{\exp\left[\frac{-2(r'-r_0')^2}{B^2}\right]\right\}\times\frac{p^2}{p^2+(z-z_0)^2}\exp(-2\alpha_{\text{eff}}z) \tag{7.23}$$

where the parameters, *B*, *p*, and α_{eff} were obtained from preliminary calibrations of the optical probe on the ZrO_2 oxide layer as 2.6 μm, 2.2 μm, and 0.075 μm^{-1}, respectively. The results of an

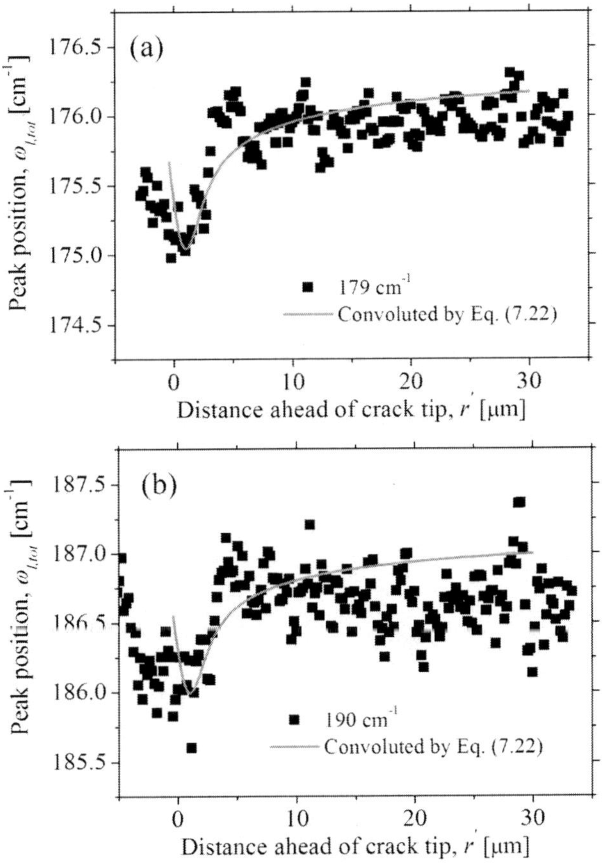

Figure 7.15 Results of Raman scans for bands located at 179 and 190 cm^{-1} (in (a) and (b), respectively), as obtained along a straight line ahead of the tip of the crack in Fig. 13(a) (i.e., 50 N-indented). Best fitting (full lines) was obtained according to Eq. (7.22).

iterative convolutive algorithm, based on Eqs. (7.22) and (7.23) and run to best fit the experimental band-shift data, are also plotted in Fig. 7.15. Best fitting could be achieved for both the investigated Raman bands with adopting an average toughness value, $K_{IC} = 2.6 \pm 0.1$ MPa × $m^{1/2}$, for the oxide film. This fracture toughness value, which is indeed in excellent agreement with the value 2.8 MPa × $m^{1/2}$ retrieved for the same crack by COD method, yet represents an extrinsic toughness parameter, since the indentation crack is arrested at an equilibrium position dictated not only by the intrinsic toughness of the film but also by the mechanical interaction between oxide film and metallic substrate. Clearly, the coating/substrate system reacts to the indentation load as an integral system with respect to the development of a plastic zone beneath the indenter. Film properties exclusively affect the developed crack length only in the case of very shallow indentations (i.e., indentation depths <7~10% of the film thickness [998, 999]), which is obviously not the case here. In this context, the fact that indentation loads >50 N produced only slightly longer crack despite a larger propagation driving force reflects a marked effect of plastic compliance in the substrate material. This extrinsic effect leads to the accumulation of increasingly larger displacements at the crack mouth, and thus to apparently higher values for the fracture toughness of the oxide film.

A method for extracting the intrinsic fracture toughness of a thin brittle film bonded to a compliant substrate has been proposed in a recent work by Demidova *et al.* [1000]. The computational algorithm of this model, which is based on a re-elaboration of the micromechanics of small Vickers indentation cracks, incorporates the effect of a mismatch in hardness between the film and the substrate. Moreover, the variation in indentation crack morphology (i.e., with respect to that developed in a bulk brittle material), which occurs in the case of a brittle film bonded on a ductile substrate, is also taken into due consideration in the model, including the possibility that the crack arrests at the bi-material interface. The intrinsic toughness of the oxide film, $K_{IC}^{(i)}$, is then expressed as

$$K_{IC}^{(i)} = 10^3 \times \chi_r Y_i \beta \frac{P_r}{c^{1.5}} \Phi(\varphi, k) \quad (\text{for: } 0 \le \varphi \le \pi) \tag{7.24}$$

where φ is a planar angle taken on the sample cross-section and comprised between a direction normal to the local crack front and the sample surface; P_r is the load transmitted on the composite structure, which is related to the indentation load, P, but affected by the geometry of the indenter (geometrical factor of the indenter, χ_r, and pyramidal indenter angle, ψ = 68°) [295] and by the "composite" hardness, H, representative of the integral film/substrate system [1001]:

$$P_r = \frac{P}{3(1-2\nu_f)} \times \left(\frac{E_f}{H}\right)^{0.5} \times \sqrt[3]{(\cot\psi)^2} \tag{7.25}$$

$$H = H_s + 3\left(\frac{2T}{D}\right)\left(\frac{H_f}{E_f}\right)^{0.5} \times (H_f - H_s)\sqrt[3]{\tan\psi} \tag{7.26}$$

$$\chi_r \approx \frac{1}{3\pi^2(1-\nu_f)} \times \left(\frac{E_f}{H}\right)^{0.5} \times \sqrt[3]{(\cot\psi)^2} \tag{7.27}$$

where H, E and ν are hardness, Young's modulus, and Poisson ratio, respectively; the subscripts "f" and "s" locate film and substrate, respectively (ν_f = 0.34 and E_f = 200 GPa for monoclinic ZrO_2; H_s = 3.5 GPa and H_f = 14 GPa for Zr-2.5%Nb alloy and monoclinic ZrO_2, respectively); and, D is the diagonal of the indentation print. The geometry of the indentation crack is that of a partly developed semi-elliptical crack, arrested at the film/metal interface. The stress intensification at the tip of such crack can be expressed by matching the Borodachev's solution [1002] for an elliptical crack under a concentrated force applied at its center (product, $\beta \times \Phi(\varphi,k)$) with an interface correction factor as expressed according to the analysis by the Noda *et al.* [1003] analysis for an elliptical crack near a bi-material interface (correction factor, Y_i):

$$\Phi(\varphi, k) = \left(1 + \frac{k^2}{1-k^2}\sin^2\varphi\right)^{0.25} \times \frac{1}{1-k^2\sin^2\varphi} \tag{7.28}$$

$$k^2 = 1 - \left(\frac{a}{c}\right)^2 \tag{7.29}$$

$$\beta = \frac{\pi}{2(1-k^2)^{0.5} \times \int_0^{\pi/2} \Phi(\varphi,k) \times \left(1+\frac{k^2}{1-k^2}\sin^2\varphi\right) d\varphi} \tag{7.30}$$

$$Y_\mathrm{i} = \frac{1+\frac{E_\mathrm{s}}{E_\mathrm{f}}\cos^{0.25}\left(\frac{\pi a \sin\varphi}{2T}\right)}{\frac{E_\mathrm{s}}{E_\mathrm{f}}+\cos^{0.25}\left(\frac{\pi a \sin\varphi}{2T}\right)} \quad (\text{for: } 0 < \varphi < \pi) \tag{7.31}$$

where a is the crack depth, which is taken here as the film thickness since the crack propagated in the brittle oxide film is arrested at the interface; and, E_s = 88 GPa. Upon indenting the OXINIUM™ surface with 10, 20, and 50 N, we obtained indentation prints with diagonal lengths, D = 85, 126, and 205 μm and crack extensions from the indentation corners of 21.3, 31.8, and 38.3 μm, respectively. Calculations of an *intrinsic* toughness value for the monoclinic ZrO_2 film using cracks propagated upon indenting with different loads and according to Eqs. (7.24)~(7.31) consistently yielded a critical stress intensity factor, $K_{IC}^{(i)}$ = 0.6 ± 0.1 MPa × $m^{1/2}$, namely a constant value four to five times smaller than the apparent toughness measured by direct crack-tip methods. A closer analysis of the dependence on elastic property mismatch between film and substrate, as expressed according to Eq. (7.31), reveals that the larger the elastic mismatch, the stronger the extrinsic (apparent) toughening effect operated by the presence of the substrate. In other words, a compliant substrate tends to pull the crack toward the interface with greatly limiting its longitudinal extension on the surface of the brittle film. This means that if the substrate is highly tough and compliant, the crack will arrest at the interface and will remain confined into limited surface regions. The substrate of OXINIUM™ femoral head components is a quite ductile Zr-2.5%Nb alloy and its fracture toughness can be estimated in the order of 75~96 MPa × $m^{1/2}$ [1004–1006], which is comparable to or even higher than steel [1007], and much higher than the surface oxide fracture toughness and of that of any bulk ceramic biomaterial so far discovered. Therefore, any crack, occasionally formed as a consequence of extrinsic factors, on the OXINIUM™ surface not only will remain confined in its depth within the oxide film but will also hardly spread through the surface of the oxide film, which proves the extremely high structural reliability of the OXINIUM^{TM} joint components.

The choice of a highly tough substrate is fully justified by the need of a high structural reliability in artificial hip joints. However, there are also structural disadvantages in this choice, since tough materials are generally also those most easily deforming in a plastic fashion. Recently, Galetz *et al.* [954] have reviewed this important point with discussing the film/substrate adhesion properties of OXINIUM^{TM} in comparison with TiN-coated CoCrMo and Zr-2.5%Nb alloys. Conical (Rockwell) indentation tests were systematically performed in order to allow for an estimation of what might happen if a large puncturing load is applied on those different samples (e.g., in the case of an hard-on-hard contact in a hip implant). Indentation tests showed that fewer (but larger) cracks were visible around indentation printed on OXINIUM^{TM} in comparison with those in TiN-coated alloys, a clear indication for the higher adhesion strength of the former sample. Our Vickers indentation data show good agreement with the Rockwell indentation data in Ref. [954], with the observation of a limited number of cracks running parallel to the indentation edges in the zone around the indentation print (cf. Fig. 7.13(a)). Moreover, no delamination of the oxide layer could be observed under any of the investigated loading conditions. As additional damage introduced by indenting hard coatings bonded to ductile substrates, shear steps on the indented surface, and edge or inclined cracks around it were reported for TiN films on steel substrate. None of the damage could be observed on the indented surface of OXINIUM^{TM}. This should be considered as a remarkable result since TiN-coated steel has long been recognized as a standard for its superior adhesion characteristics [1008, 1009]. However, unlike harder alloys such as CoCrMo, loads of even small magnitudes superimposed on the Zr-2.5%Nb alloy might result in relatively large and deep plastic hollows (i.e., depths is the order of 100 μm under 50 N indentation load). In other words, a catastrophic outcome can be foreseen in the case of repeated hard-on-hard contacts. Especially when, for any reasons, the oxide layer of OXINIUM^{TM} should fail and the bare metal become exposed, the effect on surface integrity could be devastating, as described for the rare *in vivo* cases of dislocation for femoral heads made of oxidized zirconium [949,1010]. On the other hand, we have shown that suitable gradients of oxygen off-stoichiometry and residual stress, as developed along the subsurface of the fully transformed monoclinic ZrO_2 layer, resulted in a fundamental synergism for maximizing adhesion between oxide layer and substrate. Unfortunately, extraordinary high loads can occur *in vivo* for a hard-on-hard bearing couple even under normal service conditions. From this viewpoint, the indentation print might closely simulate the kind of damage that brittle surfaces suffer from incidental contacts with hard counterparts. Since the hardness of the bulk material determines the amount of local deformation, still, the relatively soft zirconium alloy substrate remains the main weak point of OXINIUM™ joint components. Unlike the case of a soft counterpart as polyethylene, hard-on-hard coupling might lead to local deformations with the potential to cause severe damage to the ceramic layer. From this perspective, the deformation properties of the bulk Zr-2.5%Nb alloy of OXINIUM™ joint components seem yet to require a substantial improvement before allowing a safe use in hard-on-hard bearing components. Research in this direction is already ongoing, which involves the modification of the geometry of the oxide layer of OXINIUM™, as well as a modified gradient of oxygen concentration through it [1011].

7.2 Innovative Surgical Techniques and New Upcoming Biomaterials

Besides the significant improvements achieved, as summarized in Chapters 5 and 6, and in the previous section, in quality and innovation of bearing biomaterials, the last decade has also brought to us many important technical advances in the surgical methods and procedures for hip replacement. This is a quite important topic in the field of arthroplasty because it is clear that any paradigmatic improvement in hip arthroplasty will always arise from the concurrent actions of biomaterials scientists, implant designers, and medical doctors. However, a full description of the innovative surgical techniques stems somewhat at the margins of the contents of this book, dedicated to biomaterials and their analytical characterizations. Thus, the description given here will necessarily be a concise one, with the main emphasis placed on the interconnections between different surgical approaches and biomaterial properties.

An increasingly spreading trend in total hip replacement consists nowadays in minimizing surgical exposure, which in turn involves a less traumatic impact on the muscles surrounding the hip joint and greatly helps to expedite postoperative recovery. One such procedure is commonly referred to as the mini-hip incision. The major benefit of this innovative procedure, i.e., the smaller incision (10 to 12 cm in length rather than the standard 25 cm incision), also involves less blood loss, faster rehabilitation, and decreased pain. However, significant discussion has occurred over the last decade about the suitability of performing total hip replacements with using smaller incisions, because of possible post-operative complications such as a higher rate of dislocations. Basically, a less invasive implantation of the total hip components becomes possible upon the modification of different surgical hip accesses, including posterior, lateral, anterolateral and anterior approaches [1012–1014]. Moreover, approaches with both single and double incision have been explored [1015,1016]. As a consequence of using new (and quite uncommon) approaches (e.g., the double-incision technique), minimally invasive procedures might also require special training for surgeons, involving a possibly extended learning curve. Appropriate patient selection and the experience of the surgeon become then, more critically than in the case of "traditional" hip surgeries, key factors for a successful application of minimally invasive approaches. Despite the fact that such procedures are becoming increasingly popular, experts have argued that the length of the skin incision could be by far less important when compared with disruption of muscles (needed in some approach), impairment of soft-tissue, vascularization and innervation, or preservation of bone. The need of optimizing all the outputs renders the selected surgical approach an item of fundamental importance. The so-called direct anterior approach [1017,1018], independent of the length of skin incision, would require no muscular dissection in order to expose the hip joint.

Such approach represents the shortest and most direct way to the hip joint. Accordingly, no injury to hip abductor muscles occurs, as in the case of lateral or anterolateral approaches. Since the acetabulum can be clearly visualized, easy orientation is also possible, although control of the femoral implant position could result somewhat more difficult to achieve [1018]. The main negative aspect stems from the limited visibility and exposure of anatomical landmarks, which might increase the risk of implant malalignement, thus possibly leading to an inferior long-term result in terms of wear and durability. The situation could be improved by using computer navigation assistance, but navigation procedures that could be adapted to minimally invasive implantation of the hip joint appear to be yet under development [1019].

Technological advances in computed navigation and simulation techniques, as mentioned above, can lead to greater precision and accuracy in acetabular positioning and limb length management [1020–1026]. Navigation surgery can be considered as yet standing in a process of continuous evolution, aimed at rendering it highly reproducible and capable of providing more and more reliable information. Accurate registration of three-dimensional bony anatomy, coupled with real-time tracking during surgery, potentially allow optimal component placement as well as balancing of limb length to ensure optimal clinical outcome. Misalignment of the hip prosthesis, which can cause loosening and consequent revision surgery, can be conspicuously avoided by using computer-assisted total hip replacement to insure correct positioning of the total hip. The computer navigation system uses transmitters and an infrared camera, which sends messages and displays images of the patient anatomy on the computer. The use of computer navigation in hip surgery allows the surgeon to place components with a precision accuracy, which cannot be accomplished with the naked eye. In total hip arthroplasty, several navigation systems are available that offer navigated cup positioning or workflows for navigating the positions of both cup and shaft. The resulting geometry of the articulation is also displayed, while the navigation monitors acetabular cup positioning in relation to the palpation of the anterior pelvic plane. Inclination, anteversion, insertion depth and shifting of head center are displayed during acetabular reaming and cup implantation. In addition, during femoral preparation, a continuous monitoring of femoral antetorsion, lateral offset and leg length change are also displayed. The resulting range of motion is finally calculated according to the selected modular head and acetabular cup liner options. The two main options available for navigating implant positioning in total hip replacement consist in image guided procedures and kinematic navigation. The former type of system employs pre-operative CT scans or intra-operative fluoroscopy. Its disadvantages are the need for additional exposure to radiation, pre- and intra-operative time consumption and a limited accuracy. Kinematic navigation systems are instead based on the registration of intraoperative landmarks and kinematic data, which are acquired during both pre- and intra-surgical procedures. It has been developed according to a different paradigm, more based on daily routine and intuitive handling. Navigation adds to the accuracy of cup positioning even for experienced surgeons, the gain in accuracy exceeding the gain in accuracy resulting from the increasing experience of the individual surgeon. Navigation technology also comprises popular procedures in the field of total knee arthroplasty [1027–1029], for which, however, it could result easier (i.e., compared with hip arthroplasty) to define a uniform optimal implant position. The actual limitations of the hip navigation technology include the difficulty of palpation of the anterior pelvic plane especially in a lateral patient position, the additional surgical time required (10~15 min), and the fact that stem navigation is not yet fully optimized for minimally invasive surgical approaches. Nevertheless, navigation might become increasingly important upon its further development with increasing the popularity of minimal invasive approaches to hip surgery. As discussed above, such approaches mainly suffer for limitations regarding exposure of anatomical landmarks and orientation of endoprosthetic devices.

Hip resurfacing is a surgical technique that has become a popular alternative to conventional hip replacement over the last decade in young and active patients. Hip resurfacing involves replacing the femoral head surface with a metal cap, while no stem is inserted into the proximal femoral shaft. The main advantage of this type of surgery is that the femoral bone stock is preserved for possible future revisions. Moreover, by just replacing the surface, the natural biomechanical function of the joint is restored with minimal alterations. Resurfacing algorithms usually lead to a larger head size compared with conventional hip arthroplasty, in order to lower the dislocation rate. On the other hand, the acetabulum is replaced with a metal socket as during standard hip replacements. The bearing surfaces are both metallic, so no polyethylene surface is involved with the sliding process. In its early stage of development, hip resurfacing generated poor results, possibly because metal-on-plastic couples were used. On the other hand, midterm results over the last decade are showing very promising results for some commercially available implants with metal-on-metal bearings. One main concern about resurfacing surgery resides in a femoral neck fracture, which might occur post-operatively [1030]. This unfortunate event would be more common when bone density is low, i.e., in older patients, female patients or in patients having a history of inflammatory arthritis. Another concern is the possible loosening of the femoral cap because of avascular necrosis of the remaining femoral head [1031]. However, the most striking issue regarding hip resurfacing can be located in the elevation of blood metal ion levels that unavoidably occurs post-operatively as a consequence of metal-on-metal surface sliding. The fact that high concentrations of cobalt and chrome in the serum and urine of patients results from the wear of modern metal-on-metal prosthesis components indeed represents an experimental evidence that cannot be easily disregarded [1032–1037]. Savarino *et al.* [1038] recently reported significant increase of cobalt, chromium and aluminum levels in patients with metal-on-metal total hip replacement. Prospective clinical studies have also shown that an enormous increase of cobalt and chromium ions in blood and urine levels should be expected after hip resurfacing arthroplasty [1039], although no study has yet clearly located a safe or a toxic dose of cobalt or chromium in the human body [1040]. Hart *et al.* [1041] have reported that the levels of cobalt and chromium ions in blood are associated with the numbers of circulating lymphocytes. Adverse local immune responses have also been reported in association with metal-on-metal bearings [1042]. The implant options on both femoral head and acetabular sides might differ significantly in resurfacing, with direct impact on the amount of released metal ions. Despite the risks above described, marketing of hip resurfacing has been relatively aggressive around the world, pulling on the arguments that resurfacing is particularly appealing to the younger and active population. In the meanwhile, long-term results are still pending. Moreover, in 2007, analyses of data reported by the Australian National Joint Replacement Registry first suggested that the DePuy metal-on-metal ASR resurfacing hip implant (approved for use in Australia since 2004) was associated with a higher than average replacement rate. Data were put before an independent expert advisory committee, which advised that the higher rates of revision for this type of ASR hip prosthesis were most probably due to the technical complexity of correctly siting the device during surgery. It was recommended that additional training and education be provided to surgeons to fix the problem. A further recommendation was that of continuing monitoring the situation through the National Registry to verify the effectiveness of this additional training. DePuy Orthopaedics agreed to provide additional training to surgeons on the correct insertion technique. In 2009, the monitoring procedure of the performance of the ASR hip prosthesis revealed that the rate of hip revisions remained of concern. Accordingly, the ASR resurfacing hip implant was removed from the Australian market in December 2009. In August 2010, DePuy Orthopaedics recalled its hip resurfacing ASR devices after it was implanted in about 93000 people worldwide, due to a high rate of revision surgeries [1043]. The general concern was that owing to a defective design, the metal surfaces wore down at significantly accelerated rates, with metal particles being extensively released and biologically reacting with the soft tissue surrounding the joint before entering the bloodstream. Despite the quite successful application of other types of resurfacing hip devices, such painful and detrimental failures in implant design, as in the case of the ASR implant, strongly delay technological development and significantly increase the costs for developing new arthroplastic devices.

It is yet a quite common understanding in arthroplasty that there are hardly options on the type of bearing surface in hip resurfacing, surface replacement being nowadays only possible through the metal-on-metal implant technology. This belief stems from the understanding that the components involved with resurfacing implants are relatively thin compared with conventional hip components and thus require a level of structural reliability that only metals seem to guarantee at the actual technological state of material development. Ceramic-on-ceramic hip prostheses have been widely regarded as quite body-friendly implants, owing to their excellent biocompatibility and minimum wear rate upon *in vivo* loading [1044, 1045]. No toxic effect has been reported since the last 40 years of their use [421, 501, 1046–1050]. Recently, several authors have started suggesting that ceramic articulations may actually represent a valid alternative for future breakthrough develop-ments in hip resurfacing prostheses [1050–1052]. According to the need for high strength and reliability of components used in hip resurfacing implants, the use of non-oxide ceramics like silicon nitride and silicon carbide has been recommended [1053]. A preliminary study from Cappi *et al.* [1054] has shown the cytocompatibility of such high strength non-oxide ceramics, which thus makes those materials primary candidates for ceramic resurfacing hip prostheses. Silicon nitride and silicon carbide materials with engineered microstructures certainly exhibit better mechanical behavior compared with monolithic alumina [1055–1057], which is presently the most used ceramic in total hip arthroplasty. This would certainly represent a benefit for hip implant materials, explicitly in terms of an improved safety factor. However, the long-term failure probability remains an issue to be clarified, which mainly deals with the delayed-failure behavior of non-oxide materials or, more precisely, to their resistance to the subcritical growth of internal cracks propagating from pre-existing defects under the combined actions of static/dynamic load and environmental attack [1058, 1059]. Evaluations of the failure probability under subcritical crack growth conditions performed with using crack growth parameters under normal laboratory conditions (e.g., even with employing tests at 60% of relative humidity) obviously do not represent a sufficiently valid reference for hip prosthesis designs. In fact, it is known that the crack-growth parameters in non-oxide ceramics are (detrimentally) dependent on temperature and humidity according to a power exponential law [1059, 1060]. The values of the exponential and pre-exponential parameters constitutive of the crack growth law are strongly affected by humidity [1061]. The dependence of such parameters on an increase in humidity is indeed a complex one and depends on the particular material and additives used for its densification, but unavoidably it show an increase in subcritical crack growth rate, therefore it accelerates a reduction in strength with time. Moreover, we have seen in Chapter 3 through 5 that even the extremely stable surfaces of oxide ceramics can be severely affected in their local stoichiometry by the extreme environmentally driven stress-assisted phenomena occurring in a hip joint. It has been rigorously demonstrated that these surface stoichiometry effects have a direct impact on the plastic behavior of the crystalline network exposed to the surface and, consequently, on the wear behavior of the entire bearing surface [365–367, 1062]. Fisher and Tomizawa [1063] studied in detail the interaction of tribochemistry and microfracture in the friction and wear of self-mating silicon nitride. Unlike the experimental results found by Rainforth and coworkers for alumina [365–367], no evidence of plastic deformation was found for this non-oxide material. In water and humidity-saturated gases, wear predominantly occurred via a tribochemical reaction that produced an amorphous protective layer in humid gas and dissolution in liquid water. This result is in line with a detailed study by Dong and Jahanmir [1064] showing that at relatively low temperatures, the tribological behavior of silicon nitride is controlled by tribochemical reactions between the silicon nitride surface and the water vapor in the environment. In an intermediate humidity environment, wear became a combination of fracture and tribochemistry, the latter factor increasing adhesion between wear particles to form a layer of compacted wear particles on the wear track. Differences in chemical reactivity and susceptibility to stress corrosion cracking between alumina and silicon nitride might lead to fundamental differences (eventually positive for the latter materials) in wear behavior in humid environment, but such differences should yet be rigorously evaluated and interpreted with respect to arthroplastic applications. Regarding subcritical crack growth, however, the presence of an intrinsic amount of silicon oxide at the grain boundary of polycrystalline silicon nitride (i.e., a native oxide stemming since raw powder oxidation and leaching in the presence of hot steam), remains a concern in the structural reliability of the material. The native amount of amorphous silica in high-purity raw silicon carbide powders can be significantly lower than that found in silicon nitride powders of comparable purity. Therefore, the risk of leaching effects at grain boundaries in dense polycrystalline samples could be somewhat reduced in silicon carbide materials compared with silicon nitride. Nevertheless, a later experimental report by Dong *et al.* [1065] showed that at room temperature, under high loads and high environmental humidity, also the tribological behavior of sintered silicon carbide is controlled by tribochemical reactions between the silicon carbide surface and water vapor in the environment. Under low loads and at temperatures <250°C, wear occurs by ploughing and polishing. On the other hand, at temperatures >250°C and under low loads, tribo-oxidation and formation of cylindrical wear particles control the tribological behavior. Surface microfracture is the mechanism controlling wear when the load is increased above a critical value, with increasing both friction coefficient and wear coefficients. In our *in situ* spectroscopic studies of wear behavior in self-mating oxide ceramics, reported in Chapter 5, we have shown how under wear testing conditions considered standard for hip joints, quite high local temperatures and stresses can be achieved at the contact point between hard sliding surfaces. Such extreme conditions indeed appear to stand close to the thermo-mechanical threshold for tribo-oxidation and formation of wear particles assessed for silicon carbide in the wear transition map compiled by Dong *et al.* [1065]. Therefore, a validation of the suitability of such non-oxide materials is required with respect to their wear behavior in human joints. For the rich body of the above-mentioned reasons, it is quite natural that biomaterials scientists continue to skeptically look at the performance of non-oxide ceramics, with their well-known natural attitude to oxidize in the extremely severe environments as the human joints, until final experimental proofs for their environmental resistance with respect to both subcritical crack growth and chemically assisted wear behavior will be rigorously provided.

So far, while no resurfacing implant made of ceramics has yet been submitted for regulatory approval or commercialized, the ceramic implant that could be considered the most innovative from the design viewpoint is probably the so-called DeltaMotion®-System designed by (the former) Finsbury Orthopaedics [1066, 1067]. This innovative implant yet employs an oxide material, the BIOLOX®*delta* ceramic composite extensively discussed in Chapter 5 of this book. With its high strength and toughness, the BIOLOX®*delta* ceramic allowed an "aggressive" implant design including relatively thin acetabular cups, which in turn permit the introduction of larger head diameters (in the diameter range between 32 and 48 mm) in relatively small diameter liners (from 42 to 66 mm). The substantial increase in bearing size then allows larger ranges of motion and better stability of the replaced hip joint, so far only possible using large diameter metal-on-metal devices. According to the National Joint Registry of England and Wales (JREW) [1068], on a total number of 42312 cementless cup implanted in 2010, only 626 belonged to the DeltaMotion® -System. Despite the innovative design, the selection rate by UK surgeons yet remained in the order of <1%.

In Chapter 6, the clinical performance of first-generation polyethylene liners was discussed in details. The benefits of the reduction in femoral head penetration and the clinical relevance of *in vivo* oxidation and wear reduction in the long-term exposure, which are expected with the second-generation of highly cross-linked polyethylene liners, were reviewed in the light of new experimental data by confocal Raman spectroscopy. Improvements are expected according to two different stabilization strategies: addition of natural antioxidants (e.g., vitamin E) or sequential irradiation and annealing processes [847,853,1069–1072]. In sequentially annealed liners, experimental studies proved that thin components maintained a similar wear rate compared with thicker components, thus confirming that thin components should not be considered as disadvantageous under suitable processing and design formulations [1073]. This argument is quite relevant in support of the possibility of using larger heads, which, given the enlarged range of motion they might allow, presumably free the femoral head from damage by local liner impingement [1074]. In vitamin E-stabilized materials, independent of whether the antioxidant is blended with polyethylene at the time of consolidation or vitamin E diffused through the consolidated polymer, possibility has been shown for oxidation to be conspicuously controlled, as shown by experiments on materials after 36 months of artificial aging [1075]. Moreover, in such doped materials post-irradiation oxidation decreased with increasing vitamin

E concentrations [1076], while vitamin E dopant in amounts <0.1 wt.% was shown not to affect the mechanical properties of polyethylene [1077]. Besides the many encouraging results with vitamin E doping, however, new antioxidant strategies have also been paid attention to and are presently under development. Such strategies foresee the use of different free-radical scavengers, as nitroxide-2,2,6,6-tetramethylpiperidine-1-oxyl (TEMPO) [1078–1081], hindered amine light stabilizers (HALS) [1082–1085], and anthocyanin extracts [1086], which could eventually become valid antioxidant alternatives to vitamin E. Nitroxides are stable organic compounds that have a strong paramagnetic signal and are very efficient in preventing lipid peroxidation and providing radioprotection in biological tissues [1079, 1080]. Moreover, nitroxides are also quite efficient carbon-centered free radical scavengers [1081], which can suitably delay oxidation *in vivo*. Carbon-centered free radicals in UHMWPE will quite effectively combine with the nitroxide radical through the electron transfer mechanism. However, attention should be paid to the effect that the addition of TEMPO can have on the polyethylene microstructure. Similar to what we have discussed in Chapter 6 for the case of vitamin E doping [843], if UHMWPE is doped with the nitroxide before irradiation, cross-linking inhibition could occur. This has been the main argument in support of *a posteriori* infusion of the dopant into the cross-linked polymer rather than its initial blend with the polymer powder. In the case of dopant infusion, the number of existing carbon-centered free radicals, which depends on the irradiation dose, could be predicted or measured. Thus, if the residual free radical concentration is known after cross-linking, a minimal amount of TEMPO antioxidant can be infused into the polymer to scavenge the rest of the free radicals. By following the infusion approach after cross-linking and quantifying the concentration of nitroxides needed to scavenge the known concentration of alkyl, allyl, and peroxyl radicals, one could thus manage all of the infused nitroxide be consumed through radical scavenging, eliminating the concern that elution of residual antioxidant out of the prosthesis could occur in any deleterious amount. As far as HALS is concerned, its mechanism of action in the environmental stabilization of polyethylene is intrinsically different from that of the radical scavenger vitamin E [1083–1085]. As vitamin E directly reacts with alkyl radicals, it can also interfere in the cross-linking process. Because vitamin E is partly consumed during irradiation of the sample, a decreased cross-link density might result at a given radiation dose compared with an undoped material. On the other hand, HALS itself does not directly scavenge radicals, its conversion into a nitroxide being preliminary necessary to activate its radical scavenging activity. As this does not happen during radiation, HALS not only remains unconsumed during irradiation but also does not have any negative influence on cross-link density.

Additions of secondary phases to obtain nanoscale modifications are also presently researched in order to reinforce the polyethylene structure while maintaining (or even improving) its oxidation resistance. Polyethylene-matrix multiwall carbon nanoube-reinforced composites [1087–1091], addition of lanthanides to the polyethylene structure (e.g., Eu ions obtained from the addition to the polyethylene powder of Eu(II)-stearate, fabricated from sodium stearate and europium nitrate [1092]), and polyethylene grafting by means of 2-methacryloyloxyethyl-phosphorylcholine (MPC) polymer [1093–1095] represent three of the latest examples of these attempts. A brief description of the salient achievements obtained by these new processing methods is given hereafter. However, it is anticipated at the outset that all such possibly new refinements of polyethylene at the molecular scale will need strict experimental and clinical validations before their conceptual foundations could prove possessing appropriate solidity. Zoo *et al.* [1096] added multiwall carbon nanotubes to UHMWPE and investigated the impact of such addition on the tribological properties of the material by means of ball-on-disc wear testing. The results of such testing showed that the wear loss of the 0.5 wt.% nanotube-added material decreased by about 90% compared with the monolithic UHMWPE matrix. On the other hand, the coefficient of friction increased, but only slightly, as the weight percentage of nanotubes increased. The improvement in properties was ascribed to an increase in shear strength of the UHMWPE caused by addition of the stiff carbon nanotube reinforcement. In a more recent paper, also Johnson *et al.* [1097] reported decreasing wear rates with increasing nanotube content in high-density polyethylene composites, while not negatively affecting other material properties. Moreover, a reduction in the coefficient of friction could also be noticed in that same study. The next steps in developing UHMWPE-matrix carbon nanotube composites appear to necessarily involve the development of improved techniques for dispersing the nanotubes in the polymeric matrix and for molding the obtained homogeneous blend. So far unavailable determinations of material surface characteristics, including wear debris size and uniformity, and a precise evaluation of the biological reactivity of the wear debris, will then link the characterization outputs more directly to clinical applications.

The addition of elements belonging to the lanthanide group (e.g., Eu(II)) is pursued based on the hypothesis that their addition would prevent oxidation of molded polyethylene components. According to the peculiar electron configuration of such ions, one would expect that selected lanthanide ions would readily accept one electron, and therefore actively scavenge radicals in addition to hindering oxidative reactions in irradiated and successively *in vivo* exposed polyethylene. Preliminary experimental results collected by Gallardo *et al.* [1092] showed that the addition of Eu(II)-stearate effectively improved the oxidation resistance to environmental aging of UHMWPE, while also improving the mechanical performance in its load-bearing capacity (81% improvement in load to failure retention versus conventional UHMWPE), ductility (51% improvement in retention of deformation to failure with respect to conventional UHMWPE), and energy absorption (improvement of work to failure by about 60% compared with conventional UHMWPE). As in the case of carbon nanotube addition, however, the complex effects generated by adding lanthanide compounds on both homogeneous mixing and compression molding procedures need further investigations, including the determination of optimum dopant doses. Moreover, the actual antioxidation mechanism has yet to be clarified, although it has been suggested to arise from steric hindrance induced by the random allocation of europium-stearates on the free radicals produced by high-energy irradiation on the polyethylene backbone chains [1092].

MPC is a methacrylate monomer that possesses a phospholipid polar group in a side chain as found in the neutral phospholipids of biomembranes. Many polymers consisting of various MPC units have been widely used as biomaterials [1098, 1099], as well as various medical devices including MPC polymer components have already been developed and clinically approved [1099–1101]. The original idea of developing new artificial joints with highly lubricated bearing surfaces produced by photo-induced MPC radical graft polymerization [1102] is based on the double aspect of biocompatibility and hydrophilicity of this polymer. The procedure of grafting MPC directly to cross-linked polyethylene and thus forming C–C covalent bonds between the polyethylene substrate and the MPC polymer, was found to reduce by 88% the friction coefficient of cross-linked acetabular liners compared with untreated liners [1095]. Moreover, even after several millions of cycles in hip joint simulator, the wear rate of grafted polyethylene liners remained low. One important advantage of the photo-induced radical graft polymerization technique is that the grafted polymer layer produces high lubricity while only affecting the liner surface and having no effect on the bulk properties of the polyethylene component. As already discussed in some detail, a reduced production of wear particles in the hip joint is expected to eliminate bone-resorptive responses and, with it, periprosthetic osteolysis. The tribological advantages obtained through MPC grafting procedures might thus play a fundamental role in the next-generation artificial hip joint systems.

A long-standing problem in hip arthroplasty resides in the fact that all contemporary hip bearings are supported by femoral stems and acetabular shells that are very stiff with respect to adjacent bone. In the acetabulum, the presence of a stiff shell can lead to retroacetabular bone loss [1103]. Acetabular stress shielding and bone loss might indeed result inevitable with using hemispherical acetabular shells, independent of the thickness of the cup wall [1104]. Recent efforts have been focused on solving this problem by means of an approach involving both new design concepts and the employment of advanced biomaterials. A specially designed horseshoe-shaped all-polymer-made (i.e., a component consisting of a polyethylene bearing surface and a carbon fiber reinforced polybutyleneterphthalate shell with a hydroxyapatite coating) cup (Cambridge Cup; Howmedica, Staines, UK) showed an early reduction in bone loss and substantial recovery in bone density in the weight-bearing region of the acetabulum at 2 years follow-up [1105]. A further innovative design of a similar horseshoe-shaped design (MITCH™PCR Cup; Stryker SA, Montreux, Switzerland) instead foresees both hip cup structure and bearing surfaces made of carbon fiber/polyetheretherketone composite, while fixation to bone is made by means of a hydroxyapatite coating. On the other hand, the femoral head is made of a conventional alumina ceramic. A pre-clinical study with positive outputs can be found in a published literature, which has been released in 2008 by Latif *et al.* [1106]. We learn from this paper that the innovative cup is specially designed to obtain superior loading of the acetabular dome compared with a traditional hemispherical design. Clinical trials are yet under way in order to clarify its actual performance *in vivo*.

7.3 Cartilage Regeneration and the Role of Vibrational Spectroscopy

In the previous chapters, we have extensively discussed about the performance of microstructurally engineered ceramic and polyethylene materials as bearing substitutes for damaged joint cartilage. From the discussions, it has become clear that whatever the biomaterial designed for this purpose, it should meet quite severe structural requirements (i.e., bearing compressive, tensile, and shear forces in an aggressive environment, while transferring dynamic loads during motion with minimal friction), in addition to biocompatibility. Moreover, the artificial biomaterial joint component should also be capable to stand several tens of years with preserving a chemically stable surface configuration under dynamic stress conditions, while compatibly co-existing with the native tissue. A critical statement, according to the contents so far discussed in this book, could be that indeed no single product has yet been capable to meet all such requirements. Besides, it is not clear if such a "perfect" artificial biomaterial could ever be developed. This statement should also represent the opinion of a wide group of scientists and biotechnologists, who spend their full efforts in pursuing repair (rather than replacement with artificial biomaterials) of damaged cartilage. However, articular cartilage is a hydrated, avascular tissue, which possesses a very limited (intrinsic) ability of self-repairing [1107, 1108]. This makes a prompt and exhaustive strategy for cartilage repair problematic.

In this section, we briefly review the state of art of the main alternatives to joint replacement, in the field of cartilage regeneration. We thus inquire about the actual potential of the so far reached achievements in healing procedures for chronically damaged joints, in order to judge about the actual possibility of avoiding intrusive surgical procedures associated to total joint replacement.

As a consequence of the deficient self-repairing characteristics of human cartilage, damage of articular cartilage that does not penetrate down to the subchondral bone systematically fails to heal spontaneously. On the other hand, the damage that reaches the subchondral bone might engender an intrinsic repair response that generates a fibro-cartilaginous repair tissue. However, such tissue unfortunately results to be only a quite poor substitute for hyaline articular cartilage [1109,1110]. Despite this severe limitation, several arthroscopic repair strategies exist, which aim at utilizing the intrinsic repair response to induce regeneration of tissue with the same functional and mechanical properties of hyaline articular cartilage within the defect. Three main approaches have been proposed, which involve: (i) direct excision of healthy cartilage portions from regions aside of the load-bearing area and their direct surgical transfer into damaged regions (a method referred to as autologous osteochondral transfer) [1111–1113]; (ii) transplantation of expanded autologous chondrocytes (i.e., the only cells found in cartilage) from healthy cartilage to defective regions to form new repair tissue [1114,1115]; and, (iii) use of mesenchymal stem cells (as well as the combination of stem cells with biodegradable scaffolds) as a source for newly generated tissue [1116].

As already mentioned, in the case of defect with partial thickness in the articular cartilage, mature tissue does not heal spontaneously. This failure is thought to arise from a lack of penetration to the subchondral bone and, thus, from the failed access to the progenitor cells in the bone marrow space. In a fetal lamb model, spontaneous repair of superficial defects occurred with no fibrous scar [1117]. But, in mature tissue, only a limited repair process can take place in response to a trauma within the tissue immediately adjacent to the site of the defect. The cells adjacent to the wound margins undergo cell death and, after twenty-four hours, cell proliferation increases concurrent to an increase in matrix synthesis and catabolism. This response, however, is short lived and fails to repair the defect [1118]. Cells can migrate from the synovium across the articular surface to the lesion and, under the influence of growth factors, can fill the defect with repair tissue [1119, 1120]. However, in the absence of a fibrin matrix and mitogenic factors, the migrating cells fail to fill the defect in part because of the anti-adhesive properties of proteoglycans (i.e., especially small leucine-rich proteoglycans [1120]). Therefore, it is not only a lack of access to bone marrow cells that prevents the repair of partial thickness defects, but also a structural inhibition of healing mechanisms. In particular, it appears crucial to develop an improved surgical method promoting successful lateral integration between repair tissue and remaining cartilage [1121–1123]. In this latter context, several *in vitro* studies have shown that mechanical forces can greatly influence the development of cartilage (see Ref. [1124] for a review of this topic). Recently, researchers have begun to combine cell culture systems with external mechanical stimuli to improve the quality of the cartilage produced. For example, Carver *et al.* [1125] described a perfusion system, which applies intermittent hydrostatic pressure to chondrocytes embedded in polymer scaffolds. The pressurized scaffolds demonstrated better cartilage development compared with samples that were not exposed to pressure.

To this end, the regenerative method of autologous osteochondral transfer (method (i) above) has been found to provide symptomatic relief but an only partial improvement of joint functions. Chondrocyte transplantation in humans (method (ii)) was early described [1114] and recently reviewed by Brittberg [1126]. The procedure is minimally intrusive since it merely involves the excision of a healthy biopsy by arthroscopy. Results of the longest ongoing clinical study demonstrated satisfactory results after follow-up of 2~9 years in 80% of patients, with 90% of patients with femoral condylar defects showing good results [1127]. A new adapted approach also based on this procedure has also shown encouraging clinical results. Matrix-induced autologous chondrocyte implantation is now performed arthroscopically and allows the delivery of the patient's own autologous chondrocytes into deep cartilage lesions using a collagen scaffold in place of a periosteal flap [1128–1130]. This procedure allows seeding of chondrocytes onto a bilayer collagen I/III carrier membrane, which is subsequently implanted into the cartilage defect and secured in place with fibrin glue. Chondrocytes are seeded on a porous surface that when implanted, faces the bone to encourage tissue integration whilst a smooth surface acts as a natural barrier against soft tissue invasion [1131]. Mesenchymal stem cells (method (iii)) are multipotent stem cells that have the ability to self-renew and intrinsically repair and regenerate the tissue in which they reside following damage or trauma. In addition, such cells have the capacity to differentiate into a variety of other connective tissues such cartilage, bone, tendon, adipose tissue and muscle [1132–1139]. Current research focuses mainly on methods to isolate and expand these cells *in vitro*, in order to improve the functional integrity of repair tissue by delivery *via* carrier scaffolds in conjunction with specific active biomolecules such as growth factors to facilitate differentiation and maturation. While human clinical trials are yet to be performed, efforts to prevent future degeneration of repair tissue yet appear in their embryonic state.

From the above short description of the state of the art in cartilage regeneration, it appears that the achievement of the main clinical goal of avoiding intrusive surgeries with totally artificial joint components in favor of regeneration therapies, although representing a real and longed for objective, is yet far from a full realization. The success so far achieved through biological cartilage repair strategies, although providing symptomatic relief and improved joint function, is confined to local injuries and can be applied only in knee surgeries. On the other hand, all the so far applied methods yet conspicuously fail in both full regeneration and prevention of future degeneration of repair tissue and surrounding host tissue. Even when hyaline cartilage is successfully reproduced, it is often of an immature nature and does not have a true articular surface. Thus, it fails to withstand the mechanical functions of regular articular cartilage. Actually, no current experimental strategy has so far succeeded in consistently producing cartilage with no signs of degeneration after one year [1140], as well as in none of the published studies a tissue could be created that fully regenerates the natural zonal organization of articular cartilage. This demonstrates that the main hurdle to full cartilage regeneration consists in the integration of the transplanted or newly formed tissue with the existing cartilage. Without such integration, forces that occur at the bearing interface will unavoidable wear out the replacement tissue. In other words, for the time being, full cartilage replacement with synthetic materials yet appears as being the most probable choice for patients enduring chronic joint pain. However, it is also likely that future advances in the field of cartilage regeneration will cover more fundamental importance in future joint therapy research, which would strongly benefit of the capability of detect cartilage degradation at its very early stage. In other words, both therapeutic and preventive procedures should be more efficiently advanced through a combination of improved diagnostic and analytical techniques sensitive to both structural features and mechanical strain.

The employment of vibrational spectroscopy in analyzing bone tissue has been instrumental in advancing understanding of bone structure/function relations [85,100,1141]. Infrared and Raman spectra can thoroughly reflect perturbations in bone tissue that result from chemical damage, mechanical stress, or genetic defects. The micrometric spatial resolution of such spectroscopies facilitates the collection of local information on chemical processes, such as re-mineralization in bone and collagen matrix degeneration, which would otherwise remain unveiled when using other spectroscopic or biochemical analyses. Raman analyses of cartilage also possess high potential as a diagnostic tool, and the characterization of components such as collagen or hyaluronic acid provide a framework for assessing pathological changes not only in articular cartilage but also in the surrounding synovial fluid. Raman spectra complement histological or optical microscopy findings, and can be correlated to standard histological measures of cartilage tissue quality. Unlike infrared spectroscopy, Raman spectra are not obscured by water and measurements do not require direct contact with tissue. Moreover, the visible or near-infrared optics that are used by Raman instruments are compatible with fiber-optic probes widely used in clinical instruments such as arthroscopes. The Raman probe could be especially useful to distinguish between normal and pathological tissues, given the high sensitivity to subtle molecular changes. Because of these advantages, the use of Raman for tissue analysis has been widely reported [1142,1143], although Raman studies of cartilage are seldom published, possibly due to its inherently low Raman signal, which might require either long integration time or high laser power in order to obtain spectra that can be used as diagnostic fingerprints. Table 7.2 lists the origin of the numerous Raman bands detectable in cartilage tissue, which are directly related to the inherent chemical structure of collagen. Raman studies of cartilages have been greatly advanced in the research group of professor Michael Morris at the University of Michigan [1144,1145]. Beyond merely diagnostic aspects, Heger *et al.* [1146] also proposed a mechanism according to which laser-induced mineralization of treated cartilage could be responsible for long-term structural stability, the mechanism being possibly extrapolated to biological mineralization. Intracellular and extracellular laser-induced cartilage mineralization was monitored using Raman spectroscopy of a laser re-shaped rabbit (auricular) cartilage. Calcium sulfate and calcium carbonate crystals were found at intracellular sites and calcium phosphate crystals within extracellular spaces. Heger *et al.* [1146] thus proposed that in addition to stress relaxation in cartilage tissue, the laser treatment also caused apoptotic cells to release matrix vesicles and the released matrix vesicles mediated mineralization.

Table 7.2 Raman bands and respective vibrational modes in human knee cartilage

Wavenumber [cm^{-1}]	Assignment
856	ν(C–C–H) aromatic ring
875	ν(C–C)
1003	ν(C–C) aromatic ring
1241	$\sigma(NH_2)$ random coil (disordered); amide III
1269	$\sigma(NH_2)$ alpha-helix (ordered); amide III
1450	σ(C–H) protein CH_2, CH_3 scissor
1667	ν(C=O) alpha–helix; amide I
1685	ν(C=O); amide I
	$\nu \rightarrow$ stretching; $\sigma \rightarrow$ bending

More specific about the above discussion of cartilage regeneration, spectroscopic data can be used to examine cartilage in health or disease and be applied toward optimizations of engineered cartilage. Boskey and Camacho [1147] reviewed Fourier-transformed infrared spectroscopic imaging and other micro-spectroscopic methods used in the analysis of bone and cartilage. Camacho *et al.* [1148] also studied genetically modified bovine chondrocytes using spectroscopic imaging. These researchers used previously identified markers for collagen orientation and proteoglycan content in cartilage in order to examine integration of engineered cartilage-like tissue into defect sites and to reveal the native cartilage organization. Spectroscopic images showed an increase in proteoglycan production and a decrease in collagen II output, thus showing the capability to distinguish between neo-tissue and host tissue. Incomplete integration of neo-tissue could be confirmed and no conclusive evidence could be found that indicated an active role of surrounding tissues in neo-tissue integration. It was thus suggested, in agreement with the statements given in Ref. [1108], that cell-based repairs could not be achieved by simply placing engineered tissue atop of defective tissue.

As an applicative example of the high potentiality of Raman spectroscopic assessments in the field of diagnostic of soft tissue research, an investigation is shown in the remainder of this section, which aims at spectroscopically assessing pathological articular cartilage. Several samples of arthritic human tibial cartilages were examined immediately after total knee arthroplasty by means of near-infrared Raman spectroscopy excited with 647.1 nm lines of a Kr-ion laser. Healthy cartilage obtained from a cadaver donor was also examined as a control sample. Degradation severity was first visually classified into five grades (Grades 0~VI) on the surface of both medial and lateral zones (referred to as M and L locations, respectively) in each tibial plateau, according to the Collins scale. Raman spectra were then systematically collected from selected zones with different damage severity and spectral variations from bands belonging to in type II collagen related to degradation grades in Collins scale. The findings suggest that the Raman spectroscopic approach might be useful in recognizing and quantitatively assessing the degree of osteoarthritis since its early manifestation stage. Osteoarthritis is basically a degenerative disease in the synovial joint caused by an increase in fluid shear and hydrostatic pressure between two adjacent bones, which ultimately leads to severe disruption of the cartilage [1149–1151]. For its diagnosis, radiographic inspection is the most commonly conducted procedure, which main output is to confirm the presence of osteophytes at the joint margins, joint space narrowing, and subchondral bone sclerosis. Osteoarthritis severity has been long assessed by radiologists based on Kellgren-Lawrence (K/L) scores (0~4 scale), which is the most universally accepted method of radiographic classification of joint diseases [1152]. However, this technique is valid and feasible only for cartilages that entered into an advanced stage of osteoarthritis. In alternative, magnetic resonance imaging has been proposed, which is believed to be one of the most promising non-invasive technique [1153–1155]. However, this latter method still encounters problems with the reliability of diagnostic outcomes due to a lack in spatial resolution [1156]. In the clinical practice, early osteoarthritis assessments merely rely on ultrasonic analyses or "naked-eye" assessments through an endoscope and optical coherence tomography, which nevertheless are not capable to provide satisfying results for diagnosis of early OA. For macroscopic visual assessments, Collins provided a pathological grading of cartilage and bone changes due to aging or osteoarthritis [1157]. Degradation severity on the surface of human knee articular cartilage was then classified into five grades (grades 0~IV), referred to as the Collins scale. However, Collins assessments should be performed *ex vivo*, so that an accurate method for the precise diagnosis of early osteoarthritis, despite being strongly required by doctors as well as subclinical patients, is still missing.

In laboratory tests, infrared absorption spectroscopy has historically been employed (usually in Fourier-transform mode) for monitoring collagen damage in degraded cartilage based on the detection of spectral changes [1147, 1158]. However, the already mentioned influence of water on the spectrum represents a major limitation in utilizing infrared spectroscopy in cartilage studies (as well as, generally, in living tissues). Therefore, prior to collecting infrared spectra, dehydration and cutting of the sample into thin slices (~20 μm thick) are necessarily required. Due to the high water content (70~80% of the total weight of cartilage) in cartilage, sample preparation for infrared measurement unavoidably alters the chemical structures, and may lead to biases in the obtained results. To overcome these analytical limitations, near-infrared Raman spectroscopy can be applied to study cartilage diseases [1144, 1145]. The Raman technique is shown capable not only of non-destructively providing structural information in damaged cartilage, but also of allowing a high spatial resolution at the biomolecular level that can be useful in detailed microstructural analyses of cartilage diseases. The main advantage is that the water contained in the cartilage structure does not disturb the acquisition of accurate Raman spectra. Early Raman studies of mineralized tissues focused on assigning bands and determining its structure (cf. Table 7.2) [1141, 1159]. The most abundant proteins in human cartilage are members of the collagen family and have a fibrillar structure. The fibril-forming type II collagen, which is the predominant component (≥90%) of cartilage among all types of collagen, can be detected as Raman bands arising from the backbone amide groups in collagen. In the Raman spectra, vibrational modes of amide III in the spectral interval 1220~1280 cm^{-1} have been employed as a sensitive sensor for microstructural changes in collagen [1160–1164].

In this section, we take a further step along the direction indicated by previous Raman spectroscopy studies and attempt an assessment of cartilage osteoarthritis disease through linking the structural alterations generated at the molecular level with conventional macroscopic inspections used for diagnostic outcomes. A clear relationship was found between spectral changes of amide III Raman bands and pathological abnormality of human knee cartilage, which indicates the possibility to employ near-infrared Raman spectroscopy as a diagnostic tool for osteoarthritis, with tangible advantages especially in its early pathologic stage.

A total of five osteoarthritic human knee tibial plateau samples (Cases 1~5), which were obtained from right or left knee of female patients (82~87 y/o) during knee replacement surgery, were investigated in this study. As a control, normal cartilage with no macroscopic damage was also analyzed. A control sample was obtained from the right knee of a cadaveric donor (84 y/o female). Clinical information of the six cartilage samples is summarized in Table 7.3. All samples were stored in saline solution at freezer temperature immediately after harvesting cartilage from human knee, and backed into room temperature before the assessments. Knee radiographs were obtained in all patients preliminary to surgery, and the respective Kellgren-Lawrence (K/L) score [1152] determined for each patient. Knee radiographic images obtained from each patient are shown in Figs. 7.16 (a)~(f) (with the respective K/L scores listed in Table 7.3). The control sample exhibited K/L score 0 with no radiological evidence of osteoarthritis. Case 1 was in a mild stage of osteoarthritis with K/L score 2, while Cases 2~5 presented extensively narrowed joint space in the medial side with K/L score 4, which indicated an advanced and severe stage of osteoarthritis. According to radiographic features, the above five cases were considered positive for osteoarthritis, and surgical procedures were strongly recommended for Cases 2~5. On the other hand, Case 1 was in a relatively early stage of osteoarthritis and required a further independent assessment according to a different approach. Therefore, the Collins scale was also considered, which corresponds to the output of cartilage morphology and surface texture inspection after explantation. The Collins scale classifies osteoarthritis severity as Grades 0~IV, as specifically defined hereafter [1163]: Grade 0 is a normal healthy joint with smooth cartilage; Grade I corresponds to superficial flaking of cartilage in areas of pressure and frictional movement; Grade II represents a more extensive destruction of cartilage without denuding bone; Grade III refers to a total loss of cartilage in one or more pressure areas and obvious marginal osteophytes; Grade IV is comprehensive of a complete loss of cartilage from large areas with eburnation of bone and prominent osteophytes. After these macroscopic inspections, a grade according to Collins scale was assigned to each sample, and then Raman spectra systematically recorded at different zones of different osteoarthritis grades, as preliminary determined by Collins scale.

Table 7.3 Clinical data of the studied knee cartilage and Kellgren-Lawrence (K/L) score for each patient

Sample	y/o	Knee	K/L score
Control	84	Right	0
Case 1	87	Right	2
Case 2	82	Left	4
Case 3	83	Left	4
Case 4	82	Left	4
Case 5	87	Right	4

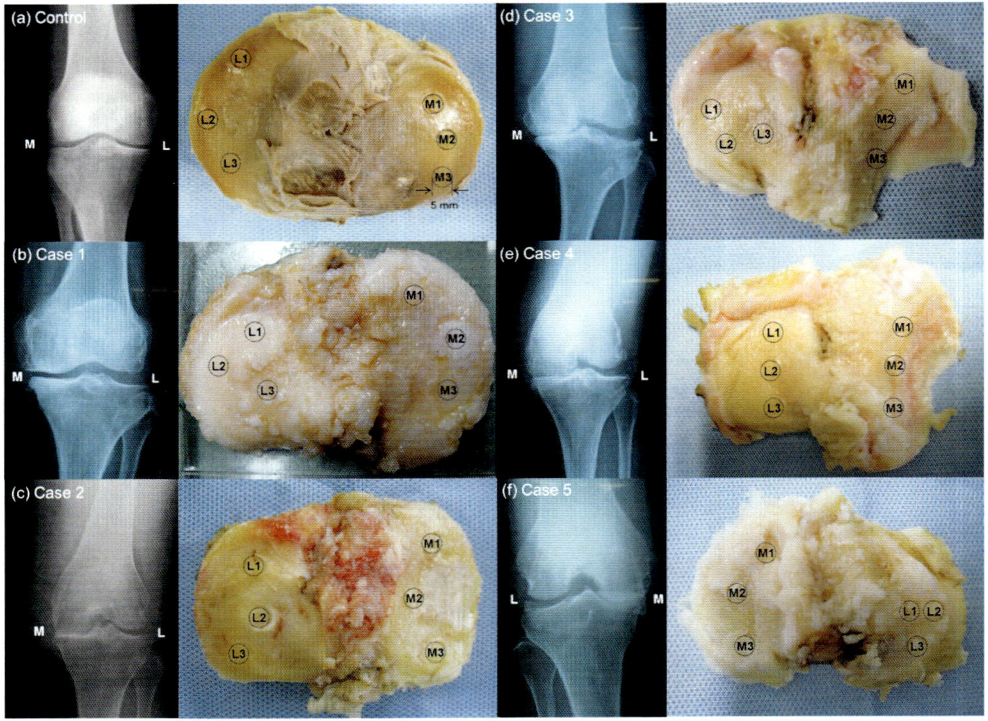

Figure 7.16 Knee radiographic images and cartilage photographs obtained from each patient before and after cartilage surgical explantation, respectively. Measurement areas are indicated in the medial (M1~3) and lateral sides (L1~3) for each cartilage sample.

Collins-scale surface severity, as classified in Grades 0–IV, is explicitly given in Table 7.4. Grade 0, which indicates no macroscopic surface damage, was seen on all surface zones of control cartilage. Grade 0 was also observed on the lateral side of Cases 1 and 2. Grades I and II were frequently observed on the lateral side, which is less frictionally exposed and can be considered yet in an early stage of progressive osteoarthritis. As a general feature, severe osteo-arthritis areas (≥Grade III) were always located at the medial zone of the cartilage surface, especially in M2 areas, which was selected at around the central region of the medial side and received the maximum dose of load and frictional sliding during deambu-lation. Grades III and IV were found only at locations in the medial side of the studied knee joints. The variety in severity depending on location can be interpreted as arising from the difference in mechanical shear and compressive stress magnitudes gene-rated at the contact between two adjacent cartilage surfaces subjected to *in vivo* loading (i.e., body weight and gait motion of the patients).

Table 7.4 Classification of osteoarthritis progression for surface areas of each articular surface

Sample	L1	L2	L3	M1	M2	M3
Control	Grade 0	Grade 0	Grade 0	Grade 0	Grade 0	Grade 0
Case 1	Grade 0	Grade 0	Grade II	Grade I	Grade III	Grade III
Case 2	Grade II	Grade I	Grade 0	Grade II	Grade III	Grade III
Case 3	Grade I	Grade I	Grade II	Grade I	Grade III	Grade III
Case 4	Grade I	Grade I	Grade I	Grade II	Grade III	Grade IV
Case 5	Grade II	Grade II	Grade II	Grade II	Grade IV	Grade II

In order to confirm the structural differences between normal and osteoarthritis cartilage, Raman spectra were collected on the surface of Grade 0~IV areas in all cartilage samples. Figure 7.17(a) shows the typical Raman spectrum of human knee cartilage recorded using near-infrared excitation at 647.1 nm. Several bands arising from the cartilage molecular structure could be detected in the spectral range of 400~3000 cm^{-1}. The Raman bands observed in the high wavenumber region mainly arose from the presence of collagen in human knee cartilage (cf. Table 7.2), which are vibrational modes of amide III structures (1220~1280 cm^{-1}), C–H bond bending mode (1447~1452 cm^{-1}), vibrational modes of amide I structures (1600~1720 cm^{-1}), and C–H bond stretching mode (2840~2986 cm^{-1}). However, other organic components in cartilage are also expected to contribute to the scattered band intensity of the C–C or C–H vibrational modes. Chi *et al.* [1160] have used these amide bands to characterize changes in the secondary structure of the proteins. Especially, the intensity change of amide III bands (NH_2 vibrations) is a quite sensitive indicator of the alterations in both ordered protein secondary structure such as α–helix or β–sheet, and disordered structure such as a random coil. The Raman peaks from amide I region are generally less intense due to the lower quantum efficiency of the CCD in the range of 1600~1720 cm^{-1}. Raman spectral patterns representing normal and the advanced osteoarthritic (Grade 4) cartilages could be extracted as shown in Figs. 7.17(b) and (c), respectively. The intensity of the amide III band located at 1241 cm^{-1} remarkably increased in going from the healthy to the diseased state. This spectral trend was also observed in a study of the sclera component from mice eyes reported by Dehring *et al.* [1161], who assessed the relative content of random coil in collagen through the analysis of relative intensity of the amide III doublet peaks. The amide III peak, located at a lower wavenumber in the range of 1230~1250 cm^{-1}, is indicative of the presence of random coil in the protein secondary structure, while the peak at a higher wavenumber in the rage of 1260~1280 cm^{-1} arises from the α–helix configuration in the protein secondary structure. Therefore, the higher relative intensity of the amide III doublet (I_{1241}/I_{1269}) represents the higher content of disordered collagen, which actually is a direct evidence for defective collagen, leading to the abnormality of the cartilage structure.

Figures 7.18(a)~(e) show data for the amide III ratio at differently damaged surfaces in medial and lateral zones of all cartilage samples. The average amide III ratio of Grade 0 obtained from control sample was 0.24, which is drawn with dotted lines in each graph. A Grade 0 area was also observed in the lateral zone of Cases 1 (L1 and L2) and 2 (L3) with ratio (0.26~0.28) comparable to that of the healthy control. However, Grade 0 on the surface of osteoarthritis cartilage exhibited slightly higher values, compared with the normal cartilage obtained from cadaver donor. The amide III ratio of Grade I area varied in the range 0.23~0.47. L1, L2 and M1 areas in Case 3, all classified as the same Grade I, showed large variations of amide III ratio in the range of 0.32~0.47 according to the microscopic assessment performed by Raman spectroscopy. It is interesting to note that the amide III ratio increases markedly in Grade II (0.41~0.76). This tendency indicates that tangible microstructural changes in human knee cartilage also occur in the early stage of osteoarthritis, namely since Grades I–II. More specifically, the relative content of disordered random coil in collagen secondary structure rapidly increased between Grades I and II. Grade III possessed a high amide III ratio from 0.62~0.86, while Grade IV showed the highest ratio (minimum 0.87, maximum 0.90) among all the areas measured in this study.

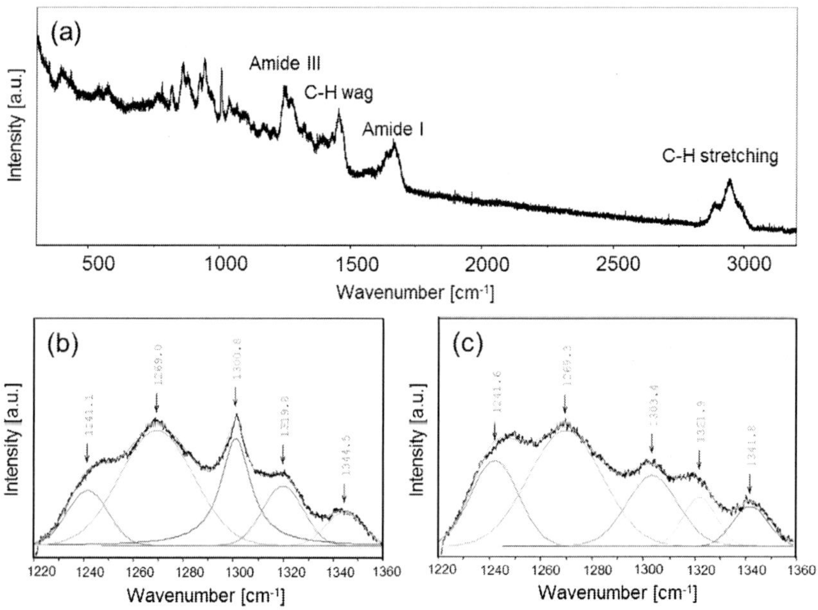

Figure 7.17 Typical near-infrared Raman spectra of human knee cartilage observed in the range of 400~3000 cm^{-1} (a), and Raman spectral patterns in amide III band regions of human knee cartilage in its normal (b) and advanced osteoarthritic (c) states.

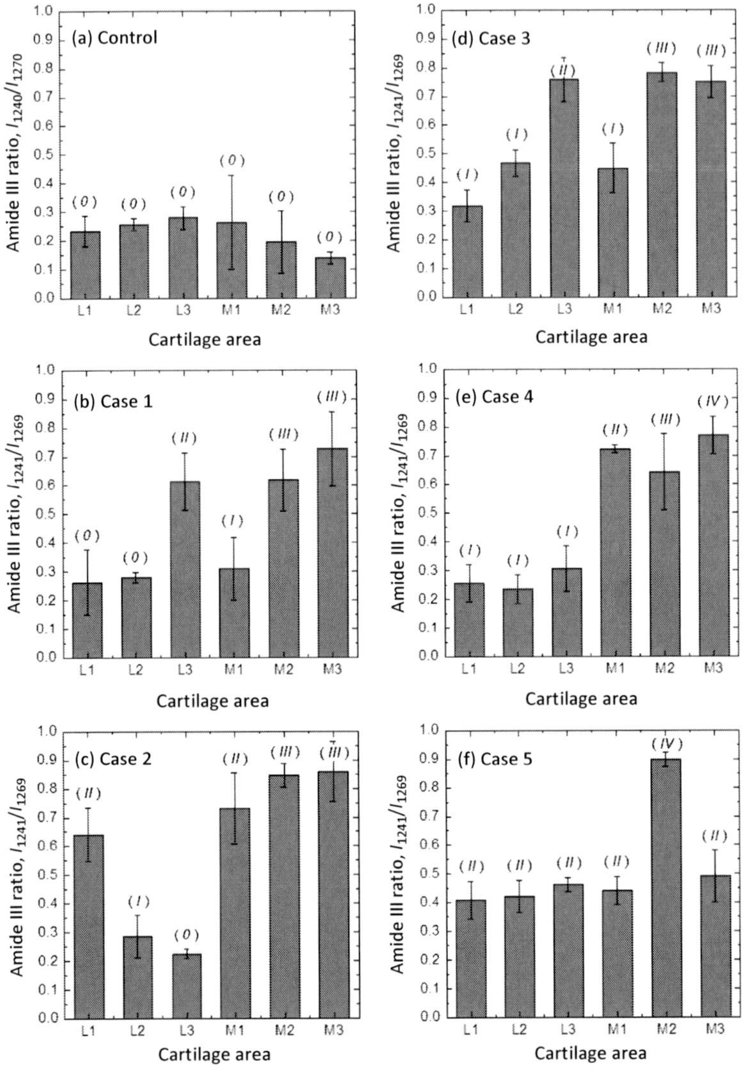

Figure 7.18 Comparison of amide III ratio (I_{1240}/I_{1269}) in medial and lateral zones of all the investigated cartilage samples. A higher relative intensity of the amide III doublet represents a higher fractional content of disordered collagen, which is in turn evidence of the defective collagen structure leading to the abnormality of cartilage.

The average values of amide III ratio among each grade are plotted in Fig. 7.19. Amide III ratio, namely the degree of disorder in collagen secondary structure, clearly increased with progressing osteoarthritis severity. The availability of a phenomenological relationship between the relative intensity of selected Raman bands and the degree of severity in cartilage osteoarthritis might play a key-role in the technological feasibility of a future diagnostic tool for early detection of osteoarthritis based on Raman spectroscopy. One important characteristic of the newly found relationship is the rapid degeneration of collagen microstructure between Grades I and II, which triggers irreversible damage on the cartilage surface and ultimately lead to severe osteoarthritis states as Grades III and IV. Such a process of collagen degeneration and cartilage damage is schematically shown in Fig. 7.20. The plot in Fig. 7.19 and the draft in Fig. 7.20 suggest that chemical, mechanical, and environmental factors all contribute to the microstructural modifications and degenerations of human cartilage. In the case of early degenerations in Grade I, biochemical or environmental effects (i.e., compositional change of synovial fluid) are likely more predominant in causing cartilage degradation than mechanical effects (i.e., contact stresses in the joint). Raman spectroscopy locates subtle differences at this early stage, were no significant difference in surface morphology can be identified only based on Collins scale criteria between Grades 0 and I. Healthy cartilage can preserve an extremely low-friction bearing surface (frictional coefficient: 0.003~0.02), but increases in frictional coefficient are expected due to initial microstructural alterations driven by biochemical and environmental effects. This will give rise to loss of a self-reparation mechanism in the vital tissue function against mechanical stresses. Beyond Grade II, mechanical effects become to gradually contribute to cartilage degeneration in the addition to biochemical effects, and the bearing surface starts to be worn out. Therefore, a rapid increase of the degree of disorder in the structure is observed beyond this stage. Severe wear, as observed in advanced stages of osteoarthritis (Grades III~IV), exacerbates upon increasing frictional coefficient, resulting in severe detachment and disruption of cartilage surface. Recent studies [1165,1166] confirmed that the coefficient of friction increased significantly with osteoarthritis progression, particularly in medial zones, due to a decrease in the concentration of lubricin, which is a hyaluronate-binding protein found in synovial fluid at the cartilage surface. In addition, surface morphological changes after Grade II are accompanied with a tangible increase of surface roughness, resulting in a substantial increase in local frictional stresses at asperity contacts, with rapid removal of the boundary lubricant [1167].

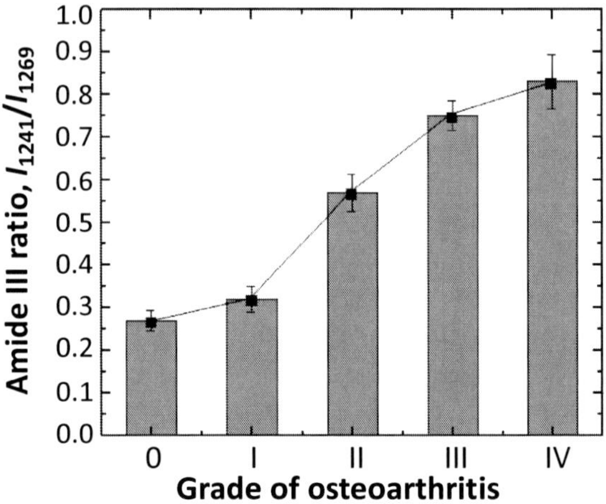

Figure 7.19 Dependence of the amide III Raman band ratio (I_{1240} / I_{1269}) as a function of osteoarthritis severity as defined according to the Collins scale.

The Raman assessments shown in this section revealed clear evidence of structural alterations at the molecular level in human knee cartilage since very early stages of osteoarthritis that cannot be clarified by conventional assessments such as radiography and endoscopy. In addition, Raman spectra could be used to link microstructural information at the molecular level with surface morphological classifications based on the conventional Collins scale. Amide III band ratio (I_{1241}/I_{1269}) can be regarded as a responsive sensor of the degree of disorder in the collagen secondary structure of human knee cartilage. In particular, we detected a clear microstructural difference in early osteoarthritis between Grades I and II. This applicative study of Raman spectroscopy to diagnostic assessments of osteoarthritis clearly shows the suitability of this method to systematic assessments of cartilage degenerations. The shown spectroscopic procedure could be implemented in the future into reaching a routine practice by conventional endoscopic inspections. Such practice could consistently contribute to a precise diagnosis of knees in their early osteoarthritis stages in subclinical patients.

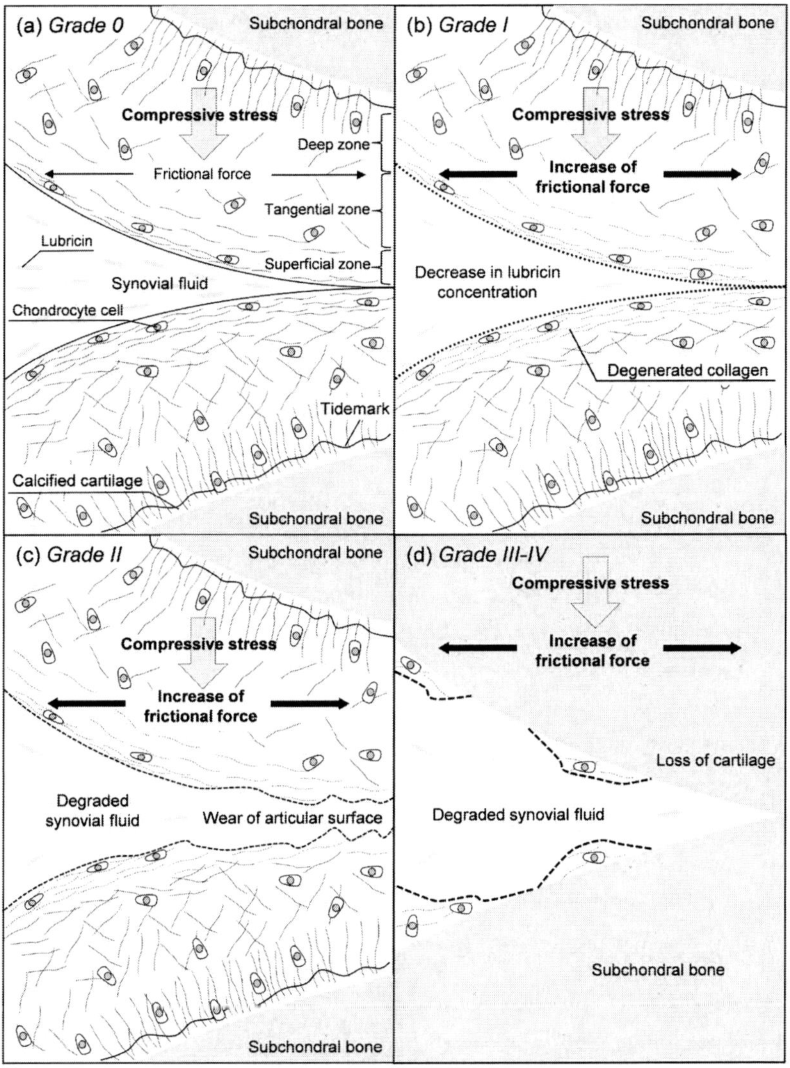

Figure 7.20 Schematic draft of the process of damage accumulation on the surface of human knee cartilage due to osteoarthritis: (a) normal healthy cartilage with extremely low friction articular surface; (b) collagen microstructural alterations driven by biochemical and environmental effects (i.e., decrease in lubricin concentration in synovial fluid), which induce frictional effects; (c) accumulation of wear damage by the combined effects of mechanical stress and environmentally-degraded synovial fluid; (d) severe disruption of cartilage with or without denuding subchondral bone.

Chapter 8

Conclusive Remarks

As nowadays statistics have reported results about the former generation implants and are showing us that wear and the associated propagation of wear debris represented the main issue in obtaining long-term durability of total hip arthroplasty, tremendous efforts have been made and successes achieved in the last decade in improving the quality of biomaterials for joint bearing surfaces. In this book, we have given a critical review starting from the formerly established to the most recently developed biomaterials, including several generations of ceramics, conventional and highly cross-linked polyethylene, and the most advanced evolution of metal implants with oxidized surfaces (cf. Chapters 3, 5, and Section 7.1). The many possible material combinations currently available in designing the sliding couple of an artificial joint provide the surgeons with a large number of choices, to be made according to personal preferences for a given surgical procedure, experience about different individual brands, and differentiation between young and middle-aged patients. Actual trends in new load-bearing biomaterials for hip joints are presently strongly influenced by a widespread quest for increasing head diameters; in order to achieve both improved range of motion and dislocation stability. Nevertheless, large head diameters have been so far a strict prerogative of metallic implants due to structural reliability

Advanced Materials for Joint Implants
Giuseppe Pezzotti

ISBN 978-981-4316-88-0 (Hardcover), 978-981-4364-39-3 (eBook)
www.panstanford.com

reasons. The available design solutions based on large ceramic head diameters are yet seldom found and ceramic resurfacing technology is yet *in embryo* (cf. Section 7.2). On the other hand, the main advantage of ceramic-on-ceramic bearings remains the fact that this type of articulation provides the lowest wear rates compared with any other material options in hip arthroplasty, even lower than ceramic versus highly cross-linked polyethylene [20]. The main disadvantage resides in a quite low (but, anyway, non-zero) risk of fracture (i.e., 2 in 10.000 or less) either for the ceramic head or for the ceramic liner. The current life expectancy for a successfully implanted hip joint can be approximately estimated to be 15 years when "standard" articulations consisting of metal/UHMWPE or alumina/UHMWPE are implanted. However, with the most recently developed alternatives of low-wear bearings, one could expect (or, at least, assertively hope) that future statistical results will show the achievement of longer lifetimes, owing to a significant decrease in the volume of wear (e.g., in the case of advanced ceramic-on-ceramic heads or ceramic composite heads sliding against UHMWPE liners with engineered structures, as described in Chapters 5 and 6, respectively). The burden to the lymphatic system could be reduced and the life expectancy for an artificial hip joint could be significantly improved as a result. The final goal in lowering wear rate at the joint surface, namely the design of a hip prosthesis that reliably experiences a longer lifetime than the patient who has received the surgery, could be closer to a satisfactory level of achievement than we could predict at the time of writing this book. Nevertheless, deeper scientific understanding and continuous technological monitoring need to be unremittingly pursued, at least for a full establishment of the clinical procedures involved with the newly developed implants.

What is next in hip bearings? This is the crucial question that we should ultimately be able to answer at the end of the dissertations given in this book. Summarizing the present situation, one could certainly state that the current generation of hard-on-soft and hard-on-hard hip bearings has become to exhibit extremely low wear when compared with traditional implants made of the cobalt–chromium alloy coupled with conventional polyethylene used in the past. At more than 10 years' clinical follow-up for hard-on-hard bearings and more than 5 years' follow-up for highly cross-linked polyethylene materials, we might soon obtain officially compiled statistics showing a significant reduction of particle-mediated osteolysis compared with the past [765,1168]. However, further issues (i.e., other than wear) certainly remain unsolved, as we have discussed them in some detail in the previous chapter. For better summarizing, in these conclusive remarks, one could say that ceramic-on-ceramic bearings are quite innovative, but also quite sensitive to cup position and neck impingement and, although in quite rare instances, could fracture. Metal-on-metal bearings are also sensitive to cup position and edge loading, including the possibility of unexpected pain, allergic reaction, soft tissue necrosis, pseudotumor, aseptic lymphocyte dominated vasculitis associated lesion (ALVAL), and metallic ion contamination (metallosis). Metal or ceramic heads on highly cross-linked polyethylene acetabular cups might appear more forgiving than hard-on-hard bearings with regard to the degree of precision required in the surgical technique. However, edge loading arising from joint laxity or component malposition might increase the actual polyethylene wear rate with these couples as well (i.e., although without emission of any detectable noise). Moreover, even in advanced polymer components, high contact stresses due to very thin liners or edge loading might ultimately lead to component fracture [1169–1173]. Several reports have detailed the cause of fracture for highly cross-linked polyethylene liners. Typically in these cases, fracture occurs in a region of thin and/or unsupported polyethylene, in association with superiorly directed edge-loading conditions, in turn associated to an excessive inclination of the implanted acetabular component. The reported cases of polyethylene liner fracture obviously have forced biomaterials scientists and technologists to give a second thought to the long-term benefit of the low wear rate obtained with highly cross-linked polyethylene. Such benefits can be achieved and exploited only if short-term mechanical failures are avoided. The potential for rim loading on thin polyethylene, particularly for patients with a relatively vertical cup orientation, is nowadays carefully assessed before considering the use of a cross-linked liner in combination with a large-size femoral head.

A further unsolved issue, which we have mentioned at the end of Section 7.2, is that contemporary hip bearings are supported by femoral stems and acetabular shells made of materials that are rather stiff with respect to adjacent bone. Such a large imbalance in stiffness between synthetic components and bone potentially leads to retroacetabular bone loss and acetabular stress shielding. We have also reported in the previous chapter that attempts to fix this long-known problem have recently been made by combining revolutionary choices for the bearing biomaterials and advances in component design. While such quite recent developments again confirm that paradigmatic progresses in hip arthroplasty cannot prescind from the development of new biomaterials, such progresses are also expected to occur in line with the long-discussed trends in developing less intrusive and more patient-friendly implants.

In the literature review necessary to compile this book, we came across an interesting analysis by Morscher [1174]. This report is indeed, for some aspects, "disconcerting" for any passionate scientist, who, as in the case of the writer, compellingly believes in innovation. In reviewing past failures and successes in total hip replacement, this researcher gives a clever disquisition on the reasons why "good ideas may not work" in joint arthroplasty. In the paper by Morscher, the analysis of the way endoprosthetic practices have progressed (and presumably will progress from now on) is presented in a realistic and overwhelming way. The main concept put forward in that analysis is that as a general issue in technological developments, "success is the greatest obstacle to further progress." From the scrutiny of past experiences, a general reasoning is given, which describes the curve of progress toward a hypothetical perfection, whatever the field of application, as a discontinuous one, definitely asymptotic in any advanced field, except for the occurrence of abrupt jumps in correspondence of discrete tipping points. This trend is qualitatively shown in Fig. 8.1, which also summarizes the discussions on future trends extensively made in the previous Chapter 7. In other words, as further progress is searched for, more efforts (and finances) become needed. According to the analysis of what might actually be feasible in the middle-range development of hip arthroplasty, and with what resources this could become available, one might come across a tangible probability that the medical device market, as presently structured, could even turn back to adopting less advanced technologies in the near future. The first step or initial development of hip arthroplastic surgery, namely what one could define the immediate achievement of short-term aims, has been fully achieved and consisted of liberating the patients from pain,

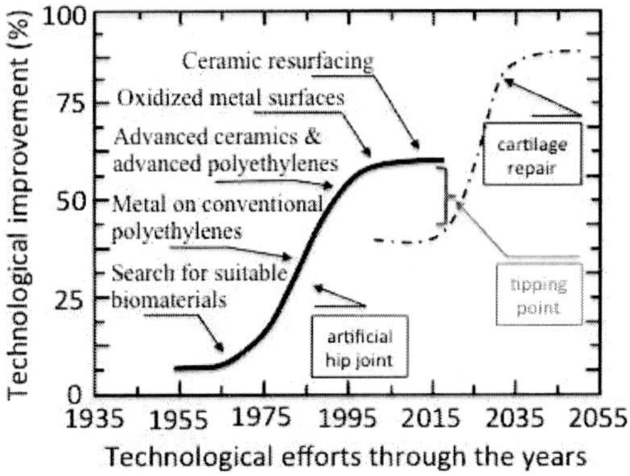

Figure 8.1 Line of development for artificial hip materials and implants and the prediction of a tipping point in surgical development reached with the establishment of cartilage healing technologies.

improving the mobility of the affected joints, and restoring the ability of the patients to stand and to walk. A subsequent progress, presently in a progressive stage in the field of arthroplasty, resides in a systematic recognition and in a responsible consideration of the risk factors that could eventually compromise the longevity of an artificial joint. Such second step has necessarily involved and continues to require reiterative developments of improved prosthetic materials (and surgical techniques) as we have described in Chapter 7, thus necessarily demanding enormous economical efforts but also resulting in a substantial decrease in the severity and frequency of surgical complications. Then, what can we expect next? According to Morscher, an innovation might solve one or more problems, but it will also definitely create a number of new problems. If this concept will prove valid, after the many innovations the arthroplasty field has reached in the last decade, we should expect a wave of new problems coming back to us in the very near future (i.e., one might even suspect that the stream of new problems has already started with the metal-on-metal resurfacing recall mentioned in the previous chapter). There is no doubt that the pioneering age of joint replacement has already come to an end, and that technological developments seem now to approach a saturated stage. However, what additional choices do we have but continue to believe in research as the only way to further progress it?

In summary, the situation we are contemplating nowadays displays a younger, more active, heavier, and longer-lived patient population placing more and more demands on the performance of joint bearings and on the structures that support them. Besides the needs of an increased range of motion and enhanced implant stability through the solution of both design and material problems, an absolute necessity in young and active patients has emerged in preserving the bone stock supporting the bearing for maximum elongation of implant survivorship. Component placement and joint laxity can also play important roles in edge loading, wear, bearing damage, and thus hip longevity. These considerations support the argument that wear reduction actually represents just the first step toward the future of joint arthroplasty, and also teach us that further developments in hip bearings need to be focused on performance issues related to the entire total hip construct rather than only to the abrasive wear resistance of the bearing couple *per se*. In the previous chapter, we have reviewed three main possible future directions for the future of total hip prostheses: (i) the development of low-friction and structurally strong coatings; (ii) the development of new tougher ceramics with minimized fracture risks to be used in ceramic-on-ceramic minimally intrusive articulations and, hopefully, for newly developing implant consisting of ceramic resurfacing; and (iii) the development of biological solutions, which could completely eliminate the need for artificial implants through healing and regenerating pathological articular cartilage. Which direction will be the most successful in a middle-term view is hard to predict. However, it is clear that the above points (i) and (ii) yet belong to the slowly saturating curve of the present joint arthroplasty pushed toward extreme sophistication, while the above point (iii) would represent what was referred to as a tipping point in the paper by Morscher, thus starting a completely new trend (cf. Fig. 8.1). It is also conceivable that the future of total hip replacement will be perceived as a divergent tendency for developed and developing countries. Advances in technology, including the development of improved materials, of improved surgical procedures, and better understanding of natural tissue reactions, will certainly result in breakthroughs in both materials and implant selections. Nevertheless, while affluent societies will continue to be capable to afford the rising costs of research and medical expenditure, developing countries will likely be ineffective in affording the expensive failures of implant surgery that we have already witnessed in the past (cf. the cases mentioned in Chapter 1) as well as those we are already witnessing while this book is being compiled (cf. Section 7.2). Due to the unpredictable occurrence of such failures, the costs of arthroplastic treatments, as they could be predicted, for example, in a decade perspective by medico-economical studies, might amount to a mere fraction of what they will actually end to be. We have also learned from our own experience that the course over time representing the development of total hip replacement has been neither harmoniously progressive nor linear in its nature, but rather discontinuous, with progress and setbacks in systematic alternation. Problems that have led to failures have often found their origin in the over-generalization of expected patient responses, in ignoring or misinterpreting past experience, in assigning wrong causes to encountered problems and, last but not least, in a lack of quality control in both manufacturing and clinical practice. Regarding the last cause in the above list, one important step beyond has been made with the introduction of the proof testing for ceramic femoral heads [306, 307], which enabled the makers to deterministically screen for potential fracture candidates among all the component released to the market, thus conspicuously eliminating from the production line flawed components and reducing the fracture probability to the minimal fraction shown by nowadays statistics. If ceramics are blamed for fracture, what about oxidation of polyethylene? It is quite surprising to this writer that no proof test has so far been developed or even proposed (i.e., either by makers before the release of the components to the market or by the hospitals directly before implantation) for screening the oxidation state of polyethylene liners. One could be tempted to believe that neither implant makers nor hospitals are the right counterparts for inquiring into such a thorough extent on biomaterials safety issues. Perhaps, as an addendum to the standard regulatory procedures and forerunner to national register-related actions, such screening should be made through the actions of an independent government-driven committee. The reason for the delay in deterministically summoning implant safety could also have resided in the unavailability of a fully non-destructive procedure for screening oxidation index in polyethylene liners (i.e., as mentioned in Chapter 2, the standard method is based on infrared spectroscopy, which necessarily requires assessments in transmission, thus destructively slicing the sample). In Chapter 6 of this book, we have shown the possibility (validated in several previously published papers [98, 99, 217]) of non-destructively checking about polyethylene oxidation by means of back-scattered Raman spectroscopy, hoping that this procedure will be adopted in the near future by joint makers and/or (at least) hospitals to avoid the release of flawed and oxidized hip liners to the orthopedics market. Short-term future developments in joint arthroplasty will continue to mandatorily deal with reliability issues for the components released to the market. For future innovative evolutions in this field, advanced Raman spectroscopic techniques could play a crucial role. It could not be otherwise, if one would just think that the fundamental knowledge on the structure of atoms or molecules that we nowadays possess is indeed mainly a result of laser spectroscopic investigations, and Raman spectroscopy allows one to derive detailed and specific information on the molecular level that other spectroscopic methods can provide only to a limited extent. Raman spectroscopy has emerged in the past years as an extremely powerful method in almost all disciplines of natural science. Although the Raman effect was discovered more than 80 years ago, its fundamental role in almost all branches of science has only been proven in the last few decades, triggered by the latest advancements in laser technology and in the development of extremely sensitive detectors. More innovation is going on. The most recent approaches adopting the resonance Raman effect [1175, 1176] can enhance the intensity of the Raman signals by several orders of magnitudes, thereby opening straight forward possibilities to a fast on-line and/or *in situ* deterministic screening of biomedical devices. Raman spectroscopy also allows for pursuing deep and specific investigations of mechanical and chemical states at the molecular level, pivotal to understanding the function of the respective molecules in a bioactive environment.

During the last five or six years, *in vivo* Raman spectroscopic investigations of biological tissues and cells have become of significant importance in the fields of medical, pharmaceutical, and biological diagnosis [1177, 1178]. In this context, the chemical composition of cell material and its dependence on exogenous factors have been shown to cover utmost importance. Therefore, it must be a main task for *in vivo* methods to provide information on the ingredients of living cells without destroying them. With the aid of microprobe Raman spectroscopy, it will be possible to resolve the submicron range and thus to record Raman spectra of single cells and thus support the development of biological solutions, which could ultimately lead to healing and regeneration of pathological articular cartilage.

Another item of fundamental technological innovation, stressed throughout this book, resides in the possibility of monitoring at the nanometer scale and, more importantly, of engineering (through doping and surface treatments) the oxygen sublattice at the bearing surfaces of ceramic joint components. The practice of altering surface stoichiometry is widely employed in other fields of materials engineering [1179, 1180] but yet scarcely attempted in bulk ceramic materials. Such practice leads to a comprehensive optimization of the environmental response of the joint surfaces and enables to maximize the wear resistance (and, thus, the lifetime) of the ceramic joint. Cathodoluminescence has been shown to provide a sensitive analytical probe of the very-near-surface region of bioceramics, and several examples of the strengths of this technique have been presented using recent data collected on alumina and zirconia materials. Analyses of monolithic and composite bioceramics have shown that by spectrally resolving data it is possible to separate the emission bands from intrinsic lattice imperfections, including oxygen vacancies and cations in various valence states, as they were introduced during processing or entered the bioceramic lattice by the effect of environmental/mechanical actions at the bearing surfaces. Correlation of cathodoluminescence data with the environmentally driven chemical evolution of bioceramic surfaces then has provided the basis for modeling the distribution and the types of defect sites, and for attempting their manipulation by processing. The possibility of using the cathodoluminescence locally emitted from oxygen-vacancy sites for surface stress analysis of ceramic bearing surfaces has also opened the way to engineering the surface stress state for optimi-zing wear resistance. Cathodoluminescence spectroscopy is a uniquely insightful tool for bridging chemistry and mechanics at the molecular scale. Its emission from an oxidized zirconia layer revealed the presence of a steep oxygen-stoichio-metry gradient capable to reduce the magnitude of thermal residual stress at the metal/ceramic interface. This work opens the possibility to engineering oxygen stoichiometry to control residual stresses on the bearing surface and subsurface, while also underpinning confidence in the method of production of oxidized metal surfaces. The observed cathodoluminescence effects were directly linked to surface wear damage, point defects and dislocations caused not only by sample preparation steps of cutting and polishing, but also by service loading *in vitro* or *in vivo*. Methods to minimize the damage, by furnace or pulsed laser annealing, and chemical routes, can now be easily and effectively figured out. Such surface preparation processes might have a profound effect on surface engineering of bioceramics for artificial joints, whether for fundamental studies or for applications. Finally, a stoichiometry route to eliminate environmental aging problems has also been rigorously demonstrated, with consequent implications on improved surface quality range of future bioceramics.

In Chapter 1, which was dedicated to a general review of the most recent trends in joint arthroplasty, we mentioned the possible misleading assertions that could be spread throughout information networks and might induce even expert audiences to retain inexact understanding. In particular, we referred to the presumed bioinertness of oxide ceramics in the human body, to the effect of zirconia phase transformation on fracture, and to the mismatch found in biomaterial degradation rate between *in vitro* experiments and *in vivo* loading. We hope that the previous chapters of this book have contributed to the process of providing clear answers to these topics, at least in partly clarifying the fundamental roles played by stoichiometry, micromechanics and molecular physics in biomaterials science. There could not be any clear understanding of biomaterials without the basic development of such advanced fields. However, in finalizing here the conceptual meaning of this book, it also appears appropriate to this writer mentioning and discussing some of the contents described in 1993 by Dr. J. W. Goodfellow in his famous Shands Memorial Lecture delivered in front of the prestigious American Academy of Orthopaedic Surgeons [1181]. In the reasoning offered at the beginning of that lecture, an item was stressed about the necessity of promoting "real science" in clinical orthopedics, in case, it "gets forgotten or continues to be over-looked," with rather sticking on "religious convictions" than on real scientific demonstrations. Such words continue to sound so appropriate even 20 years after the lecture was given that they could even be interpreted as a real prophecy. Besides the "religious convictions," we would also like to add some merely money-making-driven convictions (provided that Dr. Goodfellow would not implicitly mean those also in the meaning of the word "religious"). A further argument assessed in that Memorial Lecture dealt with the need for surgeons strongly asserting their requirements for clinical proofs of the efficacy of each new implant and/or modification of established practice based on strictly scientific arguments (and this writer would add here, rather than on merely bureaucratic regulatory procedures). There is fundamental truth in these assertions, and they could easily be extended toward a detailed demonstration of the weaknesses and the strengths of the joint arthroplasty we can observe nowadays. Again, we end up with the (perhaps obvious) observation that we have no other alternative but to continue to believe in basic research. The field of joint arthroplasty needs, nowadays as it was in 1993, to obtain the precious contributions of chemists and physicists besides the surgical experience of medical doctors, putting forward new scientific perspectives without attempting to oversimplify real situations in search for wider consensus from less specialized audiences.

In conclusion, past experiences have taught us how optimistic anticipations frequently fall short of reality in the field of joint arthroplasty. Formulating and promoting an outstanding and innovative idea could be a necessary but not sufficient prerequisite to obtain a breakthrough in this field, which is driven not only by scientific but also by economic and social driving forces. It is gradually becoming clear that new social schemes and strategies should be developed that will allow tackling the problem of a continuously increasing demand for medical services in a more simplified, reliable, and inexpensive way, since future societies (especially those of developing countries) could become less capable of absorbing new technologies in a possible future age of reduced infrastructure, lack of training, and superficially transmitted scientific and technical know-how. If this social perspective is to become the factual one in the next two decades, prevention may then become the most important factor to pursue in joint orthopedics, involving a better understanding of the significance of both appropriate dietary and life style modifications. Therefore, besides strongly believing in basic research and continuing to optimistically await the many possible and most likely astonishing breakthroughs in biomedical technology, we should also look forward to replenishing our future lives with superior judgment, understanding, and moderation.

Bibliography

1. Swedish Hip Arthroplasty Register: Annual Report 2008. Available at www.jru.orthop.gu.se.
2. Learmonth I, Young C, Rorabeck C. The operation of the century: total hip replacement. *Lancet*, 2007; **370**: 1508–1519.
3. Rahaman MN, Yao A, Sonny Bal B, Garino JP, Ries MD. Ceramics for prosthetic hip and knee joint replacement. *J. Am. Ceram. Soc.*, 2007; **90**: 1965–1988.
4. Bizot P, Banallec L, Sedel L, Nizard R. Alumina-on-alumina total hip prostheses in patients 40 years of age or younger. *Clin. Orthop. Relat. Res.*, 2000; **379**: 68–76.
5. National Joint Registry of England and Wales (NJR): 4th Annual Report 2008. Available at www.njcentre.org.uk.
6. Kurtz S, Mowat F, Ong K, Chan N, Lau E, Halpern M. Prevalence of primary and revision total hip and knee arthroplasty in the United States from 1990 through 2002. *J. Bone Joint Surg.* (*Am.*), 2005; **87**: 1487–1497.
7. Tateiwa T, Clarke IC, Williams PA, Garino J, Manaka M, Shishido T, Yamamoto K, Imakiire A. Ceramic total hip arthroplasty in the United States: safety and risk issues revisited. *Am. J. Orthop.*, 2008; **37**: E26–E31.
8. Garino J, Rahaman MN, Sonny Bal B. The reliability of modern alumina bearings in total hip arthroplasty. *Semin. Arthroplasty*, 2006; **17**: 113–119.
9. Zhu YH, Chiu KY, Tang WM. Review article: Polyethylene wear and osteolysis in total hip arthroplasty. *J. Orthop. Surg.*, 2001; **9**: 91–99.
10. Li S, Burstein AH. Current concepts review: UHMW polyethylene. *J. Bone Joint Surg.* (*Am.*), 1994; **76**: 1080–1090.
11. Gordon AC, D'Lima D, Colwell Jr. CV. Highly cross-linked polyethylene in total hip arthroplasty. *J. Am. Acad. Orthop. Surg.*, 2006; **14**: 511–523.
12. Jacobs CA, Christensen CP, Greenwald AS, McKellop H. Clinical performance of highly cross-linked polyethylenes in total hip arthroplasty. *J. Bone Joint Surg.* (*Am.*), 2007; **89**: 2779–2786.
13. Mu Z, Tian J, Wu T, Yang J, Pei F. A systematic review of radiological outcomes of highly cross-linked polyethylene versus conventional polyethylene in total hip arthroplasty. *Int. Orthop.*, 2009; **33**: 599–604.

14. Fisher J, Hailey JL, Chan KL, Shaw D, Stone M. The effect of ageing following irradiation on the wear of UHMWPE. *Trans. Orthop. Res. Soc.*, 1995; **20**: 120–128.

15. Endo MM, Barbour PS, Barton DC, Fisher J, Tipper JL, Ingham E, Stone MH. Comparative wear and wear debris under three different counterface conditions of crosslinked and non-crosslinked ultra high molecular weight polyethylene. *Biomed. Mater. Eng.*, 2001; **11**: 23–35.

16. Premnath V, Harris WH, Jasty M, Merrill EW. Gamma sterilization of UHMWPE articular implants: an analysis of the oxidation problem. *Biomaterials*, 1996; **17**: 1741–1753.

17. Oparaugo PC, Clarke IC, Malchau H, Herberts P. Correlation of wear debris-induced osteolysis and revision with volumetric wear-rates of polyethylene: A survey of 8 reports in the literature. *Acta Orthop.*, 2001; **72**: 22–28.

18. Bradford L, Baker DA, Graham J, Chawa A, Ries MD, Pruitt LA. Wear and surface cracking in early retrieved highly cross-linked polyethylene acetabular liners. *J. Bone Joint Surg.* (*Am.*), 2004; **86-A**: 1271–1282.

19. Bladen CL, Teramura S, Russell SL, Fujiwara K, Fisher J, Ingham E, Tomita N, Tipper JL. Analysis of wear, wear particles, and reduced inflammatory potential of vitamin E ultrahigh-molecular weight polyethylene for use in total joint replacement. *J. Biomed. Mater. Res. B: Appl. Biomater.*, 2013; **101**: 458–466.

20. Hannouche D, Nich C, Bizot P, Meunier A, Nizard R, Sedel L. Fractures of ceramic bearings: history and present status. *Clin. Orthop. Relat. Res.*, 2003; **417**: 19–26.

21. Allain J, Roudot-Thoraval F, Delecrin J, Anract P, Migaud H, Goutallier D. Revision total hip arthroplasty performed after fracture of a ceramic femoral head. A multicenter survivorship study. *J. Bone Joint Surg.* (*Am.*), 2003; **85**: 825–830.

22. Macirowski T, Tepic S, Mann RW. Cartilage stresses in the human hip joint. *J. Biomech. Eng.*, 1994; **116**: 10–18.

23. von Eisenhart-Rothe R, Eckstein F, Muller-Gerbl M, Landgraf J, Rock C, Putz R. Direct comparison of contact areas, contact stress and subchondral mineralization in human hip joint specimens. *Anat. Embryol.* (*Berl.*), 1997; **195**: 279–288.

24. von Eisenhart-Rothe R, Steinlechner M, Muller-Gerbl M, Eckstein F. Quantitative determination of joint incongruity and pressure distribution during simulated gait and cartilage thickness in the human hip joint. *J. Orthop. Res.*, 1999; **7**: 532–539.

25. Brown TD, Shaw DT. *In vitro* contact stress distributions in the natural human hip. *J. Biomech.*, 1983; **16**: 373–384.

26. Rushfeldt PD, Mann RW, Harris WH. Improved techniques for measuring *in vitro* the geometry and pressure distribution in the human acetabulum — I. Ultrasonic measurement of acetabular surfaces, sphericity and cartilage thickness. *J. Biomech.*, 1981; **14**: 253–260.

27. Shepherd DE, Seedhom BB. Thickness of human articular cartilage in joints of the lower limb. *Ann. Rheum. Dis.*, 1999; **58**: 27–34.

28. Konishi N, Mieno T. Determination of acetabular coverage of the femoral head with use of a single anteroposterior radiograph. A new computerized technique. *J. Bone Joint Surg.* (*Am.*), 1993; **75**: 1318–1333.

29. Adams MA, Kerin AJ, Bhatia LS, Chakrabarty G, Dolan P. Experimental determination of stress distributions in articular cartilage before and after sustained loading. *Clin. Biomech.* (*Bristol, Avon*), 1999; **14**: 88–96.

30. Adams D, Swanson SA. Direct measurement of local pressures in the cadaveric human hip joint during simulated level walking. *Ann. Rheum. Dis.*, 1985; **44**: 658–666.

31. Afoke NY, Byers PD, Hutton WC. Contact pressures in the human hip joint. *J. Bone Joint Surg.* (*Br.*), 1987; **69**: 536–541.

32. Sparks DR, Beason DP, Etheridge BS, Alonso JE, Eberhardt AW. Contact pressures in the flexed hip joint during lateral trochanteric loading. *J. Orthop. Res.*, 2005; **23**: 359–366.

33. Rushfeldt PD, Mann RW, Harris WH. Influence of cartilage geometry on the pressure distribution in the human hip joint. *Science*, 1979; **204**: 413–415.

34. Rushfeldt PD, Mann RW, Harris WH. Improved techniques for measuring *in vitro* the geometry and pressure distribution in the human acetabulum. II Instrumented endoprosthesis measurement of articular surface pressure distribution. *J. Biomech.*, 1981; **14**: 315–323.

35. Shirazi R, Shirazi-Adl A, Hurtig M. Role of cartilage collagen fibrils networks in knee joint biomechanics under compression. *J. Biomech.*, 2008; **41**: 3340–3348.

36. Mononen ME, Julkunen P, Töyräs J, Jurvelin JS, Kiviranta I, Korhonen RK. Alterations in structure and properties of collagen network of osteoarthritic and repaired cartilage modify knee joint stresses. *Biomech. Model Mechanobiol.*, 2011; **10**: 357–369.

37. Wiederhorn SM. Brittle fracture and toughening mechanisms in ceramics. *Ann. Rev. Mater. Sci.*, 1984; **14**: 373–403.

38. Gilman J. *Electronic basis of the strength of materials*. Cambridge University Press, Cambridge; 2003.

39. Peterlik H. Relationship of strength and defects of ceramic materials and their treatment by Weibull theory. *J. Ceram. Soc. Jpn.*, 2001; **109(8)**: 121–126.

40. Richter HG, Willmann G. Reliability of ceramic components for total hip endoprostheses. *Br. Ceram. Trans.*, 1999; **98(1)**: 29–34.

41. Benninghoff A. Form und bau der gelenkknorpel in ihren beziehungen zur funktion. *Z. Zellforsch. Mikrosk. Anat.*, 1925; **2**: 814–819.

42. Hu JCY, Athanasiou KA. Structure and Function of articular cartilage. In *Handbook of histology methods for bone and cartilage*. An YH, Martin KL (Eds.). Humana Press Inc., New Jersey, Chapter 4, 2003.

43. Mansfield JC, Winlove CP, Moger J, Matcher SJ. Collagen fiber arrangement in normal and diseased cartilage studied by polarization sensitive nonlinear microscopy. *J. Biomed. Opt.*, 2008; **13**: 044020-1–8.

44. Owen GRh, Kääb M, Ito K. Scanning electron microscopy examination of collagen network morphology at the cartilage, labrum, and bone interfaces in the acetabulum. *Scann. Micr.*, 1999; **13**: 83–91.

45. Kääb M, Ap Gwynn I, Nötzli HP. Collagen fibre arrangement in the tibial plateau articular cartilage of man and other mammalian species. *J. Anat.*, 1998; **193** (Pt 1): 23–34.

46. Sutula LC, Collier JP, Saum KA, Currier BH, Currier JH, Sanford WM, Mayor MB, Wooding RE, Sperling DK, Williams IR. Impact of gamma sterilization on clinical performance of polyethylene in the hip. *Clin. Orthop.*, 1995; **319**: 28–40.

47. Bapst JM, Valentine RH, Vasquez R. Wear simulation testing of direct compression molded UHMWPE irradiated in oxygenless packaging. In: *Transactions of the 23rd annual meeting of the Society for Biomaterials*, 1997; New Orleans: pp. 72–78.

48. Streicher RM. Influence of ionizing irradiation in air and nitrogen for sterilization of surgical grade PE for implants. *Radiat. Phys. Chem.*, 1988; **31**: 693–698.

49. St John KR, Takeuchi MJ, Poggie RA. Effect of radiation dose and packaging conditions on the oxidation of UHMWPE. In: *Transactions of the 23rd annual meeting of the Society for Biomaterials*, 1997; New Orleans: pp. 46–51.

50. Trieu HH, Avent R. Effect of sterilization on shelf-aged UHMWPE tibial inserts. In: *Transactions of the 21st annual meeting of the Society for Biomaterials*, 1995; San Francisco: pp. 109–114.

51. Sun DC, Wang A, Stark C, Dumbleton JH. The concept of stabilization in UHMWPE. In: *Transactions of the Society for Biomaterials, 5th World Congress*, 1996; Toronto: pp. 195–201.

52. Visentin M, Stea S, Squarzoni S, Reggiani M, Fagnano C, Antonietti B, Toni A. Isolation and characterization of wear debris generated in patients wearing polyethylene Hylamer inserts, gamma irradiated in air. *J. Biomater. Appl.*, 2005; **20**: 103–121.

53. Bargmann LS, Bargmann BC, Collier JP, Currier BH, Mayor MB. Current sterilization and packaging methods for polyethylene. *Clin. Orthop.*, 1999; **369**: 49–58.

54. Fisher J, Reeves EA, Isaac GH, Saum KA, Sanford WM. Comparison of the wear of aged and non-aged UHMWPE sterilized by gamma irradiation and by gas plasma. In: *Transactions of the Society for Biomaterials, 5th World Congress*, 1996; Toronto: pp. 971–976.

55. Clarke IC, Manaka M, Green DD, Williams P, Pezzotti G, Kim Y-H. Current status of zirconia used in total hip implants. *J. Bone Joint Surg.* (*Am.*), 2003; **85**: 73–84.

56. Chevalier J. What future for zirconia as a biomaterial? *Biomaterials*, 2006; **27**: 535–546.

57. Tateishi T, Yunoki H. Research and development of advanced biocompatible materials and applications to the artificial hip joint. *Bull. Mech. Eng.*, 1987; **45**: 1–9.

58. Brown SS, Green DD, Pezzotti G, Donaldson TK, Clarke IC. Possible triggers for phase transformation in zirconia hip balls. *J. Biomed. Mater. Res. B: Appl. Biomater.*, 2008; **85**: 444–452.

59. Heros RJ, Willman G. Ceramic in total hip arthroplasty: history, mechanical properties, clinical results, and current manufacturing state of the art. *Semin. Arthroplasty*, 1998; **9**: 114–122.

60. Hasegawa M, Sudo A, Hirata H. Ceramic acetabular liner fracture in total hip arthroplasty with a ceramic sandwich cup. *J. Arthroplasty*, 2003; **18**: 658–661.

61. Boehler M, Plenk Jr. H, Salzer M. Alumina ceramic bearings for hip endoprostheses: The Austrian experiences. *Clin. Orthop. Relat. Res.*, 2000; **379**: 85–93.

62. Ha Y-C, Kim S-Y, Kim HJ, Yoo JJ, Koo K-H. Ceramic liner fracture after cementless alumina-on-alumina total hip arthroplasty. *Clin. Orthop. Relat. Res.*, 2007; **458**: 106–110.

63. Garino JP. Modern ceramic-on-ceramic total hip systems in the United States: early results. *Clin. Orthop. Relat. Res.*, 2000; **379**: 41–47.

64. Kelley SS, Lachiewicz PF, Hickman JM, Paterno SM. Relationship of femoral head and acetabular size to the prevalence of dislocation. *Clin. Orthop.*, 1998; **355**: 163–170.

65. Hedlundh U, Ahnfelt L, Hybbinette CH, Wallinder L, Wecksreom J, Fredin H. Dislocations and the femoral head size in primary total hip arthroplasty. *Clin. Orthop. Relat. Res.*, 1996; **333**: 226–233.

66. Bader R, Scholz R, Steinhauser E, Zimmermann S, Busch R, Mittelmeier W. The influence of head and neck geometry on stability of total hip replacement: A mechanical test study. *Acta Orthop. Scand.*, 2004; **75**: 415–421.

67. Beaule P, Schmalzried T, Udomkiat P, Amstutz H. Jumbo femoral head for the treatment of recurrent dislocation following total hip replacement. *J. Bone Joint Surg.* (*Am.*), 2002; **84**: 256–263.

68. Bartz RL, Noble PC, Kadakia NR, Tullos HS. The effect of femoral component head size on posterior dislocation of the artificial joint. *J. Bone Joint Surg.* (*Am.*), 2000; **82**: 1300–1307.

69. Burroughs BR, Hallstrom B, Golladay GJ, Hoeffel D, Harris WH. Range of motion and stability in total hip arthroplasty with 28-, 32-, 38-, and 44-mm femoral head sizes. *J. Arthroplasty*, 2005; **20**: 11–19.

70. Pezzotti G, Yamada K, Porporati AA, Kuntz M, Yamamoto K. Fracture toughness analysis of advanced ceramic composite for hip prosthesis. *J. Am. Ceram. Soc.*, 2009; **92**: 1817–1822.

71. Pezzotti G, Munisso MC, Porporati AA, Lessnau K. On the role of oxygen vacancies and lattice strain in the tetragonal to monoclinic transformation in alumina/zirconia composites and improved environmental stability. *Biomaterials*, 2010; **31**: 6901–6908.

72. Lanyon LE, Rubin CT. Static vs dynamic loads as an influence on bone remodeling. *J. Biomech.*, 1984; **17**: 897–905.

73. Stein H, D'Ambrosia R. Wolff's law decoded. *Orthopedics*, 2008; **31**: 213.

74. Bradney M, Pearce G, Naughton G, Sullivan C, Bass S, Beck T, Carlson J, Seeman E. Moderate exercise during growth in prepubertal boys: Changes in one mass, size, volumetric density, and bone strength: A controlled rospective study. *J. Bone Miner. Res.*, 1998; **13**: 1814–1821.

75. Carter DR, Bouxsein ML, Marcus R. New approaches for interpreting projected bone densitometry data. *J. Bone Miner. Res.*, 1992; **7**: 137–145.

76. Hayes W, Gerhart T. Biomechanics of bone: Applications for assessment of bone strength. *J. Bone Miner. Res.*, 1985; **3**: 259–294.

77. Timlin JA, Carden A, Morris MD. Chemical microstructure of cortical bone probed by Raman transects. *Appl. Spectr.*, 1999; **53**: 1429–1435.

78. Kazanci M, Roschger P, Paschalis EP, Klaushofer K, Fratzl P. Bone osteonal tissues by Raman spectral mapping: Orientation-composition. *J. Struct. Biol.*, 2006; **156**: 489–496.

79. Morris MD. Raman spectroscopy of bone and cartilage. In *Emerging Raman applications and techniques in biomedical and pharmacetical fields*. Motousek P, Morris M (Eds.). Springer, New York, Chapter 14, 2010.

80. Kazanci M, Wagner HD, Manjubala NI, Gupta HS, Paschalis E, Roschger, Fratzl P. Raman imaging of two orthogonal planes within cortical bone. *Bone*, 2007; **41**: 456–461.

81. Morris MD, Mandair GS. Raman assessment of bone quality. *Clin. Orthop. Relat. Res.*, 2011; **469**: 2160–2169.

82. Gourion-Arsiquaud S, Boskey AL. Fourier transform infrared and Raman microspectroscopy and microscopic imaging of bone. *Curr. Opin. Orthop.*, 2007; **18**: 499–504.

83. Carden A, Rajachar RM, Morris MD, Kohn DH. Ultrastructural changes accompanying the mechanical deformation of bone tissue: A Raman imaging study. *Calcif. Tissue Int.*, 2003; **72**: 166–175.

84. Dooley KA, McCormack J, Fyhrie DP, Morris MD. Stress mapping of undamaged, strained, and failed regions of bone using Raman spectroscopy. *J. Biomed. Opt.*, 2009; **14**: 044018-1–8.

85. Pezzotti G, Sakakura S. Study of the toughening mechanisms in bone and biomimetic hydroxyapatite materials using Raman microprobe spectroscopy. *J. Biomed. Mater. Res. A*, 2003; **65**: 229–236.

86. Falgayrac G, Facq S, Leroy G, Cortet B, Penel G. New method for Raman investigation of the orientation of collagen fibrils and crystallites in the Haversian system of bone. *Appl. Spectr.*, 2010; **64**: 775–780.

87. Sundgren J-E, Bodö P, Lundström I, Berggren A, Hellem S. Auger electron spectroscopic studies of stainless-steel implants. *J. Biomed. Mater. Res. A*, 1985; **19**: 663–671.

88. Tzaphlidou M, Berillis P, Matthopoulos D. Bone calcium, phosphorus detection by Auger electron spectroscopy. *Micron*, 2005; **36**: 706–709.

89. Griesshaber E, Neuser RD, Schmahl WW. The application of EBSD analysis to biomaterials: microstructural and crystallographic texture

variations in marine carbonate shells. *Semin. Soc. Esp. Mineral.*, 2010; **7**: 20–30.

90. Tabb DL, Sevcik JJ, Koenig JL. FTIR study of the effects of irradiation on polyethylene. *J. Polym. Sci. Polym. Phys.*, 1975; **13**: 815–824.
91. Shen F-W, Yu Y-J, McKellop H. Potential errors in FTIR measurement of oxidation in ultrahigh molecular weight polyethylene implants. *J. Biomed. Mater. Res.*, 1999; **48**: 203–210.
92. James SP, Blazka S, Merrill EW, Jasty M, Lee KR, Bragdon CR, Harris WH. Challenge to the concept that UHMWPE acetabular components oxidize *in vivo*. *Biomaterials*, 1993; **14**: 643–647.
93. Lipiński P, Bieliński D, Okrój W, Jakubowski W, Klimek L, Jagielski J. Biomedical aspects of ion bombardment of polyethylene. *Vacuum*, 2009; **83** (Suppl.): S200–S203.
94. Stern T, Cohn D. Surface tailoring of biomedical polymers: An FTIR study. *J. Appl. Polym. Sci.*, 2001; **81**: 2203–2209.
95. Dadsetan M, Christenson EM, Unger F, Ausborn M, Kissel T, Hiltner A, Anderson JM. *In vivo* biocompatibility and biodegradation of poly(ethylene carbonate). *J. Control. Release*, 2003; **93**: 259–270.
96. Bruni P, Conti C, Corvi A, Rocchi M, Tosi G. Damaged polyethylene acetabular cups microscopy FT-IR and mechanical determinations. *Vibrat. Spectr.*, 2002; **29**: 103–107.
97. Rocha MF, Mansur AAP, Mansur HS. FTIR investigation of UHMWPE oxidation submitted to accelerated aging procedure. *Macromol. Symp.*, (Special Issue: *Modern Trends in Polymer Science*) 2010; **296**: 487–492.
98. Pezzotti G, Kumakura T, Yamada K, Tateiwa T, Puppulin L, Zhu W, Yamamoto K. Confocal Raman spectroscopic analysis of cross-linked ultra-high molecular weight polyethylene for application in artificial hip joints. *J. Biomed. Opt.*, 2007; **12**: 014011-1–14.
99. Pezzotti G. Stress microscopy and confocal Raman imaging of load-bearing surfaces in artificial hip joints. *Expert Rev. Med. Devices*, 2007; **4**: 165–189.
100. Pezzotti G. Raman piezo-spectroscopic analysis of natural and synthetic biomaterials. *Anal. Bioanal. Chem.*, 2005; **381**: 577–590.
101. Kalin M, Novak S, Vizintin J. Wear and friction behavior of alumina ceramics in aqueous solutions with different pH. *Wear*, 2003; **254**: 1141–1146.
102. Ramer BD. Characterization of biomaterial surfaces. *Cardiovasc. Pathol.*, 1993; **2**: 875–1005.

103. Hall SR, Fischer TE, Gruffel P, Carry C. Effect of grain boundary dopants an mean grain size on tribomechanical behavior of highly purified α-alumina in the mild wear regime. *Wear*, 1995; **181–183**: 165–167.

104. West GD, Perkins JM, Lewis MH. The effect of rare earth dopants on grain boundary cohesion in alumina. *J. Eur. Ceram. Soc.*, 2007; **27**: 1913–1918.

105. Raghavan S, Wang H, Porter WD, Dinwiddie RB, Mayo MJ. Thermal properties of zirconia co-doped with trivalent and pentavalent oxides. *Acta Mater.*, 2001; **49**: 169–179.

106. Guo X, Wang Z. Effect of niobia on the defect structure of yttria-stabilized zirconia. *J. Eur. Ceram. Soc.*, 1998; **18**: 237–240.

107. Hall RM, Siney P, Unsworth A, Wroblewski BM. The effect of surface topography of retrieved femoral heads on the wear of UHMWPE sockets. *Med. Eng. Phy.*, 1997; **19**: 711–719.

108. Puloski SKT, McCalden RW, MacDonald SJ, Bourne RB, Rorabeck CH. Surface analysis of posterior stabilized femoral components used in total knee arthroplasty. *J. Arthroplasty*, 2003; **18**: 822–826.

109. Lakdawala A, Todo S, Scott G. The significance of surface changes on retrieved femoral components after total knee replacement. *J. Bone Joint Surg.* (*Br.*), 2005; **87-B**: 796–799.

110. Pezzotti G, Saito T, Padeletti G, Cossari P, Yamamoto K. Nano-scale topography of bearing surface in advanced alumina/zirconia hip joint before and after severe exposure in water vapor environment. *J. Orthop. Res.*, 2010; **28**: 762–766.

111. Williams SR, Wu JJ, Unsworth A, Khan I. Tribological and surface analysis of 38 mm alumina–as-cast Co–Cr–Mo total hip arthroplasties. *Proc. Inst. Mech. Eng. H*, 2009; **223**: 941–954.

112. Currier BH, Currier JH, Mayor MB, Kimberly AL, Collier JP, Van Citters DW. Evaluation of oxidation and fatigue damage of retrieved crossfire polyethylene acetabular cups. *J. Bone Joint Surg.* (*Am.*), 2007; **89**: 2023–2029.

113. Currier BH, Van Citters DW, Currier JH, Collier JO. *In vivo* oxidation in remelted highly cross-linked retrievals. *J. Bone Joint Surg.* (*Am.*), 2010; **92**: 2409–2418.

114. Taddei P, Affatato S, Fagnano C, Toni A. Oxidation in ultrahigh molecular weight polyethylene an cross-linked polyethylene acetabular cups tested against roughened femoral heads in a hip joint simulator. *Biomacromolecules*, 2006; **7**: 1912–1920.

115. Chenery DH. Detection of peroxy species in ultra-high-molecular weight polyethylene by Raman spectroscopy. *Biomaterials*, 1997; **18**: 415–419.

116. Kumakura T, Puppulin L, Yamamoto K, Takahashi Y, Pezzotti G. In depth oxidation and strain profiles in UHMWPE acetabular cups non-destructively studied by confocal Raman microprobe spectroscopy. *J. Biomater. Sci. Polym. Ed.*, 2009; **20**: 1809–1822.

117. Pezzotti G, Porporati AA. Raman spectroscopic analysis of phase-transformation and stress patterns in zirconia hip joints. *J. Biomed. Opt.*, 2004; **9**: 372–384.

118. Simon V, Popa C, Muresan D, Simon S. Vibrational investigation of sintered titanium biomaterials. *J. Optoelectron. Adv. Mater.*, 2006; **8**: 540–542.

119. Hill MR, Catledge SA, Konovalov V, Clem WC, Chowdhury SA, Etheridge BS, Stanishevsky A, Lemons JE, Vohra YK, Eberhardt AW. Tribological evaluation of nanostructured diamond coatings and CoCr against ultra-high molecular weight polyethylene. *J. Biomed. Mater. Res. B: Appl. Biomater.*, 2008; **85**: 140–148.

120. Pezzotti G, Tateiwa T, Zhu W, Kumakura T, Yamada K, Yamamoto K. Fluorescence spectroscopic analysis of surface and subsurface residual stress fields in alumina hip joints. *J. Biomed. Opt.*, 2006; **11**: 024009-1–09.

121. Tateiwa T, Clarke IC, Pezzotti G, Sedel L, Kumakura T, Shishido T, Yamamoto K. Surface micro-analyses of long-term worn retrieved "Osteal™" alumina ceramic total hip replacement. *J. Biomed. Mater. Res. B*, 2007; **83-B**: 562–570.

122. Pezzotti G, Munisso MC, Lessnau K, Zhu W. Quantitative assessments of residual stress fields at the surface of alumina hip joints. *J. Biomed. Mater. Res. B*, 2010; **95B**: 250–262.

123. Puppulin L. Takahashi Y, Zhu W, Sugano N, Pezzotti G. Polarized Raman analysis of the molecular and residual strain on the surface of retrieved polyethylene tibial plates. *Acta Biomater.*, 2011; **7**: 1150–1159.

124. Takahashi Y, Puppulin L, Zhu W, Pezzotti G. Raman tensor analysis of ultra-high molecular weight polyethylene and its application to study retrieved hip joint components. *Acta Biomater.*, 2010; **6**: 3583–3594.

125. Wan K, Zhu W, Pezzotti G. Determination of in-depth probe response function using spectral perturbation methods. *J. Appl. Phys.*, 2005; **98**: 113101-1–7.

126. Zhu W, Zhu JL, Ge WY, Pezzotti G. A photo-stimulated spectroscopic method for spatially resolved stress analysis in hetero-epitaxial films. *J. Phys. D: Appl. Phys.*, 2009; **42**: 015505-1–8.

127. Caspers PJ, Lucassen GW, Puppels GJ. Combined *in vivo* confocal Raman spectroscopy and confocal microscopy of human skin. *Biophys. J.*, 2003; **85**: 572–580.

128. Hirotani H, Ito T. Scanning electron microscopy of the articular surfaces of the hip joint disorders. *Anat. Anz.*, 1975; **138**: 29–38.

129. Cullen JC, Tietjens BR, Poon J, Gavin JB. A scanning electron microscopic study of wear in the plastic components of prosthetic knee and hip joints. *Aust. N. Zeal. J. Surg.*, 1977; **47**: 189–192.

130. McCall J. Scanning electron microscopy study of articular cartilage. *Lancet*, 1968; **2**: 1194.

131. Clarke IC. Surface characteristics of human articular cartilage — a scanning electron microscope study. *J. Anat.*, 1971; **108**: 23–30.

132. Cameron HU, Macnab I, Anderson W. Hemiarthroplasty: A histological and scanning electron microscope study. *J. Biomed. Mater. Res.*, 1974; **8**: 221–230.

133. Sammons R, Marquis P. Application of the low vacuum scanning electron microscope to the study of biomaterials and mammalian cells. *Biomaterials*, 1997; **18**: 81–86.

134. Curtis ASG. Cell reactions with biomaterials: the microscopies. *Eur. Cells Mater.*, 2001; **1**: 59–65.

135. Richards RG, Gwynn I. Backscattered electron imaging of the undersurface of resin-embedded cells by field emission scanning electron microscopy. *J. Microsc.*, 1995; **177**: 43–52.

136. Richards RG, Gwynn I, Bundy KJ, Rahn BA. Microjet impingement followed by scanning electron microscopy as a qualitative technique to compare cellular adhesion to various biomaterials. *Cell Biol. Int.*, 1995; **19**: 1015–1024.

137. Ramer BD. Surface characterization of Biomaterials, by electron spectroscopy for chemical analysis. *Ann. Biomed. Eng.*, 1983; **11**: 313–336.

138. Godec M, Kocijan A, Dolinar D, Mandrino D, Jenko M, Antolič V. An investigation of the aseptic loosening of an AISI 316L stainless steel hip prosthesis. *Biomed. Mater.*, 2010; **5**: 045012-1–08.

139. Gordin DM, Gloriant T, Bohn M, Guillou A, Thibon I, Ansel D. Characterization of a laser-nitride titanium alloy by electron backscattered diffraction and electron probe microanalysis. *Surf. Interf. Anal.*, 2005; **37**: 1161–1167.

140. Checa AG, Okamoto T, Ramirez J. Organization pattern of nacre in Pteriidae (Bivalvia: Mollusca) explained by crystal competition. *Proc. Biol. Sci.*, 2006; **273**: 1329–1337.

141. MacDonald J, Freer A, Cusack M. Alignment of crystallographic *c*-axis throughout the four distinct microstructural layers of the oyster *Crassostrea gigas*. *Cryst. Growth Des.*, 2010; **10**: 1243–1246.

142. Goetze J, Heimann RB, Hildebrandt H, Gburek U. Microstructural investigation into calcium phosphate biomaterials, by spatially resolved cathodoluminescence. *Mat.-wiss. u. Werkstofftech.* 2001; **32**: 130–136.

143. Sprio S, Pezzotti G, Celotti G, Landi E, Tampieri A. Raman and cathodoluminescence spectroscopies of magnesium-substituted hydroxyapatite powders. *J. Mater. Res.*, 2005; **20**: 1009–1016.

144. Gross KA, Phillips MR. Identification and mapping of the amorphous phase in plasma-sprayed hydroxyapatite coatings using scanning cathodoluminescence microscopy. *J. Mater. Sci. Mater. Med.*, 1998; **9**: 797–802.

145. Zhu W, Munisso MC, Matsutani A, Ge W, Pezzotti G. Stress perturbation method for the assessment of cathodoluminescence probe response functions. *Appl. Spectr.*, 2009; **63**: 185–191.

146. Boyde A, Reid SA. New methods for cathodoluminescence in the scanning electron microscope. *Scan. Electron Microsc.*, 1983; **4**: 1803–1814.

147. Ritter E, Greenspan DC, Palmer RA, Hench LL. Use of fracture mechanics theory in lifetime predictions for alumina and bioglass-coated alumina. *J. Biomed Mater. Res.*, 1979; **13**, 251–263.

148. Lychkovs'kyl EI. Evaluation of the service life of a hip joint made of 08Kh18N10T steel by the methods of fracture mechanics. *Mater. Sci.*, 2005; **41**: 247–252.

149. Ritchie RO. Fatigue and fracture of pyrolytic carbon: a damage-tolerant approach to structural integrity and life prediction in "ceramic" heart valve prostheses. *J. Heart Valve Dis.*, 1996; **5** (suppl. I): S9–S31.

150. McKellop H, Clarke IC, Markolf KL, Amstutz HC. Wear characteristics of UHMWPE polyethylene: A method for accurately measuring extremely low wear rates. *J. Biomed. Mater. Res.*, 1978; **12**: 895–927.

151. Bowsher JG. A hip simulator study of the influence of patient activity level on the wear of crosslinked polyethylene under smooth and roughened femoral conditions. *Wear*, 2001; **250**: 167–179.

152. Morrison DE. A prototype scanning stylus profilometer for rapid measurement of small surface areas. *Int. J. Machine Tools Manuf.*, 1995; **35**: 325–331.

153. Poon CY, Bhushan B. Comparison of surface roughness measurements by stylus profiler, AFM and non-contact optical profiler. *Wear*, 1995; **190**: 76–88.

154. Wyant JC, Koliopoulos CL, Bhushan B, Basila D. Development of a three-dimensional noncontact digital optical profiler. *ASME J. Tribol.*, 1986; **108**: 1–8.

155. Bhushan B, Wyant JC, Koliopoulos CL. Measurement of surface topography of magnetic tapes by Mirau interferometry. *Appl. Opt.*, 1985; **24**: 1489–1897.

156. Bhushan B, Wyant JC, Koliopoulos CL. A new three-dimensional digital optical profiler. *Wear*, 1988; **122**: 301–312.

157. Lange SR, Bhushan B. Use of two- and three-dimensional noncontact surface profiler for tribology application. *Surf. Topograp.*, 1988; **1**: 277–290.

158. Wang SH, Quan C, Tay CJ, Shang HM. Surface roughness measurement in the submicrometer range using laser scattering. *Opt. Eng.*, 2000; **39**: 1597–1601.

159. Tortonese M, Barrett RC, Quate CF, Edward L. Atomic resolution with an atomic force microscope using piezoresistive detection. *Appl. Phys. Lett.*, 1993; **62**: 834–836.

160. Giessibl FJ, Quate CF. Exploring the nanoworld with atomic force microscopy. *Phys. Today*, 2006; **59**: 44–50.

161. Wade LA, Shapiro IR, Ma Z, Quake SR, Collier CP. Correlating AFM probe morphology to image resolution for single-wall carbon nanotube tips. *Nano Lett.*, 2004; **4**: 725–731.

162. Velegol SB, Pardi S, Li X, Velegol D, Logan BE. AFM imaging artifacts due to bacterial cell height and AFM tip geometry. *Langmuir*, 2003; **19**: 851–857.

163. Emerson RJ, Camesano TA. On the importance of precise calibration techniques for an atomic force microscope. *Ultramicroscopy*, 2006; **106**: 413–422.

164. Wenzler LA, Moyes GL, Raikar GN, Hansen RL, Harris JM, Beebe Jr. TP. Measurements of single-molecule bond-rupture forces between self-assembled monolayers of organosilanes with the atomic force microscope. *Langmuir*, 1997; **13**: 3761–3768.

165. Butt H-J, Kappl M, Mueller H, Paiteri R, Meyer W, Ruhe J. Steric forces measured with the atomic force microscope at various temperatures. *Langmuir*, 1999; **15**: 2559–2565.

166. Burnham NA, Colton RJ. Measuring the nanomechanical properties and surface forces of materials using an atomic force microscope. *J. Vacuum Sci. Tech.*, 1989; **7**: 2906–2913.

167. Burnham NA, Colton RJ, Pollock HM. Interpretation of force curves in atomic force microscopy. *Nanotechnology*, 1993; **4**: 64–80.

168. Burnham NA, Gremaud G, Kulik AJ, Gallo P-J, Oulevey F. Materials' properties measurements: Choosing the optimal scanning probe microscope configuration. *J. Vacuum Sci. Tech.*, 1996; **14**: 1308–1312.

169. Landman U, Luedtke WD, Burnham NA, Colton RJ. Atomistic mechanisms and dynamics of adhesion, nanoindentation and fracture. *Science*, 1990; **248**: 454–461.

170. Todd BA, Eppell SJ, Zypman FR. Squeezing out hidden force information from scanning force microscopes. *Appl. Phys. Lett.*, 2001; **79**: 1888–1890.

171. Burnham NA, Kulik AJ. Surface forces and adhesion. In Bhushan B (Ed.) *Handbook of micro/nano tribology*, CRC Press, Boca Raton, 2nd Edition, pp. 247–271, 1999.

172. Lee S-W, Sigmund WM. AFM study of repulsive van der Waals forces between Teflon AFTM thin film and silica or alumina. *Colloids Surf. A*, 2002; **204**: 43–50.

173. Dufrene YF, Boonaert CJP, van der Mei HC, Busscher HJ, Rouxhet PG. Probing molecular interactions and mechanical properties of microbial cell surfaces by atomic force microscopy. *Ultramicroscopy*, 2001; **86**: 113–120.

174. Touhami A, Hoffmann B, Vasella A, Denis FA, Dufrene YF. Probing specific lectin-carbohydrate interactions using atomic force microscopy imaging and force measurements. *Langmuir*, 2003; **19**: 1745–1751.

175. Lee GU, Chrisey LA, Colton RJ. Direct measurement of the forces between complementary strands of DNA. *Science*, 1994; **266**: 771–773.

176. Li X, Logan BE. Analysis of bacterial adhesion using a gradient force analysis and colloid probe atomic force microscopy. *Langmuir*, 2004; **20**: 8817–8822.

177. Ong Y-L, Razatos A, Georgiou G, Sharma MM. Adhesion forces between *E. coli* bacteria and biomaterial surfaces. *Langmuir*, 1999; **15**: 2719–2725.

178. Razatos A, Ong Y-L, Boulay F, Elbert DL, Hubbell JA, Sharma MM, Georgiou G. Force measurements between bacteria and poly(ethylene glycol)-coated surfaces. *Langmuir*, 2000; **16**: 9155–9158.

179. Schwarz UD, Hoelscher H, Wiesendanger R. Atomic resolution in scanning force microscopy: Concepts, requirements, contrast mechanisms, and image interpretation. *Phys. Rev. B*, 2000; **62**: 13089–13097.

180. Burnham NA, Chen X, Hodges CS, Matei GA, Thoreson EJ, Roberts CJ, Davies MC, Tendler SJB. Comparison of calibration methods for atomic-force microscopy cantilevers. *Nanotechnology*, 2003; **14**: 1–6.

181. Cappella B, Dietler G. Force-distance curves by atomic force microscopy. *Surf. Sci. Rep.*, 1999; **34**: 1–104.

182. Cleveland JP, Manne S, Bocek D, Hansma PK. A nondestructive method for determining the spring constant of cantilevers for scanning force microscopy. *Rev. Sci. Instr.*, 1993; **64**: 403-405.

183. Torii A, Sasaki M, Hane K, Okuma S. A method for determining the spring constant of cantilevers for atomic force microscopy. *Meas. Sci. Technol.*, 1996; **7**: 179–184.

184. Ratner BD, Hoffman AS, Schoen FJ, Lemons JE. *Biomaterials, science: an introduction to materials in medicine.* Academic Press, California, 1996, p. 23–28, pp. 447–449.

185. Stout KJ, Blunt L. Applications of 3-D topography to bio engineering. *Int. J. Mach. Tools Manufact.*, 1995; **35**: 219–229.

186. Stout KJ, Blunt L. Nanometres to micrometres: three-dimensional surface measurement in bio-engineering. *Surf. Coating Tech.*, 1995; **71**: 69–81.

187. Tayebi N, Polycarpou AA. Modeling the effect of skewness and kurtosis on the static friction coefficient of rough surfaces. *Tribol. Int.*, 2004; **37**: 491–505.

188. Vahabi M, Jafari GR, Mansour N, Karimzadeh R, Zamiranvari J. Stochastic features of rough surfaces: analysis of laser-induced silicon surface modifications. *J. Stat. Mech.*, 2008; **2008**: 03002-1–6.

189. Dong WP, Sullivan PJ, Stout KJ. Comprehensive study of parameters for characterizing three-dimensional surface topography III: Parameters for characterizing amplitude and some functional properties. *Wear*, 1994; **178**: 29–35.

190. Long DA. *The Raman effect: A unified treatment of the theory of Raman scattering by molecules.* John Wiley & Sons. Ltd., New York (2002).

191. Penel G, Delfosse C, Descamps M, Leroy G. Composition of bone and apatitic Biomaterials, as revealed by intravital Raman micro-spectroscopy. *Bone*, 2005; **36**: 893–901.

192. Davies MC, Binns JS, Melia CD, Bourgeois D. Fourier transform Raman spectroscopy of polymeric Biomaterials, and drug delivery systems. Spectrochim. *Acta Part A: Molec. Spectr.*, 1990; **46**: 277–283.

193. Duraipandian S, Zheng W, Ng J, Low JJ, Ilancheran A, Huang Z. Simultaneous fingerprint and high wavenumber confocal Raman spectroscopy enhances early detection of cervical precancer *in vivo*. *Anal. Chem.*, 2012; **84**: 5913–5919.

194. Shin WS, Li XF, Schwartz B, Wunder SL, Baran GR. Determination of the degree of cure of dental resins using Raman and FT-Raman spectroscopy. *Dent. Mater.*, 1993; **9**: 317–324.

195. Swain RJ, Stevens MM. Raman microspectroscopy for non-invasive biochemical analysis of single cells. *Biochem. Soc. Trans.*, 2007; **35**: 544–549.

196. de Carmejane O, Morris MD, Davis MK, Stixrude L, Tecklenburg M, Rajachar RM, Kohn DH. Bone chemical structure response to mechamical stress studied by high pressure Raman spectroscopy. *Calcif. Tissue Int.*, 2005; **76**: 207–213.

197. Duncan D, Reintjes J, Manuccia TJ. Scanning coherent anti-Stokes Raman microscope. *Opt. Lett.*, 1982; **7**: 350–352.

198. Cheng J-X, Book LD, Xie XS. Polarization coherent anti-Stokes Raman scattering microscopy. *Opt. Lett.*, 2001; **26**: 1341–1343.

199. Kee TW, Cicerone MT. Simple approach to one-laser, broadband coherent anti-Stokes Raman scattering microscopy. *Opt. Lett.*, 2004; **29**: 2701–2703.

200. Kneipp, K., Wang Y, Kneipp H, Perelman LT, Itzkan I, Dasari RR, Feld MS. Single molecule detection using surface-enhanced Raman scattering (SERS). *Phys. Rev. Lett.*, 1997; **78**: 1667–1670.

201. Vannier C, Yeo B-S, Melanson J, Zenobi R. Multifunctional microscope for far-field and tip-enhanced Raman spectroscopy. *Rev. Sci. Instr.*, 2006; **77**: 023104-1–5.

202. Lipkin DM, Clarke DR. Sample-probe interactions: Sampling microscopic property gradients. *J. Appl. Phys.*, 1995; **77**: 1855–1863.

203. Atkinson A, Jain SC. Spatially resolved stress analysis using Raman spectroscopy. *J. Raman Spectrosc.*, 1999; **30**: 885–891.

204. Onorato RM, Muraki N, Knutsen KP, Saykally RJ. Chirped coherent anti-Stokes Raman scattering as a high-spectral- and spatial-resolution microscopy. *Opt. Lett.*, 2007; **32**: 2858–2860.

205. Tabaksblat R, Meier RJ, Kip BJ. Confocal Raman microspectroscopy: Theory and application to thin polymer samples. *Appl. Spectrosc.*, 1992; **46**: 60–68.

206. Williams KPJ, Pitt GD, Batchelder DN, Kip BJ. Confocal Raman microspectroscopy using a stigmatic spectrograph and CCD detector. *Appl. Spectrosc.*, 1994; **48**: 232–235.

207. Pezzotti G, Sueoka H, Porporati AA, Manghnani M, Zhu W. Raman tensor elements for wurtzitic GaN and their application to assess crystallographic orientation at film/substrate interfaces. *J. Appl. Phys.*, 2011; **110**: 013527-1-10.

208. Wan K, Tochino S, Zhu W, Ohtsuka S, Pezzotti G. Quantitative evaluation of probe response functions for Raman and fluorescence bands of single-crystalline and polycrystalline Al_2O_3. *J. Phys. D: Appl. Phys.*, 2010; **43**: 205501–205508.

209. Turrell G. Analysis of polarization measurements in Raman micro-spectroscopy. *J. Raman Spectrosc.*, 1984; **15**: 103–108.

210. Fukatsu K, Zhu W, Pezzotti G. Raman tensor analysis of baddeleyte single-crystal and its application to define crystallographic domains in polycrystalline zirconia. *Phys. Status Solidi* (*b*), 2010; **247**: 278–287.

211. Munisso MC, Zhu W, Pezzotti G. Raman tensor analysis of sapphire single crystal and its application to define crystallographic orientation in polycrystalline alumina. *Phys. Status Solidi* (*b*), 2009; **246**: 1893–1900.

212. Takahashi Y, Puppulin L, Pezzotti G. Raman tensor analysis of ultra-high molecular weight polyethylene and its application to study retrieved hip-joint components. *Acta Biomater.*, 2010; **6**: 3583–3594.

213. Jones JR, Vats A, Notingher L, Gough JE, Tolley NS, Polak JM, Hench LL. *In situ* monitoring of chondrocyte response to bioactive scaffolds using Raman spectroscopy. *Bioceramics*, 2005; **17**: 623–626.

214. Nalla RK, Kruzic JJ, Kirmey JH, Balooch M, Ager JW, Ritchie RO. Role of microstructure in the aging-related deterioration of the toughness of human cortical bone. *Mater. Sci. Eng. C*, 2006; **26**: 1251–1260.

215. Galetz MC, Glatzel U. Molecular deformation mechanisms in UHMWPE during tribological loading in artificial joints. *Tribol. Lett.*, 2010; **38**: 1–13.

216. Pezzotti G. Severe evaluation of mechanical properties and phase stability in advanced ceramic composite for artificial joints. *J. Bone Joint Surg.* (*Br.*), 2010; **92-B** (Suppl. I): 167–172.

217. Pezzotti G, Takahashi Y, Takamatsu S, Puppulin L, Nishii T, Miki H, Sugano N. Non-destructively differentiating the roles of creep, wear and oxidation in long-term *in vivo* exposed polyethylene cups. *J. Biomater. Sci. Polym. Ed.*, 2011; **22**: 2165–2184.

218. Bertoluzza A, Fagnano C, Monti P, Simoni R, Tinti A, Tosi MR, Caramazza R. Raman spectroscopy in the study of biocompatibility. *Clin. Mater.*, 1992; **9**: 49–68.

219. Bertoluzza A, Monti P, Arciola R, Pizzoferrato A. Structural properties and biocompatibility of polymers used in ophthalmology. *Clin. Mater.*, 1991; **8**: 165–169.

220. Reggiani M, Tinti A, Taddei P, Visentin M, Stea S, De Clerico M, Fagnano C. Phase transformation in explanted highly crystalline UHMWPE acetabular cups and debris after *in vivo* wear. *J. Mol. Struct.*, 2006; **785**: 98–105.

221. Affatato S, Bersaglia G, Emiliani D, Foltran I, Taddei P, Reggiani M, Ferrieri P, Toni A. The performance of gamma- and EtO-sterilised UHMWPE acetabular cups tested under severe simulator conditions. Part 2: wear particle characteristics with isolation protocols. *Biomaterials*, 2003; **24**: 4045–4055.

222. Abbiss JB, Heeg B. Imaging piezospectroscopy. *Rev. Sci. Instr.*, 2008; **79**: 123105-1–9.

223. Zhu W, Pezzotti G. Raman analysis of three-dimensionally graded stress tensor components in sapphire. *J. Appl. Phys.*, 2011; **109:** 073502-1-13.

224. He J, Clarke DR. Determination of the piezospectroscopic coefficients for chromium-doped sapphire. *J. Am. Ceram. Soc.*, 1995; **78**: 1347–1353.

225. Gallas MR, Chu YC, Piermarini GJ. Calibration of the Raman effect in α-Al_2O_3 ceramic for residual stress measurements. *J. Mater. Res.*, 1995; **10**: 2817–2822.

226. Pezzotti G, Müller WH. Micromechanics of fracture in a ceramic/metal composite studied by *in situ* fluorescence spectroscopy I: Foundations and stress analysis. *Continuum Mech. Therm.*, 2002; **14**: 113–126.

227. Clarke DR, Adar F. Measurement of the crystallographically transformed zone produced by fracture in ceramics containing tetragonal zirconia. *J. Am. Ceram. Soc.*, 1982; **65**: 284–288.

228. Kalasinsky VF. Biomedical applications of infrared and Raman microscopy. *Appl. Spectr. Rev.*, 1996; **31**: 193–249.

229. Liza S, Haseeb ASMA, Masjuki HH, Abbas AA. The wear behavior of cross-linked UHMWPE under dry and bovine calf serum-lubricated conditions. *Tribol. Trans.*, 2013; **56**: 130–140.

230. Okubo Y, Teramura S, Niwa Y, Ibaraki K, Murata K, Hyon S-H, Pezzotti G, Tomita N. Strain-induced crystallization and orientation of vitamin E-blended ultrahigh molecular weight polyethylene. *Biomed. Mater. Eng.*, 2009; **19**: 431–439.

231. Puértolas JA, Martínez-Nogués V, Martínez-Morlanes MJ, Mariscal MD, Medel FJ, López-Santos C, Yubero F. Improved wear performance of ultra high molecular weight polyethylene coated with hydrogenated diamond like carbon. *Wear*, 2010; **269**: 458–465.

232. Bell LD, Kaiser WJ. Ballistic-electron-emission microscopy: a nanometer-scale probe of interfaces and carrier transport. *Annu. Rev. Mater. Sci.*, 1996; **26**: 189–222.

233. Pezzotti G. Spatially resolved Raman and cathodoluminescence probes in electronic materials: basics and applications. *Phys. Status Solidi (a)*, 2011; **208**: 976–999.

234. Fisher PJ, Wessels WS, Dietz AB, Prendergast FG. Enhanced biological cathodoluminescence. *Opt. Comm.*, 2008; **281**: 1901–1908.

235. Waychunas GA. Luminescence, X-ray emission and new spectroscopies. *Rev. Miner.*, 1988; **18**: 639–698.

236. Remond G, Cesbron F, Chapoulie R, Ohnenstetter D, Rouques-Carmes C, Schvoerer M. Cathodoluminescence applied to the microcharacterization of mineral materials: a present status in experimentation and interpretation. *Scanning Microsc.*, 1992; **6**: 23–69.

237. Marfunin AS. *Advanced Mineralogy. Vol. 2 — Methods and instrumentations: Results and recent developments.* Springer: Berlin, Heidelberg, New York (1995).

238. Marfunin AS. *Spectroscopy, luminescence and radiation centres in minerals.* Translated from Russian by Schiffer VV. Springer: Berlin (1979).

239. Richter DK, Goette Th, J. Goetze, Neuser RD. Progress in application of cathodoluminescence (CL) in sedimentary petrology. *Mineral. Petrol.*, 2003; **79**: 127–166.

240. Gillhaus A, Habermann D, Meijer J, Richter DK. Cathodoluminescence spectroscopy and micro-PIXE: combined high resolution Mn-analyses in dolomites — First results. *Nucl. Instr. Meth. Phys. Res. Section B*, 2000; **161–163**: 842–845.

241. Salh R, von Czarnowski A, Fitting H-J. Cathodoluminescence of non-stoichiometric silica: The role of oxygen. *J. Non-Cryst. Solids*, 2007; **353**: 546–549.

242. Heimke G, Griss P. Ceramic implant materials. *Med. Biol. Eng. Comp.* 1980; **18**: 503–510.

243. Liu D, Robertson J. Oxygen vacancy levels and interfaces of Al_2O_3. *Microelectr. Eng.*, 2009; **66**: 1668–1671.

244. Duwez P, Brown Jr. FH, Odell F. The zirconia-yttria system. *J. Electrochem. Soc.*, 1951; **98**: 356–362.

245. Lange FF. Transformation toughening: Part 3, experimental observations in the ZrO_2–Y_2O_3 system. *J. Mater. Sci.*, 1982; **17**: 240–247.

246. Fabris S, Paxton AT, Finnis MW. A stabilization mechanism of zirconia based on oxygen vacancies only. *Acta Mater.*, 2002; **50**: 5171–5178.

247. Suresh A, Mayo MJ, Porter D. Thermodynamics of the tetragonal-to-monoclinic phase transformation in fine and nanocrystalline yttria-stabilized zirconia powders. *J. Mater. Res.*, 2003; **18**: 2912–2921.

248. Badwal SPS. Zirconia-based solid electrolytes: microstructure, stability and ionic conductivity. *Solid State Ionics*, 1992; **52:** 23–32.

249. Jurado E, Bouvier P, Lucazeau G. Crystallite size effect on the tetragonal–monoclinic transition of undoped nano-crystalline zirconia studied by XRD and Raman spectrometry. *J. Solid State Chem.*, 2000; **149**: 399–407.

250. Pezzotti G, Saito T, Takahashi Y, Fukatsu K, Sugano N. Surface topology of advanced alumina/zirconia composite femoral head as compared with commercial femoral heads made of monolithic zirconia. *J. Am. Ceram. Soc.*, 2011; **94**: 945–950.

251. Chowdhury S, Vohra YK, Lemons JE, Ueno M, Ikeda J. Accelerating aging of zirconia femoral head implants: Change of surface structure and mechanical properties. *J. Biomed. Mater. Res. B*, 2007; **81B**: 486–492.

252. Adams BL, Wright SI, Kunze K. Orientation imaging: the emergence of a new microscopy. *Metall. Trans.*, 1993; **24A**: 819–831.

253. Dingley DJ. On-line determination of crystal orientation and texture determination in an SEM. *Proc. Royal Microsc. Soc.*, 1984; **19**: 74–75.

254. Dingley DJ. Progressive steps in the development of electron backscatter diffraction and orientation imaging microscopy. *J. Microsc.*, 2004; **213**: 214–224.

255. Humphreys FJ. Review: Grain and subgrain characterisation by electron backscatter diffraction. *J. Mat. Sci.*, 2001; **36**: 3833–3854.

256. Chen J, Browne M, Taylor M, Gregson PJ. Application of an interface failure model to predict fatigue crack growth in an implanted metallic femoral stem. *Computer Meth. Progr. Biomed.*, 2004; **73**: 249–256.

257. Wang SC, Browne M, Ubhi HS, Starink MJ. Determination of the fatigue fracture planes of Co–Cr–Mo biomedical alloys using electron backscatter diffraction. *J. Microsc.*, 2005; **217**:118–121.

258. Randle V. A methodology for grain boundary plane assessment by single-section trace analysis. *Script Mater.*, 2001; **44**: 2789–2794.

259. Wang SC, Aindow M, Starink MJ. Effect of self-accommodation on α/α boundary populations in pure titanium. *Acta Mater.*, 2003; **51**: 2485–2503.

260. Wang SC, Starink MJ. A simple approach to the determination of the crystallographic orientation: applications and accuracy. *J. Microsc.*, 2003; **211**: 130–136.

261. Sun D, Wharton JA, Wood RJK. Micro-abrasion mechanisms of cast CoCrMo in simulated body fluids. *Wear*, 2009; **267**: 1845–1855.

262. Weibull W. A statistical distribution of wide applicability. *J. Appl. Mech.*, 1951; **18**: 293–297.

263. Kovarik RE, Ergle JW, Fairhurst CW. Effects of specimen geometry on the measurement of fracture toughness. *Dent. Mater.*, 1991; **7**: 166–169.

264. Taira M, Nomura Y, Wakasa K, Yamaki M, Matsui A. Studies on fracture toughness of dental ceramics. *J. Oral Rehab.*, 1990; **17**: 551–563.

265. Fujishima A, Ferracane JL. Comparison of four modes of fracture toughness testing for dental composites. *Dent. Mater.*, 1996; **12**: 38–43.

266. Brown WF, Srawley JE. Plane strain crack toughness testing of high strength metallic materials. *ASTM Spec. Tech. Publ.*, 1967; **410**: 13–14.

267. White SN, Luo W, Paine ML, Fong H, Sarikaya M, Snead ML. Biological organization of hydroxyapatite crystallites into a fibrous continuum toughens and controls anisotropy in human enamel. *J. Dent. Res.*, 2001; **80**: 321–326.

268. Nalla RK, Kinney JH, Ritchie RO. On the fracture of human dentin: Is it stress- or strain-controlled? *J. Biomed. Mater. Res. A*, 2003; **67A**: 484–495.

269. Kahler B, Swain MV, Moule A. Fracture-toughening mechanisms responsible for differences in work to fracture of hydrated and dehydrated dentine. *J. Biomech.*, 2003; **36**: 229–237.

270. Needleman A, van der Giessen E. Micromechanics of fracture: Connecting physics to engineering. *MRS Bull.*, 2001; **26**: 211–214.

271. De Aza AH, Chevalier J, Fantozzi G, Schehl M, Torrecillas R. Crack growth resistance of alumina, zirconia and zirconia toughened alumina ceramics for joint prostheses. *Biomaterials*, 2002; **23**: 937–945.

272. Nalla RK, Kruzic JJ, Ritchie RO. On the origin of the toughness of mineralized tissue: microcracking or crack bridging? *Bone*, 2003; **34**: 790–798.

273. Garvie RC, Hannink RH, Pascoe RT. Ceramic steel? *Nature*, 1975; **258**: 703–704.

274. Hannink RH, Kelly PM, Muddle BC. Transformation toughening in zirconia-containing ceramics. *J. Am. Ceram. Soc.*, 2000; **83**: 461–487.

275. Stevens R, Evans P. Transformation toughening by dispersed polycrystalline zirconia. *Br. Ceram. Trans. J.*, 1984; **83**: 28–31.

276. Steinbrech RW. Toughening mechanisms for ceramic materials. *J. Eur. Ceram. Soc.*, 1992; **10**: 131–142.

277. Becher PF. Microstructural design of toughened ceramics. *J. Am. Ceram. Soc.*, 1991; **74**: 255–269.

278. Li C-W, Lui S-C, Goldacker J. Relation between strength, microstructure, and grain-bridging characteristics in *in situ* reinforced silicon nitride. *J. Am. Ceram. Soc.*, 1995; **78**: 449–459.

279. Sanchis-Alfonso V. Severe metallosis after unicompartmental knee arthroplasty. Knee Surg. *Sports Traumatol. Arthrosc.*, 2007; **15**: 361–364.

280. Coleman RF, Herrington, J, Scales JT. Concentration of wear products in hair, blood, and urine after hip replacement. *Br. Med. J.*, 1973; **1**: 527–529.

281. Pandit H, Glyn-Jones S, McLardy-Smith P, Gundle R, Whitwell D, Gibbons CL, Ostlere S, Athanasou N, Gill HS, Murray DW. Pseudotumours associated with metal-on-metal resurfacings. *J. Bone Joint Surg.* (*Br.*), 2008; **90**: 847–851.

282. Pezzotti G. *In situ* study of fracture mechanisms in advanced ceramics using fluorescence and Raman microprobe spectroscopy. *J. Raman Spectr.*, 1999; **30**: 867–875.

283. Fett T, Munz D, Kounga Njiwa AB, Rödel J, Quinn GD. Bridging stresses in sintered reaction-bonded Si_3N_4 from COD measurements. *J. Eur. Ceram. Soc.*, 2005; **25**: 29–36.

284. Padture NP. *In situ*-toughened silicon carbide. *J. Am. Ceram. Soc.*, 1994; **77**: 519–523.

285. ISO 13356:1997. Implants for surgery — Ceramic materials based on yttria-stabilized tetragonal zirconia (Y-TZP); 1997.

286. ISO 7206-10:2003. Implants for surgery — Partial and total hip prostheses — Part 10: Determination of resistance to static load of modular femoral heads; 2003.

287. Japanese Standards Association. *Test method for impact resistance of ceramic femoral head for hip-joint prostheses*. Japan Industrial Standard, JIS T 0308:2008. Japanese Standards Association, Tokyo, Japan, 2008.

288. Japanese Standards Association. *Testing methods for fracture toughness on high performance ceramics*. Japan Industrial Standard, JIS R 1607. Japanese Standards Association, Tokyo, Japan, 1990.

289. Munz D. Effect of specimen type on the measured values of fracture toughness of brittle ceramics. In *Fracture Toughness of Ceramics*, Bradt RC, Evans AG, Hasselman DPH, Lange FF (Eds.). Plenum Press, New York, Vol. 6. pp. 1–26, 1983.

290. Nishida T, Hanaki Y, Pezzotti G. Effect of notch-root radius on the fracture toughness of a fine grained alumina. *J. Am. Ceram. Soc.*, 1994; **77**: 606–608.

291. Kruzic JJ, Kim DK, Koester KJ, Ritchie RO. Indentation techniques for evaluating the fracture toughness of biomaterials and hard tissues. *J. Mech. Behav. Biomed. Mater.* 2008; **2**: 384–395.

292. Sakar-Deliormanli A, Guden M. Microhardness and fracture toughness of dental materials by indentation method. *J. Biomed. Mater. Res. B*, 2006; **76B**: 257–264.

293. Cook RF, Pharr GM. Direct observation and analysis of indentation cracking in glasses and ceramics. *J. Am. Ceram. Soc.*, 1990; **73**: 787–817.

294. Anstis GR, Chantikul P, Lawn BR, Marshall DB. A critical evaluation of indentation techniques for measuring fracture toughness. I. Direct crack measurements. *J. Am. Ceram. Soc.*, 1981; **64**: 533–538.

295. Lawn BR, Evans AG, Marshall DB. Elastic/plastic indentation damage in ceramics: The median/radial crack system. *J. Am. Ceram. Soc.*, 1980; **63**: 574–581.

296. Rödel J, Kelly JF, Lawn BR. *In situ* measurements of bridged crack interfaces in the SEM. *J. Am. Ceram. Soc.*, 1990; **73**: 3313–3318.

297. Fett T, Kounga AB, Rödel J. Stresses and stress intensity factor from COD of Vickers indentation cracks. *J. Mater. Sci.*, 2004; **39**: 2219–2221.

298. Fett T, Njiwa ABK, Rödel J. Crack opening displacements of Vickers indentation cracks. *Eng. Fract. Mech.*, 2005; **72**: 647–659.

299. Meschke F, Raddatz O, Kolleck A, Schneider GA. *R*-curve behavior and crack-closure stresses in barium titanate and (Mg,Y)-PSZ ceramics. *J. Am. Ceram. Soc.*, 2000; **83**: 353–361.

300. Marshall DB, Lawn BR. Residual stress effects in sharp-contact cracking: I. *J. Mater. Sci.*, 1979; **14**: 2001–2012.

301. Burghard Z, Zimmermann A, Rödel J, Aldinger F, Lawn BR. Crack opening profiles of indentation cracks in normal and anomalous glasses. *Acta Mater.* 2004; **52**: 293–297.

302. ISO 6474-1:2010. Implants for surgery — Ceramic materials — Part 1: Ceramic materials based on high purity alumina; 2010.

303. ISO 6474-2: under development. Implants for surgery — Ceramic materials — Part 2: Composite materials based on a high purity alumina matrix with zirconia reinforcement; June 2010 (Enquiry state, full report circulated).

304. Weisse B, Zahner M, Weber W, Rieger W. Improvement of the reliability of ceramic hip joint implants. *J. Biomech.*, 2003; **36**: 1633–169.

305. Willman G. Ceramic femoral head retrieval data. *Clin. Orthop. Relat. Res.*, 2000; **379**: 22–28.

306. Pfaff H-G. Ceramic component failure and the role of proof testing. *Clin. Orthop. Relat. Res.*, 2000; **379**: 29–33.

307. Weisse B, Affolter C, Koller RE, Stutz A. Proof testing of ceramic femoral heads for hip joint implants. *Proc. Inst. Mech. Eng. H*, 2010; **224**: 1051–1059.

308. Kuntz M. Validation of a new high performance alumina matrix composite for use in total joint replacement. *Semin. Arthroplasty*, 2006; **17**: 141–145.

309. Piconi C, Maccauro G, Muratori F, Brach del Prever E. Alumina and zirconia ceramics in joint replacements. *J. Appl. Biomater. Biomech.*, 2003; **1**: 19–32.

310. Maher SA, Lipman JD, Curley LJ, Gilchrist M, Wright TM. Mechanical performance of ceramic acetabular liners under impact conditions. *J. Arthroplasty*, 2003; **18**: 936–941.

311. Willmann G, Kramer U. Ceramic cups for hip endoprostheses: Consideration of designs. *Biomed. Tech.* (*Berl.*), 1998; **43**: 342–349.

312. Hench LL. Bioceramics: from concept to clinic. *J. Am. Ceram. Soc.*, 1991; **74**: 1487–1510.

313. Nair RP, Griffin D, Randall NX. The use of the pin-on-disk tribology test method to study three unique industrial applications. *Wear*, 2009; **267**: 823–827.

314. Korres S, Dienwiebel M. Design and construction of a novel tribometer with online topography and wear measurement. *Rev. Sci. Instrum.*, 2010; **81**: 063904-1–7.

315. Zemzemi F, Bensalem W, Rech J, Dogui A, Kapsa P. New tribometer designed for the characterization of the friction properties at the tool/chip/workpiece interface in machining. *Tribotest*, 2008; **14**: 11–25.

316. Patton S, Zabinski JS. Advanced tribometer for *in situ* studies of friction, wear, and contact condition — Advanced tribometer for friction and wear studies. *Tribol. Lett.*, 2002; **13**: 263–273.

317. Saikko V. A 12-station anatomic hip joint simulator. *Proc. Inst. Mech. Eng. H*, 2005; **219**: 437–448.

318. Goldsmith AA, Dowson D. A multi-station hip joint simulator study of the performance of 22 mm diameter zirconia-ultra-high molecular weight polyethylene total replacement hip joints. *Proc. Inst. Mech. Eng. H*, 1999; **213**: 77–90.

319. Maletsky LP, Hillberry BM. Simulating dynamic activities using a five-axis knee simulator. *J. Biomech. Eng.*, 2005; **127**: 123–133.

320. McKellop HA, D'Lima D. How have wear testing and joint simulator studies helped to discriminate among materials and designs? *J. Acad. Orthop. Surg.* 2008; **16** (Suppl. 1): S111–S119.

321. Ramamurti BS, Estok DM, Jasty M, Harris WH. Analysis of the kinematics of different hip simulators used to study wear of candidate materials for the articulation of total hip arthroplasties. *J. Orthop. Res.* 1998; **16**: 365–369.

322. Harris SJ, Krauss GG. Improved technique for measuring the ball volume removed in a ball-on-disk test. *Tribol. Lett.*, 2001; **10**: 187–188.

323. Bragdon CR, O'Connor DO, Lowenstein JD, Jasty M, Biggs SA, Harris WH. A new pin-on-disk wear testing method for simulating wear of polyethylene on cobalt-chrome alloy in total hip arthroplasty. *J. Arthroplasty*, 2001; **16**: 658–665.

324. Cho HJ, Wei WJ, Kao HC, Cheng CK. Wear behavior of UHMWPE sliding on artificial hip arthroplasty materials. *Mater. Chem. Phys.* 2004; **88**: 9–16.

325. Wang A, Stark C, Dumbleton JH. Mechanistic and morphologic origins of ultra-high molecular weight polyethylene wear debris in total

joint replacement prostheses. *Proc. Inst. Mech. Eng. H*, 1996; **210**: 141–155.

326. Livermore J, Ilstrup D, Morrey B. Effect of femoral head size on wear of the polyethylene acetabular component. *J. Bone Joint Surg.*, 1990; **72A**: 518–528.

327. Magnissalis EA, Xenakis TA, Zacharis C. Wear of retrieved ceramic THA components — four matched pairs retrieved after 5–13 years in service. *J. Biomed. Mater. Res. A*, 2001; **58**: 593–598.

328. Landy MM, Walker PS. Wear of ultra-high-molecular-weight polyethylene components of 90 retrieved knee prostheses. *J. Arthroplasty*, 1988; **3** (Suppl.): S73–S85.

329. Gunter J, Rose RM. Long-term performance and wear of ultrahigh-molecular-weight polyethylene in total joint replacement prostheses: a brief overview and perspective. *J. Long Term Eff. Med. Implants*, 1994; **4**: 157–175.

330. Goldsmith AA, Dowson D, Isaac GH, Lancaster JG. A comparative joint simulator study of the wear of metal-on-metal and alternative material combinations in hip replacements. *Proc. Inst. Mech. Eng. H*, 2000; **214**: 39–47.

331. Dowson D. New joints for the Millennium: wear control in total replacement hip joints. *Proc. Inst. Mech. Eng. H*, 2001; **215**: 335–358.

332. Kerkwijk B, Garcia M, van Zyl WE, Winnubst AJA, Mulder EJ, Schipper DJ, Verweij H. Friction behaviour of solid oxide lubricants as second phase in α-Al_2O_3 and stabilized ZrO_2 composites. *Wear*, 2004; **256**: 182–189.

333. Kerkwijk B, Winnubst AJA, Verweij H, Metselaar HSC, Mulder EJ, Schipper DJ. Tribological properties of nanoscale alumina–zirconia composites. *Wear*, 1999; **225–229**: 1293–1302.

334. Stachowiak GW, Stachowiak GB. Unlubricated wear and friction of toughened zirconia ceramics at elevated temperatures. *Wear*, 1991; **143**: 277–295.

335. Sasaki S. The effects of the surrounding atmosphere on the friction and wear of alumina, zirconia, silicon carbide and silicon nitride. *Wear*, 1989; **134**: 185–200.

336. Dey AK, Biswas K. Dry sliding wear of zirconia-toughened alumina with different metal oxide additives. *Ceram. Int.* 2009; **35**: 997–1002.

337. Conoci S, Melandri C, De Portu G. Wear of 3Y-TZP containing compressive residual stresses at the surface. *J. Mater. Sci.*, 1999; **34**: 1009–1015.

338. Agraït N, Rubio G, Vieira S. Plastic deformation in nanometer scale contacts. *Langmuir*, 1996; **12**: 4505–4509.

339. Guicciardi S, Sciti D, Melandri C, Pezzotti G. Dry sliding wear behavior of nano-sized SiC pins against SiC and Si_3N_4 discs. *Wear*, 2007; **262**: 529–535.

340. Nakayama K, Martin J-M. Tribochemical reactions at and in the vicinity of a sliding contact. *Wear*, 2006; **261**: 235–240.

341. Singer IL. Mechanics and chemistry of solids in sliding contact. *Langmuir*, 1996; **12**: 4486–4491.

342. Singer IL, Dvorak SD, Wahl KJ, Scharf TW. Third body processes and friction of solid lubricants studied by *in situ* optical and Raman tribometry. *Tribol. Series*, 2001; **40**: 327–336.

343. Belin M, Martin JM. Triboscopy, a new approach to surface degradations of thin films. *Wear*, 1992; **156**: 151–160.

344. Bair S, Green I, Bhushan B. Measurements of asperity temperatures of a read/write head slider bearing in hard magnetic recording disks. *J. Tribol.*, 1991; **113**: 547–554.

345. Cann PM, Spikes HA. In-contact IR spectroscopy of hydrocarbon lubricants. *Tribol. Lett.*, 2005; **19**: 289–297.

346. Cheng CU, Stair PC. *In situ* study of multialkylated cyclopentane and perfluoropolyalkyl ether chemistry in concentrated contacts using ultraviolet Raman spectroscopy. *Tribol. Lett.*, 1998; **4**: 163–170.

347. Berthier Y, Godet M, Brendle M. Velocity accommodation in friction. *Tribol. Trans.* 1989; **32**: 490–496.

348. Sliney H. Dynamics of solid lubrification as observed by optical microscopy. *ASLE Trans.* 1977; **21**: 109–117.

349. Jullien A, Meurisse MH, Berthier Y. Determination of tribological history and wear through visualisation in lubricated contacts using a carbon-based composite. *Wear*, 1996; **194**: 116–125.

350. Israelachvili JN, Tabor D. The shear properties of molecular films. *Wear*, 1973; **24**: 386–390.

351. Donnet C. In *Handbook of Surface and Interface Analysis*. Riviere JC, Myhra S. (Eds.). Marcel Dekker, Inc., Chapter 16, pp. 697–745, 1998.

352. Joly-Pottuz L, Martin JM, Belin M, Dassenoy F. Study of inorganic fullerenes and carbon nanotubes by *in situ* Raman tribometry. *Appl. Phys. Lett.* 2007; **91**: 153107-1–3.

353. Cherif K, Gueroult B, Rigaud M. Al_2O_3–ZrO_2 debris life cycle during wear: effects of the third body on wear and friction. *Wear*, 1997; **208**: 161–168.

354. DIN 50 324:1992. *Testing of friction and wear*; 1992.

355. ASTM G 133–195:1996. *Standard test method for linearly reciprocating ball-on-flat sliding wear* (re-approved), 2002.

356. ASTM G 99–05:2010. *Standard test method for wear testing with a pin-on-disk apparatus*, 2010.

357. Buescher R, Taeger G, Dudzinski W, Gleising B, Wimmer MA, Fisher A. Subsurface microstructure of metal-on-metal hip joints and its relationship to wear particle generation. *J. Biomed. Mater. Res. B*, 2004; **72B**: 206–214.

358. Wimmer MA, Loos J, Heitkemper M, Fischer A. The acting wear mechanisms on metal-on-metal hip joint bearings — *In vitro* results. *Wear*, 2001; **250**: 129–139.

359. Wimmer MA, Sprecher C, Hauert R, Taeger G, Fischer A. Tribochemical reactions on metal-on-metal hip joint bearings — A comparison between *in vitro* and *in vivo* results. *Wear*, 2003; **255**: 1007–1014.

360. Kinbrum A, Vasilliou K, Lee SM, Unsworth A. A tribological and particle debris study of as-cast and heat treated CoCrMo alloy. *J. Bone Joint Surg.* (*Br.*), 2010; **92B** (Supp. 1): 101.

361. Sinnett-Jones PE, Wharton JA, Wood RJK. Micro-abrasion-corrosion of a CoCrMo alloy in simulated artificial hip joint environments. *Wear*, 2005; **259**: 898–909.

362. Bowsher JG, Nevelos J, Williams PA, Shelton JC. "Severe" wear challenge to "as-cast" and "double heat-treated" large-diameter metal-on-metal hip bearings. *Proc. Inst. Mech. Eng. H*, 2006: **220**: 135–143.

363. Bowsher JG, Hussain A, Williams PA, Shelton JC. Metal-on-metal hip simulator study of increased wear particle surface area due to "severe" patient activity. *Proc. Inst. Mech. Eng. H*, 2006: **220**: 279–287.

364. Suh NP. An overview of the delamination theory of wear. *Wear*, 1977; **44**: 1–16.

365. Rainforth WM. The wear behaviour of oxide ceramics — a review. *J. Mater. Sci.*, 2004; **39**: 6705–6721.

366. Zeng P, Inkson BJ, Rainforth WM, Stewart T. Characterisation of alumina hip-joint wear by FIB microscopy. *J. Phys.: Conf. Ser.*, 2006; **26**: 343–346.

367. Barceinas-Sanchez JDO, Rainforth WM. On the role of plastic deformation during the mild wear of alumina. *Acta Mater.*, 1998; **46**: 6475–6483.

368. Hockey BJ. Plastic deformation of aluminium oxide by indentation and abrasion. *J. Am. Ceram. Soc.*, 1971; **54**: 223–231.

369. Inkson BJ. Dislocations and twinning activated by the abrasion of Al_2O_3. *Acta Mater.*, 2000; **48**: 1883–1895.

370. Lagerlöf KPD, Heuer AH. Slip and twining in sapphire (α-Al_2O_3). *J. Am. Ceram. Soc.*, 1994; **77**: 385–397.

371. Brown TD, Stewart KJ, Niemen JC, Pedersen DR, Callaghan JJ. Local head roughening as a factor contributing to variability of total hip wear: a finite element analysis. *J. Biomech. Eng.*, 2002; **124**: 691–698.

372. Callaghan JJ, Dysart SH, Savory CF, Hopkinson WJ. Assessing the results of hip replacement. A comparison of five different rating systems. *J. Bone Joint Surg.* (*Br.*), 1990; **72-B**: 1008–1009.

373. Murray DW, Carr AJ, Bulstrode CJ. Which primary total hip replacement? *J. Bone Joint Surg.* (*Br.*), 1995; **77-B**: 520–527.

374. Boutin P. The classic: Total hip arthroplasty using a ceramic prosthesis. *Clin. Orthop.*, 2000; **379**: 3–11.

375. Boutin P. Arthroplastie total de la hanche par prosthese on alumine frittee. *Rev. Chirurgie Orthop.*, 1972; **58**: 229–246.

376. Hamadouche M, Meunier A, Nizard R, Hannouche D, Bizot P, Sedel L. Alumina-on-alumina articulation in total hip arthroplasty: from bench-side to bedside. *Semin. Arthroplasty*, 2006; **17**: 125–133.

377. Murphy SB, Ecker T, Tannast M, Bierbaum B, Garino J, Howe J, Hume E, Jones R, Keggi K, Kress K, Phillips D, Zann R. Experience in the United States with alumina ceramic-ceramic total hip arthroplasty. *Semin. Arthroplasty*, 2006; **17**: 120–124.

378. Sedel L, Raould A. Engineering aspect of alumina on alumina hip prosthesis. *Proc. Inst. Mech. Eng. H*, 2007; **221**: 21–27.

379. Antonov PI, Bakholdin SI, Galaktionov EV, Tropp EV, Nikanorov SP. Anisotropy of thermoelastic stresses in shaped sapphire single crystals. *J. Cryst. Growth*, 1981; **52** Part 1: 404–410.

380. Clarke DR. Microfracture in brittle solids resulting from anisotropic shape changes. *Acta Metall.*, 1980; **28**: 913–924.

381. Ortiz M, Suresh S. Statistical properties of residual stresses and intergranular fracture in ceramic materials. *J. Appl. Mech.*, 1993; **60**: 77–84.

382. Evans AG. Microfracture from thermal expansion anisotropy — I. Single phase systems. *Acta Metall.*, 1978; **26**: 1845–1853.

383. Krell A, Teresiak A, Schaefer D. Grain size dependent residual microstresses in submicron Al_2O_3 and ZrO_2. *J. Eur. Ceram. Soc.*, 1996; **16**: 803–811.

384. Rice RW, Pohanka RC. Grain size dependence of spontaneous cracking in ceramics. *J. Am. Ceram. Soc.*, 1979; **62**: 559–563.

385. Pezzotti G. Internal friction of polycrystalline ceramic oxides. *Phys. Rev. B*, 1999; **60**: 4018–4029.

386. Gates RS, Hsu SM, Klaus EE. Tribochemical mechanism of alumina with water. *Tribol. Trans.*, 1989; **32**: 357–363.

387. Eshelby JD. The determination of the elastic field of an ellipsoidal inclusion and related problems. *Proc. Roy. Soc.*, 1957; **A241**: 376–396.

388. Sternitzke M. Structural ceramic nanocomposites. *J. Eur. Ceram. Soc.*, 1997; **17**: 1061–1082.

389. Evans AG, Clarke DR. Residual stresses and microcracking induced by thermal contraction inhomogeneity. In *Thermal stresses in severe environments*. Hasselman DPH, Heller RA (Eds.). Plenum Press, New York, 1980, pp. 629–648.

390. Mura T, Lin TY, Qin S. Thermal stress in triangular and rectangular inclusion. *Thermoelasticity*, 1995; **1**: 207–210.

391. Boutin P, Christel P, Dorlot J-M, Meunier A, de Roquancourt A, Blanquaert D, Herman S, Sedel L, Witvoet J. The use of dense alumina-alumina ceramic combination in total hip replacement. *J. Biomed. Mater. Res. A*, 1988; **22**: 1203–1232.

392. Bennison SJ, Harmer MP. Effect of MgO solute on the kinetics of grain growth in Al_2O_3. *J. Am. Ceram. Soc.*, 1983; **66**: C90–C92.

393. Bennison SJ, Harmer MP. Grain-growth kinetics for alumina in the absence of a liquid phase. *J. Am. Ceram. Soc.*, 1985; **68**: C22–C24.

394. Handwerker CA, Morris PA, Coble RL. Effects of Chemical Inhomogeneities on Grain Growth and Microstructure in Al_2O_3. *J. Am. Ceram. Soc.*, 1989; **72**: 130–136.

395. Yoshida H, Ikuhara Y, Sakuma T, Sakurai M, Matsubara E. XAFS study on the fine structure of lutetium segregated at grain boundaries in fine-grained polycrystalline alumina. *Phil. Mag.*, 2004; **84**: 865–876.

396. Kara H, Roberts SG. Wet erosion behaviour of low SiC alumina-SiC nanocomposites. *J. Mat. Sci.*, 2002; **37**: 2421–2426.

397. Wu HZ, Roberts SG, Möbus G, Inkson BJ. Subsurface damage analysis by TEM and 3D FIB crack mapping in alumina and alumina/5 vol.% SiC nanocomposites. *Acta Mater.*, 2003; **51**: 149–163.

398. Pezzotti G, Mueller WH. Strengthening mechanisms in Al_2O_3/SiC nanocomposites. *Comput. Mater. Sci.*, 2001; 22: 155–168.

399. Ferroni LP, Pezzotti G. Evidence for bulk residual stress strengthening in Al_2O_3/SiC nanocomposites. *J. Am. Ceram. Soc.*, 2002; **85**: 2033–2038.

400. Sternitzke M, Derby B, Brook RJ. Alumina/silicon carbide nanocomposites by hybrid polymer/powder processing: Microstructures and mechanical properties. *J. Am. Ceram. Soc.*, 1998; **81**: 41–48.

401. Perez-Rigueiro J, Pastor JY, Llorca J, Elices M, Miranzo P, Moya JS. Revisiting the mechanical behavior of alumina silicon carbide nanocomposites. *Acta Mater.*, 1998; **15**: 5399–5411.

402. Levin I, Kaplan WD, Brandon DG. Effect of SiC submicrometer particle-size and content on fracture toughness of alumina-SiC nonocomposites. *J. Am. Ceram. Soc.*, 1995; **78**: 254–256.

403. Pezzotti G, Sergo V, Ota K, Sbaizero O, Muraki N, Nishida T, Sakai M. Residual stresses and apparent strengthening in ceramic-matrix nanocomposites. *J. Ceram. Soc. Jpn.*, 1996; **104**: 497–503.

404. Bae SI, Baik S. Sintering and grain growth of ultrapure alumina. *J. Mater. Sci.*, 1993; **28**: 4197–4204.

405. Zhang S, Garofalini SH. Molecular dynamics simulations of the effect of the composition of calcium alumino-silicate intergranular films on alumina grain growth. *J. Phys. Chem. B*, 2006; **110**: 2233–2240.

406. Suárez M, Fernández A, Menéndez JL, Ramírez-Rico J, Torrecillas R. Blocking of grain reorientation in self-doped alumina materials. *Scripta Mater.*, 2011; **64**: 517–520.

407. Jung J, Baik S. Abnormal grain growth of alumina: CaO effect. *J. Am. Ceram. Soc.*, 2003; **86**: 644–649.

408. Bae SI, Baik S. Determination of critical concentration of silica and/or calcia for abnormal grain growth in alumina. *J. Am. Ceram. Soc.*, 1993; **76**: 1065–1067.

409. Brydson R, Chen S, Riley FL, Milne SJ, Pan X, Rühle M. Microstructure and chemistry of intergranular glassy films in liquid-phase-sintered alumina. *J. Am. Ceram. Soc.*, 1998; **81**: 369–379.

410. Baik S, White CL. Anisotropic Ca segregation to the surface of alumina. *J. Am. Ceram. Soc.*, 1987; **70**: 682–688.

411. Litton DA, Garofalini SH. Atomistic structure of sodium and calcium silicate intergranular films in alumina. *J. Mater. Res.*, 1999; **14**: 1418–1429.

412. West GD, Perkins JM, Lewis MH. The effect of rare earth dopants on grain boundary cohesion in alumina. *J. Eur. Ceram. Soc.*, 2007; **27**: 1913–1918.

413. Chantikul P, Bennison SJ, Lawn BR. Role of grain size in the strength and *R*-curve properties of alumina. *J. Am. Ceram. Soc.*, 1990; **73**: 2419–2427.

414. Burgos-Montes O, Moreno R, Baudin C. Effect of mullite additions on the fracture mode of alumina. *J. Eur. Ceram. Soc.*, 2010; **30**: 857–863.

415. Buban JP, Matsunaga K, Chen J, Shibata N, Ching WY, Yamamoto T, Ikuhara Y. Grain boundary strengthening in alumina by rare earth impurities. *Science*, 2006; **311**: 212–215.

416. Béguin B, Garbowski E, Primet M. Stabilization of alumina by addition of lanthanum, *Appl. Catal.*, 1991; **75**: 119–132.

417. Williams DF, Black J, Doherty PJ. Second consensus conference on definitions in biomaterials. in: *Biomaterials–tissue interfaces*. Doherty PJ, Williams RL, Williams DF, Lee AIJ (eds.). Elsevier, Amsterdam, pp. 525–533, 1992.

418. Williams DF. Biomaterials, and biocompatibility. *Med. Prog. Technol.*, 1976; **20**: 31–42.

419. Dörre E, Hübner H. Alumina. Springer Verlag (Heidelberg, Germany) 1984; p. 235.

420. Takami Y, Yamane S, Makinouchi K, Otsuka G, Glueck J, Benkowski R, Nose Y. Protein adsorption onto ceramic surfaces. *J. Biomed. Mater. Res.*, 1998; **40**: 24–30.

421. Christel P. Biocompatibility of surgical-grade dense polycrystalline alumina. *Clin. Orthop.*, 1992; **282**: 10–18.

422. Griss P, von Adrian-Werburg HV. Biological activity and histo-compatibility of dense Al_2O_3–MgO ceramic implants in rats. *J. Biomed. Mater. Res.*, 1973; **7**: 453–462.

423. Torricelli P, Verne E, Brovarone CV, Appendino P, Rustichelli F, Krajewski A, Ravaglioli A, Pierini G, Fini M, Giavaresi G, Giardino R. Biological glass coating on ceramic materials: *in vitro* evaluation using primary osteoblast cultures from healthy and osteopenic rat bone. *Biomaterials*, 2001; **22**: 2535–2543.

424. Novak S, Kalin M, Kosmac T. Chemical aspects of wear of alumina ceramics. *Wear*, 2001; **250**: 318–321.

425. Novak S, Kalin M. The effect of pH on the wear of water-lubricated alumina and zirconia ceramics. *Tribol. Lett.*, 2004; **17(4)**, 727–732.

426. Mahoney OM, Dimon JH. Unsatisfactory results with a ceramic total hip prosthesis. *J. Bone Joint Surg.* (*Am.*), 1990; **72**: 663–671.

427. Mittelmeier TH, Walter A. The influence of prosthesis design on wear and loosening phenomena. *Crit. Rev. Biocompat.*, 1987; **3**: 319.

428. Yoon TR, Sung MR, Sung TJ, Kwang JS, Maloney WJ. Osteolysis in association with a total hip arthroplasty with ceramic bearings surfaces. *J. Bone Joint Surg.* (*Am.*), 1998; **80**: 1459–1468.

429. Charnley J, Halley DK. Rate of wear in total hip replacement. *Clin. Orthop. Relat. Res.* 1975; **112**: 170–179.

430. Tanaka K, Tamura J, Kawanabe K, Shimizu M, Nakamura T. Effect of alumina femoral heads on polyethylene wear in cemented total hip arthroplasty. *J. Bone Joint Surg.* (*Br.*), 2003; **85-B**: 655–660.

431. Pattyn C, De Smet KA. Primary ceramic-on-ceramic total hip replacement versus metal-on-metal hip resurfacing in young active patients. *Orthopedics*, 2008; **31**: 1078.

432. Yamamoto K, Shishido T, Tateiwa T, Katori Y, Masaoka T, Imakiire A, Clarke IC. Failure of ceramic THR with liner dislocation — a case report. *Acta Orth. Scand.*, 2004; **75**: 500–502.

433. Hwang DS, Kim YM, Lee CH. Alumina femoral head fracture in uncemented total hip arthroplasty with a ceramic sandwich cup. *J. Arthroplasty*, 2007; **22**: 468–471.

434. Kircher J, Bader R, Schroeder B, Mittelmeier W. Extremely high fracture rate of a modular acetabular component with a sandwich polyethylene ceramic insertion for THA: a preliminary report. *Arch. Orthop. Trauma Surg.*, 2009; **129**: 1145–1150.

435. Heisel C, Silva M, Schmalzried TP. Bearing surface options for total hip replacement in young patients. *Instr. Course Lect.*, 2004; **53**: 49–65.

436. Masson B. Emergence of the alumina matrix composite in total hip arthroplasty. *Int. Orthop.*, 2009; **33**: 359–363.

437. Nevelos J, Ingham E, Doyle C, Streicher R, Nevelos A, Walter W, Fisher J. Microseparation of the centers of alumina-alumna artificial hip joints during simulator testing produces clinically relevant wear and patterns. *J. Arthroplasty*, 2000; **15**: 793–795.

438. Williams S, Steward TD, Ingham E, Stone MH, Fisher J. Influence of microseparation and joint laxity on wear of ceramic on polyethylene, ceramic on ceramic and metal on metal total hip replacements. *J. Bone Joint Surg.* (*Br.*), 2003; **85-B** (Supp. I): 57.

439. Williams S, Butterfield M, Steward T, Ingham E, Stone M, Fisher J. Wear and deformation of ceramic-on-polyethylene total hip replacements with joint laxity and swing phase microseparation. *Proc. Inst. Mech. Eng. H*, 2003; **217**: 147–153.

440. Jin ZM, Dowson D, Fisher J. Analysis of fluid film lubrication in artificial hip joint replacements with surfaces of high elastic modulus. *Proc Inst. Mech. Eng. H*, 1997; **211**: 247–256.

441. Schaefer R, Soltesz U, Bernard P-F. Friction in hip-joint prostheses and its influence on the fixation of the artificial head. *J. Mater. Sci.: Mater. Med.* 1998; **9**: 687–690.

442. Wang A, Essner A, Klein, R. Effect of contact stress on friction and wear of ultra-high molecular weight polyethylene in total hip replacement. *Proc. Inst. Mech. Eng. H*, 2001; **215**: 133–139.

443. Tuke MA, Scott G, Roques A, Hu XQ, Taylor A. Design considerations and life prediction of metal-on-metal bearings: The effect of clearance. *J. Bone Joint Surg.* (*Am.*), 2008; **90**: 134–141.

444. Clarke IC, Manley MT. How do alternative bearing surfaces influence wear behavior? *J. Am. Acad. Orthop. Surg.*, 2008; **16** (Supp. 1): S86–S93.

445. Kamali A, Daniel JT, Javid SF, Youseffi M, Band T, Ashton R, Hussain A, Li CX, Daniel J, McMinn DJW. The effect of cup deflection on friction in metal-on-metal bearings. *J. Bone Joint Surg.* (*Br.*), 2008; **90-B** (Supp. 3): 552.

446. Nevelos JE, Ingham E, Doyle C, Nevelos AB, Fisher J. Wear of HIPed and non-HIPed alumina-alumina hip joints under standard and severe simulator testing conditions. *Biomaterials*, 2001; **22**: 2191–2197.

447. Nevelos JE, Ingham, Doyle C, Nevelos AB, Fisher J. The influence of acetabular cup angle on the wear of "BIOLOX Forte" alumina ceramic bearing couples in a hip joint simulator. *J. Mater. Sci.: Mater. Med.* 2001; **12**: 141–144.

448. Oonishi H, Clarke IC, Good V, Amino H, Ueno M. Alumina hip joints characterized by run-in wear and steady-state wear to 14 million cycles in hip-simulator model. *J. Biomed. Mater. Res. A*, 2004; **70-A**: 523–532.

449. Widmer KH, Zurfluh B. Compliant positioning of total hip components for optimal range of motion. *J Orthop Res.*, 2004; **22**: 815–821.

450. Murray DW. The definition and measurement of acetabular orientation. *J. Bone Joint Surg.* (*Br.*), 1993; **75**: 228–232.

451. Shishido T, Clarke IC, Williams P, Boehler M, Asano T, Shoji H, Masaoka T, Yamamoto K, Imakiire A. Clinical and simulator wear study of alumina ceramic THR to 17 years and beyond. *J. Biomed. Mater. Res. B*, 2003; **67-B**: 638–647.

452. Manaka M, Clarke IC, Yamamoto K, Shishido T, Gustafson A, Imakiire A. Stripe wear rates in alumina THR — comparison of microseparation simulator study with retrieved implants. *J. Biomed. Mater. Res. B*, 2004;

69-B: 149–157.

453. Chen Y, Huang W. Numerical simulation of the geometrical factors affecting surface roughness measurements by AFM. *Meas. Sci. Tech.*, 2004; **15**: 2005–2010.

454. Barbour PSM, Stone MH, Fisher J. A hip joint simulator study using new and physiologically scratched femoral heads with ultra-high molecular weight polyethylene acetabular cups. *Proc. Inst. Mech. Eng. H*, 2000; **214**: 569–576.

455. Eberhardt AW, McKee RT, Cuckler JM, Peterson DW, Beck PR, Lemons JE. Surface roughness of CoCr and ZrO_2 femoral heads with metal transfer: A retrieval and wear simulator study. *Int. J. Biomater.*, 2009; **2009**: 185456-1–6.

456. Dowson D, Hardaker C, Flett M, Isaac GH. A hip joint simulator study of the performance of metal-on-metal joints, Part II: design. *J. Arthroplasty*, 2004; **19** (Suppl. 3): 124–130.

457. Stewart TD, Tipper J, Streicher R, Ingham E, Fisher J. Long-term wear of HIPed alumina on alumina bearings for THR under microseparation conditions. *J. Mater. Sci.: Mater. Med.*, 2001; **12**: 1053–1056.

458. Affatato S, Traina F, Toni A. Microseparation and stripe wear in alumina-on-alumina hip implants. *Int. J. Artif. Organs*, 2011; **34**: 506–512.

459. Muller U, Gautier E, Roeder C, Busato A. The relationship between cup design and the radiological signs of aseptic loosening in total hip arthroplasty. *J. Bone Joint Surg.* (*Br.*), 2003; **85-B**: 31–36.

460. Duisabeau L, Combrade P, Forest B. Environmental effect on fretting of metallic materials for orthopaedic implants. *Wear*, 2004; **256**: 805–816.

461. Sundfeldt M, Carlsson LV, Johansson CB, Thomsen P, Gretzer C. Aseptic loosening, not only a question of wear: a review of different theories. *Acta Orthop.*, 2006; **77**: 177–197.

462. Affatato S, Spinelli M, Zavalloni M, Mazzega-Fabbro C, Viceconti M. Tribology and total hip joint replacement: Current concepts in mechanical simulation. *Med. Eng. Phys.*, 2008; **30**: 1305–1317.

463. Grabner L. Spectroscopic technique for the measurement of residual stress in sintered Al_2O_3. *J. Appl. Phys.*, 1978; **49**: 580–583.

464. Munisso MC, Zhu W, Leto A, Pezzotti G. Stress dependence of sapphire cathodoluminescence from optically active oxygen defects as a function of crystallographic orientation. *J. Phys. Chem. A*, 2007; **111**: 3526–3533.

465. Leto A, Munisso MC, Porporati AA, Zhu W, Pezzotti G. Stress dependence of paramagnetic point defects in amorphous silicon oxide. *J. Phys. Chem. A*, 2008; **112** (17): 3927–3934.

466. Leto A, Porporati AA, Zhu W, Green M, Pezzotti G. High-resolution stress assessments of interconnect/dielectric electronic patterns using optically active point defects of silica glass as a stress sensor. *J. Appl. Phys.*, 2007; **101**: 093514-1–14.

467. McClure DS. Optical spectra of transition-metal ions in corundum. *J. Chem. Phys.*, 1962; **36**: 2757–2779.

468. Poole Jr. CP. The optical spectra and color of chromium containing solids. *J. Phys. Chem. Solids*, 1964; **25**: 1169–1182.

469. Porto SPS, Krishnan RS. Raman effect of corundum. *J. Chem. Phys.*, 1967; **47**: 1009–1012.

470. Krishnan RS. Raman spectrum of alumina and the luminescence of ruby. *Proc. Math. Sci.* (*Indian Acad. Sci. A*), 1947; **26**: 450–459.

471. Lee KH, Krawford JH. Luminescence of the F center in sapphire. *Phys. Rev. B*, 1979; **19**: 3217–3221.

472. Draeger BG, Summers GP. Defects in unirradiated α-Al_2O_3. *Phys. Rev. B*, 1979; **19**: 1172–1177.

473. Wan KS, Tochino S, Zhu W, Ohtsuka S, Pezzotti G. Quantitative evaluation of probe response functions for Raman and fluorescence bands of single-crystalline and polycrystalline Al_2O_3. *J. Phys. D: Appl. Phys.*, 2010; **43**: 205501-1–10.

474. Fitting H-J, Glaefeke H, Wild W. Electron penetration and energy transfer in solid targets. *Phys. Status Solidi* (*a*), 1977; **43**: 185–190.

475. Kanaya K, Okayama S. Penetration and energy-loss theory of electrons in solid targets. *J. Phys. D: Appl. Phys.*, 1972; **5**: 43–58.

476. Grellner F, Hoescheler S, Greil P, Sindel J, Petschelt A. Residual stress measurements of computer aided design/computer aided manufacturing (CAD/CAM) machined dental ceramics. *J. Mater. Sci.*, 1997; **32**: 6235–6242.

477. Sparks RG, Paesler MA. Depth profiling of residual stress along interrupted test cuts in machined germanium crystals. *J. Appl. Phys.*, 1992; **71**: 891–897.

478. Vedula VR, Glass SJ, Saylor DM, Rohrer GS, Carter WC, Langer SA, Fuller Jr. ER. Residual-stress predictions in polycrystalline alumina. *J. Am. Ceram. Soc.*, 2001; **84**: 2947–2954.

479. Ma Q, Clarke DR. Piezospectroscopic determination of residual stresses in polycrystalline alumina. *J. Am. Ceram. Soc.*, 1994; **77**: 298–302.

480. Hsu YC, Forman RG. Elastic-plastic analysis of an infinite sheet having a circular hole under pressure. *Trans. ASME: J. Appl. Mech.*, 1975; **42**: 347–352.

481. Ball DL, Lowry DR. Experimental investigation on the effects of cold expansion of fastener holes. *Fatigue Fract. Eng. Mater. Struct.*, 1998; **21**: 17–34.

482. Che Z, Xiong L, Shi T, Cheng H, Yang L. Experimental analysis of microscale laser shock processing on metallic material using excimer laser. *J. Mater. Sci. Technol.*, 2009; **25**: 829–834.

483. Bhuvaraghan B, Srinivasan RM, Maffeo B. Optimization of the fatigue strength of materials due to shot peening: A survey. *Int. J. Struct. Changes — Solids*, 2010; **2**: 33–63.

484. Jahanmir S. Tribological applications of advanced ceramics. *Mat. Res. Soc. Symp. Proc.*, 1989; **140**: 285–291.

485. Xiong F, Manory RR, Ward L, Terheci M, Lathabai S. Effect of grain size and test configuration on the wear behavior of alumina. *J. Am. Ceram. Soc.*, 1997; **80**: 1310–1312.

486. Chen YM, Rigaut B. Friction and wear of alumina ceramics at high sliding speed. *Lubr. Eng.*, 1990; **47**: 531–537.

487. Dong X, Jahanmir S, Hsu SM. Tribological characteristics of α-alumina at elevated temperature. *J. Am. Ceram. Soc.*, 1991; **74**: 1036–1044.

488. Esposito L, Tucci A, Solomah AG, Palmonari C. Effects of temperature and sliding velocity an the dry tribological characteristics of high purity, high density polycrystalline aluminium oxides. *Wear*, 1992; **153**: 351–360.

489. Perez-Unzueta AJ, Beynon JH, Gee MG. The effect of surrounding atmosphere on the sliding wear of alumina. *Wear*, 1991; **146**: 179–196.

490. Andersson P. Water lubricated pin-on-disc tests with ceramics. *Wear*, 1992; **154**: 37–47.

491. Wang Y, Hsu SM. The effect of operating parameters and environment on the wear and wear transition of alumina. *Wear*, 1996; **195**: 90–99.

492. Mukhopadhyay AK, Mai YW. Grain size effect on abrasive wear mechanisms in alumina ceramics. *Wear*, 1993; **162–164**: 258–268.

493. Zum Gahr KH, Bundschuh W, Zimmerlin B. Effect of grain size on friction and sliding wear of oxide ceramics. *Wear*, 1993; **162–164**: 269–279.

494. Malkin S, Ritter JE. Grinding mechanisms and strength degradation for ceramics. *J. Eng. Ind.*, 1989; **111**: 167–174.

495. Mukherji J, Das PK. Wear of some advanced ceramics under a sharp indenter in unidirectional sliding. *J. Am. Ceram. Soc.*, 1993; **76**: 2376–2378.

496. Ajayi OO, Ludema KC. The effect of microstructure on wear modes of ceramic materials. *Wear*, 1992; **154**: 371–385.

497. Hokkirigawa K. Wear mode map of ceramics. *Wear*, 1991; **151**: 219–228.

498. Cutter LA, McPherson R. Plastic deformation of Al_2O_3 during abrasion. *J. Am. Ceram. Soc.*, 1973; **56**: 266–269.

499. Gilbert CJ, Petrany RN, Ritchie RO, Dauskardt RH, Steinbrech RW. Cyclic fatigue in monolithic alumina: mechanisms for crack advance promoted by frictional wear of grain bridges. *J. Mater. Sci.*, 1995; **30**: 643–654.

500. Gee MG. The formation of aluminium hydroxide in the sliding wear of alumina. *Wear*, 1992; **153**: 201–227.

501. Li J, Liu Y, Hermansson L, Soremark R. Evaluation of biocompatibility of various ceramic powders with human fibroblasts *in vitro*. *Clin. Mater.*, 1993; **12:** 197–201.

502. Khanna R, Basu B. Low friction and severe wear of alumina in cryogenic environment: A first report. *J. Mater. Res.*, 2006; **21**: 832–843.

503. Jamari J, de Rooij MB, Schipper DJ. Plastic deterministic contact of rough surfaces. *J. Tribol.*, 2007; **129**: 957–962.

504. Gao YF, Lucas BN, Hay JC, Oliver WC, Pharr GM. Nanoscale incipient asperity sliding at interface micro-slip assessed by the measurement of tangential contact stiffness. *Scripta Mater.*, 2006; **55**: 653–656.

505. Tipper JL, Hatton A, Nevelos JE, Ingham E, Doyle C, Streicher R, Nevelos AB, Fisher J. Alumina-alumina artificial hip joints. Part II: characterization of the wear debris from *in vitro* hip joint simulations. *Biomaterials*, 2002; **23**: 3441–3448.

506. Nevelos A, Evans PA, Harrison P, Rainforth WM. Examination of alumina ceramic components from total hip arthroplasties. *Proc. Inst. Mech. Eng. H*, 1993; **207**: 155–162.

507. Lagerlöf KPD, Mitchel TE, Heuer AH, Riviere JP, Cadoz J, Castaing J, Phillips DS. Stacking fault energy in sapphire (α-Al_2O_3). *Acta Metall.*, 1984; **32**: 97–105.

508. Jahanmir S. Wear of ceramics: wear transitions and tribochemical reactions. In Stachowiak GW (Ed.). *Wear — Materials, mechanisms and practice*. John Wiley & Sons Ltd, Chichester, pp. 167–189, 2005.

509. Jeng MC, Yan LY. Environmental effects on wear behavior of alumina. *Wear*, 1993; **161**: 111–119.

510. Mori S. The lubrication of ceramics — adsorption and chemical reaction. *Tribol. J. Jpn. Soc. Tribol.*, 1991; **36**: 130–134.

511. Shapovalov V, Truong TN. *Ab initio* study of water adsorption on α-Al_2O_3 (0001) crystal surface. *J. Phys. Chem. B*, 2000; **104**: 9859–9866.

512. Fernandez EM, Eglitis RI, Borstel G, Balbas LC. *Ab initio* calculations of H_2O and O_2 adsorption on Al_2O_3 substrates. *Comput. Mater. Sci.*, 2007; **39**: 587–592.

513. Zeng H, Chittur KK, Lacefield WR. Analysis of bovine serum albumin adsorption on calcium phosphate and titanium surfaces. *Biomaterials*, 1999; **20**: 377–384.

514. Garrett Q, Griesser HJ, Milthorpe BK, Garrett RW. Irreversible adsorption of human serum albumin to hydrogel contact lenses: A study using electron spin resonance spectroscopy. *Biomaterials*, 1999; **20**: 1345–1356.

515. Mishina H, Kojima M. Changes in human serum albumin on arthroplasty frictional surfaces. *Wear*, 2008; **265**: 655–663.

516. Nevelos JE, Prudhommeaux F, Hamadouche M, Doyle C, Ingham E, Meunier A, Nevelos AB, Sedel L, Fisher J. Comparative analysis of two different types of alumina-alumina hip prosthesis retrieved for aseptic loosening. *J. Bone Joint Surg.* (*Br.*), 2001; **83-B**: 598–603.

517. Deckman DE, Jahanmir S. Wear mechanisms of alpha alumina lubricated with a paraffin oil. *Wear*, 1991; **149**: 155–168.

518. Dahl LB, Dahl IM, Engström-Laurent A, Granath K. Concentration and molecular weight of sodium hyaluronate in synovial fluid from patients with rheumatoid arthritis and other arthropathies. *Ann. Rheum. Dis.*, 1985; **44**: 817–822.

519. Ghamnia M, Jardin C, Bouslama M. Luminescence centres F and F^+ in α-alumina detected by cathodoluminescence technique. *J. Electron Spectr. Rel. Phenom.*, 2003; **133**: 55–63.

520. Brandt G, Mikus M. An electron microprobe and cathodoluminescence study of chemical reactions between tool and workpiece when turning steel with alumina-based ceramics. *Wear*, 1987; **115**: 243–263.

521. Surdo AI, Pustarov VA, Kortov VS, Kishka AS, Zinin EI. Luminescence in anion-defective α-Al_2O_3 crystals over the nano- micro- and millisecond intervals. *Nucl. Instr. Meth. A*, 2005; **543**: 234–238.

522. Boumasa A, Djelloul A, Guerrab F. Specific signatures of α-alumina powders prepared by calcination of bohemite or gibbsite. *Powd. Tech.*, 2010; **201**: 177–180.

523. Stathopoulos AY, Pells GP. Damage in the cation sublattice of α-Al_2O_3 irradiated in an HVEM. *Philos. Mag. A*, 1983; **47**: 381–394.

524. Dubinko VI, Turkin AA, Vainshtein DI, den Hartog HW. New mechanism for radiation defect production and aggregation in crystalline ceramics. *J. Nucl. Mater.*, 2001; **289**: 86–95.

525. Oda K, Yoshio T. Hydrothermal corrosion of alumina ceramics. *J. Am. Ceram. Soc.*, 1997; **80**: 3233–3236.

526. Bennison SJ, Harmer MP. Swelling of hot-pressed Al_2O_3. *J. Am. Ceram. Soc.*, 1985; **68**: 591–597.

527. Jonnard P, Bonnelle C, Blaise G, Remond G, Roques-Carmes C. F^+ and F centers in α-Al_2O_3 by electron-induced X-ray emission spectroscopy and cathodoluminescence. *J. Appl. Phys.*, 2000; **88**: 6413–6417.

528. Stoyanovskii VO, Snytnikov VN. Laser-induced luminescence associated with surface hydroxide groups in Al_2O_3. *Kinet. Catal.*, 2009; **50**: 470–475.

529. Wiederhorn SM. Moisture assisted crack growth in ceramics. *Int. J. Fract. Mech.*, 1968; **4**: 171–177.

530. Castaing J, Kronenberg AK, Kirby SH, Mitchell TE. Hydrogen defects in α-Al_2O_3 and water weakening of sapphire and alumina ceramics between 600 and 1000°C — II. Mechanical properties. *Acta Mater.*, 2000; **48**: 1495–1504.

531. Mainprice D, Taki S, Hosaka M. Water in hydrothermally grown sapphire (α-Al_2O_3). In Boland JN, Fitz Gerald JD (Eds.). *Defects and processes in the solid state: geoscience applications, the McLaren volume*. Elsevier Science Publishers, Amsterdam and New York, pp. 347–358, 1993.

532. Lam DCC, Lange FF, Evans AG. Mechanical properties of partially dense alumina produced from powder compacts. *J. Am. Ceram. Soc.*, 1994; **77**: 2113–2117.

533. Ostrowski T, Ziegler A, Bordia RK, Rödel J. Evolution of Young's modulus, strength and microstructure during liquid phase sintering. *J. Am. Ceram. Soc.*, 1998; **81**: 1852–1860.

534. Ostrowski T, Rödel J. Evolution of mechanical properties of porous alumina during free sintering and hot pressing. *J. Am. Ceram. Soc.*, 1999; **82**: 3080–3086.

535. Baratta FI. Refinement of stress intensity factor estimates for a peripherally cracked spherical void and a hemispherical surface pit. *J. Am. Ceram. Soc.*, 1981; **64**: C3–C4.

536. Evans AG, Biswas DR, Fulrath RM. Some effects of cavities on the fracture of ceramics: II, spherical cavities. *J. Am. Ceram. Soc.*, 1979; **62**: 101–106.

537. Kingery WD, Francois B. Sintering of crystalline oxides, I. Interaction between grain boundaries and pores. In *Sintering and related phenomena*. Kuczynski GC, Hooton NA, Gibbon GF (Eds.). Gordon Breach, New York, pp. 471–498, 1967.

538. Kellett BJ, Lange FF. Experiments on pore closure during hot isostatic pressing and forging. *J. Am. Ceram. Soc.*, 1988; **71**: 7–12.

539. Oh K-S, Kim D-Y, Cho S-J. Shrinkage of large isolated pores during hot isostatic pressing of presintered alumina ceramics. *J. Am. Ceram. Soc.*, 1995; **78**: 2537–2540.

540. Evans AG, Hsueh CH. Behavior of large pores during sintering and hot pressing. *J. Am. Ceram. Soc.*, 1986; **69**: 444–448.

541. Flinn BD, Bordia RK, Rödel J. Evolution of strength determining flaws during sintering. In *Sintering technology*. German RM, Messing GL, Cornwall RG (Eds.). Marcel Dekker, New York, pp. 13–20, 1996.

542. Fett T, Munz D, Seidel J, Stech M, Rödel J. Correlation between long and short crack R-curves in alumina using the crack opening displacement and fracture mechanical weight function approach. *J. Am. Ceram. Soc.*, 1996; **79**: 1189–1196.

543. Zimmermann A, Hoffman M, Flinn BD, Bordia RK, Chuang T-J, Fuller ER, Rödel J. Fracture of alumina with controlled pores. *J. Am. Ceram. Soc.*, 1998; **81**: 2449–2457.

544. Seidel J, Claussen N, Rödel J. Reliability of alumina ceramics: I, Effect of grain size. *J. Eur. Ceram. Soc.*, 1995; **15**: 395–404.

545. Seidel J, Rödel J. Measurement of crack tip toughness in alumina as a function of grain size. *J. Am. Ceram. Soc.*, 1997; **80**: 433–438.

546. Velamakanni BV, Lange FF, Zok FW, Pearson DS. Influence of inter-particle forces on the rheological behavior of pressure-consolidated alumina particle slurries. *J. Am. Ceram. Soc.*, 1994; **77**: 216–220.

547. Heinrich J, Munz D. Strength of reaction-bonded silicon nitride with artificial pores. *Bull. Am. Ceram. Soc.*, 1980; **59**: 1221–1222.

548. Irwin GR. Analysis of stresses and strains near the end of a crack transversing a plate. *J. Appl. Mech. Trans. ASME*, 1957; **79**: 361–364.

549. Fett T. An extension of the Newman-Raju formula. *Int. J. Fracture*, 1987; **33**: R47–R50.

550. Jayatilaka ADeS, Trustrum K. Statistical approach to brittle fracture. *J. Mater. Sci.*, 1977; **12**: 1426–1430.

551. Trustrum K, Jayatilaka ADeS. On estimating the Weibull modulus for a brittle material. *J. Mater. Sci.*, 1979; **14**: 1080–1084.

552. Nakamura S, Tanaka S, Furushima R, Sato K, Uematsu K. Estimation of Weibull modulus from coarser defect distribution in dry-pressed alumina ceramics. *J. Ceram. Soc. Jpn.*, 2009; **117**: 742–747.

553. Tinschert J, Zwez D, Marx R, Anusavice KJ. Structural reliability of alumina-, feldspar-, leucite-, mica- and zirconia-based ceramics. *J. Dentistry*, 2000; **28**: 529–535.

554. Meyers MA, Chawla KK. *Mechanical behavior of materials* (2nd Edition). Cambridge University Press, Cambridge, p. 453, 2009.

555. Tuan WH, Kuo JC. Effect of grinding parameters on the reliability of alumina. *Mater. Chem. Phys.*, 1998; **52**: 41–45.

556. Gong J. Correlation between Weibull moduli for tensile and bending strength of brittle ceramics: A numerical simulation analysis based on a three-parameter Weibull distribution. *J. Mater. Sci.*, 2003; **38**: 2541–2545.

557. Ruff O, Ebert F. Beiträge zur Keramik hochfeuerfeste Stoffe. I. Die Formen des Zirkondioxyds. *Z. Anorg. Allg. Chem.*, 1929; **180**: 19–41.

558. Strickler DW, Carlson WG. Ionic conductivity of cubic solid solutions in the system $CaO–Y_2O_3–ZrO_2$. *J. Am. Ceram. Soc.*, 1964; **47**: 122–127.

559. Dixon JM, LaGrange LD, Merten U, Miller CF, Porter II JT. Electrical resistivity of stabilized zirconia at elevated temperatures. *J. Electrochem. Soc.*, 1963; **110**: 276–280.

560. Cales B. Zirconia as a sliding material: Histologic, laboratory, and clinical data. *Clin. Orthop. Relat. Res.*, 2000; **379**: 94–112.

561. Piconi C, Maccauro G. Zirconia as a ceramic biomaterial. *Biomaterials*, 1999; **20**: 1–25.

562. Nernst W. Über die Elektrolytische Leitung fester Koerper bei sehr hohen Temperaturen. *Z. Elektrochem.*, 1899; **6**: 41–43.

563. Teufer G. The crystal structure of tetragonal ZrO_2. *Acta Crystallogr.* 1962; **15**: 1187.

564. Orlando R, Pisani C, Poetti C, Stefanovich E. *Ab initio* Hartree–Fock study of tetragonal and cubic phases of zirconium dioxide. *Phys. Rev. B*, 1992; **45**: 596–601.

565. Patil RN, Subbarao EC. Axial thermal expansion of ZrO_2 and HfO_2 in the range room temperature to 1400°C. *J. Appl. Crystallogr.*, 1969; **2**: 281–288.

566. Patil RN, Subbarao EC. Monoclinic-tetragonal phase transition in zirconia: Mechanism, pretransformation and coexistence. *Acta Crystallogr. A*, 1970; **26**: 535–542.

567. Deville S. Guenin G., Chevalier J. Martensitic transformation in zirconia Part I. Nanometer scale prediction and measurement of transformation induced relief. *Acta Mater.*, 2004; **52**: 5697–5707.

568. Frey F, Boysen H, Vogt T. Neutron powder investigation of the monoclinic to tetragonal phase transformation in undoped zirconia. *Acta Crystallogr. B*, 1990; **46**: 724–730.

569. Subbarao EC, Maiti HS, Srivastava KK. Martensitic transformation in zirconia. *Phys. Status Solidi (a)*, 1974; **21**: 9–40.

570. Bansal G, Heuer AH. On a martensitic phase transformation in zirconia (ZrO_2) — I. Metallographic evidence. *Acta Metall.*, 1972; **20**: 1281–1289.

571. Bansal G, Heuer AH. On a martensitic phase transformation in zirconia (ZrO_2) — II. Crystallographic aspects. *Acta Metall.*, 1974; **22**: 409–417.

572. Chen M, Hallstedt B, Gauckler LJ. Thermodynamic modeling of the ZrO_2-$YO_{1.5}$ system. *Solid State Ionics*, 2004; **170**: 255–274.

573. Garvie RC. The occurrence of metastable tetragonal zirconia as a crystallite size effect. *J. Phys. Chem.*, 1965; **69**: 1238–1243.

574. Hund F. Anomale Mischkristalle im System ZrO_2–Y_2O_3. Kristallbau der Nernst-Stifte. *Zeitschrift. Elektrochem. Angew. Phys. Chem.*, 1951; **55**: 363–366.

575. Kröger FA, Vink HJ. Relations between the concentrations of imperfections in solids. *J. Phys. Chem. Solids*, 1958; **5**: 208–223.

576. Grain CF. Phase Relations in the ZrO_2–MgO System. *J. Am. Ceram. Soc.*, 1967; **50**: 288–290.

577. Stubican VS, Ray SP. Phase equilibria and ordering in the system ZrO_2–CaO. *J. Am. Ceram. Soc.*, 1977; **60**: 534–537.

578. Goff JP, Hayes W, Hull S, Hutchings MT, Clausen KN. Defect structure of yttria-stabilized zirconia and its influence on the ionic conductivity at elevated temperatures. *Phys. Rev. B*, 1999; **59**: 14202–14219.

579. Stefanovich EV, Shluger AL, Catlow CRA. Theoretical study of the stabilization of cubic-phase ZrO_2 by impurities. *Phys. Rev. B*, 1994; **49**: 11560–11571.

580. Tuilier MH, Dexpert-Ghys J, Dexpert H, Lagarde PJ. X-ray absorption study of the ZrO_2–Y_2O_3 system. *Solid State Chem.*, 1987; **69**: 153–161.

581. Morikawa H, Shimizugawa Y, Marumo F, Harasawa T, Ikawa H, Tohji K, Udagawa Y. Local structures around Y atoms in Y_2O_3-stabilized tetragonal ZrO_2. *J. Jpn. Ceram. Soc.*, 1988; **96**: 253–258.

582. Steele D, Fender BEF. The structure of cubic ZrO_2:$YO_{1.5}$ solid solutions by neutron scattering. *J. Phys. C: Solid State Phys.*, 1974; **7**: 1–11.

583. Catlow CRA, Chadwick AV, Greaves GN, Moroney LM. EXAFS study of yttria-stabilized zirconia. *J. Am. Ceram. Soc.*, 1986; **69**: 272–277.

584. Veal BW, Mckale AG, Paulikas AP, Rothman SJ, Nowicki LJ. EXAFS study of yttria-stabilized cubic zirconia. *Physica B*, 1988; **150**: 234–240.

585. Komyoji D, Yoshiasa A, Moriga T, Emura S, Kanamaru F, Koto K. EXAFS study of the fluorite-type compounds in the systems $(1 - x)ZrO_2$–$xYbO_{1.5}$ ($x = 0.18 \leq x \leq 0.5$) and $Zr_2Ln_2O_7$ (Ln = Tb, Dy, Ho, Er, and Yb). *Solid State Ionics*, 1992; **50**: 291–301.

586. Kushima A, Yildiz B. Oxygen ion diffusivity in strained yttria stabilized zirconia: where is the fastest strain? *J. Mater. Chem.*, 2010; **20**: 4809–4819.

587. Li P, Chen I-W, Penner-Hahn JE. Effect of dopants on zirconia stabilization — an X-ray-absorption study. 3. Charge-compensating dopants. *J. Am. Ceram. Soc.*, 1994; **77**: 1289–1295.

588. Stapper G, Bernasconi M, Nicoloso N, Parrinello M. *Ab initio* study of structural and electronic properties of yttria-stabilized cubic zirconia. *Phys. Rev. B*, 1999; **59**: 797–810.

589. Bogicevic A, Wolverton C, Crosbie GM, Stechel EB. Defect ordering in aliovalently doped cubic zirconia from first principles. *Phys. Rev. B*, 2001; **64**: 14106-1–14.

590. Howard CJ, Hill RJ, Reichert BE. Structures of the ZrO_2 polymorphs at room temperature by high-resolution neutron powder diffraction. *Acta Crystallogr.*, 1988; **B44**: 116–120.

591. Morterra C, Cerrato G, Ferroni L, Montanari L. Surface characterization of yttria-stabilized tetragonal ZrO_2. Part 1. Structural, morphological, and surface hydration features. *Mat. Chem. Phys.*, 1994; **37**: 243–257.

592. de Ridder M, Vervoort AGJ, van Welzenis RG, Brongersma HH. The limiting factor for oxygen exchange at the surface of fuel cell electrolytes. *Solid State Ionics*, 2003; **156**: 255–262.

593. de Ridder M, van Welzenis RG, Brongersma HH, Kreissig U. Oxygen exchange and diffusion in the near surface of pure and modified yttria-stabilised zirconia. *Solid State Ionics*, 2003; **158**: 67–77.

594. Bernasik A, Kowalski K, Sadowski A. Surface segregation in yttria-stabilized zirconia by means of angle resolved X-ray photoelectron spectroscopy. *J. Phys. Chem. Solids*, 2002; **63**: 233–239.

595. Zhu J, van Ommen JG, Henny J, Bouwmeester M, Lefferts LJ. Activation of O_2 and CH_4 on yttrium-stabilized zirconia for the partial oxidation of methane to synthesis gas. *J. Catal.*, 2005; **233**: 434–441.

596. Ballabio G, Bernasconi M, Pietrucci F, Serra S. *Ab initio* study of yttria-stabilized cubic zirconia surfaces. *Phys. Rev. B*, 2004; **70**: 075417-1–6.

597. Eichler A, Kresse G. First-principles calculations for the surface termination of pure and yttria-doped zirconia surfaces. *Phys. Rev. B*, 2004; **69**: 045402-1–17.

598. Rieth PH, Reed JS, Naumann AW. Fabrication and flexural strength of ultra-fine grained yttria-stabilised zirconia. *Bull. Am. Ceram. Soc.*, 1976; **55**: 717–721.

599. Christel P, Meunier A, Heller M, Torre JP, Peille CN. Mechanical properties and short-term *in-vivo* evaluation of yttrium-oxide partially-stabilized zirconia. *J. Biomed. Mater. Res.*, 1989; **23**: 45–61.

600. Tateishi T, Yunoki H. Research and development of alumina and zirconia artificial hip joint. *Clin. Mater.*, 1993; **12**: 219–225.

601. Piconi C, Burger W, Richter HG, Cittadini A, Maccauro G, Covacci V, Bruzzese N, Ricci GA, Marmo E. Y-TZP ceramics for artificial joint replacements. *Biomaterials*, 1998; **19**: 1489–1494.

602. Medical Devices Agency — Adverse Incident Centre. Zirconia ceramic heads for modular total hip femoral components: advice to users on re-sterilization. Safety Notice MDA SN 9617, UK Government, June 1996.

603. Guo X. Roles of alumina in zirconia for functional applications. *J. Am. Ceram. Soc.*, 2003; **86**: 1867–1873.

604. Guo X. On the degradation of zirconia ceramic during low-temperature annealing in water or water vapor. *J. Phys. Chem. Solids*, 1999; **60**: 539–546.

605. Matsui K, Ohmichi N, Ohgai M, Enomoto N, Hojo J. Sintering kinetics at constant rates of heating: Effect of Al_2O_3 on the initial sintering stage of fine zirconia powder. *J. Am. Ceram. Soc.*, 2005; **88**: 3346–3352.

606. Matsui K, Yamakawa T, Uehara M, Enomoto N, Hojo J. Mechanism of alumina-enhanced sintering of fine zirconia powder: Influence of alumina concentration on the initial stage sintering. *J. Am. Ceram. Soc.*, 2008; **91**: 1888–1897.

607. Li JF, Watanabe R. Influence of a small amount of Al_2O_3 addition on the transformation of Y_2O_3-partially stabilized ZrO_2 during annealing. *J. Mater. Sci.*, 1997; **32**: 1149–1153.

608. Mullens S, Cooymans J, Smolders C, Luyten J. Processing oxide-based nanocomposites. *Am. Ceram. Soc. Bull.*, 2005; **84**: 9101–9103.

609. Chen C-C, Hsiang H-I, Hsu S-W. Preparation and characterization of Y-TZP powders coated with alumina. *J. Ceram. Proc. Res.*, 2008; **9**: 131–134.

610. Burger W, Richter HG, Piconi C, Vatteroni R, Cittadini A, Boccalari M. New Y-TZP powders for medical grade zirconia. *J. Mater. Sci. Mat. Med.*, 1997; **8**: 113–118.

611. Watanabe M, Iio S, Fukuura I. Aging behavior of Y-TZP. In *Advances in ceramics, Vol. 12, Science and technology of zirconia II*. Claussen N, Rühle M, Heuer AH (Eds.). The American Ceramic Society, Inc., Columbus, OH, pp. 391–398, 1984.

612. Chung TJ, Song H, Kim GH, Kim DY. Microstructure and phase stability of yttria-doped tetragonal zirconia polycrystals heat treated in nitrogen atmosphere. *J. Am. Ceram. Soc.*, 1997; **80**: 2607–2612.

613. Hernandez MT, Jurado JR, Duran P, Fierro JLG. Subeutectoid degradation of yttria-stabilized tetragonal zirconia polycrystal and ceria-doped yttria-stabilized tetragonal zirconia polycrystal ceramics. *J. Am. Ceram. Soc.*, 1991; **74**: 1254–1258.

614. Sato T, Ohtaki S, Endo T, Shimada M. Improvement of thermal stability of yttria-doped tetragonal zirconia polycrystals by doping CeO_2 on the surface. *J. Mat. Sci. Lett.*, 1986; **5**: 1140–1142.

615. Evans AG, Perspective on the development of high-toughness ceramics. *J. Am. Ceram. Soc.*, 1990; **73**: 187–206.

616. McMeeking, RM, Evans AG. Mechanics of transformation toughening in brittle materials. *J. Am. Ceram. Soc.*, 1982; **65**: 242–246.

617. Nalla RK, Kruzic JJ, Kinney JH, Ritchie RO. Mechanistic aspects of fracture and R-curve behavior in human cortical bone. *Biomaterials*, 2005; **26**: 217–231.

618. Kulin RM, Jianf F, Vecchio KS. Loading effects on the R-curve behavior of cortical bone. *Acta Biomater.*, 2011; **7**: 724–732.

619. Rose LRF, Swain MV. Two R curves for partially stabilized zirconia. *J. Am. Ceram. Soc.*, 1986; **69**: 203–207.

620. Li CW, Yamanis J. Super-tough silicon nitride with R-curve behavior. *Ceram. Eng. Sci. Proc.*, 1989; **10**: 632–645.

621. Marshall DB, Shaw MC, Dauskardt RH, Ritchie RO, Readey MJ, Heuer AH. Crack-tip transformation zones in toughened zirconia. *J. Am. Ceram. Soc.*, 1990; **73**: 2659–2666.

622. Shimozono T, Ikeda J, Pezzotti G. Evaluation of transformation zone around propagating cracks in zirconia biomaterials using Raman microprobe spectroscopy. *Key Eng. Mater.*, 2006; **309–311**: 1207–1210.

623. Ohtsuka S, Zhu W, Tochino S, Sekiguchi Y, Pezzotti G. In depth analysis of residual stress in an alumina coating on silicon nitride substrate using confocal Raman piezo-spectroscopy. *Acta Mater.*, 2007; **55**: 1129–1135.

624. Rice JR. Some remarks on elastic crack — tip stress fields. *Int. J. Solids Struct.*, 1972; **8**: 751–758.

625. Evans AG, Heuer AH. Review — Transformation toughening in ceramics: Martensitic transformations in crack-tip stress fields. *J. Am. Ceram. Soc.*, 1980; **63**: 241–248.

626. Kouroulis GA, Liarokapis E. Pressure and temperature dependence of the Raman spectra of zirconia and hafnia. *J. Am. Ceram. Soc.*, 1991; **74**: 520–530.

627. Milman V, Perlov A, Refson K, Clark SJ, Gavartin J, Winkler B. Structural, electronic and vibrational properties of tetragonal zirconia under pressure: a density functional theory study. *J. Phys.: Condens. Matter*, 2009; **21**: 485404-1-12.

628. Sato T, Shimada M. Transformation of yttria-doped tetragonal zirconia polycrystals by annealing in water. *J. Am. Ceram. Soc.*, 1985; **68**; 356–359.

629. Yoshimura M, Noma T, Kawabata K, Somiya S. Role of water on the degradation process of Y-TZP yttrium-doped tetragonal zirconia. *J. Mater. Sci. Lett.*, 1987; **6**: 465–467.

630. Schmauder S, Schubert H. Significance of internal stresses for the martensitic transformation in yttria-stabilized tetragonal zirconia polycrystals during degradation. *J. Am. Ceram. Soc.*, 1986; **69**: 534–540.

631. von Schewelov, Sanzén L, Önsten I, Carlsson A, Besjakov J. Total hip replacement with a zirconium oxide ceramic femoral head. A randomized Roentgen stereophotogrammetric study. *J. Bone Joint Surg. (Br.)*, 2005; **87-B**: 1631–1635.

632. Kraay MJ, Thomas RD, Rimnac CM, Fitzgerald SJ, Goldberg VM. Zirconia versus Co–Cr femoral heads in total hip arthroplasty: Early assessment of wear. *Clin. Orthop. Relat. Res.*, 2006; **453**: 86–90.

633. Hall RM, Unsworth A. Friction in hip prostheses. *Biomaterials*, 1997; **18**: 1017–1026.

634. Clarke IC, Pezzotti G, Sakakura S, Sugano N. Phase transformation and residual stresses in retrieved zirconia ball implant. *Key Eng. Mater.*, 2003; **240–242**: 781–784.

635. Katagiri G, Ishida H, Ishitani A, Masaki T. Direct determination by Raman microprobe of the transformation zone size in Y_2O_3 containing tetragonal ZrO_2 polycrystals. In *Advances in ceramics, Vol. 24, Science and technology of zirconia III*. Somiya S, Yamamoto N, Yanagida H (Eds.). The American Ceramic Society, Columbus, OH, pp. 537–544, 1988.

636. Munoz-Saldana J, Balmori-Ramirez H, Jaramillo-Vigueras D, Iga T, Schneider GA. Mechanical properties and low-temperature aging of tetragonal zirconia polycrystals processed by hot isostatic pressing. *J. Mater. Res.*, 2003; **18**: 2415–2426.

637. Masonis JL, Bourne RB, Ries MD, McCalden RW, Salehi A, Kelman DC. Zirconia femoral head fractures: a clinical and retrieval analysis. *J. Arthroplasty*, 2004; **19**: 898–905.

638. Hellmann JR, Stubican VS. Stable and metastable phase relations in the system zirconia-calcia. *J. Am. Ceram. Soc.*, 1983; **66**: 260–264.

639. Roy ME, Whiteside LA, Katerberg BJ, Steiger JA. Phase transformation, roughness, and microhardness of artificially aged yttria- and magnesia-stabilized zirconia femoral heads. *J. Biomed. Mater. Res A*, 2007; **83-A**: 1096–1102.

640. Roy ME, Whiteside LA, Katerberg BJ, Steiger JA, Nayfeh TA. Not all zirconia femoral heads degrade *in vivo*. *Clin. Orthop. Relat. Res.*, 2007; **465**: 220–226.

641. Roy ME, Whiteside LA. Clinical comparison of polyethylene wear with zirconia or cobalt-chromium femoral heads. *Clin. Orthop. Relat. Res.* 2010; 468: 624–625.

642. Shimizu K, Oka M, Kumar P, Kotoura Y, Yamamuro T, Makinouchi K, Nakamura T. Time-dependent changes in the mechanical properties of zirconia ceramic. *J. Biomed. Mater. Res.*, 1993; **27**: 729–734.

643. Makinouchi K, Yanagida T, Shimizu K. Development of zirconia ceramic for implants. *Orthop. Ceram. Implant Jpn.*, 1992; **8**: 173–177.

644. Johnson W, Mehl R. Reaction kinetics in processes of nucleation and growth. *Trans. Am. Inst. Min. Metall. Pet. Eng.*, 1939; **135**: 416–441.

645. Chevalier J, Cales B, Drouin JM. Low temperature aging of Y-TZP ceramics. *J. Am. Ceram. Soc.*, 1999; **82**: 2150–2154.

646. Yashima M, Yoshimura M. Phase formation in rapidly quenched rare earths doped zirconia melts. In *Zirconia ceramics 12*. Masaki T, Yoshimura M. (Eds.). Japan Materials Research Society, Uchida Rokakuho, Tokyo, Japan, pp. 21–46, 1992.

647. Kim D-J, Park I-S, Lee K-Y, Chevalier J, Attaoui H, Han J-S. Subcritical crack growth resistance of low temperature degradation free zirconia/alumina composite for medical applications. *Key Eng. Mater.*, 2005; **284–286**: 1007–1010.

648. Ohmichi N, Kamioka K, Ueda K, Matsui K, Ogai M. Phase transformation of zirconia ceramics by annealing in hot water. *J. Ceram. Soc. Jpn.*, 1999; **107**: 128–133.

649. Matsui K, Horikoshi H, Ohmichi Y, Ohgai M, Yoshida H, Ikuhara Y. Cubic-formation and grain — growth mechanisms in tetragonal zirconia polycrystal. *J. Am. Ceram. Soc.*, 2003; **86**: 1401–1408.

650. Yamashita I, Tsukuma K. Phase separation and hydrothermal degradation of 3 mol% Y_2O_3–ZrO_2 ceramics. *J. Ceram. Soc. Jpn.*, 2005; **113**: 530–533.

651. Chevalier J, Deville S, Münch E, Jullian R, Lair F. Critical effect of cubic phase on aging 3 mol% yttria-stabilized zirconia ceramics for hip replacement prosthesis. *Biomaterials*, 2004; **25**: 5539–5545.

652. Michel D, Van Den Borre MT, Ennaciri A. Vibrational spectra and force fields of tetragonal zirconia and zirconium germanates. *Advances in ceramics 24: Science and technology of zirconia III*. Somiya S, Yamamoto N, Yanagida H (Eds.). The American Ceramic Society, Columbus, OH, pp. 555–562, 1988.

653. Howard CJ, Hunter BA. Oxygen position and bond length from lattice parameters in tetragonal zirconias. *J. Am. Ceram. Soc.*, 1998; **81**: 241–243.

654. Igawa N, Ishii Y. Crystal structure of metastable tetragonal zirconia up to 1473 K. *J. Am. Ceram. Soc.*, 2001; **84**: 1169–1171.

655. Kim D-J, Jang J-W, Lee H-L. Effect of tetravalent dopants on Raman spectra of tetragonal zirconia. *J. Am. Ceram. Soc.*, 1997; **80**: 1453–1461.

656. Kim D-J, Jung H-J. Raman spectroscopy of tetragonal zirconia solid solution. *J. Am. Ceram. Soc.*, 1993; **76**: 2106–2108.

657. Yashima M, Ishizawa N, Yoshimura M. Application of an ion-packing model based on defect clusters to zirconia solid solutions. *J. Am. Ceram. Soc.*, 1992; **75**: 1541–1549.

658. Zhao X, Vanderbilt D. Phonons and lattice dielectric properties of zirconia. *Phys. Rev. B*, 2002; **65**: 075105-1–10.

659. Ohmichi N, Kamioka K, Ueda K, Matsui K. Phase transfromation of zirconia ceramic by annealing in hot water. *J. Ceram. Soc. Jpn.*, 1999; **107**: 128–133.

660. Ma Q, Pompe W, Clarke DR. Residual stress in Al_2O_3–ZrO_2 composites: A test of stochastic stress models. *Acta Metall. Mater.*, 1994; **42**: 1673–1681.

661. Lawson S. Environmental degradation of zirconia ceramics. *J. Eur. Ceram. Soc.*, 1995; **15**: 485–502.

662. Seung KL, Rajan T, Readey MJ, Lawn BR. Scratch damage in zirconia ceramics. *J. Am. Ceram. Soc.*, 2000; **83**: 1428–1432.

663. Lu X, Liang K, Gu S, Zheng Y, Fang H. Effect of oxygen vacancies on transformation of zirconia at low temperatures. *J. Mater. Sci.*, 1997; **32**: 6653–6656.

664. Petrik NG, Taylor DP, Orlando TM. Laser-stimulated luminescence of yttria-stabilized cubic zirconia crystals. *J. Appl. Phys.*, 1999; **85**: 6770–6776.

665. Li P, Chen I-W, Penner-Hahn JE. X-ray-absorption studies of zirconia polymorphs. I. Characteristic local structures. *Phys. Rev. B*, 1993; **48**: 10063–10073.

666. Smits K, Grigorjeva L, Qojkowski W, Fidelus JD. Luminescence of oxygen related defects in zirconia nanocrystals. *Phys. Status Solidi* (*c*), 2007; **4**: 770–773.

667. Gholinia A, Leach C. Cathodoluminescence microscopy of impurity phases in ZrO_2/Ni nano-composites. *J. Mater. Sci.*, 1997; **32**: 6625–6628.

668. Shibano T, Takigawa Y, Uesugi T, Higashi K. Effect of second phase particles on phase stability of zirconia in hot water. *Adv. Mater. Res.*, 2007; **26–28**:781–784.

669. Chevalier J, Grandjean S, Kuntz M, Pezzotti G. Activation energy for polymorphic transformation in an advanced alumina/zirconia composite for arthroplastic applications. *Biomaterials*, 2009; **30**: 5279–5282.

670. Liang B, Kawanabe K, Ise K, Iida H, Nakamura T. Polyethylene wear against alumina and zirconia heads in cemented total hip arthroplasty. *J. Arthroplasty*, 2007; **22**: 251–257.

671. Lu Z, McKellop H. Frictional heating of bearing materials tested in a hip joint wear simulator. *Proc. Inst. Mech. Eng. H*, 1997; **211**: 101–108.

672. Kim YH, Kim JS, Cho SH. A comparison of polyethylene wear in hips with cobalt-chrome or zirconia heads. A prospective, randomised study. *J. Bone Joint Surg.* (*Br.*), 2001; **83**: 742–750.

673. Trunec M. Effect of grain size on mechanical properties of 3Y-TZP ceramics. *Ceramics — Silikáty*, 2008; **52**: 165–171.

674. Shevchenko AV, Ruban AK, Dudnik EV. High-technology ceramics based on zirconium dioxide. *Ogneup. Tekh. Keram.*, 2000; **9**: 2–8.

675. Pezzotti G, Matsutani A, Zhu W. Spectroscopic assessments of domain texture in barium titanate: I. Confocal Raman polarization analysis. *J. Am. Ceram. Soc.*, 2010; **93**: 256–264.

676. Tang X, Zheng X. Raman scattering and *t*-phase lattice vibration of 3% (mole fraction) Y_2O_3–ZrO_2. *J. Mater. Sci. Technol.*, 2004; **20**: 485–489.

677. Sobukawa H. Development of ceria-zirconia solid solutions and future trends. R&D Review Toyota CRDL 2002; **37(4)**: 1–5.

678. Pushkarev VV, Kovalchuk VI, d'Itri JL. Probing defect sites on the CeO_2 surface with dioxygen. *J. Phys. Chem. B*, 2004; **108**: 5341–5348.

679. Chevalier J, Gremillard L, Virkar AV, Clarke DR. The tetragonal-monoclinic transformation in zirconia: lessons learned and future trends. *J. Am. Ceram. Soc.*, 2009; **92**: 1901–1920.

680. Eichler A. Tetragonal Y-doped zirconia: Structure and ion conductivity. *Phys. Rev. B*, 2001; **64**: 174103-1–8.

681. Bonanos N, Butler EP. Ionic conductivity of monoclinic and tetragonal yttria-zirconia single crystals. *J. Mater. Sci. Lett.*, 1985; **4**; 561–564.

682. Badwal SPS. Zirconia-based solid electrolytes: Microstructure, stability and ionic conductivity. *Solid State Ionics*, 1992; **52**: 23–32.

683. Filal M, Petot C, Petot-Ervas G, Amamra MC, Carpentier JL, Dellis JL. Influence of the dopants and of the microstructure on the ionic conductivity of zirconia. *J. Phys. IV*, 1993; **3**: C7-1463–1466.

684. Marro FG, Valle J, Mestra A, Anglada M. Improvement of 3Y-TZP hydrothermal degradation resistance by surface modification with ceria without impairing mechanical properties. *IOP Conf. Series: Mater. Sci. Eng.*, 2009; **5**: 012015-1–8.

685. Claussen N. Microstructural design of zirconia-toughened ceramics ZTC. In: *Advances in Ceramics, Vol. 12: Science and Technology of*

Zirconia II (Claussen N, Rühle M, Heuer AH, eds). (American Ceramic Society, Westerville, Ohio 1984); pp. 325–351.

686. Rieu J, Goeuriot P. Ceramic composites for biomedical applications. *Clin. Mater.* 1993; **12**: 211–217.
687. Affatato S, Testoni M, Cacciari GL, Toni A. Mixed-oxide prosthetic ceramic ball heads. *Biomaterials*, 1999; **20**: 1925–1929.
688. Bartolomé JF, De Aza AH, Martín A, Pastor JY, Llorca J, Torrecillas R, Bruno G. Alumina/zirconia micro/nanocomposites: A new material for biomedical applications with superior sliding wear resistance. *J. Am. Ceram. Soc.*, 2007; **90**: 3177–3184.
689. Burger W. Umwandlungs- und plateletverstärkte Aluminiumoxid-Matrixwerkstoffe (Teil 1). *Keram. Z.*, 1997; **49**: 1067–1070.
690. Burger W, Richter HG. High strength and toughness alumina matrix composites by transformation toughening and "*in situ*" platelet reinforcement (ZPTA). *Key Eng. Mater.*, 2001; **192–195**: 545–548.
691. Deville S, Chevalier J, Fantozzi G, Bartolomé JF, Requena J, Moya JS, Díaz LA, Torrecillas R. Low-temperature ageing of zirconia-toughened alumina ceramics and its implication in biomaterial implants. *J. Eur. Ceram. Soc.*, 2003; **23**: 2975–2982.
692. Affatato S, Goldoni M, Testoni M, Toni A. Mixed oxides prosthetic ceramic ball heads. Part III: Effect of the ZrO_2 fraction on the wear of ceramic on polyethylene joints. A long-term *in vitro* wear study. *Biomaterials*, 2001; **22**: 717–723.
693. Stewart TP, Tipper JL, Insley G, Streicher RM, Ingham E, Fisher J. Long-term wear of ceramic-matrix composite material for hip prostheses under severe swing phase microsimulation. *J. Biomed. Mater. Res. Appl. Biomater.*, 2003; **66B**: 567–573.
694. Chang J-D, Kamdar R, Yoo J-H, Hur M, Lee S-S. Third generation ceramic-on-ceramic bearing surfaces in revision total hip arthroplasty. *J. Arthroplasty*, 2010; **24**: 1231–1235.
695. Hamilton WG, McAuley J, P, Dennis DA, Murphy JA, Blumenfeld TJ, Politi J. THA with Delta ceramic on ceramic. *Clin. Orthop.*, 2010; **468**: 358–366.
696. Sornakumar T, Krishnamurthy R, Gokularathnam CV. Machining performance of phase transformation toughened alumina and partially stabilized zirconia composite cutting tools. *J. Eur. Ceram. Soc.*, 1993; **12**: 455–460.
697. Kumar AS, Durai AR, Sornakumar T. Machinability of hardened steel using alumina based ceramic cutting tools. *Int. J. Refractory Met. Hard Mater.*, 2003; **21**: 109–117.

698. Taya M, Hayashi S, Kobayashi AS, Yoon HS. Toughening of a particulate-reinforced ceramic-matrix composite by thermal residual stress. *J. Am. Ceram. Soc.*, 1990; **73**: 1382–1391.

699. Mori T, Tanaka K. Average stress in matrix and average energy of materials with misfitting inclusions. *Acta Metall.*, 1973; **21**: 571–574.

700. Akiniwa Y, Tanaka K, Minakawa N, Morii Y. Neutron diffraction study of thermal residual stress in ceramic composite mater. *Sci. Res. Int.*, 2000; **6**: 281–286.

701. Harlan NR, Merino RI, Peña JI, Larrea A, Orera VM, González C, Poza P, LLorca J. Phase distribution and residual stresses in melt-grown Al_2O_3-$ZrO_2(Y_2O_3)$ eutectics. *J. Am. Ceram. Soc.*, 2002; **85**: 2025–2032.

702. Bobet JL, Ji N, LeBrun JL. The X-ray measurement of axial and hoop residual stresses in microcomposite specimens. *J. Thermal Stresses*, 1998; **21**: 743–749.

703. Ma Q. Pompe W, French JD, Clarke DR. Residual-stresses in Al_2O_3-ZrO_2 composites — a test of stochastic stress models. *Acta Metall. Mater.*, 1994; **42**: 1673–1681.

704. Garvie RC, Goss MF. Intrinsic size dependence of the phase transformation temperature in zirconia microcrystals. *J. Mater. Sci.*, 1986; 21: 1253–1257.

705. Sergo V, Wang X-L, Clarke DR, Becher PF. Residual stress in alumina/ceria-stabilized zirconia composites. *J. Am. Ceram. Soc.*, 1995; **78**: 2213–2214.

706. Heuer AH, Claussen N, Kriven WM, Rühle M. Stability of tetragonal ZrO_2 particles in ceramic matrices. *J. Am. Ceram. Soc.*, 1982; **65**: 642–650.

707. Takao Y, Taya M. Thermal expansion coefficients and thermal stresses in an aligned short fiber composite with application to a short carbon fiber/aluminum. *J. Appl. Mech.*, 1985; **52**: 806–810.

708. Orera VM, Cemborain R, Merino RI, Peña JI, Larrea A. Piezo-spectroscopy at low temperatures: residual stresses in Al_2O_3-$ZrO_2(Y_2O_3)$ eutectics measured from 77 to 350 K. *Acta Mater.*, 2001; **50**: 4677–4686.

709. Budiansky B, Hutchinson J, Lambropoulos J. Continuum theory of dilatant transformation toughening in ceramics. *Int. J. Solids Struct.*, 1983; **19**: 337–355.

710. Amazigo JC, Budiansky B. Steady-state crack growth in supercritically transforming materials. *Int. J. Solids Struct.*, 1988; **24**: 751–755.

711. Ikeda J, Mabuchi M, Nakanishi T, Miyaji F, Ueno M, Pezzotti G. Phase stability and fracture toughness of zirconia toughened alumina for joint replacement. *Key Eng. Mater.*, 2008; **361–363:**: 767–770.

712. Tuan WH, Chen RZ, Wang TC, Cheng CH, Kuo PS. Mechanical properties of Al_2O_3/ZrO_2 composites. *J. Eur. Ceram. Soc.*, 2002; **22**: 2827–2833.

713. Tuan W-H, Chen J-R, Ho C-J. Critical zirconia amount to enhance the strength of alumina. *Ceram. Int.*, 2008; **34**: 2129–2135.

714. Rao PG, Iwasa M, Tanaka T, Kondoh I, Inoue T. Preparation and mechanical properties of Al_2O_3-15 wt.% ZrO_2 composites. *Scripta Mater.*, 2003; **48**: 437–441.

715. Szutkowska M. Fracture resistance beuhavior of alumina-zirconia composites. *J. Mater. Proc. Tech.*, 2004; **153–54**: 868–874.

716. Shin YS, Rhee YW, Kang SJ. Experimental evaluation of toughening mechanism in alumina-zirconia composites. *J. Am. Ceram. Soc.*, 1999; **82**: 1229–1232.

717. Kuntz M, Masson B, Pandorf T. Current state of the art of the ceramic composite material BIOLOX®*delta*. In: *Strength of Materials.* (Mendes G, Lago B, eds) (Nova Science Publishers, Inc., Huntington, New York, 2009); pp. 133–155.

718. Nakanishi T, Sasaki M, Ikeda J, Miyaji F, Kondo M. Mechanical and phase stability of zirconia toughened alumina. *Key Eng. Mater.*, 2007; **330–332**: 1267–1270.

719. Sergo V, Clarke DR. Deformation bands in ceria-stabilized tetragonal zirconia/alumina: II, Stress-induced aging at room temperature. *J. Am. Ceram. Soc.*, 1995; **78**: 641–644.

720. Sergo V, Lipkin DM, De Portu G, Clarke DR. Edge stresses in ceramics laminate composites. *J. Am. Ceram. Soc.*, 1997; **80**: 1633–1639.

721. Sergo V. Room-temperature aging of laminate composites of alumina/3-mol%-yttria-stabilized tetragonal zirconia polycrystals. *J. Am. Ceram. Soc.*, 2004; **87**: 247–253.

722. Deville S, Chevalier J, Dauvergne CH, Fantozzi G, Bartolomé JF, Moya JS, Torrecillas R. Microstructural investigation of the aging behavior of (3Y-TZP)-Al_2O_3 composites. *J. Am. Ceram. Soc.*, 2005; **88**: 1273–1280.

723. ASTM F2033–05. Standard specification for total hip joint prosthesis and hip endoprosthesis bearing surfaces made of metallic, ceramic, and polymeric materials. In: *Book of Standards*, Vol. 13.01 (West Conshohocken, PA: ASTM International, 2005).

724. Pulliam IT, Trousdale RT. Fracture of a ceramic femoral head after a revision operation. A case report. *J. Bone Joint Surg.* (*Am.*), 1997; **79**: 118–121.

725. Pfaff H-G, Rack R, Willmann G. Long-term performance of a transformation toughened platelet reinforced alumina matrix composite. *Bioceramics*. 2001; **14**: 541–542.

726. Insleyand G, Steicher R. Next generation ceramics based on zirconia toughened alumina for hip joint prostheses. *Key Eng. Mater.* 2004; **254–256**: 675–678.

727. Rühle M, Heuer AH, Claussen N. Transformation and microcrack toughening as complementary processes in zirconia-toughened alumina. *J. Am. Ceram. Soc.*, 1986; **69**: 195–197.

728. Claussen NJ, Fracture toughness of Al_2O_3 with an unstable ZrO_2 dispersed second phase. *J. Am. Ceram. Soc.*, 1976; **61**: 49–51.

729. Nojima T, Nakai O. Stable crack extension of an alumina ceramic in three point bending test. (in Jpn.) *J. Soc. Mater. Sci. Jpn.*, 1993; **42**, 142–148.

730. Srawley JE. Wide range stress intensity factor expressions for ASTM E399 Standard Fracture Toughness Specimens. *Int. J. Fract.*, 1976; **12**: 475–476.

731. Kruzic J, Ritchie O. Determining the toughness of ceramics from Vickers indentations using the crack-opening displacements: An experimental study. *J. Am. Ceram. Soc.*, 2003; **86**: 1433–1436.

732. Chevalier J, Deville S, Fantozzi G, Bartolomé JF, Pecharroman C, Moya JS, Diaz LA, Torrecillas R. Nanostructured ceramic oxides with a slow crack growth resistance close to covalent materials. *Nano Lett.*, 2005; **5**: 1297–1310.

733. Benzaid R, Chevalier J, Saâdaoui M, Fantozzi G, Nawa M, Diaz LA, Torrecillas R. Fracture toughness, strength and slow crack growth in a ceria stabilized zirconia–alumina nanocomposite for medical applications. *Biomaterials*, 2008; **29**: 3636–3641.

734. Akimov GYa, Timchenko VM. Effect of strain rate and preloading on the fracture toughness of ZrO_2-based ceramics. *Strength Mater.*, 2002; **34**: 514–517.

735. Pezzotti G, Okamoto Y, Nishida T, Sakai M. On the near-tip toughening by crack-face bridging in particulate and platelet-reinforced ceramics. *Acta Mater.*, 1996; **44**: 899–914.

736. Novak S, Kalin M, Lukas P, Anne G, Vleugels J, Van Der Biest O. The effect of residual stresses in functionally graded alumina-ZTA composites on their wear and friction behavior. *J. Eur. Ceram. Soc.*, 2007; **27**: 151–156.

737. Yueh HK, Cox B. Luminescence properties of zirconium oxide films. *J. Nucl. Mater.*, 2003; **323**: 57–67.

738. Xu J, Mao HK, Bell PM. High-pressure ruby and diamond fluorescence: Observations at 0.21 to 0.55 terapascal. *Science*, 1986: **232**: 1404–1406.

739. Mikhailik VB, Di Stefano PCF, Henry S, Kraus H, Lynch A, Tsybulskyi V, Verdier MA. Studies of concentration dependences in the luminescence of Ti-doped Al_2O_3. *J. Appl. Phys.*, 2011; **109**: 053116-1–6.

740. Lee CH, Kröger FA. Electrical conductivity of polycrystalline Al_2O_3 doped with silicon. *J. Am. Ceram. Soc.*, 1985; **68**: 92–99.

741. Lushchik A, Lushchik Ch., Kirm M, Nagirnyi V, Savikhin F, Vasil'chenko E. Defect creation caused by the decay of cation excitons and hot electron-hole recombination in wide-gap dielectrics. *Nucl. Instr. Meth. B*, 2006; **250**: 330–336.

742. Mohapatra SK, Kröger FA. Defect structure of α–Al_2O_3 doped with titanium. *J. Am. Ceram. Soc.*, 1977; **60**: 381–387.

743. Guo X. Property degradation of tetragonal zirconia induced by low-temperature defect reaction with water molecules. *Chem. Mater.*, 2004; **16**: 3988–3994.

744. Schubert H, Frey F. Stability of Y-TZP during hydrothermal treatment: Neutron experiments and stability considerations. *J. Eur. Ceram. Soc.*, 2005; **25**: 1597–1602.

745. Pezzotti G, Takahashi Y, Zhu W. In-depth profiling of elastic residual stress and the *in vivo* wear mechanism of self-mating alumina hip joints. *Wear*, 2012; **284–285**: 91–97.

746. Kreher W, Pompe W. *Internal Stresses in Heterogeneous Solids*. Akademie Verlag: Berlin (1988).

747. Gregori G, Burger W, Sergo V. Piezo-spectroscopic analysis of the residual stresses in zirconia-toughened alumina ceramics: The influence of the tetragonal-to-monoclinic transformation. *Mater. Sci. Eng. A*, 1999; **271**: 401–406.

748. Larché F, Cahn JW. The interactions of composition and stress in crystalline solids. *Acta Metall.*, 1985; **33**: 331–357.

749. Pezzotti G, Yamada K, Sakakura S, Pitto RP. Raman spectroscopic analysis of advanced ceramic composite for hip prosthesis. *J. Am. Ceram. Soc.*, 2008; **91**: 1199–1206.

750. Puchin VE, Gale JD, Shluger AL, Kotomin EA, Günster J, Brause M, Kempter V. Atomic structure of the (0001) corundum surface. *Surf. Sci.*, 1997; **370**: 190–200.

751. Zhu W, Puppulin L, Leto A, Takahashi Y, Sugano N, Pezzotti G. *In situ* measurements of local temperature and contact stress magnitude during wear of ceramic-on-ceramic hip joints. *J. Mech. Behavior Biomater.* DOI: 10.1016/j.jmbbm.2013.01.018.

752. Mc Cumber DE, Sturge MD. Linewidth and temperature shift of the *R* lines in ruby. *J. Appl. Phys.*, 1963; **34**: 1682–1684.

753. Huber MT. Zur Theorie der Berührung fester elastischer Körper. *Ann. Phys.*, 1904; **14**: 153–163.

754. Deeg EW. New algorithms for calculating Hertzian stresses, deformations, and contact zone parameters. *AMP J. Tech.*, 1992; **2**: 14–24.

755. Clarke IC, Green D, Williams P, Donaldson T, Pezzotti G. US perspective on hip simulator wear testing of BIOLOX®*delta* in "severe" test modes. In: *Bioceramics and Alternative Bearings in Joint Arthroplasty.* (Benazzo F, Falez F, Dietrich M, eds) (Steinkopff Verlag, Darmstadt, Germany, 2006); pp. 189–205.

756. Harris WH. The problem is osteolysis. *Clin. Orthop.*, 1995; **311**: 46–53.

757. Fisher J. Biomedical Applications. Modern Tribology Handbook, Vol. Two: Materials, Coating and Industrial Applications, (Bharat Bhushan. Florida: CRC Press, Boca Raton; 2001, pp. 1593–1609.

758. Green TR, Fisher J, Stone MH, Wroblewski BM, and Ingham E. Polyethylene particles of a "critical size" are necessary for the induction of cytokines by macrophages *in vitro*. *Biomaterials*, 1998; **19**: 2297–2302.

759. Semlitsch M, Lehmann M, Weber H, Doerre E, Willert HG. New prospects for a prolonged functional life span of artificial hip joints by using the material combination polyethylene/aluminum oxide ceramic metal. *J. Biomed. Mater. Res.*, 1977; **11**: 537–552.

760. Oonishi H, Kuno M, Tsuji E, Fujiwara A. The optimum dose of gamma radiation-heavy doses to low wear to low wear polyethylene in total hip prostheses. *J. Mater. Sci.: Mater. Med.*, 1997; **8**: 11–18.

761. Scott M, Morrison M, Mishra SR, Jani S. Particle analysis for the determination of UHMWPE wear. *J. Biomed. Mater. Res. B*, 2005; **73**: 325–337.

762. McKellop H, Shen F, Lu B, Campbell P, Salovey R. Development of an extremely wear-resistant ultra high molecular weight polyethylene for total hip replacement. *J. Orthop. Res.*, 1999; **17**: 157–167.

763. Oonishi H, Saito M, Kadoya Y. Wear of high-dose gamma irradiated polyethylene in total joint replacement-Long term radiological evaluation. In: *Transaction of the 44th Annual Meeting of the Orthopaedic Research Society*, New Orleans, LA, March 16–19, 1998; 97: 17.

764. Digas G, Kärrholm J, Thanner J, Malchau H, Herberts P. The Otto Aufranc Award. Highly cross-linked polyethylene in total hip arthroplasty: Randomized evaluation of penetration rate in cemented and uncemented sockets using radiostereometric analysis. *Clin. Orthop. Relat. Res.*, 2004; **429**: 6–16.

765. Dorr LD, Wan Z, Shahrdar C, Sirianni L, Boutary M, Yun A. Clinical performance of a Durasul highly corss-linked polyethylene acetabular liner for total hip arthroplasty at five years. *J. Bone Joint Surg.*, (*Am.*) 2005; **87**: 1816–1821.

766. Zhao Y, Luo YX, Jiang BZ. Effect of irradiation on crystallinity and mechanical properties of ultrahigh molecular-weight polyethylene. *J. Appl. Polym. Sci.*, 1993; **50**: 1797–1801.

767. Lewis G. Properties of crosslinked ultra-high-molecular-weight polyethylene. *Biomaterials*, 2001; **22**: 371–401.

768. Oral E, Malhi AS, Muratoglu OK. Mechanism of decrease in fatigue crack propagation resistance in irradiated and melted UHMWPE. *Biomaterials*, 2006; **27**: 917–925.

769. Eyerer P, Ke YC. Property changes of UHMW polyethylene hip cup endoprostheses during implantation. *J. Biomed. Mater. Res.*, 1984; **18**: 1137–1151.

770. Fouad H. Effect of long-term aging on the thermal, mechanical, and viscoelastic behavior of biomedical grade of ultra high molecular weight polyethylene. *J. Appl. Polym. Sci.*, 2010; **118**: 17–24.

771. Oral E, Godleski Beckos C, Bassem W, Ghali BW, Lozynsky AJ, Muratoglu OK. Effect of crosslink density on the high pressure crystallization of UHMWPE. *J. Biomed. Mater. Res. B: Appl. Biomater.*, 2009; **90**: 720–729.

772. Bellare A, Cohen RE. Morphology of rod stock and compression-moulded sheets of ultra-high-molecular-weight polyethylene used in orthopaedic implants. *Biomaterials*, 1996; **17**: 2325–2333.

773. Edidin AA, Pruitt L, Jewett CW, Crane DJ, Roberts D, Kurtz SM. Plasticity-induced damage layer is a precursor to wear in radiation-cross-linked UHMWPE acetabular components for total hip replacement. *J. Arthroplasty.*, 1999: **14**: 616–627.

774. Dumbleton JH, D'Antonio JA, Manley MT, Capello WN, Wang A. The basis for a second-generation highly cross-linked UHMWPE. *Clin. Orthop. Relat. Res.*, 2006; **453**: 265–271.

775. Campbell DG, Field JR, Stuart AC. Second-generation highly cross-linked X3TM polyethylene wear: A preliminary radiostereometric analysis study. *Clin. Orthop. Relat. Res.*, 2010; **468**: 2704–2709.

776. Bellare A, Schnablegger H, Cohen RE. A small-angle X-ray scattering study of high-density polyethylene and ultra-high molecular weight polyethylene. *Macromolecules*, 1995; **17**: 2325–2333.

777. Jaynes ET. Information theory and statistical mechanics. *Phys. Rev.*, 1957; **106**: 620–630.

778. Pérez R, Banda S, Ounaies Z. Determination of the orientation distribution function in aligned single wall nanotube polymer composites by polarized Raman spectroscopy. *J. Appl. Phys.*, 2008; **103**: 074302-1–14.

779. Roe RJ. Orientation distribution function of statistical segments in deformed polymer networks. *J. Appl. Phys.*, 1964; **35**: 2215–2219.

780. Wang A, Polineni VK, Essner AP, Sokol M, Sun DC, Stark C, Dumbleton JH. The significance of nonlinear motion in the wear screening of orthopaedic implant materials. *J. Test. Eval.*, 1997; **25**: 239–245.

781. Oonishi H, Takayama Y, Tsuji E. Improvement of polyethylene by irradiation in artificial joints, Radiat. *Phys. Chem.*, 1992; **39**: 495–504.

782. Wroblewski GM. Siney PD, Dowson D, Collins SN. A prospective clinical and joint simulator study of the performance of 22 mm alumina ceramic heads and polyethylene acetabular cups in total hip arthroplasty. *J. Bone Joint Surg.* (*Br.*), 1996; **78**: 280–285.

783. Sambasivan S, Fischer DA, Hsu SM. Effect of cross-linking ultrahigh molecular weight polyethylene: Surface molecular orientation and wear characteristics. *J. Vac. Sci. Technol. A*, 2007; **25**: 932–937.

784. Popli R, Mandelkern L. Influence of structural and morphological factors on the mechanical properties of the polyethylenes. *J. Polym. Sci. Polym. Phys. Edn.*, 1987; **25**: 441–483.

785. Williamson GR, Wright B, Haward RN. The preparation and properties of fractions from high density polyethylenes. *J. Appl. Chem.*, 1964; **14**: 131–140.

786. Fleissner M. Die Spezifische Bruchenergie von Polyethylen in Abhängigkeit von Structurellen Parametern. *Die Angew: Macromol. Chem.*, 1982; **105**: 167–185.

787. Lu X, Qian R, Brown N. The effect of crystallinity on fracture and yielding of polyethylenes. *Polymer*, 1995; **36**: 4239–4244.

788. Lin L, Argon AS. Review Structure and plastic deformation of polyethylene. *J. Mater. Sci.*, 1994; **29**: 294–323.

789. Philip M, Ward IM, Parsons B. A comparison of tensile, compressive and torsional creep in isotropic and oriented polyethylene. *J. Mater. Sci.*, 1986; **21**: 879–886.

790. Bartczak Z. Effect of chain entanglements on plastic deformation behavior of ultra-high molecular weight polyethylene. *J. Polym. Sci., Part B: Polym. Phys.*, 2010; **48**: 276–285.

791. Lee KY, Pienkowski D. Compressive creep characteristics of extruded ultrahigh-molecular weight polyethylene. *J. Biomed. Mater. Res.*, 1998; **39**: 261–265.

792. Collier JP, Currier BH, Kennedy FE, Currier JH, Timmins GS, Jackson SK, Brewer RL. Comparison of cross-linked polyethylene materials for orthopaedic applications. *Clin. Orthop. Relat. Res.*, 2003; **414**: 289–304.

793. Wang A, Zeng H, Yau S-S, Essner A, Manely M, Dumbleton J. Wear, oxidation and mechanical properties of a sequentially irradiated and annealed UHMWPE in total joint replacement. *J. Phys. D: Appl. Phys.*, 2006; **39**: 3213–3219.

794. Barron D, Birkinshaw C. On the morphology of some irradiated ultra high molecular weight polyethylenes. *Polym. Degradation and Stability*, 2009; **94**: 1621–1631.

795. Moonen JAHM, Roovers WAC, Meier RJ, Kip, BJ. Crystal and molecular deformation in strained high-performance polyethylene fibers studied by wide-angle X-ray scattering and Raman spectroscopy. *J. Polym. Sci.: Part B: Polym. Phys.*, 1992; **30**: 361–372.

796. Tashiro K, Wu G, Kobayashi M. Morphological effect on the Raman frequency shift induced by tensile stress applied to crystalline polyoxymethylene and polyethylene: Spectroscopic support for the idea of an inhomogeneous stress distribution in polymer material. *Polymer*, 1988; **29**: 1768–1783.

797. Yeh WY, Young RJ. Deformation processes in poly(ethylene terephthalate) fibers. *J. Macromol. Sci. — Phys.*, 1998; **B37**: 83–118.

798. Bartczak Z, Argon AS, Cohen RE. Deformation mechanisms and plastic resistance in single-crystal-textured high-density polyethylene. *Macromolecules*, 1992; **25**: 5036–5053.

799. Galeski A, Bartczak Z, Argon AS, Cohen RE. Morphological alterations during texture-producing plastic plane strain compression of high-density polyethylene. *Macromolecules*, 1992; **25**: 5705–5718.

800. Boontongkong Y, Cohen RE, Spector M, Bellare A. Orientation of plane strain-compressed ultra-high-molecular-weight polyethylene. *Polymer*, 1998; **39**: 6391–6400.

801. Wroblewski B. Direction and rate of socket wear in Charnley low friction arthroplasty. *J. Bone Joint Surg.* (*Br.*), 1985; **67**: 757–761.

802. McDonald MD, Bloebaum RD. Distinguishing wear and creep in clinically retrieved polyethylene inserts. *J. Biomed. Mater. Res.*, 1995; **29**: 1–7.

803. Huber J, Walter A, Plitz W, Refior HJ. Effect of the manufacturing process on creep and wear properties of UHMWPE (ultra-high molecular weight polyethylene). *Biomed. Tech.* (*Berl.*), 1995; **40**: 88–92.

804. Taddei P, Affatato S, Fagnano C, Bordini B, Tinti A, Toni A. Vibrational spectroscopy of ultra-high molecular weight polyethylene hip prostheses: Influence of the sterilization method on crystallinity and surface oxidation. *J. Mol. Struct.*, 2002; **613**: 121–129.

805. Goldman M, Gronsky R, Ranganathan R, Pruitt L. The effects of gamma radiation sterilization and ageing on the structure and morphology of medical grade ultra high molecular weight polyethylene. *Polymer*, 1996; **37**: 2909–2913.

806. Heisel C, Silva M, dela Rosa MA, and Schmalzried TP. Short-term *in vivo* wear of cross-linked polyethylene. *J. Bone Joint Surg.* (*Am.*), 2004; **86**: 748–751.

807. Gomez-Barrena E, Li S, Furman BS, Masri BA, Wright TM, Salvati EA. Role of polyethylene oxidation and consolidation defects in cup performance. *Clin. Orthop. Relat. Res.*, 1998; **352**: 105–117.

808. Stea S, Antonietti B, Baruffaldi F, Visentin M, Bordini B, Sudanese A, Toni A. Behavior of Hylamer polyethylene in hip arthroplasty: Comparison of two gamma sterilization techniques. *Int. Orthop.*, 2006; **30**: 35–38.

809. Williams S, Isaac G, Porter P, Fisher J, Older J. Long-term radiographic assessment of cemented polyethylene acetabular cups. *Clin. Orthop. Relat. Res.*, 2008; **466**: 366–372.

810. Affatato S, Bersaglia G, Rocchi M, Taddei P, Fagnano C, Toni A. Wear behaviour of cross-linked polyethylene assessed *in vitro* under severe conditions. *Biomaterials*, 2005; **26**: 3259–3267.

811. McKellop HA, Campbell P, Park SH, Schmalzried TP, Grigoris P, Amstutz HC, Sarmiento A. The origin of submicron polyethylene wear debris in total hip arthroplasty. *Clin. Orthop.*, 1995; **311**: 3–20.

812. Kabo J, Gebhard S, Loren G, Amstutz HC. *In vivo* wear of polyethylene acetabular components. *J. Bone Joint Surg.* (*Br.*), 1993; **75**: 254–258.

813. Lewis G, Carroll M. Effect of crosslinking UHMWPE on its tensile and compressive creep performance. *Bio-Med. Mater. Eng.*, 2001; **11**: 167–183.

814. Galvin AL, Ingham E, Stone MH, Fisher J. Penetration, creep and wear of highly crosslinked UHMWPE in a hip joint simulator. *J. Bone Joint Surg.* (*Br.*), 2006; **88** (Suppl. II): 236–241.

815. Digas G, Thanner J, Nivbrant B, Rohrl S, Strom HC, Karrholm J. Increase in early polyethylene wear after sterilization with ethylene oxide: Radiostereometric analyses of 201 total hips. *Acta Orthop., Scand.*, 2003; **74**: 531–541.

816. Rose RM, Goldfarb EV, Ellis E, Crugnola AN. Radiation sterilization and the wear rate of polyethylene. *J. Orthop. Res.*, 2005; **2**: 393–400.

817. Dowson D, Jobbins B. Design and development of a versatile hip joint simulator and a preliminary assessment of the wear and creep in Charnley total replacement hip joints. *Engng. Med.*, 1988; **17**: 111–117.

818. Tarantili PA, Andreopoulos AG, Galiotis C. Real-time micro-Raman measurements on stressed polyethylene fibers. 1. Strain rate effects and molecular stress redistribution. *Macromolecules*, 1998; **31**: 6964–6976.

819. Wool RP, Bretzlaff RS, Li BY, Wang CH, Boyd RH. Infrared and Raman spectroscopy of stressed polyethylene. *J. Polym. Sci. Part B: Polym. Phys.*, 1986; **24**: 1039–1066.

820. Wong WF, Young RJ. Molecular deformation processes in gel-spun polyethylene fibres using Raman spectroscopy. *J. Mater. Sci.*, 1994; **29**: 510–519.

821. Rull F, Prieto AC, Casado JM, Sobron F, Edwards HGM. Estimation of crystallinity in polyethylene by Raman spectroscopy. *J. Raman Spectrosc.*, 1993; **24**: 545–550.

822. Kyomoto M, Miwa Y, Pezzotti G. Strain in UHMWPE for orthopaedic use studied by Raman microprobe spectroscopy. *J. Biomater. Sci. Polym. Ed.*, 2007; **18**: 165–178.

823. Hiss R, Hobeika S, Lynn C, Strobl G. Network stretching, slip processes, and fragmentation of crystallites during uniaxial drawing of polyethylene and related copolymers. A comparative study. *Macromolecules*, 1999; **32**: 4390–4403.

824. Bell C, Walker P, Abeysundera M, Simmons J, King P, Blunn G. Effect of oxidation on delamination of ultrahigh-molecular-weight polyethylene tibial components. *J. Arthroplasty*, 2009; **13**: 280–290.

825. Muratoglu OK, Mark A, Vittetoe DA, Harris WH, Rubash HE. Polyethylene damage in total knees and use of highly crosslinked polyethylene. *J. Bone Joint Surg.* (*Am.*), 2003; **85**: S7–S13.

826. Daly BM, Yin J. Subsurface oxidation of polyethylene. *J. Biomed. Mater. Res.*, 1998; **42**: 523–529.

827. Jacob RJ, Pienkowski D, Lee KY, Hamilton DM, Schroeder D, and Higgins J. Time- and depth-dependent changes in crosslinking and oxidation of shelf-aged polyethylene acetabular liners. *J. Biomed. Mater. Res.*, 2001; **56**: 168–176.

828. Glyn-Jones S, McLardy-Smith P, Gill HS, Murray DW. The creep and wear of highly cross-linked polyethylene. *J. Bone Joint Surg.* (*Br.*), 2008; **90**: 556–561.

829. Bewill SL, Bevill GR, Penmetsa JR, Petrella AJ, Rullkoetter PJ. Finite element simulation of early creep and wear in total hip arthroplasty. *J. Biomech.*, 2005; **38**: 2365–2374.

830. Plank GR, Estok II DM, Muratoglu OK, O'Connor DO, Burroughs BR, Harris WH. Contact stress assessment of conventional and highly crosslinked ultra high molecular weight polyethylene acetabular liners with finite element analysis and pressure sensitive films. *J. Biomed. Mater. Res. Part B: Appl. Biomater.*, 2006; **80B**: 1–10.

831. Medel FJ, Rimnac CM, Kurtz SM. On the assessment of oxidative and microstructural changes after *in vivo* degradation of historical UHMWPE knee components by means of vibrational spectroscopies and nanoindentation. *J. Biomed. Mater. Res. Part B: Appl. Biomater.*, 2008; **89A**: 530–538.

832. Hood RW, Wright TM, Burstein AH. Retrieval analysis of total knee prostheses: A method and its application to 48 total condylar prostheses. *J. Biomed. Mater. Res.*, 1983; **17**: 829–842.

833. Buchanan FJ, White JR, Simand B, Downes S. The influence of gamma irradiation and aging on degradation mechanisms of ultra-high molecular weight polyethylene. *J. Mater. Sci. Mater. Med.*, 2001; **12**: 29–37.

834. Buchanan FJ, Simand B, Downes S. Effect of sterilisation and ageing on UHMWPE used in medical implants. *Plastics Rubber Compd. Process. Appl.*, 1998; **27**: 148–153.

835. Costa L, Bracco P, Brach del Prever E, Luda MP, Trossarelli L. Analysis of products diffused into UHMWPE prosthetic components *in vivo*. *Biomaterials*, 2001; **22**: 307–315.

836. Oral E, Ghali BW, Neils A, Muratoglu OK. A new mechanism of oxidation in ultrahigh molecular weight polyethylene caused by squalene absorption. *J. Biomed. Mater. Res. Part B: Appl. Biomater.*, 2012; **100B**: 742–751.

837. Amstutz HC, Campbell P, Kossovsky N, Clarke IC. Mechanism and clinical significance of wear debris-induced osteolysis. *Clin. Orthop.*, 1992; **276**: 7–18.

838. Oral E, Muratoglu OK. Radiation cross-linking in ultra-high molecular weight polyethylene for orthopaedic applications. *Nucl. Instrum. Methods Phys. Res. B*, 2007; **265**: 18–22.

839. Baker DA, Bellare A, Pruitt L. The effects of degree of crosslinking on the fatigue crack initiation and propagation resistance of orthopedic-grade polyethylene. *J. Biomed. Mater. Res.*, 2003; **66A**: 146–154.

840. Gencur SJ, Rimnac CM, Kurtz SM. Failure micromechanisms during uniaxial tensile fracture of conventional and highly crosslinked ultra-high molecular weight polyethylenes used in total joint replacements. *Biomaterials*, 2003; **24**: 3947–3954.

841. Muratoglu OK, Merrill EW, Bragdon CR, O'Connor D, Hoeffel D, Burroughs B, Jasty M, Harris WH. Effect of radiation, heat, and aging on *in vitro* wear resistance of polyethylene. *Clin. Orthop. Relat. Res.*, 2003; **417**: 253–262.

842. Wannomae K, Bhattacharyya S, Freiberg A, Estok D, Harris WH, Muratoglu O. *In vivo* oxidation of retrieved cross-linked ultra-high-molecular-weight polyethylene acetabular components with residual free radicals. *J. Arthopl.*, 2006; **21**: 1005–1011.

843. Oral E, Wannomae KK, Hawkins NE, Harris WH, Muratoglu OK. α-Tocopherol doped irradiated UHMWPE for high fatigue resistance and low wear. *Biomaterials*, 2004; **25**: 5515–5522.

844. Oral E, Muratoglu OK. Vitamin E diffused, highly crosslinked UHMWPE: A review. *Int. Orthop.*, 2011; **35**: 215–223.

845. Kurtz SM, Bracco P, Costa L. *Vitamin E blended UHMWPE biomaterials*. In: Kurtz SM, editor. UHMWPE Biomaterials, Handbook. 2nd ed. (Elsevier; Amsterdam, 2009). pp. 237–246.

846. Lerf R, Zurbrügg D, Delfosse D. Use of vitamin E to protect cross-linked UHMWPE from oxidation. *Biomaterials*, 2010; **31**: 3643–3648.

847. Bracco P, Brunella V, Zanetti M, Luda MP, Costa L. Stabilisation of ultra-high molecular weight polyethylene with vitamin *E*. *Polym. Degrad. Stab.*, 2007; **92**: 2155–2162.

848. Burton G, Ingold K. Autoxidation of biological molecules. 1. The antioxidant activity of vitamin E and related chain-breaking phenolic antioxidants *in vitro*. *J. Am. Chem. Soc.*, 1981; **103**: 6472–6477.

849. Kamal-Eldin A, Appelqvist L. The chemistry and antioxidant properties of tocopherols and tocotrienols. *Lipids*, 1996; **31**: 671–701.

850. Strobl GR, Hagedorn W. Raman spectroscopic method for determining the crystallinity of polyethylene. *J. Polym. Sci. Polym. Phys. Ed.*, 1978; **16**: 1181–1193.

851. Maxfield J, Stein RS, Chen MC. Polarized Raman studies of crystalline and amorphous orientation in polyethylene. *J. Polym. Sci. Polym. Phys. Ed.*, 1978; **16**: 37–48.

852. Nylor CC, Meier RJ, Kip BJ, Williams KPJ, Mason SM, Conroy N, Gerrard DL. Raman spectroscopy employed for the determination of the intermediate phase in polyethylene. *Macromolecules*, 1995; **28**: 2969–2978.

853. Oral E, Wannomae KK, Rowell SL, Muratoglu OK. Diffusion of vitamin E in ultra-high molecular weight polyethylene. *Biomaterials*, 2007; **28**: 5225–5237.

854. Wolf C, Maninger J, Lederer K, Fruhwirth-Smounig H, Gamse T, Marr R. Stabilisation of crosslinked ultra-high molecular weight polyethylene (UHMW-PE)-acetabular components with α-tocopherol. *J. Mater. Sci. Mater. Med.*, 2006; **17**: 1323–1331

855. Li DS, Garmestani H, Davis SC, Moss LK, Siddiqi AK, Guthrie JB, Johansen N, Matrisciano L. Wear resistance and texture evolution of ultra high molecular weight polyethylenes during uniaxial compression. *Ceramic Transactions*, 2009; **201**: 595–603.

856. Wang A, Sun DC, Yau S-S, Edwards B, Sokol M, Essner A, Polineni VK, Stark C, Dumbleton JH. Orientation softening in the deformation and wear of ultra-high molecular weight polyethylene. *Wear*, 1997; **203–204**: 230–241.

857. http://www.biometeurope.fr/userfiles/files/Technologies/E1BiometLab-Paper.pdf.

858. Birkinshaw C, Buggy M, Daly S, O'Neill M. The effect of gamma radiation on the physical structure and mechanical properties of ultrahigh molecular weight polyethylene. *J. Appl. Polym. Sci.*, 1989; **38**: 1967–1973.

859. Hozack WJ, Mesa JJ, Carey C, Rothman RH. Relationship between polyethylene wear, pelvic osteolysis and clinical symptomatology in patients with cementless acetabular components. *J. Arthroplasty*, 1996; **11**: 769–772.

860. Campbell P, Ma S, Yeom B. Isolation of predominantly submicron-sized UHMWPE wear particles from periprosthetic tissues. *J. Biomed. Mater. Res.*, 1995; **29**: 127–131.

861. Yeom B, Yu Y-J, McKellop HA, Salovey R. Profile of oxidation in irradiated polyethylene. *J. Polym. Sci.: Part A: Polym. Chem.*, 1998; **36**: 329–339.

862. Fagnano C, Rossi M, Porter RS, Ottani S. A study on solid-state drawn fibers of polyethylene by confocal Raman microspectrometry: Evaluation of the orientation profiles of amorphous and crystalline phases across the fiber section. *Polymer*, 2001; **42**: 5871–5883.

863. Ratner S, Moret PM, Wachtel E, Marom G. New lnsights into lamellar twisting in transcrystalline polyethylene. *Macromol. Chem. Phys.*, 2005; **206**: 1183–1189.

864. Pigeon M, Prud'homme RE, Pézolet M. Characterization of molecular orientation in polyethylene by Raman spectroscopy. *Macromolecules*, 1991; **24**: 5687–5694.

865. Citra MJ, Chase DB, Ikeda RM, Gardner KH. Molecular orientation of high-density polyethylene fibers characterized by polarized Raman spectroscopy. *Macromolecules*, 1995; **28**: 4007–4012.

866. Nikolaeva GY, Semenova LE, Prokhorov KA, Gordeyev SA. Quantitative characterization of macromolecules orientation in polymers by micro Raman spectroscopy. *Laser Phys.*, 1997; **7(2)**: 403–415.

867. Bower DI. Investigation of molecular orientation distributions by polarized Raman scattering and polarized fluorescence. *J. Polym. Sci. Polym. Phys. Ed.*, 1972; **10**: 2135–2153.

868. Frisk S, Ikeda RM, Chase DB, Rabolt JF. Determination of the molecular orientation of poly(propylene terephthalate) fibers using polarized Raman spectroscopy: A comparison of methods. *Appl. Spectrosc.*, 2004; **58**: 279–286.

869. Minn M, Sinha SK. Molecular orientation, crystallinity, and topographical changes in sliding and their frictional effects for UHMWPE film. *Tribol. Lett.*, 2009; **34**: 133–140.

870. Heo SJ, Jang I, Barry PR, Phillpot SR, Perry SS, Sawyer WG, Sinnott SB. Effect of the sliding orientation on the tribological properties of polyethylene in molecular dynamics simulations. *J. Appl. Phys.*, 2008; **103**: 083502-1–6.

871. Sambasivan S, Fischer DA, Shen MC, Hsu SM. Molecular orientation of ultrahigh molecular weight polyethylene induced by various sliding motions. *J. Biomed. Mater. Res.*, 2004; **70**: 273–285.

872. Gurp MV. The use of rotation matrices in the mathematical description of molecular orientations in polymers. *Colloid Polym. Sci.*, 1995; **273**: 607–625.

873. Bower DI. Orientation distribution functions for biaxially oriented polymers. *Polymer*, 1982; **23**: 1251–1255.

874. McBrierty VJ. Use of rotation operators in the general description of polymer properties. *J. Chem. Phys.*, 1974; **61**: 872–882.

875. Mutter R, Stille W, Strobl G. Transition regions and surface melting in partially crystalline polyethylene: A Raman spectroscopic study. *J. Polym. Sci.: Part B: Polym. Phys.*, 1993; **31**: 99–105.

876. Bergstrom JS, Rimnac C, Kurtz SM. Molecular chain stretch is a multiaxial failure criterion for conventional and highly crosslinked UHMWPE. *J. Orthop. Res.*, 2005; **23**: 367–375.

877. Kurtz SM, Muhlstein C, Edidin AA. Surface morphology and wear mechanisms of four clinically relevant biomaterials after hip simulator testing. *J. Biomed. Mater. Res. A*, 2000; **52**: 447–459.

878. Bankston AB, Cates H, Ritter MA, Keating EM, Faris PM. Polyethylene wear in total hip arthroplasty. *Clin Orthop.*, 1995; **317**: 7–13.

879. Kurtz SM. Stress in UHMWPE tibial and patellar components for TKR. In: Kurtz SM editor. The UHMWPE Handbook, Ultra-High-Molecular-Weight-Polyethylene in Total Joint Replacement. (New York: Elsevier Academic Press; 2002); pp. 100–102.

880. Bartel DL, Rawlinson VL, Burstein AH, Ranawat CS, Flynn Jr WF. Stress in polyethylene components of contemporary total knee replacements. *Clin. Orthop.*, 1995; **380**: 76–82.

881. Olley RH, Hosier IL, Bassett DC, Smith NG. On morphology of consolidated UHMWPE resin in hip cups. *Biomaterials*, 1999; **20**: 2037–2046.

882. Li DS, Garmestani H, Alamo RG, Kalidindi SR. The role of crystallinity in the crystallographic texture evolution of polyethylenes during tensile deformation. *Polymer*, 2003; **44**: 5355–5367.

883. Song HH, Argon AS, Cohen RE. Morphology of highly textured high-density polyethylene. *Macromolecules*, 1990; **23**: 870–876.

884. Bartczak Z, Cohen RE, Argon AS. Evolution of the crystalline texture of high-density polyethylene during uniaxial compression. *Macromolecules*, 1992; **25**: 4692–4704.

885. Atkinson JR, Dowling JM, Cicek RZ. Materials for internal prostheses: The present position and possible future developments. *Biomaterials*, 1980; **1**: 89–96.

886. Edidin AA, Herr MP, Villarraga ML, Muth J, Yau SS, Kurtz SM. Accelerated ageing studies of UHMWPE. 1. Effect of resin, processing, and radiation environment on resistance to mechanical degradation. *J. Biomed. Mater. Res.*, 2002; **61**: 312–322.

887. Muratoglu OK, O'Connor DO, Bragdon CR, Delaney J, Jasty M, Harris WH, Merrill E, Venugopalan P. Gradient crosslinking of UHMWPE using irradiation in molten state for total joint arthroplasty. *Biomaterials*, 2002; **23**: 717–724.

888. Muratoglu OK, Bragdon CR, O'Connor DO, Jasty M, Harris WH, Gul R, McGarry F. Unified wear model for highly crosslinked ultra-high molecular weight polyethylenes (UHMWPE). *Biomaterials*, 1999; **20**: 1463–1470.

889. Hamadouche M, Boutin P, Daussange J, Bolander ME, Sedel L. Alumina-on-alumina total hip arthroplasty: A minimum 18.5-year follow-up study. *J. Bone Joint Surg.* (*Am.*), 2002; **84**: 69–77.

890. Sedel L. Evolution of alumina-on-alumina implants: A review. *Clin. Orthop. Relat. Res.*, 2000; **379**: 48–54.

891. Huo MH, Martin RP, Zatorski LE, Keggi KJ. Total hip replacements using the ceramic Mittelmeier prosthesis. *Clin. Orthop.*, 1996; **332**: 143–150.

892. Peiro A, Pardo J, Navarrete R, Rodriguez-Alonso L, Martos F. Fracture of the ceramic head in total hip arthroplasty: Report of two cases. *J. Arthroplasty*, 1991; **6**: 371–374.

893. Cameron HU. Ceramic head implantation failures. *J. Arthroplasty.*, 1991; **6**:185–188.

894. Oonishi H. New design feature of high-quality alumina-alumina ceramic. combination in total hip replacement. *Bioceramics*, 1992; **5**: 403–408.

895. Suzuki K, Matsubara M, Morita S, Muneta T, Shinomiya K. Fracture of a ceramic acetabular insert after ceramic-on-ceramic THA — a case report. *Acta Orthop. Scand.*, 2003; **74**: 101–103.

896. Amino H. Ceramic on ceramic total hip arthroplasty in Japan. (in Japanese) Pharm. *Medica*, 2002; **20**: 19–25.

897. Kitajima S, Hotokebuchi T. Ceramic on ceramic total hip arthroplasty. (in Japanese) *J. Joint Surg.*, 2003; **22**: 85–89.

898. Park YS, Hwang SK, Choy WS, Kim YS, Moon YW, Lim SJ. Ceramic failure after total hip arthroplasty with an alumina-on-alumina bearing. *J. Bone Joint Surg.* (*Am.*), 2006; **88**: 780–787.

899. Krikler SJ. Fracture of a ceramic femoral head after a revision operation. A case report. *J. Bone Joint Surg.* (*Am.*), 1997; **79A**: 118–121.

900. Maccauro G, Piconi C. Ceramic femoral head fracture in total hip replacement. *Int. Orthop.*, 2000; **24**: 239–243.

901. McLean CR, Dabis H, Mok D. Delayed fracture of the ceramic femoral head after trauma. *J. Arthroplasty*, 2002; **17**: 503–504.

902. Piconi C, Labanti M, Magnani G, Caporale M, Maccauro G, Magliocchetti G. Analysis of a failed alumina THR ball head. *Biomaterials*, 1999; **20**: 1637–1646.

903. Lewinnek GE, Lewis JL, Tarr R, Compere CL, Zimmerman JR. Dislocations after total hip-replacement arthroplasties. *J. Bone Joint Surg.* (*Am.*), 1978; **60**: 217–220.

904. Messieh M, Mattingly DA, Turner RH, Scott R, Fox J, Slater J. Wear debris from bipolar femoral neck-cup impingement: A cause of femoral stem loosening. *J. Arthroplasty*, 1994; **9**: 89–93.

905. Kaku N, Tsumura H, Yorisu T. Qualitative analysis of polyethylene wear in a bipolar femoral prosthesis: A case report. *J. Orthop. Surg.*, 2001; **9**: 71–76.

906. Yamaguchi M, Akisue T, Bauer TW, Hashimoto Y. The spatial location of impingement in total hip arthroplasty. *J. Arthroplasty*, 2000; **15**: 305–313.

907. Coventry MB. Late dislocations in patients with Charnley total hip arthroplasty. *J. Bone Joint Surg.* (*Am.*), 1985; **67**: 832–841.

908. McCollum DE, Gray WJ. Dislocation after total hip arthroplasty: Causes and prevention. *Clin. Orthop. Relat. Res.*, 1990; **261**: 159–170.

909. Woo RY, Morrey BF. Dislocations after total hip arthroplasty. *J. Bone Joint Surg.* (*Am.*), 1982; **64**: 1295–1306.

910. Dalla Pria P, Zagra L, Esopi P, Masoni D. Breakage and noises in ceramic on ceramic couplings. *Eur. Orthop. Traumatol.*, 2010; **1**: 53–59.

911. Sariali E, Stewart T, Mamoudy P, Jin Z, Fisher J. Undetected fracture of an alumina ceramic on ceramic hip prosthesis. *J. Arthroplasty*. 2009; **25**: 658.E1–E5.

912. Willmann G. Retrieved ceramic wear couple: unexpected findings. In: *Bioceramics in Joint Arthroplasty: Proceedings of the 6th BIOLOX®*Symposium. (Toni A, Willmann G, eds). (Georg Thieme Verlag, Stuttgart, Germany, 2001) pp. 63–65.

913. Hasegawa M, Sudo A, Uchida A. Cobalt-chromium head wear following revision hip arthroplasty performed after ceramic fracture — a case report. *Acta Orthop.*, 2006; **77**: 833–835.

914. Rudas M, Qasim T, Bush MB, Lawn BR. Failure of curved brittle layer systems from radial cracking in concentrated surface loading. *J. Mater. Res.*, 2005; **20**: 2812–2819.

915. Espinosa HD, Zavattieri PD, Dwivedi SK. A finite deformation continuum/discrete model for the description of fragmentation and damage in brittle materials. *J. Mech. Phys. Solids*, 1998; **46**: 1909–1942.

916. Zavattieri PD, Espinosa HD. Grain level analysis of crack initiation and propagation in brittle materials. *Acta Mater.*, 2001; **49**: 4291–4311.

917. Uribe J, Hausselle J, Geringer J, Forest B. Finite element modeling of shock-induced damages on ceramic hip prostheses. *ISRN Mater. Sci.*, 2011; **121**, 486-1–14.

918. Evans AG, Crumley GB, Demaray RE. On the mechanical behavior of brittle coatings and layers. *Oxidation Met.*, 1983; **20**: 193–216.

919. Teixeira V. Residual stress and cracking in thin PVD coatings. *Vacuum*, 2002; **64**: 393–399.

920. Jha SK, Sohn YH, Sastri S, Gunda N, Haynes JA. Al-O-N based duplex coating system for improved oxidation resistance of superalloys and NiCrAlY coatings. *Surf. Coatings Tech.*, 2004; **183**: 224–232.

921. Gu T, Xiong W, Ning C, Zhang J. Residual stresses in microarc oxidation ceramic coatings on biocompatible AZ31 magnesium alloys. *J. Mater. Eng. Performance*, 2012; **21**: 1085–1090.

922. Pang X, Gao K, Yang H, Qiao L, Wang Y, Volinsky AA. Interfacial microstructure of chromium oxide coatings. *Adv. Eng. Mater.*, 2007; **9**: 594–599.

923. Ohno K, Uchiyama H, Kozuka H. Understanding of the development of the in-plane residual stress in sol–gel-derived metal oxide thin films. *J. Appl. Phys.*, 2012; **111**: 014910-1–9.

924. Sue JA. X-ray elastic constants and residual stress of textured titanium nitride coating. *Surf. Coatings Tech.*, 1992; **54–55**: 154–159.

925. Leoni M, Scardi P, Rossi S, Fedrizzi L, Massiani Y. (Ti,Cr)N and Ti /TiN PVD coatings on 304 stainless steel substrates: Texture and residual stress. *Thin Solid Films* 1999; **345**: 263–269.

926. Shieu FS, Cheng LH, Shiao MH, Lin SH. Effects of Ti interlayer on the microstructure of ion-plated TiN coatings on AISI 304 stainless steel. *Thin Solid Films*, 1997; **311**: 138–145.

927. Agarwal A, Dahotre NB, Sudarshan TS. Evolution of interface in pulsed electrode deposited titanium diboride on copper and steel. *J. Surf. Eng.*, 1999; **15**: 27–32.

928. Tomsia AP, Launey ME, Lee JS, Mankani MH, Wegst UGK, Saiz E. Nanotechnology approaches for better dental implants. *Int. J. Oral Maxillofac. Implants*, 2011; **26** (Suppl.): 25–49.

929. Moon H, Lange FF. Strengthening with a uniform compressive layer produced by a dip-coating: A study of processing variables. *J. Am. Ceram. Soc.*, 2010; **93**: 1264–1269.

930. Fu Y, Loh NL, Batchelor AW, Liu D, Zhu X, He J, Xu K. Improvement in fretting wear and fatigue resistance of Ti–6Al–4V by application of several surface treatments and coatings. *Surf. Coatings Tech.*, 1998; **106**: 193–197.

931. Mao WG, Dai CY, Zhou YC, Liu QX. An experimental investigation on thermo-mechanical buckling delamination failure characteristic of air plasma sprayed thermal barrier coatings. *Surf. Coatings Tech.*, 2007; **201**: 6217–6227.

932. Chen J, Bull SJ. Approaches to investigate delamination and interfacial toughness in coated systems: An overview. *J. Phys. D: Appl. Phys.*, 2011; **44**: 34001-1–35.

933. Rühle M, Evans AG. Structure and chemistry of metal/ceramic interfaces. *Mater. Sci. Eng. A*, 1989; **A107**: 187–197.

934. Beltran JI, Gallego S, Cerda J, Munoz MC. Oxygen vacancies at Ni/c-ZrO_2 interfaces. *J. Eur. Ceram. Soc.*, 2003; **23**: 2737–2740.

935. Parise M, Touet I, Sicardy O. Oxidation of zirconium alloys. Crystallographic texture of zirconia: Interpretation and mechanical consequences. *Textures Microstr.*, 1998; **30**: 247–263.

936. Hobbs LW, Benezra Rosen V, Mangin SP, Treska M. Oxidation microstructures and interfaces in the oxidized zirconium knee. *Int. J. App. Ceram. Technol.*, 2005; **2**: 221–246.

937. Ries MD, Salehi A, Widding K, Hunter G. Polyethylene wear performance of oxidized zirconium and cobalt-chromium knee components

under abrasive conditions. *J. Bone Joint Surg.* (*Am.*), 2002; **84A** (Suppl. 2): 129–135.

938. Davidson JA, Asgian CM, Mishra AK, Kovaks P. Zirconia (ZrO_2)-coated zirconium-2.5Nb alloy for prosthetic knee bearing applications. *Bioceramics*, 1992; **5**: 389–401.

939. Mishra AK, Davidson JA. Zirconia/zirconium: A new abrasion resistant material for orthopaedic applications. *Mater. Technol.*, 1993; **8**: 16–21.

940. Laskin RS. An oxidized Zr ceramic surfaced femoral component for total knee arthroplasty. *Clin. Orthop. Relat. Res.*, 2003; **416**: 191–196.

941. Patel AM, Spector M. Oxidized zirconia for hemiarthroplasty: An *In vitro* assessment. *Biomaterials*, 1995; **8**: 169–175.

942. White SE, Whiteside LA, McCarthy DS, Anthony M, Poggie RA. Simulated wear with cobalt-chromium and oxidized zirconium knee femoral component. *Clin. Orthop.*, 1994; **309**: 176–184.

943. Laskin RS, Davis J. Total knee replacement using the Genesis II prosthesis: A 5-year follow-up study of the first 100 consecutive cases. *Knee*, 2005; **12**: 163–167.

944. National Joint Registry of England and Wales: NJR Prostheses used 2010; p. 84. Available from: URL: www.njcentre.org.uk

945. National Joint Registry of England and Wales: 8th Annual Report 2011; p. 160. Available from: URL:.www.njcentre.org.uk

946. Australian Orthopaedic Association National Joint Replacement Registry: Annual Report 2011, Hip and Knee Arthroplasty; p. 65. Available from: URL: www.dmac.adelaide.edu.au/aoanjrr/index.jsp.

947. Hunter G, Long M. Abrasive wear of oxidized Zr-2.5Nb, CoCrMo and Ti–6Al–4V against bone cement. In: *Proceedings of the 6th World Biomaterials, Congress*. (Trans. Society for Biomaterials; Minneapolis, MN, 2000). p. 835.

948. Gotman I, Gutmanas EY, Hunter G. Wear-resistant ceramic films and coatings. *Comprehensive Biomater.*, 2011; **1**: 127–155.

949. Kop AM, Whitewood C, Johnston DJL. Damage of Oxinium femoral heads subsequent to hip arthroplasty dislocation. Three retrieval case studies. *J. Arthroplasty*, 2007; **22**: 775–779.

950. McCalden RW, Charron KD, Davidson RD, Teeter MG, Holdsworth DW. Damage of an Oxinium femoral head and polyethylene liner following "routine" total hip replacement. *J. Bone Joint Surg.* (*Br.*), 2011; **93B**: 409–413.

951. Godlewski J, Gros JP, Lambertin M, Wadier JF, Weidinger H. Raman spectroscopy study of the tetragonal-to-monoclinic transition in zirconium oxide scales and determination of overall oxygen diffusion by nuclear microanalysis of O^{18}. *ASTM Special Technical Publications*, 1991; **1132**: 416–436.

952. Cox B, Wu C. Dissolution of zirconium oxide films in 300°C LiOH. *J. Nucl. Mater.*, 1993; **199**: 272–284.

953. Barberis P, Merle-Mejean T, Quintard P. On Raman spectroscopy of zirconium oxide films. *J. Nucl. Mater.*, 1997; **246**: 232–243.

954. Galetz MC, Fleischmann EW, Konrad CH, Schuetz A, Glatzel U. Abrasion resistance of oxidized zirconium in comparison with CoCrMo and titanium nitride coatings for artificial knee joints. *J. Biomed. Mater. Res. B*, 2010; **93B**: 244–251.

955. Guo X. Effect of Nb_2O_5 on the space charge conduction of Y_2O_3 stabilized ZrO_2. *Solid State Ionics*, 1997; **99**: 137–142.

956. Vidyavathy SM, Kamaraj V. Microwave sintering of niobium co-doped yttria stabilized zirconia. *Mod. Appl. Sci.*, 2009; **3**: 102–105.

957. Bartolomé JH, Gutierrez-Gonzales CF, Pecharroman C, Moya JS. Synergetic toughening mechanism in 3Y-TZP/Nb composites. *Acta Mater.*, 2007; **55**: 5924–5933.

958. Kim DJ. Effect of Ta_2O_5, Nb_2O_5, and HfO_2 alloying on the transformability of Y_2O_3-stabilized tetragonal ZrO_2. *J. Am. Ceram. Soc.*, 1990; **73**: 115–120.

959. Wachsman ED, Jiang N, Frank CW, Mason DM, Stevenson DA. Spectroscopic investigation of oxygen vacancies in solid oxide electrolytes. *Appl. Phys. A*, 1990; **50**: 545–549.

960. Matsui K, Yoshida H, Ikuhara Y. Phase-transformation and grain-growth kinetics in yttria-stabilized tetragonal zirconia polycrystal doped with a small amount of alumina. *J. Eur. Ceram. Soc.*, 2010; **30**: 1679–1690.

961. Alonso PJ, Alcalá R, Casas-Gonzales J, Cases R, Orera VM. Spectroscopy of chromium (III) in yttrium-stabilized ZrO_2. *J. Phys. Chem. Solids*, 1989; **50**: 1185–1191.

962. Chang S-M, Doong R-A. The effect of chemical states of dopants on the microstructures and band gaps of metal-doped ZrO_2 thin films at different temperatures. *J. Phys. Chem. B*, 2004; **108**: 18098–18103.

963. Berry FJ, Loretto MH, Smith MR. Iron-zirconium oxide: An investigation of structural transformations by X-ray diffraction,

electron diffraction, and iron-57 Mössbauer spectroscopy. *J. Solid State Chem.*, 1989; **83**: 91–99.

964. Nakajima H, Ishihara H, Shen Q, Toyoda T, Itoh K, Kaneko H, Tamaura Y. Effect of Fe doping on photoluminescence of yttria-stabilized zirconia. *J. Alloys Comp.*, 2007; **441**: 255–258.

965. Foster AS, Sulimov VB, Lopez Gejo F, Shluger AL, Nieminen RM. Structure and electrical levels of point defects in monoclinic zirconia. *Phys. Rev. B*, 2001; **64**: 224108-1–10.

966. Emeline A, Kataeva GV, Litke AS, Rudakova AV, Ryabchuk VK, Serpone N. Spectroscopic and photoluminescence studies of a wide-band gap insulating material: Powdered and colloidal ZrO_2 sols. *Langmuir*, 1998; **14**: 5011–5022.

967. Petrik NG, Alexandrov AB, Vall AI. Interfacial energy transfer during gamma radiolysis of water on the surface of ZrO_2 and some other oxides. *J. Phys. Chem. B*, 2001; **105**: 5935–5944.

968. Foster AS, Shluger AL, Nieminem RM. Mechanisms of interstitial oxygen diffusion in hafnia. *Phys. Rev. Lett.*, 2002; **89**: 225901-1–4.

969. Howard CJ, Hill RJ, Reichert BE. Structures of the ZrO_2 polymorphs at room temperature by high-resolution neutron powder diffraction. *Acta Cryst. B*, 1988; **B44**: 116–120.

970. Zacate MO, Minervini L, Bradfield DJ, Grimes RW, Sickafus KE. Defect cluster formation in M_2O_3-doped cubic ZrO_2. *Solid State Ionics* 2000; **128**: 243–254.

971. Minervini L, Zacate MO, Grimes RW. Defect cluster formation in M_2O_3-doped CeO_2. *Solid State Ionics*, 1999; **116**: 339–349.

972. Stefanovich EV, Shluger AL, Catlow CRA. Theoretical study of the stabilization of cubic-phase ZrO_2 by impurities. *Phys. Rev. B*, 1994; **49**: 560–571.

973. Konttinen YT, Takagi M, Mandelin J, Lassus J, Salo J, Ainola M, Li T-F, Virtanen I, Liliesträm M, Sakai H, Kobayashi Y, Sorsa T, Lappalainen R, Demulter A, Santavirta S. Acid attack and cathepsin K in bone resorption around total hip replacement prosthesis. *J. Bone Miner. Res.*, 2001; **16**: 1780–1786.

974. Li CW, McKerns MM, Fultz B. A Raman spectrometry study of phonon anharmonicity of zirconia at elevated temperatures. *J. Am. Ceram. Soc.*, 2011; **94**: 224–229.

975. McBride JR, Hass KC, Poindexter BD, Weber WH. Raman and x-ray studies of $Ce_{1-x}RE_xO_{2-y}$, where RE=La, Pr, Nd, Eu, Gd, and Tb. *J. Appl. Phys.*, 1994; **76**: 2435–2441.

976. Namavar F, Cheung CL, Sabirianov RF, Mei WN, Zeng XC, Wang G, Haider H, Garvin KL. Lotus effect in engineered zirconia. *Nano Lett.*, 2008; **8**: 988–996.

977. Namavar F, Wang G, Cheung CL, Sabirianov RF, Zeng XC, Mei WN, Bai J, Brewer JR, Haider H, Garvin KL. Thermal stability of nanostructurally stabilized zirconium oxide. *Nanotechnology*, 2007; **18**: 415702-1–9.

978. Liu D, Lord O, Flewitt PE. Calibration of Raman spectroscopy in the stress measurement of air-plasma-sprayed yttria-stabilized zirconia. *Appl. Spectrosc.*, 2012; **66**: 1204–1209.

979. Bouvier P, Lucazeau G. Raman spectra and vibrational analysis of nanometric tetragonal zirconia under high pressure. *J. Phys. Chem. Solids*, 2000; **61**: 569–578.

980. Balzaretti NM, da Jornada JAH. Pressure dependence of the refractive index of monoclinic and yttria-stabilized cubic zirconia. *Phys. Rev. B*, 1995; **52**: 9266–9269.

981. Tanaka K, Ishihara K, Akiniwa Y, Ohta H. Residual stress of aluminium thin films measured by X-ray and curvature methods. *Mater. Sci. Res. Int.*, 1996; **2**: 153–159.

982. Taylor CA, Wayne MF, Chiu WKS. Residual stress measurement in thin carbon films by Raman spectroscopy and nanoindentation. *Thin Solid Films*, 2003; **429**: 190–200.

983. Im SH, Huang R. Wrinkle patterns of anisotropic crystal films on viscoelastic substrates. *J. Mech. Phys. Solids*, 2008; **56**: 3315–3330.

984. Kharton VV, Yaremchenko AA, Patrakeev MV, Naumovich EN, Marques FMB. Thermal and chemical induced expansion of $La_{0.3}Sr_{0.7}(Fe,Ga)O_{3-\delta}$ ceramics. *J. Eur. Ceram. Soc.*, 2003; **23**: 1417–1426.

985. Hayashi H, Watanabe M, Ohuchida M, Inaba H, Hiei Y, Yamamoto T, Mori M. Thermal expansion of $La_{1-x}Sr_xCrO_{3-\delta}$. *Solid State Ionics*, 2001; **144**: 301–313.

986. Evans AG, Hutchinson JW. On the mechanics of delamination and spalling in compressed films. *Int. J. Solids Structures*, 1984; **20**: 455–466.

987. Evans AG, Mumm DR, Hutchinson JW, Meier GH, Pettit FS. Mechanisms controlling the durability of thermal barrier coatings. *Progress Mater. Sci.*, 2001; **46**: 505–553.

988. Hutchinson JW, Suo Z. Mixed mode cracking in layered materials. *Adv. Appl. Mech.*, 1991; **29**: 63–191.

989. Drory MD, Hutchinson JW. Measurement of the adhesion of a brittle film on a ductile substrate by indentation. *Proc. R. Soc. London A*, 1996; **452**: 2319–2341.

990. Pezzotti G, Okai K, Zhu W. Stress tensor dependence of the polarized Raman spectrum of tetragonal barium titanate. *J. Appl. Phys.*, 2012; **111**: 013504-1–16.

991. Miyatake T, Pezzotti G. Validating Raman spectroscopic calibrations of phonon deformation potentials in silicon single crystal: A comparison between ball-on-ring and micro-indentation methods. *J. Appl. Phys.*, 2011; **110**: 093511-1–13.

992. Zhu W, Wan K, Pezzotti G. Methods of piezo-spectroscopic calibration on thin film materials: II. Tensile stress field at indentation crack tip. *Meas. Sci. Technol.*, 2006; **17**: 191–198.

993. Fett T. *Computation of the crack opening displacements for Vickers indentation cracks.* Report FZKA 6757; Forschungszentrum Karlsruhe, Karlsruhe, Germany, 2002.

994. Gruniger MF, Lawn BR, Farabaugh EN, Wachtman JB. Measurement of residual stresses in coatings on brittle substrates by indentation fracture. *J. Am. Ceram. Soc.*, 1987; **70**: 344–348.

995. Miller KJ, Kfouri AP. An elastic-plastic finite element analysis of crack tip fields under biaxial loading conditions. *Int. J. Fracture*, 1974; **10**: 393–404.

996. Haerle AG, Cannon WR, Denda M. Direct measurement of crack tip stresses. *J. Am. Ceram. Soc.*, 1991; **74**: 2897–2901.

997. Denda M, Mattingly E. The singular crack element for 2-d boundary element analysis of multiple straight cracks in the general anisotropic solids. Electronic *J. Boundary Elements*, 2003; **1**: 404–417.

998. Puchi-Cabrera ES. A new model for the computation of the composite hardness of coated systems. *Surf. Coat. Technol.*, 2002; **160**: 177–186.

999. Malzbender J, den Toonder JMJ, Balkenende AR, de With G. Measuring mechanical properties of coatings: A methodology applied to nano-particle-filled sol–gel coatings on glass. *Mater. Sci. Eng.*, 2002; **R36**: 47–103.

1000. Demidova NV, Wu XJ, Liu R. A fracture toughness model for brittle coating on ductile substrate under indentation loading. *Eng. Fracture Mech.*, 2012; **82**: 17–28.

1001. Ichimura H, Rodriguez FM, Rodrigo A. The composite and film hardness of TiN coatings prepared by cathodic arc evaporation. *Surf. Coat. Technol.*, 2000; **127**: 138–143.

1002. Borodachev N. An elliptical crack under point forces applied to its surface. *J. Appl. Math. Mech.*, 1998; **64**: 477–483.

1003. Light TR, Keggi KJ. Anterior approach to hip arthroplasty. *Clin. Orthop. Relat. Res.*, 1980; **152**: 255–260.

1004. Walker TJ. Characterization of the fracture toughness of zircaloy. *Nucl. Technol.* 1972; **16**: 509–520.

1005. Coleman CE, Cheadle BA, Causey AR, Chow PEK, Davies PH, McManus MD, Rodgers DK, Sagat S, van Drunen G. Evaluation of Zircaloy-2 pressure tubes from NPD. Solid State Ionics ASTM Special Technical Publications, **1023**, 1989; pp. 35–49.

1006. Wallace AC, Gordon KS, Lepik OE. Effects of hydride morphology on Zr-2.5Nb fracture toughness. ASTM Special Technical Publications, **1023**, 1989; pp. 66–88.

1007. Roy H, Parida N, Sivaprasad S, Tarafder S, Rayc KK. Acoustic emissions during fracture toughness tests of steels exhibiting varying ductility. *Mater. Sci. Eng.*, 2008; **A486**: 562–571.

1008. Bhowmick S, Kale AN, Jayaram V, Biswas SK. Contact damage in TiN coatings on steel. *Thin Solid Films*, 2003; **436**: 250–258.

1009. Zhang S. TiN coating of tool steels: A review. *J. Mater. Processing Technol.*, 1993; **39**: 165–177.

1010. Evangelista GT, Fulkerson E, Kummer F, DiCesare PD. Surface damage to an oxinium femoral head prosthesis after dislocation. *J. Bone Joint Surg.*, 2007; **89**: 535–537.

1011. Pawar V, Weaver C, Jani S. Physical characterization of a new composition of oxidized zirconium-2.5 wt% niobium produced using a two step process for biomedical applications. *Appl. Surf. Sci.*, 2011; **257**: 6118–6124.

1012. Jerosch J, Theising C, Fadel ME. Antero-lateral minimal invasive (ALMI) approach for total hip arthroplasty technique and early results. *Arch. Orthop. Trauma Surg.*, 2006; **126**: 164–173.

1013. Light TR, Keggi KJ. Anterior approach to hip arthroplasty. *Clin. Orthop. Relat. Res.*, 1980; **152**: 255–260.

1014. Rittmeister M, Peters A. A posterior mini-incision for total hip arthroplasty — results of 76 consecutive cases. *Z. Orthop. Ihre Grenzgeb.*, 2005; **143**: 403–411.

1015. Keggi KJ, Huo MH, Zatorski LE. Anterior approach to total hip replacement: Surgical technique and clinical results of our first one thousand cases using non-cemented prostheses. *Yale J. Biol. Med.*, 1993; **66**: 243–256.

1016. Kennon RE, Keggi JM, Wetmore RS, Zatorski LE, Huo MH, Keggi KJ. Total hip arthroplasty through a minimally invasive anterior surgical approach. *J. Bone Joint Surg.* (*Am.*), 2003; **85** (Suppl. 4): 39–48.

1017. Krismer M, Nogler M, Rachbauer F. Direct, anterior, single incision approach. In: *Minimal Invasive Joint Arthroplasty*. Hozak WJ, Krismer M, Nogler M, Bonutti PM, Rachbauer F, Schaffer JL, Donelly WJ (Eds.): (Springer, Heidelberg, NewYork, Tokyo, 2004). pp. 4–10.

1018. Oinuma K, Eingartner C, Saito Y, Shiratsuchi H. Total hip arthroplasty by direct anterior approach. *Operat. Orthop. Traumatol.*, 2007; **19**: 310–326.

1019. Nogler M. Navigated minimal invasive total hip arthroplasty. *Surg., Technol. Int.*, 2004; **12**: 259–262.

1020. Lucas DH, Scott RD. The Ranawat sign. A specific maneuver to assess component positioning in total hip arthroplasty. *J. Orthop. Tech.*, 1994; **2**: 59–61.

1021. White TO, Dougall TW. Arthroplasty of the hip: Leg length is not important. *J. Bone Joint Surg.* (*Br.*), 2002; **84**: 335–338.

1022. Honl M, Schwieger K, Salineros M, Jacobs J, Morlock M, Wimmer M. Orientation of the acetabular component. A comparison of five navigation systems with conventional surgical techniques. *J. Bone Joint Surg.* (*Br.*), 2006; **88**:1401–1405.

1023. Noble PC, Sugano N, Johnston JD, Thompson MT, Conditt MA, Engh A, Mathis KB. Computer simulation: How can it help the surgeon optimize implant position? *Clin. Orthop. Relat. Res.*, 2003; **417**: 242–252.

1024. Lazovic D, Kaib N. Results with navigated Bicontact total hip arthroplasty. *Orthopedics*, 2005; **28** (Suppl. 10): 1227–1233.

1025. Parratte S, Argenson JN. Validation and usefulness of a computer assisted cup positioning system in THA. A prospective, randomized, controlled study. *J. Bone Joint Surg.* (*Am.*), 2007; **89**: 494–499.

1026. Dorr LD. *Hip arthroplasty: minimally invasive techniques and computer navigation*. Saunders Elsevier, Philadelphia, 2006.

1027. Haaker RG, Stockheim M, Kamp M, Proff G, Breitenfelder J, Ottersbach A. Computer-assisted navigation increases precision of component placement in total knee arthroplasty. *Clin. Orthop. Relat. Res.*, 2005; **433**: 152–159.

1028. Stulberg SD, Loan P, Sarin V. Computer-assisted navigation in total knee replacement: Results of an initial experience in thirty-five patients. *J. Bone Joint Surg.*, 2002; **84**: S90–S98.

1029. Pitto RP, Graydon AJ, Bradley L, Malak SF, Walker CG, Anderson IA. Accuracy of a computer-assisted navig264ation system for total knee replacement. *J. Bone Joint Surg.* (*Br.*), 2006; **88**: 601–605.

1030. Shimmin AJ, Back D. Femoral neck fractures following Birmingham hip resurfacing: A national review of 50 cases. *J. Bone Joint Surg.* (*Br.*), 2005; **87**: 463–464.

1031. Grammatopolous G, Pandit H, Kwon Y-M, Gundle R, McLardy-Smith P, Beard DJ, Murray DW, Gill HS. Hip resurfacings revised for inflammatory pseudotumour have a poor outcome. *J. Bone Joint Surg.* (*Br.*), 2009; **91**: 1019–1024.

1032. Grigoris P, Roberts P, Panousis K, Jin Z. Hip resurfacing arthroplasty: The evolution of contemporary designs. *Proc. Inst. Mech. Eng. H.*, 2006; **220**: 95–105.

1033. Goebel S, Blanke M, Hendrich C. Surface replacement of the hip: Contra. In: *Proceedings of the 9th BIOLOX®*Symposium. (Lazennec JY, Dietrich M, eds). (Steinkopff Verlag, Darmstadt, Germany, 2004). pp. 119–126.

1034. Clarke MT, Lee PTH, Arora A, Villar RN. Levels of metal ions after small- and large-diameter metal-on-metal hip arthroplasty. *J. Bone Joint Surg.* (*Br.*) 2003; **85**: 913–917.

1035. Jacobs JJ, Skipor AK, Doorn PF, Campbell PA, Schmalzried TP, Black J, Amstutz HC. Cobalt and chromium concentrations in patients with metal on metal total hip replacement. *Clin. Orthop. Relat. Res.*, 1996; **329**: S256–S263.

1036. Jacobs JJ, Skipor AK, Patterson LM, Hallab NJ, Paprosky WG, Black J, Galante JO. Metal release in patients who have had a primary total hip arthroplasty. A prospective, controlled, longitudinal study. *J. Bone Joint Surg.* (*Am.*), 1998; **80**:1447–1458.

1037. Savarino L, Granchi D, Ciapetti G, Cenni E, Greco M, Rotini R, Veronesi CA, Baldini N, Giunti A. Ion release in stable hip arthroplasties using metal-on-metal articulating surfaces: A comparison between short- and medium-term results. *J. Biomed. Mater. Res.*, 2003; **66A**: 450–456.

1038. Savarino L, Greco M, Cenni E, Cavasinni L, Rotini R, Baldini N, Giunti A. Differences in ion release after ceramic-on-ceramic and metal-on-metal total hip replacement, medium-term follow-up. *J. Bone Joint Surg.* (*Br.*), 2006; **88**: 472–476.

1039. Daniel J, Ziaee H, Pradhan C, Pynsent PB, McMinn DJ. Blood and urine metal ion levels in young and active patients after Birmingham hip resurfacing arthroplasty: Four-year results of a prospective longitudinal study. *J. Bone Joint Surg.* (*Br.*), 2007; **89**: 169–173.

1040. Mont MA, Schmalzried TP. Modern metal-on-metal hip resurfacing: Important observations from the first ten years. *J. Bone Joint Surg.* (*Am.*), 2008; **90**: 3–11.

1041. Hart AJ, Skinner JA, Winship P, Faria N, Kulinskaya E, Webster D, Muirhead-Allwood S, Aldam CH, Anwar H, Powell JJ. Circulating levels of cobalt and chromium from metal-on-metal hip replacement are associated with CDT-cell lymphopenia. *J. Bone Joint Surg.* (*Br.*), 2009; **91**: 835–842.

1042. Willert HG, Buchhorn GH, Fayyazi A, Flury R, Windler M, Koester G, Lohmann CH. Metal-on-metal bearings and hyper-sensitivity in patients with artificial hip joints. A clinical and histomorphological study. *J. Bone Joint Surg.* (*Am.*), 2005; **87**: 28–36.

1043. Available from: URL: www.tga.gov.au/newsroom/btn-dupuy-recall.htm.

1044. Griss P, Werner E. Alumina ceramic, bioglass and silicon nitride. A comparative biocompatibility study. In: *Mechanical Properties of Biomaterials*. (Hastings GW, Williams DF, eds) (John Wiley & Sons Ltd., London, 1980). pp. 217–225.

1045. Willmann G. Survival rate and reliability of ceramic femoral heads for total hip arthroplasty. *Mat.-wiss. U. Werkstofftech.*, 1998; **29**: 595–604.

1046. Takami Y, Nakazawa T, Makinouchi K, Glueck J, Nose Y. Biocompatibility of alumina ceramic and polyethylene as materials for pivot bearings of a centrifugal blood pump. *J. Biomed. Mater. Res.*, 1997; **36**: 381–386.

1047. Dorlot JM. Long-term effects of alumina components in total hip prostheses. *Clin. Orthop.*, 1992; **282**: 47–52.

1048. Jazrawi LM, Kummer FJ, DiCesare PE. Alternative bearing surfaces for total joint arthroplasty. *J. Am. Acad. Orthop. Surg.*, 1998; **6**: 198–203.

1049. Granchi D, Savarino L, Ciapetti G, Cenni E, Rotini R, Mieti M, Baldini N, Giunti A. Immunological changes in patients with total joint replacement following idiopathic osteoarthritis of the hip. *J. Bone Joint Surg.* (*Br.*), 2003; **85**: 758–764.

1050. Bizot P, Nizard R, Hamadouche M, Hannouche D, Sedel L. Prevention of wear and osteolysis: Alumina-on-alumina bearing. *Clin. Orthop.*, 2001; **393**: 85–93.

1051. Shimmin A, Beaule PE, Campbell P. Metal-on-metal hip resurfacing arthroplasty. *J. Bone Joint Surg.* (*Am.*), 2008; **90**: 637–654.

1052. Ong KL, Manley MT, Kurtz SM. Have contemporary hip resurfacing designs reached maturity? A review. *J. Bone Joint Surg.* (*Am.*), 2008; **90**: 81–88.

1053. Zhang W, Titze M, Cappi B, Wirtz DC, Telle R, Fischer H. Improved mechanical long-term reliability of hip resurfacing prostheses by using silicon nitride. *J. Mater. Sci. Mater. Med.*, 2010; **21**: 3049–3057.

1054. Cappi B, Neuss S, Salber J, Telle R, Knuechel R, Fischer H. Cytocompatibility of high strength non-oxide ceramics. *J. Biomed. Mater. Res. A*, 2009; **93**: 67–76.

1055. Becher PF, Sun EY, Plucknett KP, Alexander KB, Hsueh C-H, Lin H-T, Waters SB, Westmoreland CG, Kang E-S, Hirao K, Brito ME. Microstructural design of silicon nitride with improved fracture toughness: 1. Effects of grain shape and size. *J. Am. Ceram. Soc.*, 1998; **81**: 2821–2830.

1056. Sun EY, Becher PF, Plucknett KP, Hsueh C-H, Alexander KB, Waters SB, Hirao K, Brito ME. Microstructural design of silicon nitride with improved fracture toughness: 2. Effects of yttrial and alumina additives. *J. Am. Ceram. Soc.*, 1998; **81**: 2831–2840.

1057. Padture N. *In situ*-toughened silicon carbide. *J. Am. Ceram. Soc.*, 1994; **77**: 519–523.

1058. Gilbert CJ, Dauskardt RH, Ritchie RO. Behaviour of cyclic fatigue cracks in monolithic silicon nitride. *J. Am. Ceram. Soc.*, 1995; **78**: 2291–2298.

1059. Lancaster JK. A review of the influence of environmental humidity and water on friction, lubrication and wear. *Tribol. Int.*, 1990; **23**: 371–389.

1060. Tanaka I, Pezzotti G. Evaluation of slow crack growth resistance in ceramics for high-temperature applications. *J. Am. Ceram. Soc.*, 1992; **75**: 772–777.

1061. Munz D, Fett T. Ceramics: *Mechanical Properties, Failure Behaviour, Materials Selection* (1st ed.). Springer: Berlin (1999).

1062. Takahashi Y, Zhu W, Sugano N, Pezzotti G. On the role of oxygen vacancies, aliovalent ions and lattice strain in the *in vivo* wear behavior of alumina hip joints. *J. Mech. Behav. Biomed. Mater.*, 2011; **4**: 993–1003.

1063. Fischer TE, Tomizawa H. Interaction of tribochemistry and microfracture in the friction and wear of silicon nitride. *Wear*, 1985; **105**: 29–45.

1064. Dong X, Jahanmir S. Wear transition diagram for silicon nitride. *Wear*, 1993; **165**: 169–180.

1065. Dong X, Jahanmir S, Ives LK. Wear transition diagram for silicon carbide. *Tribol. Int.*, 1995; **28**: 559–572.

1066. Wilson K, Roques A, Dickinson A, Mathias R, Taylor A, Holland J. Initial fixation of a pre-assembled cup system. In: *Proceedings of the 13th Biolox Symposium 2009, Bioceramics and Alternative Bearings in Joint Arthroplasty*, Vol. 13. (Cobb JP, ed) (Springer; Berlin, 2010).

1067. Pandorf T. Delta motion monoblock cup system: What can we expect? *J. Bone Joint Surg.* (*Br.*), 2010; **92-B** (Suppl. I): 98.

1068. *National Joint Registry of England and Wales*: NJR Prostheses used 2010; p. 8. Available from: URL: www.njcentre.org.uk.

1069. Oral E, Rowell SL, Muratoglu OK. The effect of alpha-tocopherol on the oxidation and free radical decay in irradiated UHMWPE. *Biomaterials*, 2006; **27**: 5580–5587.

1070. Kurtz SM, Dumbleton J, Siskey RS, Wang A, Manley M. Trace concentrations of vitamin E protect radiation crosslinked UHMWPE from oxidative degradation. *J. Biomed. Mater. Res. A*, 2009; **90**: 549–563.

1071. Wang AG, Yau SS, Essner A, Herrera L, Manley M, Dumbleton J. A highly crosslinked UHMWPE for CR and PS total knee arthroplasties. *J. Arthroplasty*, 2008; **23**: 559–566.

1072. Kurtz SM, Mazzucco D, Rimnac CM, Schroeder D. Anisotropy and oxidative resistance of highly crosslinked UHMWPE after deformation processing by solid-state ram extrusion. *Biomaterials*, 2006; **27**: 24–34.

1073. Herrera L, Essner A, Loving L, Wang A. Hip simulator evaluation of the effect of liner thickness on the wear of sequentially crosslinked acetabular liners. In: *Transactions of the 55th Annual Meeting of the Orthopaedic Research Society*; Las Vegas, NV, 2009; p. 2336.

1074. Kelly NH, Rajadhyaksha AD, Wright TM, Maher SA, Westrich GH. The effect of liner thickness on the wear of highly cross-linked polyethylene acetabular components under "near-impingement" conditions. In: *Transactions of the 55th Annual Meeting of the Orthopaedic Research Society*; 2009; Las Vegas, NV, 2009; p. 2315.

1075. Rowell SL, Oral E, Muratoglu OK. Three-Year Real-Time Aging of vitamin E-diffused, Radiation Cross-linked UHMWPE. In: *Transactions of the 55th Annual Meeting of the Orthopaedic Research Society*; Las Vegas, NV, 2009; p. 21.

1076. Costa L, Bracco PM, Carpentieri I, V.; B, Brach del Prever EM. On post-irradiation oxidation of vitamin E-stabilized UHMWPE. In: *Transactions of the 55th Annual Meeting of the Orthopaedic Research Society*; Las Vegas, NV, 2009; p. 461.

1077. Yau S-S, Le K-P, Wang A. Doping vitamin E by diffusion deteriorates properties of crosslinked UHMWPE: Verified by experiments. In: *Transactions of the 55th Annual Meeting of the Orthopaedic Research Society*; Las Vegas, NV, 2009; p. 458.

1078. Chumakov MC, Silverman J, Al-Sheikhly M. The novel scavenging of free radicals in UHMWPE with TEMPO, a nitroxide antioxidant. In: *Transactions of the 55th Annual Meeting of the Orthopaedic Research Society*; Las Vegas, NV 2009; p. 453.

1079. Soule PB. The chemistry and biology of nitroxide compounds. *Free Radical Biol. Med.*, 2007; **42**: 1632–1650.

1080. Samuni A, Goldstein S, Russo A, Mitchell JB, Krishna MC, Neta P. Kinetics and mechanism of hydroxyl radical and OH-adduct radical reactions with nitroxides and with their hydroxylamines. *J. Am. Chem. Soc.*, 2002; **124**: 8719–8724.

1081. Beckwith ALJ, Bowry VW. Ingold KU. Kinetics of nitroxide radical trapping. 1. Solvent effect. *J. Am. Chem. Soc.*, 1992; **114**: 4983–4992.

1082. Gijsman P, Smelt HJ, Schumann D. Hindered amine light stabilizers: An alternative for radiation cross-linked UHMWPE implants. *Biomaterials*, 2010; **31**: 6685–6691.

1083. Gijsman P, Gitton M. Hindered amine stabilisers as long-term heat stabilisers for polypropylene. *Polym. Degradation Stability*, 1999; **66**: 365–371.

1084. Gijsman P, Hamskog M. Mechanism of action of hindered amines as long term heat stabilizers. *ACS Symp. Ser.*, 2007; **978**: 48–58.

1085. Klemchuk PP, Gande ME, Cordola E. Hindered Amine. Mechanisms: Part III — Investigations using isotopic labeling. *Polym. Degradation Stability*, 1990; **27**: 65–74.

1086. He S, Le K-P, Blitz JW, Yau S-S, Korduba LA, A. W. Anthocyanin doped UHMWPE: Oxidation, wear and mechanical properties. In: *Transactions of the 55th Annual Meeting of the Orthopaedic Research Society*; Las Vegas, NV 2009; p. 451.

1087. Bakshi SR, Tercero JE, Agarwal A. Synthesis and characterization of multiwalled carbon nanotube reinforced ultra high molecular weight polyethylene composite by electrostatic spraying technique. *Composites: Part A*, 2007; **38**: 2493–2499.

1088. Tang W, Santare MH, Advani SG. Melt processing and mechanical property characterization of multi-walled carbon nanotube/high density polyethylene (MWNT/HDPE) composite films. *Carbon*, 2003; **41**: 2779–2785.

1089. Ruan SL, Gao P, Yang XG, Yu TX. Toughening high performance ultrahigh molecular weight polyethylene using multiwalled carbon nanotubes. *Polymer*, 2003; **44**: 5643–5654.

1090. Wang Y, Cheng R, Liang L, Wang Y. Study on the preparation and characterization of ultra-high molecular weight polyethylene–carbon nanotubes composite fiber. *Compos. Sci. Technol.*, 2005; **65**: 793–797.

1091. Xue Y, Wu W, Jacobs O, Schadel B. Tribological behaviour of UHMWPE /HDPE blends reinforced with multi-wall carbon nanotubes. *Polym. Test.*, 2005; **25**: 221–229.

1092. Gallardo LA, Carpentieri I, Laurent MP, Costa L, Wimmer MA. Europium stearate additives delay oxidation of UHMWPE for orthopaedic applications: A pilot study. *Clin. Orthop. Relat. Res.*, 2011; **469**: 2294–2301.

1093. Moro T, Takatori Y, Ishihara K, Konno T, Takigawa Y, Matsushita T, Chung U-I, Nakamura K, Kawaguchi H. Surface grafting of artificial joints with a biocompatible polymer for preventing periprosthetic osteolysis. *Nat. Mater.*, 2004; **3**: 829–836.

1094. Kyomoto M, Moro T, Konno T, Takadama H, Yamawaki N, Kawaguchi H, Takatori Y, Nakamura K, Ishihara K. Enhanced wear resistance of modified cross-linked polyethylene by grafting with poly(2-methacryloyloxyethyl phosphorylcholine). *J. Biomed. Mater. Res.*, 2007; **82A**: 10–17.

1095. Kyomoto M, Moro T, Konno T, Takadama H, Kawaguchi H, Takatori Y, Nakamura K, Yamawaki N, Ishihara K. Effects of photo-induced graft polymerization of 2-methacryloyloxyethyl phosphorylcholine on physical properties of cross-linked polyethylene in artificial hip joints. *J. Mater. Sci.: Mater. Med.*, 2007; **18**: 1809–1815.

1096. Zoo YS, An JW, Lim DP, Lim DS. Effect of carbon nanotube addition on tribological behavior of UHMWPE. *Tribol. Lett.*, 2004; **16**: 305–309.

1097. Johnson BB, Santare MH, Novotny JE, Advani SG. Wear Behavior of carbon nanotube/high density polyethylene composites. *Mech. Mater.*, 2009; **41**: 1108–1115.

1098. Ishihara K, Ziats NP, Tierney BP, Nakabayashi N, Anderson JM. Protein adsorption from human plasma is reduced on phospholipid polymers. *J. Biomed. Mater. Res. Part A*, 1991; **25**: 1397–1407.

1099. Kuiper KJ, Nordrehaug JE. Early mobilization after protamine reversal of heparin following implantation of phosphorylcholine-coated stents in totally occluded coronary arteries. *Am. J. Cardiol.*, 2000; **85**: 698–702.

1100. Galli M, Sommariva L, Prati F, Zerboni S, Politi A, Bonatti R, Mameli S, Butti E, Pagano A, Ferrari G. Acute and mid-term results of phosphorylcholine-coated stents in primary coronary stenting for acute myocardial infarction. *Cathet. Cardiovasc. Intervent.*, 2001; **53**: 182–187.

1101. Lewis AL, Tolhurst LA, Stratford PW. Analysis of a phosphorylcholine-based polymer coating on a coronary stent pre- and post-implantation. *Biomaterials*, 2002; **23**: 1697–1706.

1102. Ishihara K, Aragaki R, Ueda T, Watanabe A, Nakabayashi N. Reduced thrombogenicity of polymers having phospholipid polar groups. *J. Biomed. Mater. Res.*, 1990; **24**: 1069–1077.

1103. Wright JM, Pellicci PM, Salvati EA, Ghelman B, Roberts MM, Koh JL. Bone density adjacent to press-fit acetabular components: A prospective analysis with quantitative computed tomography. *J. Bone Joint Surg.* (*Am.*), 2001; **83**: 529–536.

1104. Manley MT, Ong KL, Kurtz SM. The potential for bone loss in acetabular structures following THA. *Clin. Orthop. Relat. Res.*, 2006; **453**: 246–253.

1105. Field RE, Cronin MD, Singh PJ, Burtenshaw C, Rushton N. Bone remodeling around the Cambridge cup: A DEXA study of 50 hips over 2 years. *Acta Orthop.*, 2006; **77**: 726–732.

1106. Latif AMH, Mehats A, Elcocks M, Rushton N, Field RE, Jones E. Pre-clinical studies to validate the MITCH PCR^{TM} Cup: A flexible and anatomically shaped acetabular component with novel bearing characteristics. *J. Mater. Sci. Mater. Med.*, 2008; **19**: 1729–1736.

1107. Hunziker EB. Articular cartilage repair: Basic science and clinical progress. A review of the current status and prospects. *Osteoarthritis Cartilage*, 2002; **10**: 432–463.

1108. Redman SN, Oldfield SF, Archer CW. Current strategies for articular cartilage repair. *Eur. Cell. Mater.*, 2005; **9**: 23–32.

1109. Kaul G, Cucchiarini M, Remberger K, Kohn D, Madry H. Failed cartilage repair for early osteoarthritis defects: A biochemical, histological and immunohistochemical analysis of the repair tissue after treatment with marrow-stimulation techniques. *Knee Surg. Sports Traumatol. Arthrosc.*, 2012; **20**: 2315–2324.

1110. Felson DT, Zhang Y. An update on the epidemiology of knee and hip osteoarthritis with a view to prevention. *Arthritis Rheum.*, 1998; **41**: 1343–1355.

1111. Hangody L, Vasárhelyi G. Autologous osteochondral grafting — technique and long-term results. *Injury*, 2008; **39** (Suppl.): 32–39.

1112. LaPrade R, Botker JC. Donor-site morbidity after osteochondral autograft transfer procedures. *Arthrosc. J. Arthrosc. Rel. Surg.*, 2004; **20**: e69–e73.

1113. Nho SJ, Green DM, Shindle MK, Carter T, Williams III RJ, Wickiewicz TL. Patellofemoral osteochondral autologous transfer. *Tech. Knee Surg.*, 2006; **5**: 134–137.

1114. Brittberg M, Lindahl A, Nilsson A, Ohlsson C, Isaksson O, Peterson L. Treatment of deep cartilage defects in the knee with autologous chondrocyte transplantation. *New Engl. J. Med.*, 1994; **331**: 889–895.

1115. Marlovits S, Zeller P, Singer P, Resinger C, Vécsei V. Cartilage repair: Generations of autologous chondrocyte transplantation. *Eur. J. Radiol.*, 2006; **57**: 24–31.

1116. Djouad F, Bouffi C, Ghannam S, Noël D, Jorgensen C. Mesenchymal stem cells: Innovative therapeutic tools for rheumatic diseases. *Nat. Rev. Rheumatol.*, 2009; **5**: 392–399.

1117. Namba RS, Meuli M, Sullivan KM, Le AX, Adzick NS. Spontaneous repair of superficial defects in articular cartilage in a fetal lamb model. *J. Bone Joint Surg.* (*Am.*), 1998; **80**: 4–10.

1118. Mankin HJ. The response of articular cartilage to mechanical injury. *J. Bone Joint Surg.* (*Am.*), 1982; **64**: 460–466.

1119. Hunziker EB. Growth-factor-induced healing of partial-thickness defects in adult articular cartilage. *Osteoarthritis Cartilage*, 2001; **9**: 22–32.

1120. Hunziker EB, Rosenberg LC. Repair of partial-thickness defects in articular cartilage: Cell recruitment from the synovial membrane. *J. Bone Joint Surg.* (*Am.*), 1996; **78**: 721–733.

1121. Jakob RP, Franz T, Gautier E, Mainil-Varlet P. Autologous osteochondral grafting in the knee: Indication, results, and reflections. *Clin. Orthop. Relat. Res.*, 2002; **401**: 170–184.

1122. O'Driscoll SW. The healing and regeneration of articular cartilage. *J. Bone Joint Surg.* (*Am.*), 1998; **80**: 1795–1812.

1123. Minas T. The role of cartilage repair techniques, including chondrocyte transplantation, in focal chondral knee damage. *AAOS Inst. Course Lect.*, 1999; **48**: 629–643.

1124. Heath CA, Magari SR. Mini-review: Mechanical factors affecting cartilage regeneration *in vitro*. *Biotechnol. Bioeng.*, 1996; **50**: 430–437.

1125. Carver SE, Heath CA. Semi-continuous perfusion system for delivering intermittent physiological pressure to regenerating cartilage. *Tissue Eng.*, 1999; **5**: 1–11.

1126. Brittberg M. Autologous chondrocyte transplantation. *Clin. Orthop.*, 1999; **367**: S147–S155.

1127. Peterson L, Minas T, Brittberg M, Nilsson A, Sjogren-Jansson E, Lindahl A. Two- to 9-year outcome after autologous chondrocyte transplantation of the knee. *Clin. Orthop.*, 2000; **374**: 212–234.

1128. Bachmann G, Basad E, Lommel D, Steinmeyer J. MRI in the follow-up of matrix-supported autologous chondrocyte transplantation (MACI) and microfracture. *Radiologe*, 2004; **44**: 773–782.

1129. Behrens P, Ehlers EM, Kochermann KU, Rohwedel J, Russlies M, Plotz W. New therapy procedure for localized cartilage defects. Encouraging results with autologous chondrocyte implantation. *MMW Fortschr. Med.*, 1999; **141**: 49–51.

1130. Ronga M, Grassi FA, Bulgheroni P. Arthroscopic autologous chondrocyte implantation for the treatment of a chondral defect in the tibial plateau of the knee. *Arthroscopy*, 2004; **20**: 79–84.

1131. Vibe-Hansen R, Aesculai S. Methods, instruments and kit for autologous chondrocyte transplantation. *Patent WO* 98/08469 (1998).

1132. Barry FP. Biology and clinical applications of mesenchymal stem cells. *Birth Defects Res., C Embryo Today*, 2003; **69**: 250–256.

1133. Barry FP. Mesenchymal stem cell therapy in joint disease. *Novartis Found. Symp.*, 2003; **249**: 86–96.

1134. Caplan AI. Mesenchymal stem cells. *J. Orthop. Res.*, 1991; **9**: 641–650.

1135. Gao J, Caplan AI. Mesenchymal stem cells and tissue engineering for orthopaedic surgery. *Chir. Organi Mov.*, 2003; **88**: 305–316.

1136. Minguell JJ, Erices A, Conget P. Mesenchymal stem cells. *Exp. Biol. Med.*, (*Maywood*) 2001; **226**: 507–520.

1137. Pittenger MF, Mackay AM, Beck SC, Jaiswal RK, Douglas R, Mosca JD, Moorman MA, Simonetti DW, Craig S, Marshak DR. Multilineage potential of adult human mesenchymal stem cells. *Science*, 1999; **284**: 143–147.

1138. Prockop DJ. Marrow stromal cells as stem cells for nonhematopoietic tissues. *Science*, 1997; **276**: 71–74.

1139. Roufosse CA, Direkze NC, Otto WR, Wright NA. Circulating mesenchymal stem cells. *Int. J. Biochem. Cell. Biol.*, 2004; **36**: 585–597.

1140. Temenoff JS, Mikos AG. Review: Tissue engineering for regeneration of articular cartilage. *Biomaterials*, 2000; **21**: 431–440.

1141. Carden A, Morris MD. Application of vibrational spectroscopy to the study of mineralized tissues (review). *J. Biomed. Opt.*, 2000; **5**: 259–268.

1142. Mahadevan-Jansen A. Raman spectroscopy: From benchtop to bedside. In: *Biomedical Photonics Handbook*. (Vo-Dinh T, ed) (CRC Press; Boca Raton, 2003).

1143. Puppels GJ. *In vivo* Raman spectroscopy. In: *Handbook of Raman Spectroscopy: From the Research Laboratory to the Process Line*. (Lewis IR, Edwards HGM, eds) (Marcel Dekker; New York, 2001).

1144. Morris M. Raman spectroscopy of bone and cartilage. In: *Emerging Raman Applications and Techniques in Biomedical and Pharmaceutical Fields*. (Matousek P, Morris M, eds) (Springer-Verlag; Berlin, 2010). Chapter 14.

1145. Esmonde-White K, Mandair GS, Morris M, Raaii F, Jacobson JA, Miller BS, Urquhart AG, Roessler BJ. Raman spectroscopy of synovial fluid as a tool for diagnosing osteoarthritis. *J. Biomed. Opt.*, 2009; **14**: 034013-1–9.

1146. Heger M, Mordon S, Leroy G, Fleurisse L, Creusy C. Raman microspectrometry of laser-reshaped rabbit auricular cartilage: Preliminary study on laser-induced cartilage mineralization. *J. Biomed. Opt.*, 2006; **11**: 024003-1–8.

1147. Boskey A, Camacho NP. FT-IR imaging of native and tissue-engineered bone and cartilage. *Biomaterials*, 2007; **28**: 2465–2478.

1148. Camacho NP, West P, Griffith MH, Warren RF, Hidaka C. FT-IR imaging spectroscopy of genetically modified bovine chondrocytes. *Mater. Sci. Eng.*, 2001; **C17**: 3–9.

1149. Obeid EM, Adams MA, Mewman JH. Mechanical properties of articular cartilage in knees with unicompartmental osteoarthritis. *J. Bone Joint Surg.* (*Br.*), 1994; **76**: 315–319.

1150. Kuettner KE, Cole AA. Cartilage degeneration in different human joints. *Osteoarthritis Cartilage*, 2005; **13**: 93–103.

1151. Thambyah A, Broom N. On how degeneration influences load-bearing in the cartilage-bone system: A microstructural and micro-mechanical study. *Osteoarthritis Cartilage*, 2007; **15**: 1410–1423.

1152. Kellgren JH, Lawrence JS. Radiological assessments of osteo-arthrosis. *Ann. Rheum. Dis.*, 1957; **16**: 494–502.

1153. Xia Y. Magic-angle effect in magnetic resonance imaging of articular cartilage: A review. *Invest. Radiol.*, 2000; **35**: 602–621.

1154. Alhadlaq HA, Xia Y, Moody JB, Matyas JR. Detecting structural changes in early experimental osteoarthritis of tibial cartilage by microscopic magnetic resonance imaging and polarised light microscopy. *Ann. Rheum. Dis.*, 2004; **63**: 709–717.

1155. Goodwin DW, Wadghiri YZ, Zhu H, Vinton CJ, Smith ED, Dunn JF. Macroscopic structure of articular cartilage of the tibial plateau: Influence of a characteristic matrix architecture on MRI appearance. *Am. J. Roentgenol.*, 2004; **182**: 311–318.

1156. Mansfield P, Glover P. Limits to magnetic resonance microscopy. *Rep. Prog. Phys.*, 2002; **65**: 1489–1511.

1157. Collins DH, McElligott TF. Sulphate ($35SO_4$) uptake by chondrocytes in relation to histological changes in osteo-arthritic human articular cartilage. *Ann. Rheum. Dis.*, 1960; **19**: 318–330.

1158. West PA, Bostrom MPG, Torzilli PA, Camacho NP. Fourier transform infrared spectral analysis of degenerative cartilage: An Infrared fiber optic probe and imaging study. *Appl. Spectrosc.*, 2004; **58**: 376–381.

1159. Frushour BG, Koenig JL. Raman scattering of collagen, gelatin, and elastin. *Biopolymers*, 1975; **14**: 379–391.

1160. Chi Z, Chen XG, Holtz JSW, Asher SA. UV resonance Raman-selective amide vibrational enhancement: Quantitative methodology for determining protein secondary structure. *Biochemistry*, 1998; **37**: 2854–2864.

1161. Dehring KA, Smukler AR, Roessler BJ, Morris MD. Correlating changes in collagen secondary structure with aging and defective type II collagen by Raman spectroscopy. *Appl. Spectrosc.*, 2006; **60**: 366–372.

1162. Dehring KA, Crane NJ, Smukler AR, McHugh JB, Roessler BJ, Morris MD. Identifying chemical changes in subchondral bone taken from murine knee joints using Raman spectroscopy. *Appl. Spectrosc.*, 2006; **60**: 1134–1141.

1163. Ignatieva N, Zakharkina O, Leroy G, Sobol E, Vorobieva N, Mordon S. Molecular processes and structural alterations in laser redhaping of cartilage. *Laser Phys. Lett.*, 2007; **10**: 749–753.

1164. Lim NS, Hamed Z, Yeow CH, Chan C, Huang Z. Early detection of biomolecular changes in disrupted porcine cartilage using polarized Raman spectroscopy. *J. Biomed. Opt.*, 2012; **16**: 017003-1–10.

1165. Teeple E, Elsaid KA, Fleming BC, Jay GD, Aslani K, Crisco JJ, Mechrefe AP. Coefficients of friction, lubricin, and cartilage damage in the anterior cruciate ligament-deficient guinea pig knee. *J. Orthop. Res.*, 2008; **26**: 231–237.

1166. Neu CP, Reddi AH, Komvopoulos K, Schmid TM, Di Cesare PE. Friction coefficient and superficial zone protein are increased in patients with advanced osteoarthritis. *Arthritis Rheum.*, 2010; **62**: 2680–2687.

1167. Mow VC, Ratcliffe A, Poole RA. Cartilage and diarthrodial joints as paradigms for hierarchical materials and structures. *Biomaterials*, 1992; **13**: 67–97.

1168. D'Antonio JA, Manley MT, Capello WN, Bierbaum BE, Ramakrishnan R, Naughton M, Sutton K. Five-year experience with crossfire highly crosslinked polyethylene. *Clin. Orthop. Relat. Res.*, 2005; **441**: 143–150.

1169. Duffy GP, Wannomae KK, Rowell SL, Muratoglu OK. Fracture of a cross-linked polyethylene liner due to impingement. *J. Arthroplasty*, 2009; **24**: 158.e15–19.

1170. Tower SS, Currier JH, Currier BH, Lyford KA, Van Citters DW, Mayor MB. Rim cracking of the cross-linked longevity polyethylene acetabular liner after total hip arthroplasty. *J. Bone Joint Surg.* (*Am.*), 2007; **89**: 2212–2217.

1171. Moore KD, Beck PR, Petersen DW, Cuckler JM, Lemons JE, Eberhardt AW. Early failure of a cross-linked polyethylene acetabular liner. Acase report. *J. Bone Joint Surg.* (*Am.*), 2008; **90**: 2499–2504.

1172. Blumenfeld TJ, McKellop HA, Schmalzried TP, Billi F. Fracture of a cross-linked polyethylene liner: A multifactorial issue. *J. Arthroplasty*, 2011; **26**: 666.e5–8.

1173. Waewsawangwong W, Goodman SB. Unexpected failure of highly cross-linked polyethylene acetabular liner. *J. Arthroplasty*, 2012; **27**: 323. e1–4.

1174. Morscher EW. Failures and successes in total hip replacement — why good ideas may not work. *Scand. J. Surg.*, 2003; **92**: 113–120.

1175. Loudon R. Theory of the resonance Raman effect in crystals. *J. Phys.*, 1965; **26**; 677–683.

1176. Browne WR, McGarvey JJ. The Raman effect and its application to electronic spectroscopies in metal-centered species: Techniques and investigations in ground and excited states. *Coordination Chem. Rev.*, 2007; **251**: 454–473.

1177. Williams AC, Edwards HGM, Lawson EE, Barry BW. Molecular interactions between the penetration enhancer 1,8-cineole and human skin. *J. Raman Spectrosc.*, 2006; **37**: 361–366.

1178. Krafft C, Sobottka SB, Schackert G, Salzer R. Near infrared Raman spectroscopic mapping of native brain tissue and intracranial tumors, *Analyst*, 2005; **130**: 1070–1077.

1179. Ip K, Baik KH, Overberg ME, Lambers ES, Heo YW, Norton DP, Pearton SJ, Ren F, Zavada JM. Effect of high-density plasma etching on the optical properties and surface stoichiometry of ZnO. *Appl. Phys. Lett.*, 2002; **81**: 3546–3548.

1180. Goslowsky H, Kühne H-M, Neff H, Kötz R, Lewerenz HJ. The influence of chemical surface alteration on photoresponse of polycrystalline $CuInS_2$ electrodes. *Surf. Sci.*, 1985; **149**: 191–208.

1181. Goodfellow JW. The new Esperanto. *J. Bone Joint Surg.* (*Am.*), 1993; **75(A)**: 1423–1426.

Index